NEUROENDOCRINOLOGY AND PSYCHIATRIC DISORDER

Neuroendocrinology and Psychiatric Disorder

Editors

Gregory M. Brown, M.D., Ph.D.
Professor and Chairman, Department of Neurosciences
Professor, Department of Psychiatry
McMaster University
Hamilton, Canada

Stephen H. Koslow, Ph.D.
Chief, Neurosciences Research Branch
National Institute of Mental Health
Rockville, Maryland

Seymour Reichlin, M.D., Ph.D.
Professor of Medicine, Tufts University School of Medicine
Chief, Endocrinology Division
New England Medical Center, Inc.
Boston, Massachusetts

Raven Press ■ New York

Raven Press, 1140 Avenue of the Americas, New York, New York 10036

Made in the United States of America

Library of Congress Cataloging in Publication Data
Main entry under title:

Neuroendocrinology and psychiatric disorder.

Proceedings of the Psychoneuroendocrinology Symposium held at McMaster University, Canada, sponsored by the National Institute of Mental Health.
Includes bibliographical references and index.
1. Mental illness—Physiological aspects–Congresses.
2. Neuroendocrinology—Congresses. I. Brown, Gregory M.
II. Koslow, Stephen H. III. Reichlin, Seymour.
IV. Psychoneuroendocrinology Symposium (1983: McMaster University) V. National Institute of Mental Health (U.S.)
[DNLM: 1. Endocrinology—Congresses. 2. Neurology—Congresses. 3. Mental disorders—Congresses. WL 100 N4927 1981]
RC455.4.B5N46 1984 616.89 84-4727
ISBN 0-89004-742-1

Papers or parts thereof have been used as camera-ready copy as submitted by the authors whenever possible; when retyped, they have been edited by the editorial staff only to the extent considered necessary for the assistance of an international readership. The views expressed and the general style adopted remain, however, the responsibility of the named authors. Great care has been taken to maintain the accuracy of the information contained in the volume. However, neither Raven Press nor the editors can be held responsible for errors or for any consequences arising from the use of information contained herein.

The use in this book of particular designations of countries or territories does not imply any judgment by the publisher or editors as to the legal status of such countries or territories, of their authorities or institutions or of the delimitation of their boundaries.

Some of the names of products referred to in this book may be registered trademarks or proprietary names, although specific reference to this fact may not be made: however, the use of a name with designation is not to be construed as a representation by the publisher or editors that it is in the public domain. In addition, the mention of specific companies or of their products or proprietary names does not imply any endorsement or recommendation on the part of the publisher or editors.

Authors were themselves responsible for obtaining the necessary permission to reproduce copyright material from other sources.

*This volume is dedicated to the memory of Edward J. Sachar,
a pioneer in the field of psychoneuroendocrinology
who was instrumental in the planning and conceptualization
of this conference.*

Preface

Discovery of the chemistry of three major hypothalamic hormones in the early 1970s formally confirmed psychoneuroendocrinology as a legitimate field of scientific endeavor after decades of conceptual and experimental development in both basic and clinical spheres. At the same time, important developments were also being made in clinical psychiatric research. In particular, major progress in the definition of clinical entities and in the development of universal diagnostic tools enabled researchers throughout the world to achieve a reasonable consensus regarding the populations and disorders that they were describing and investigating. Simultaneous efforts were being expended by basic psychologists and physiologists to understand related neural, endocrine, and behavioral factors in animal models.

These parallel developments contributed to the emergence of an interdisciplinary network of specialties, each moving toward the evolution of a psychoneuroendocrine strategy, that hypothesizes that endocrine function may be used as an index of psychopathology and of central nervous system dysfunction. Today, this hypothesis stands as the cornerstone of psychoneuroendocrine research, which, in turn, has assumed increasing prominence among competing research strategies.

While the pace of developments in the field comprising psychoneuroendocrinology has been rapid and often dramatic, it has become increasingly evident that: (a) progress in the various disciplines is proceeding at an unequal rate, particularly at the juncture of basic research and clinical application and (b) the field as a whole has remained multidisciplinary rather than truly interdisciplinary. Disciplinary approaches, methodologies, and research strategies still have not been integrated. In order to address these issues and others dealing with administration, such as evaluation and the public need for research accountability, this volume presents a state-of-the-art assessment as a joint project between leading investigators in the field and the National Institute of Mental Health.

An adequate state-of-the-art assessment requires the expert and objective scrutiny of a specific scientific area with appraisal of past performance, current status, and future directions. This book was developed to provide such an assessment. Its goals are to identify areas of greatest potential, to focus on gaps in existing knowledge, and to formulate research issues and priorities that require further attention and/or emphasis.

Attention is focused on four major research areas to provide a comprehensive review of research data and a full consideration of all relevant issues.

Affective Disorders. This area has received the most research attention over the past decade. Numerous endocrine findings have been reported during this period and a detailed evaluation analyzing the significance of these findings, long overdue, is presented.

Schizophrenia. Research on schizophrenia has yielded few findings of relevance to the neuroendocrine field. A design for future research directions constitutes a requirement.

Anorexia nervosa. Researchers have detailed numerous endocrine abnormalities associated with anorexia nervosa and the underlying causes of these abnormalities also have been hypothesized. It therefore represents a condition of particular interest to the psychiatrist and endocrinologist, and holds considerable promise as a research model for the more-difficult-to-research diagnostic entities.

Stress and stress-related disorders. Disorders in this category have been intensively studied from biological, psychological, and behavioral perspectives. The field presents complexities as well as gaps in theory and data that constitute major stumbling blocks for psychoneuroendocrine research.

This volume presents information from scientists engaged in psychoneuroendocrine research and scientists working in related basic research fields. For each topic, the research data base was reviewed by an acknowledged authority in psychoneuroendocrinology, and critical issues characterizing the field are presented. This review is followed by a critical evaluation of the overview and finally by a detailed discussion by basic and clinical experts in the fields of psychoneuroendocrinology, neuroendocrinology, psychiatry, psychology, biochemistry, physiology, and anatomy. This book provides the opportunity for a synthesis and resolution of complex research issues. It combines a number of evaluative approaches and thus capitalizes on the advantages of each, enabling a comprehensive and objective review of the field. In addition, this volume provides for focused discussion between clinical and basic researchers.

This volume provides workers in the field as well as staff of the Neurosciences Research Branch, National Institute of Mental Health, with an exhaustive and critical evaluation of the field of neuroendocrinology as it has developed in relation to psychiatry.

Herbert Pardes, M.D.
Director, National Institute of Mental Health

Acknowledgment

This volume presents the proceedings of the Psychoneuroendocrinology Symposium held at McMaster University, Canada, that was sponsored by the National Institute of Mental Health.

Contents

Contributors

Catherine F. Allen-Rowlands
Division of Biology and Medicine
Section of Surgery
Brown University
Rhode Island Hospital
593 Eddy Street
Providence, Rhode Island 02902

Josephine Arendt, Ph.D.
Department of Biochemistry
University of Surrey
Guildford, England

David A. Bereiter, Ph.D.
Division of Biology and Medicine
Section of Surgery
Brown University
Rhode Island Hospital
593 Eddy Street
Providence, Rhode Island 02902

Francesca Brambilla, M.D., Prof.
Centro di Psicoendocrinologia
Ospedale Psichiatrico Paolo Pini
Via Ippocrate 45
Milan Afford, Italy

Gregory M. Brown, M.D., Ph.D.
Department of Neurosciences
McMaster University
1200 Main Street West
Hamilton, Ontario, L8N 3Z5 Canada

Stuart Checkley, B.A.,B.M.,C.Ch., M.R.C.P.
The Maudsley Hospital
Denmark Hill
London SE5 8AZ, United Kingdom

John M. Davis, M.D.
Illinois State Psychiatric Institute
1601 West Taylor Street
Chicago, Illinois 60612

K.T. Demarest
Department of Pharmacology and Toxicology
Michigan State University
East Lansing, Michigan 48824

William S. Evans
Department of Internal Medicine
University of Virginia School of Medicine
Charlottesville, Virginia 22908

Lawrence A. Frohman, M.D.
Division of Endocrinology and Metabolism
Department of Medicine
231 Bethesda Avenue, Mail Location 547
Cincinnati, Ohio 45267

Donald S. Gann, M.D.
Division of Biology and Medicine
Section of Surgery
Brown University
Rhode Island Hospital
593 Eddy Street
Providence, Rhode Island 02902

William F. Ganong, M.D.
Department of Physiology, S-762
University of California, San Francisco
3rd and Parnassus Street
San Francisco, California 94143

Paul E. Garfinkel, M.D. M.S.C., F.R.C.P. (C)
Toronto General Hospital; and Department of Psychiatry
University of Toronto
101 College Street
Toronto, Ontario M5G 1L7 Canada

Robert Gibbons, Ph.D.
Illinois State Psychiatric Institute
1601 West Taylor Street
Chicago, Illinois 60612

Joel A. Grinker, Ph.D.
The Rockefeller University
1230 York Avenue
New York, New York 10021

O. Hornykiewicz, M.D.
Institute of Biochemical Pharmacology
University of Vienna
Borschkegasse 8a
A-1090 Vienna, Austria

Ivor M.D. Jackson, M.B., Ch.B. M.R.C.P. F.R.C.P. Ed. F.A.C.P.
Tufts University School of Medicine; and Division of Endocrinology
Department of Medicine
New England Medical Center
171 Harrison Avenue
Boston, Massachusetts 02111

John W. Kendall, M.D.
Research Service
Portland Veterans Administration Medical Center
Portland, Oregon 97201

S.H. Koslow, Ph.D.
Neurosciences Research Branch
National Institute of Mental Health
5600 Fishers Lane, Rm. 10C-23B
Rockville, Maryland 20857

L.C. Krey, Ph.D. Assoc. Prof.
The Rockefeller University
1230 York Avenue
New York, New York 10021

Lewis Landsberg, M.D.
Department of Medicine
Harvard Medical School
Beth Israel Hospital
330 Brookline
Boston, Massachusetts 02215

Sarah Fryer Leibowitz, B.A., Ph.D.
Department of Physiology and Psychology
The Rockefeller University
1230 York Avenue
New York, New York 10021

Seymour Levine, Ph.D.
Department of Psychiatry and Behavioral Sciences
Stanford University School of Medicine
Stanford, California 94305

Peter T. Loosen, M.D.
Clinical Research Unit
Dorothea Dix Hospital
Raleigh, North Carolina 27611

Herbert Y. Meltzer, M.D.
Illinois State Psychiatric Institute; and Department of Psychiatry
University of Chicago
Pritzker School of Medicine
950 East 59 Street
Chicago, Illinois 60637

K.E. Moore, Ph.D.
Department of Pharmacology and Toxicology
Michigan State University
East Lansing, Michigan 48824

Eugenio E. Müller, M.D.
Istituto di Farmacologia
Facolta di Medicina e Chirurgia
Universitá degli Studi di Milano
Via Vanvitelli 32
20129 Milan, Italy

R.C.C. Murison, Ph.D.
Institute of Physiological Psychology
University of Bergen
Arstadveien 21
5000 Bergen, Norway

Ivan Pavkovic, M.D.
Illinois Department of Mental Health and Developmental Disabilities
Chicago, Illinois 60612

Paul M. Plotsky, Ph.D.
Division of Biology and Medicine
Section of Surgery
Brown University
Rhode Island Hospital
593 Eddy Street
Providence, Rhode Island 02902

Russell E. Poland, Ph.D.
Department of Psychiatry
Harbor U.C.L.A. Medical Center
Torrance, California 90509

Arthur J. Prange, Jr., M.D.
Department of Psychiatry
University of North Carolina at Chapel Hill
School of Medicine
Biological Sciences Research Center 220H
Chapel Hill, North Carolina 27514

M.E. Quigley, B.A., M.D., F.R.C.S.(C), F.A.C.O.G.
Department of Reproductive Medicine
University of California
550 Washington Street, Suite 529
San Diego, California 92103

Seymour Reichlin, M.D., Ph.D.
New England Medical Center Inc.
Endocrinology Division Box 275
171 Harrison Avenue
Boston, Massachusetts 02111

Robert M. Rose, M.D.
Department of Psychiatry and Behavioral Sciences
The University of Texas Medical Branch
Room 1.200 Graves Building
Galveston, Texas 77550

Robert T. Rubin, M.D., Ph.D.
Division of Biological Psychiatry
Department of Psychiatry
Harbor U.C.L.A. Medical Center
Torrance, California 90509

Benjamin Rusak, B.A., Ph.D.
Department of Psychology
Life Sciences Center
Dalhousie University
Halifax, Nova Scotia, Canada B3H 4J1

Barry M. Sherman, M.D.
Department of Internal Medicine
The Clinical Research Center
University of Iowa
University Hospitals
Iowa City, Iowa 52240

L. Cass Terry, M.D., Ph.D.
Department of Neurology
University of Michigan Medical Center
Veterans Administration
2215 Fuller Road
Ann Arbor, Michigan 48105

Michael O. Thorner, M.B., M.R.C.P.
University Medical Center
University of Virginia
Box 511
Charlottesville, Virginia 22908

G. Tolis, M.D.
Royal Victoria Hospital
687 Pine Avenue W.
Montreal, P.Q., Canada H3A 1A1

Holger Ursin, dr. Med.
Institute of Physiological Psychology
University of Bergen
Arstadveien 21
5000 Bergen, Norway

Robert A. Vigersky, M.D.
Endocrine-Metabolic Service, 7D
Department of Medicine
Walter Reed Army Medical Center
Washington, D.C. 20012

Caryn Vogel
Illinois State Psychiatric Institute
1601 West Taylor Street
Chicago, Illinois 60612

James B. Young, M.D.
Department of Medicine
Harvard Medical School
Beth Israel Hospital
330 Brookline
Boston, Massachusetts 02215

M. Zhang, M.D.
Illinois State Psychiatric Institute
1601 West Taylor Street
Chicago, Illinois 60612

Neuroendocrinology and Psychiatric Disorder,
edited by G. M. Brown, et al.
Raven Press, New York 1984.

Neuroendocrine Abnormalities in Schizophrenia: Prolactin, Growth Hormone, and Gonadotrophins

Herbert Y. Meltzer

Extensive investigation of the possible role of endocrine dysfunction in schizophrenia took place between 1940 and 1970 (11). Evidence for the relationship of hypo- or hyperfunction of the adrenal, thyroid, the gonads, pineal and pituitary glands to schizophrenia was sought by investigating: 1) the levels of target organ products - e.g., serum cortisol, urinary free cortisol, serum thyroxine, testosterone, estradiol, etc.; 2) administration of trophic hormones, or other stimuli to endocrine secretion, such as insulin-induced hypoglycemia, to examine target organ responsiveness and effect upon clinical state, and even; 3) surgical removal of the target organ, e.g. adrenalectomy. No definitive understanding of the role of the endocrine system in the etiology of schizophrenia or the extent of endocrine dysfunction in schizophrenia emerged from this research. As reviewed by Brambilla and Penati (11), evidence for hypo- and hyperfunction of the adrenal, pituitary, thyroid and gonads was sometimes found when small groups of chronically hospitalized, usually drug-free patients, were compared to normal controls. Many, but not all of these studies, were conducted in the era prior to neuroleptic drug use, so some of the reported abnormalities could have been due to neuroleptic action. Moreover, these studies took place prior to the current emphasis on distinguishing schizophrenia from manic-depressive illness and various organic illnesses, so that the ever present problem of accurate diagnosis and heterogeneity of the patient population were even more of an issue in those studies than they are today.

With these caveats aside, this large body of research found that endocrinopathies, in the classic sense of markedly diminished or excessive secretion of target organ products, were only rarely present in schizophrenic patients and that schizophreniform psychopathology is the exception rather than the rule in disorders of the pituitary, adrenal, thyroid or gonads. During five years in which we have assessed pituitary function in 125-150 patients who fulfill the Research Diagnostic Criteria (85) for schizophrenia we have found one case of borderline hypopituitarism and one with a probable prolactin secreting pituitary adenoma. In neither instance was there any apparent relationship between psychopathology and the pituitary dysfunction. Schizophreniform psychopathology may be found in patients with abnormalities of the thyroid or adrenal glands but such symptoms generally remit following appropriate treatment (11). While the psychopathology in such cases may be attributable to the endocrine dysfunction, it is clear that endocrine dysfunction of this type is not usually causally involved in schizophrenia.

As the role of neurotransmitters in the regulation of pituitary hormone release via the hypothalamic releasing or inhibiting hormones became clarified (40), neuroendocrine studies of schizophrenia increasingly have had as their goal, the use of pituitary hormone secretion as an index of the function of those neurotransmitters which were known to affect hormone secretion. Thus, since prolactin (PRL) release is known to be inhibited by dopamine (DA) from the tuberoinfundibular DA (TIDA) neurons acting on the pituitary lactotrophs (47), serum PRL levels have been studied in order to investigate whether there is increased activity of the TIDA neurons or increased responsiveness of pituitary DA receptors to DA or DA agonists in schizophrenia. The absence of an abnormal finding (e.g. low serum PRL levels) would not rule out increased DA-dependent activity elsewhere in the nervous system, but finding such an abnormality would certainly supply strong impetus to the DA hypothesis of schizophrenia (59, 84) and a relatively simple and convenient way to study that hypothesis further.

This review will cover studies of basal and stimulated growth hormone (GH), PRL, follicle stimulating hormone (FSH), luteinizing hormone (LH) and gonadal steroid hormone levels in schizophrenic patients with the aim of assessing the state of our knowledge in these areas and providing suggestions for future research. We will not discuss studies of the effect of chronic neuroleptic treatment on serum PRL levels in relation to clinical response. This has been reviewed by us elsewhere (51, 54) and is discussed elsewhere in this symposium. Several recent studies on adrenal androgens and antidiuretic hormone (ADH) will also be cited. We will also not review studies of β-endorphin or adrenal corticoids in schizophrenia. These have been reviewed elsewhere (11, 98).

Schizophrenia: Diagnosis and Course

Before presenting our review of the endocrine data concerning schizophrenia, a few comments upon the diagnosis and course of schizophrenia will be provided for the benefit of endocrinologists who may not be familiar with this syndrome. In the United States, the diagnosis of schizophrenia is now based upon the Research Diagnostic Criteria (RDC) (85) which have been incorporated into the Diagnostic Statistical Manual, Third Edition of the American Psychiatric Association. The diagnosis of schizophrenia is made in a patient who presents with one or more specific psychotic symptoms, such as bizarre delusions (e.g., thoughts being inserted or withdrawn from the mind), auditory hallucinations (e.g., two or more voices commenting on the individual's behaviour) or impaired thinking, in the absence of a primary mood disorder or organic psychosis. The illness must be present at least 6 months and should be associated with deterioration in social functioning. However, there are alternative criteria to diagnose schizophrenia, some broadening the syndrome, others narrowing it. In the absence of a pathognomonic symptom cluster or biological markers, it is inevitable that diagnosis will remain controversial. Prior to 1975, many patients were diagnosed as "acute" schizophrenics who would now be classified as having an affective psychosis, i.e., mania or melancholia. The diagnosis of chronic schizophrenia in the earlier literature had a higher probability of identifying patients who would meet modern criteria for schizophrenia. Most populations of individuals diagnosed as having schizophrenia will include some patients with occult CNS degenerative disorders, e.g., temporal lobe epilepsy, presenile dementia or metabolic disturbances.

There is ample indirect evidence to support the conlusion that the diagnosis of schizophrenia is based upon a series of phenotypes which could be the result of a number of different biological defects. Further the diverse clinical states that one observes in chronic schizophrenics ranging from residual states with minimal delusions and hallucinations but with flat affect and severe impairment in cognitive and social functioning, to superimposed florid psychoses with more or less continuous hallucinations, pervasive, bizarre delusions and severe thought disorder clearly impacts upon biological studies. It is difficult to assemble a phenomenologically homogeneous clinical population for research studies so that the lack of agreement between studies of biological parameters in schizophrenia may result from differences in clinical state as well as differences in clinical populations due to true heterogeneity (different classes of patients).

Growth Hormone (GH)

Basal GH Levels

There is no clinical evidence which suggests hypo- or hypersecretion of growth hormone (GH) in schizophrenic patients nor is psychopathology a major feature of abnormalities in GH secretion, as it often is in disorders of thyroid or adrenal secretion. Basal serum GH levels in schizophrenics have been found not to be increased in a large number of studies (3, 10, 29, 55, 65, 67, 76, 77, 88). No significant difference has been found in the serum GH levels in samples obtained in mid-morning via indwelling venous catheter in 24 drug-free schizophrenic patients and 16 normal controls: 1.54 ± 1.63 ($\bar{x} \pm$ S.D.) vs 3.28 ± 1.30, p = NS (Meltzer and Fang, unpublished data). There are no studies of 24 hr secretory patterns of GH release in schizophrenic patients.

L-Dopa and Apomorphine Stimulation Studies

A large number of studies have compared the increase in GH and decrease in PRL following administration of L-dopa, the precursor of DA and norepinephrine (NE), or apomorphine, a direct acting DA agonist, in schizophrenic patients and normal controls. The discussion of the PRL results in these studies will follow. The L-dopa-induced increase in GH is probably not based upon a dopaminergic mechanism since it is not inhibited by treatment with pimozide, a potent DA receptor blocker with minimal anti-adrenergic effects (20, 49). However, pimozide does block the NE-induced stimulation of the activity of rat limbic forebrain adenylate cyclase (6). This suggests the possibility that a mechanism other than NE might be involved in the L-dopa action or, more likely, that the NE receptor which mediates the release of GH releasing factor or somatostatin is not coupled to an adenylate cyclase. Extensive additional evidence that L-dopa stimulates GH secretion by an α-adrenergic mechanism was summarized by Muller et al. (61) and Langer et al. (43). However, it is still possible that L-dopa stimulates GH secretion by a dopaminergic or non-catecholaminergic mechanism. In contrast to L-dopa, pimozide, as well as a variety of other dopamine receptor blockers, inhibits the apomorphine-induced increase in GH in man (42, 50).

The rationale for the administration of single doses of L-dopa or apomorphine to schizophrenic patients to stimulate GH has been the attempt to test the hypothesis that there might be altered noradrenergic or dopaminergic receptor sensitivity in some schizophrenic patients as indicated by an increased or decreased GH response to the noradrenergic-based stimulation of GH by L-dopa or the dopamine-dependent stimulation of GH by apomorphine. We have reviewed the majority of these studies in detail elsewhere (50, 51) and will only highlight some of these studies here, report some of our most recent results, and discuss some of the problems with this approach.

Meltzer et al. (55) reported that the peak GH response following apomorphine, 0.75 mg subcutaneously, in 10 unmedicated chronic schizophrenic patients, was not significantly different from that of 7 normal controls. We also found that the GH response to the same dose of apomorphine was not altered in a systetmatic way after a two week period of treatment with chlorpromazine, (CPZ), followed by withdrawal of the neuroleptic for 5-7 days. This study was designed to determine if the hypothalamic or possibly pituitary dopamine receptor which regulates GH secretion would become supersensitive following withdrawal of neuroleptic medication. We concluded that they did not. However, it should be realized that the patient population in that and all subsequent studies to be discussed included a majority of patients who have had prolonged treatment with neuroleptic and other psychotropic drugs, followed by a period of withdrawal of variable duration, ranging from weeks to years.

A number of investigators have now reported that some chronic schizophrenic patients have a decreased GH response to apomorphine or L-dopa whereas some acute schizophrenic patients have an enhanced response to apomorphine or L-dopa. Thus, Ettigi et al. (29) found an inadequate GH response following apomorphine (9 ng/ml) in eight of 17 schizophrenic patients who had been withdrawn from neuroleptic treatment 2-15 weeks prior to study and 0 of 21 normal controls. The lowest GH response was noted in patients with tardive dyskinesia, a disorder believed to be associated with supersensitive striatal DA receptors (79). Ettigi et al. (29) found a significant negative relationship between duration of neuroleptic treatment and peak GH response ($r = -0.48$, $p < 0.05$) and a nearly significant negative relationship between duration of psychosis and peak GH response ($r = 0.45$, $p < 0.10$).

Rotrosen et al. (75, 77, 77b) studied the GH response following apomorphine in a group of recently admitted, floridly psychotic, chronic schizophrenic patients. They found no difference in mean GH peak in 22 schizophrenic and 9 control subjects who were given 0.5 mg of apomorphine subcutaneously. However, the distribution of the GH responses in the schizophrenic subjects showed greater variability than that for controls and appeared bimodal. In agreement with Ettigi et al. (29), Rotrosen et al. (77b) found a negative relationship between GH response to apomorphine and years of neuroleptic treatment, though they did not state that this finding was or was not statistically significant. A weak negative relationship between GH response to apomorphine and age was also found (77b). No relationship between GH response to L-dopa and age was found. An inverse relationship between the GH response to L-dopa and apomorphine in normal subjects was found (77). In their initial study, high GH response was associated with failure to respond to a subsequent course of neuroleptic treatment whereas a low GH response was seen in subsequent neuroleptic responders. In their subsequent reports (75, 76), they found no relationship between clinical response and GH response to apomorphine.

Tamminga et al. (91) reported significantly decreased GH response to L-dopa in 9 drug-free patients compared to 11 controls and a nonsignificant trend toward a decreased GH response to apomorphine in 11 chronic schizophrenic patients who were compared to five controls. Seven of the schizophrenic patients had tardive dyskinesia. In a somewhat larger study, the same group (67) reported that acute schizophrenic patients given apomorphine, 0.75 mg, had a significantly larger increase in GH compared to normal controls (N=8) and chronic schizophrenics (N=15). There was a non-significant tendency for chronic schizophrenics to have a smaller GH peak than in the normal controls. There was no difference in the GH response of chronic schizophrenics with and without tardive dyskinesia. The acute schizophrenic patients in this study had been ill for one year or less. No relationship between GH response and age in the normal controls was found.

Brambilla et al. (7) studied GH secretion in 10 chronic schizophrenic patients (duration of illness 4-32 years) who had been drug free for at least 10 days. Basal GH levels were within normal limits. L-Dopa stimulation tests, using 500 mg L-dopa orally plus carbidopa, 100 mg, were carried out before readministering haloperidol, in doses up to 10 mg per day for 30 days, and again 3 and 6 days after stopping the haloperidol. The GH response to L-dopa was normal in all patients before beginning the haloperidol therapy. The patients were further subdivided into those with and without the HLA-1 antigen. The five HLA-1 positive patients showed no significant difference in the GH response to L-dopa stimulation before and after haloperidol therapy, while the five HLA-1 negative patients had a non-significant tendency towards an enhanced GH response following withdrawal of haloperidol. The HLA-1 positive patients had a better clinical response to haloperidol than the HLA-1 negative patients. Thus, in this study, patients with a poorer clinical response to neuroleptics showed a larger GH response to L-dopa. Rotrosen et al. (77) found no such relationship between the L-dopa-induced GH response and clinical response but did not separate patients by HLA type. There was no evidence of a relationship between duration of illness and the magnitude of the GH response to L-dopa. Brambilla et al. (7) speculated that the difference in response to L-dopa and haloperidol in the two groups might be due to differences in the ability of DA receptors to modify their sensitivity following exposure to DA agonists and antagonists. This study requires confirmation in a larger sample. Should it be confirmed, it indicates the importance of controlling the duration of the drug-withdrawal period in studies of chronic schizophrenic patients and the need to examine multiple factors, including HLA antigen pattern, in analyzing the sources of variance in the GH response to DA agonists. HLA antigen patterns have shown a significant number of relationships to biological variables in schizophrenic patients. Multiple dosages of L-dopa or other DA agonists would have to be administered to test for a shift in DA receptor sensitivity.

We recently reported the interim results of a large scale ongoing study of the GH response to apomorphine, 0.75 mg subcutaneously, in schizophrenic patients and normal controls in relation to duration of illness and treatment response. We will review our current results as the study is now completed and the final results vary somewhat from the interim results of the earlier progress report.

The subjects for this study were patients admitted to wards of the Laboratory of Biological Psychiatry at the Illinois State Psychiatric Institute. Patients were diagnosed according to Research Diagnostic Criteria (85) utilizing information obtained by standardized interview schedules (99). The control group consisted of 24 normal volunteers who had no history of medical or psychiatric illness that was known to affect GH secretion. The mean age of the patients and controls was not significantly different. The majority of the subjects were between 21 and 45 years old. Subjects were in a fasting state from midnight prior to the study and throughout the study which took place in the morning.

They were kept in bed throughout the study. A 19 gauge venous catheter or butterfly infusion set was inserted into an arm vein between 9:15 and 10:15 am. Blood was withdrawn 30 and 15 min as well as just prior to injection of apomorphine 0.75 mg subcutaneously into the upper arm. Blood samples were drawn again at 1/2, 1, 1 1/2, and 2 hours after the injection. Serum GH levels were determined by the double antibody radioimmunoassay using the antisera produced by one of us (VSF). ^{125}I-GH was purchased from Abbott Laboratories, North Chicago, Ill. The GH working standard is NIH hGH-HS 2002F. Results are expressed as ng of standard/ml of plasma. The assay sensitivity is 0.5 ng/ml. Psychopathology was assessed on all subjects using the Brief Psychiatric Rating Scale (66). Other means of symptom assessment were used for different subgroups of subjects and will be discussed elsewhere. All subjects were drug free for at least one week before entering the study. Subjects were excluded if they had had fluphenazine decanoate, a long-acting neuroleptic, within 10 weeks of apomorphine administration because we have recently found a small number of sjubjects with elevated serum prolactin levels for up to 8 weeks after FD administration (Meltzer et al., unpublished data). Subjects were eliminiated from the data analysis if they had serum GH levels greater than 6 ng/ml prior to administration of apomorphine. The area under the GH curve (AUC) during the two hours after apomorphine administration was calculated using Simpson's method.

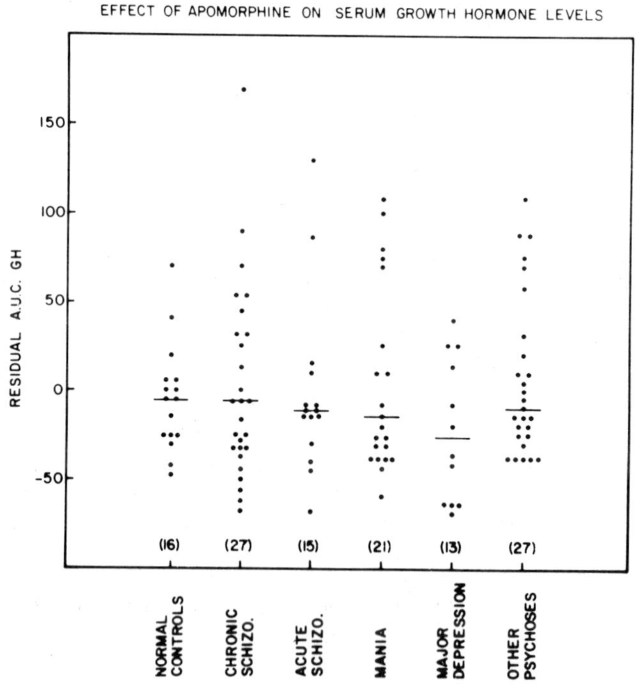

FIG. 1. Residual GH area under the curve (AUC) with sex effect covaried out for normal controls and five groups of psychiatric patients. The other psychotic group consisted predominantly of schizo-affective and atypical psychotic patients. (N-number of subjects).

TABLE 1. APOMORPHINE-INDUCED GROWTH HORMONE AREA UNDER THE CURVE

	Area Under the Curve	
	Male	Female
Chronic Schizophrenics	77.5 (14)[x]	32.3 (13)
Acute Schizophrenics	59.9 (9)	48.5 (6)
Manic Depressive, Manic	79.5 (10)	39.3 (11)
Major Depressive Disorder	26.2 (6)	37.8 (7)
Other Psychoses	71.7 (12)	50.1 (15)
Controls	58.7 (8)	40.2 (8)

[x](N)

The results are given in Fig. 1 and Table 1. Since we found, as did Ettigi et al. (28), that females had a significantly smaller GH response to apomorphine than males, the effect of sex was removed statistically. An analysis of variance (ANOVA) (Table 2) demonstrated no significant difference between the GH AUC for normal controls, chronic schizophrenics, acute schizophrenics, manic patients, patients with major depression and patients with other psychiatric illnesses (predominantly patients with other psychiatric disorders and unspecified atypical functional psychoses). When the schizophrenic patients were divided into those ill less than or more than four years, an ANOVA indicated significant differences between the two groups of schizophrenics and normal controls (Table 3). This division into those ill less than or more than 4 years was determined empirically in our previous studies (50) and is here confirmed.

The magnitude of the GH response in the schizophrenics ill less than four years is approximately 1 1/2 times that of the normal controls and three times that of schizophrenics ill 4 or more years (Fig. 2, Table 4). The difference between the two groups of schizophrenics was significant ($p < .05$) but the difference between either group and normal controls was not.

The magnitude of the GH response to apomorphine among schizophrenic patients was significantly correlated with duration of illness for males

TABLE 2. EFFECT OF DIAGNOSIS AND SEX ON APOMORPHINE-INDUCED GROWTH HORMONE AREA UNDER THE CURVE

ANOVA

	df	Sum of Square	Mean Square	F	p
Diagnosis	5	8470	1694.0	0.77	.578
Sex	1	11846	11846	5.36	.023
Diagnosis x Sex	5	9193	1838.6	0.83	.531
Error	10	236329	2208.7		

TABLE 3. EFFECT OF SEX AND DIAGNOSIS ON APOMORPHINE-INDUCED GROWTH HORMONE AREA UNDER THE CURVE, DIVIDING SCHIZOPHRENICS BY DURATION OF ILLNESS

ANOVA Table

Source	Sum of Squares	df	Mean Square	F	p
Sex	8094.26	1	8094.26	4.43	.04
Duration of illness	22958.79	2	11479.40	6.29	.004
Sex x duration of illness	3715.46	2	1857.73	1.02	.37
Error	94971.13	52	1826.37		

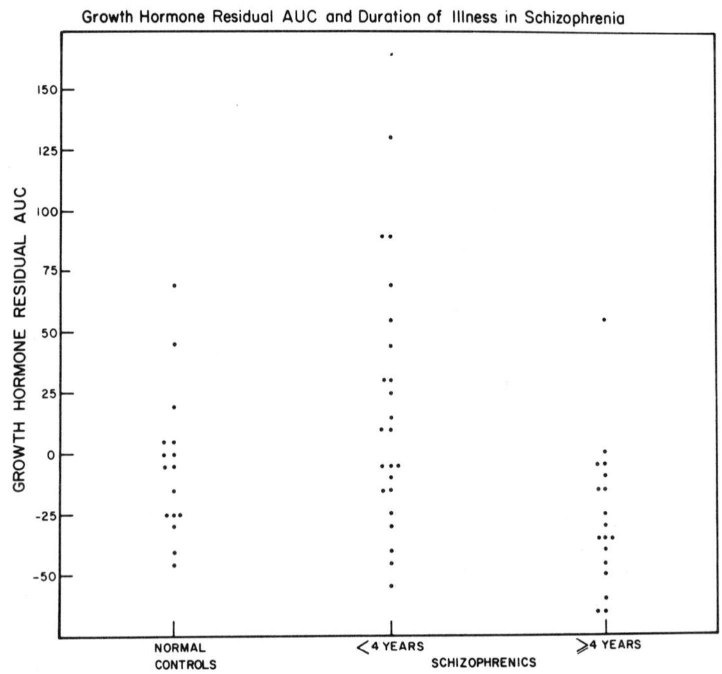

FIG. 2. Residual GH area under the curve (AUC) with sex effect covaried out for normal controls and schizophrenic patients divided into those with duration of illness less than 4 years and equal to or greater than 4 years.

TABLE 4. APOMORPHINE-INDUCED GROWTH HORMONE ARE UNDER THE CURVE, DIVIDING SCHIZOPHRENICS BY DURATION OF ILLNESS

Group	Male	Female
Schizophrenics ill 4 years	96.28 (14)*	51.20 (10)
Schizophrenics ill 4 years	30.66 (9)	22.09 (9)
Controls	58.68 (8)	40.16 (8)

*(N)

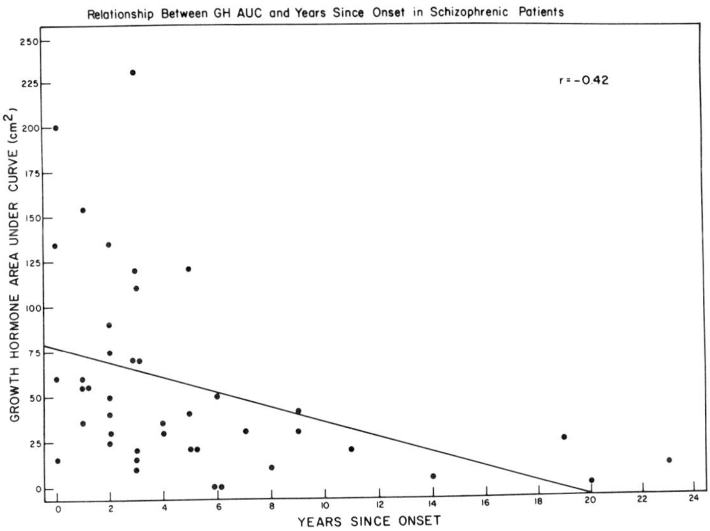

FIG. 3. Linear regression of GH area under the curve (AUC) and years since onset in schizophrenic patients.

($r = 0.43$, $N = 23$, $p < .05$) and females ($r = -0.50$, $N = 19$, $p < .05$) as was the partial correlation between GH response and duration of illness controlling for sex ($r = 0.42$, $N = 42$, $p < .01$, Fig. 3).

Since age and duration of illness were highly correlated among schizophrenics ($r = 0.78$, $N = 42$, $p < .0001$), and since age and GH response were significantly negatively correlated, multiple regression analyses were performed, removing the effects of age (and sex) to further explore the relationship between duration of illness and GH response. After removal of the effect of age and sex, the relationship of duration of illness and magnitude of GH response in the schizophrenic patients was no longer statistically significant ($p = 0.155$).

We also found that for the 60 non-schizophrenic patients, for whom duration of illness and age were less strongly correlated ($r = 0.35$, $N = 60$, $p < .001$), duration of illness and the magnitude of the GH response were significantly correlated even after covarying out sex and age ($r = 0.39$, $p = .002$, $N = 60$, Fig. 4). This indicates that the relationship between GH response and duration of illness is not unique to schizophrenia and is probably not due to neuroleptic treatment since the majority of these patients were patients with affective disorders who had only brief periods of treatment with neuroleptic drugs.

We found no relationship between the apomorphine-induced increase in GH and psychopathology at admission, discharge, or for the change scores in BPRS total or subscales between admission and discharge. However, a significant positive correlation was found between the magnitude of the PRL response to apomorphine and the admission BPRS depression subscale ratings for the group of schizophrenics and affective psychoses ($r = 0.46$, $N = 75$, $p < .0001$). This data will be presented in detail elsewhere.

In summary, earlier small scale studies have reported a negative relationship between diminished GH response to apomorphine or L-dopa and clinical response. No such relationship was found in our study which

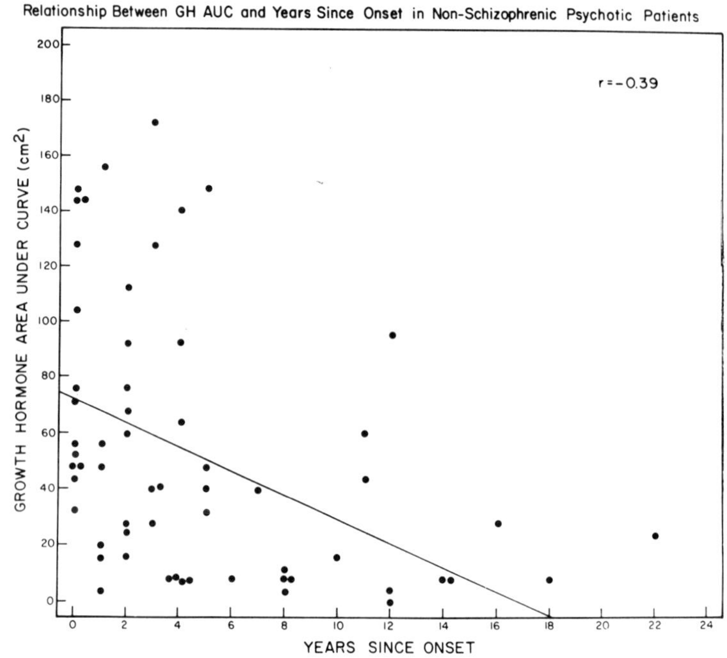

FIG. 4. Linear regression of GH area under the curve (AUC) and years since onset in schizophrenic patients.

is the largest to date. There is, however, general agreement that increased duration of schizophrenic psychopathology is associated with diminished GH response to apomorphine or L-dopa (29, 50, 77). This does not appear to be due to neuroleptic treatment since it was also observed in non-schizophrenic patients who were treated with a variety of psychotropic drugs, especially lithium and antidepressant drugs. It is possible that there is diminished GH secretion due to pharmacokinetic factors affecting the availability of apomorphine or l-dopa, decreased sensitivity of DA or NE receptors to DA or NE respectively, decreased GH reserve in the pituitary or increased metabolism of GH. Examination of the data in Fig. 1 indicates that a number of the acute schizophrenics as well as patients with affective illness and other psychoses have relatively low GH responses to apomorphine. It is possible that such diminished GH responses early in the course of illness may predict chronicity.

Effect of d-Amphetamine on GH

Langer et al. (43) studied the GH response to i.v. d-amphetamine, 0.1 mg/kg, in 5 acute paranoid schizophrenics and 3 chronic schizophrenic patients and 21 normal subjects. No significant difference was noted but the size of the schizophrenic group is quite small.

Effect of TRH and LRH on GH Levels

In conjunction with Prange and colleagues (70), we studied the effect of TRH, 500 μg i.v. on GH levels in 17 schizophrenic patients and 17 normal controls. At 45 and 90 min after TRH, there was no significant change in GH level in either group. However, Gil-Ad et al. (33) recently reported that six schizophrenic adolescent male patients (15 years, 8 ± 4 months) had an abnormal GH response following TRH 200 μg i.v. There was no difference in baseline GH levels between the patients and nine age-matched normal controls but four of the six patients had an increase in plasma GH levels 15-60 min after TRH administration whereas none of the control did. Four of the patients had a repeat study following chlorpromazine treatment and three of them continued to show a significant rise in GH levels after TRH. Eight schizophrenic boys were also given luteinizing hormone-releasing hormone (LRH) (50 g/m2 body surface i.v.). None of the nine controls had any change in GH levels after LRH. However, seven of the eight schizophrenia patients had a marked increase in GH levels 45-90 min after LRH. LRH was administered again after treatment; four patients who had shown a marked elevation of plasma GH in the pretreatment LRH test showed a blunted response; one had a persistently positive GH response and the other showed no response in either of the LRH tests. As noted by Gil-Ad et al. (33), an abnormal release of GH induced by TRH has already been reported in acromegaly, endogenous depression, anorexia nervosa, renal failure and severe liver disease. A GH response after LRH has also been reported in acromegaly and gigantism and in a few cases of anorexia nervosa. The authors raised the possibility that these abnormal responses to hypothalamic releasing hormones may reflect abnormalities in brain neurotransmitter systems or in the ability of pituitary cell membranes to selectively respond to hypothalamic releasing hormones. They suggest that stress was not a likely explanation because basal levels of GH and cortisol were normal in the schizophrenic patients and because of the dissociation between the responses to LRH and TRH after the antipsychotic treatment. However, episodic "spontaneous" GH secretion is so common that further verification is required before accepting the results of this and similar studies. Thus, further study of the GH response of adolescent and adult schizophrenics to TRH and LRH appears indicated. These results point out the need to consider both age of onset and duration of illness as separate variables in studying biological measures in schizophrenic patients.

Insulin-Induced Hypoglycemia and GH

There are conflicting data concerning the normality of the GH response to insulin-induced hypoglycemia in schizophrenic patients and the effect of neuroleptics on the GH response due to hypoglycemia. Schimmelbusch et al. (81) found a blunted GH response to an insulin tolerance test in a small number of chronically hospitalized unmedicated schizophrenic patients compared with those receiving neuroleptics and normal controls. However, Takahashi et al. (90) reported normal GH response to insulin in schizophrenic patients. Brambilla et al. (10) studied the GH response to insulin in 15 hebephrenic and 6 paranoid schizophrenic patients who had been drug free for at least 10 days prior to study. The GH response was normal in all subjects on first testing but was blunted in one-third of the hebephrenic patients on a repeat test 48 hours later. The mean GH response to insulin was not significantly affected in most of the chronic patients when retested during haloperidol treatment but some showed blunted or exaggerated responses. The hypo- and hypersecretory episodes in response to insulin on retesting were variable in each patient from experiment to experiment. No relationships between age, sex, duration of illness and GH response were found but the age of onset did correlate with the diminished GH response on repeat testing and variable response during haloperidol. The hebephrenic patients who have an earlier age of onset than the paranoid patients were the ones with the irregular GH response while subjects with onset of the disease in adulthood, i.e., the paranoid patients, did not. Brambilla et al. (10) reported that the diminished GH response to insulin was associated with defect symptoms such as severe negativism, withdrawal from reality and apathy, whereas GH hypersecretion was associated with psychomotor excitement and hostility. The differences between the hebephrenic and paranoid patients were attributed to relative deficiencies in the noradrenergic pathways mediating GH release in the hebephrenic patients.

Beg et al. (3) also reported no significant difference in the peak GH response to insulin in drug-free and chlorpromazine-treated schizophrenic patients and normal controls. No significant relationship was found between the peak GH response and duration of illness, duration of chlorpromazine administration, and drug dosage in that study. Two other studies (65, 81) have also reported no difference in the insulin-induced increase in GH with and without neuroleptic treatment. However, Chalmers et al. (18) reported that a single injection of fluphenazine decanoate significantly inhibited the insulin-induced increase in GH. The reason for these discrepancies is not apparent. It does not appear to be a simple function of the type of neuroleptic used.

There is some evidence that the increase in GH following insulin-induced hypoglycemia is mediated through a noradrenergic mechanism (61). Thus, the findings of Schimmelbusch et al. (81) and Brambilla et al. (10) of abnormalities in the GH response following insulin-induced hypoglycemia in schizophrenia are of interest in light of subsequent studies of brain and CSF NE and 3-methoxy-4-hydroxyphenylglycol (MHPG) levels in the urine of schizophrenic patients. Relatively increased levels of NE have been reported in the limbic forebrains of chronic paranoid schizophrenic patients (31). Kleinman et al. (39) found very elevated NE levels in the nucleus accumbens of two paranoid schizophrenic patients although no difference was found for four other schizophrenic patients. There was also no difference in the levels of MHPG in the brain of these patients in comparison with controls. However, increased free MHPG and decreased conjugated MHPG levels were found in the hypothalamus of the schizophrenic patients. Increased NE levels were also reported in the caudate nucleus of decreased "nuclear" schizophrenics (37) which could correspond to the hebephrenic patients. A non-significant trend towards increased NE levels in the nucleus accumbens and anterior perforated substance was also reported by Bird et al. (5). No difference in NE in 10 brain areas of schizophrenics and controls was reported by Bucht et al. (16). Differences in dissection and postmortem intervals may account for the discrepancies in these studies and make interpretation of these studies difficult.

Increased levels of NE have also been reported in the cerebrospinal fluid (CSF) of schizophrenic patients in two studies (34, 41). One (41) found the increased CSF NE levels in paranoid patients but normal NE levels in undifferentiated schizophrenic patients. However, the undifferentiated patients had the highest pulse and psychosis scores on the Bunney-Hamburg psychosis rating. The other study (34) reported increased NE and cyclic adenosine monophosphate (cAMP) in chronic but not acute schizophrenic patients. Taube et al. (92) reported that there was a very strong relationship between agitation and urinary MHPG in schizophrenic but not depressed patients. Joseph et al. (37) reported a strong negative correlation between severity of illness in a group of 18 unmedicated chronic schizophrenic patients and their 24-hr excretion of MHPG-sulfate but not of MHPG-glucuronide or vanillylmandelic acid (VMA). No consider-action was given to the issue of agitation or paranoia in that study. Taken together these results suggest the importance of further investigating noradrenergic mechanisms, especially in paranoid schizophrenia, in relation to GH secretion following insulin, L-dopa, or d-amphetamine.

Growth Hormone Secretion During Sleep

There have been surprisingly few studies of GH secretion during sleep in schizophrenic patients. GH is released during slow wave sleep shortly after sleep onset; further episodes of GH secretion may not occur during later periods of slow wave sleep (89). Neuroleptic drugs do not affect GH secretion during sleep (19). Vigneri et al. (97) studied the GH secretory pattern during sleep in four drug-free schizophrenic patients 21-37 years old. All had had a clear GH rise following insulin-induced hypoglycemia. All four patients showed decreased stage III and IV slow wave sleep. One of the patients, an acute schizophrenic, had two clear GH rises during episodes of slow wave sleep on both study nights. The three chronic schizophrenic patients had no increase in GH during both nights of the study. According to Brambilla and Penati (11), similar findings were made by Murri et al. (62, 63). Subsequently, Syvalahti and Pekkarinen (88) studied ten schizophrenic patients, ages not specified, who were treated with antipsychotic drugs. Four of the schizophrenic patients had a high sleep-related peak of GH, four had a moderate peak, while two had no increase in GH secretion. Meltzer et al. (54) reported no increase in GH during EEG-monitored sleep in two neuroleptic-treated chronic schizophrenic patients, ages 27 and 31. Thus, there are conflicting data on a relatively small number of schizophrenic patients with regard to the preservation of the sleep-related surge in GH secretion in chronic schizophrenic patients. Further research is clearly indicated in this area. However, there was evidence of an absence in sleep-related GH secretion in 15 patients (ages 23-59) with endogenous depression (80), so this abnormality may be another nonspecific indication of dysregulation of pituitary hormone secretion in patients with severe psychopathology. Since exogenous corticosteroids can interfere with the sleep-related increase in GH (60), it will be necessary to consider hypersecretion of cortisol as a factor in disrupted GH secretion in patients with affective disorders and possible schizophrenic patients in an acute exacerbation.

Conclusions

There is an intriguing but by no means definitive body of literature pointing towards a relationship between GH secretion and certain important dimensions of the schizophrenic syndrome. Early age of onset of the disorder may be associated with abnormal GH response to TRH and LRH. The magnitude of the apomorphine-induced increase in GH appears to fall off as a function of age or duration of illness, but this does not appear to be specific for schizophrenia since the same relationship was found in other types of psychoses. The insulin-induced increase in GH may develop a kind of tachyphylaxis in hebephrenic patients and also become more variable following neuroleptic-treatment in such patients compared to paranoid schizophrenics. The L-dopa-induced GH response may be genetically influenced because of the reported association with HLA antigens. Since hebephrenic patients often have an earlier age of onset as compared to paranoid schizophrenic patients, there may be an important interaction between this symptom pattern and age of onset.

Some sleep studies suggest impaired GH secretion along with diminished slow wave sleep.

It would be of great value to relate neurotransmitter mechanisms to these signs of dysregulation of GH. GH secretion is enhanced by noradrenergic and dopaminergic mechanisms, possibly by serotonin as well. Insulin-induced hypoglycemia appears to stimulate a noradrenergic-based increase in GH secretion. There is evidence for noradrenergic abnormalities in schizophrenic patients as revealed by studies of postmortem brain NE levels, CSF NE levels and urinary MHPG. As yet, there has been no study in schizophrenic patients integrating the GH response to insulin, ampomorphine, or a noradrenergic drug such as d-amphetamine or clonidine, with CSF or urinary measures of noradrenergic function. Such studies might examine the hypothesis that paranoid schizophrenic patients have a relatively normal GH response to insulin or apomorphine but an exaggerated response to d-amphetamine or clonidine and increased NE levels in CSF or increased urinary MHPG. Non-paranoid patients might have abnormal GH responses to insulin or relatively diminished responses to apomorphine, normal responses to d-amphetamine or clonidine and relatively low urinary MHPG and CSF NE.

Prolactin (PRL) Studies

Introduction

There is extensive direct evidence that DA produced by the TIDA neurons reaches the pituitary via the hypothalamic hypophysial portal circulation where it inhibits the release of PRL through an action on DA receptors. DA receptors which share some of the properties of postsynatpic DA receptors in the striatum, limbic and cortical dopaminergic areas have been identified in the anterior lobe of pituitary by use of ^{3}H-haloperidol or ^{3}H-spiroperidol (17, 21, 32). The DA receptor which inhibits the secretion of PRL in the pituitary gland does not appear to be coupled to a DA-sensitive adenylate cyclase (71), although there is still controversy about this issue (1). Kebabian and Calne (38) have named this DA receptor the D-2 receptor to distinguish it from the postsynaptic DA receptors in the forebrain which they have called the D-1 receptor. We have suggested that there may be another DA receptor in the pituitary which has a high affinity for sulpiride and related drugs and may also contribute to the ability of classical neuroleptic drugs to block the inhibitory effects of DA on PRL release (58). The ability of neuroleptic drugs to stimulate PRL secretion *in vivo* is highly correlated with their antipsychotic potency and their ability to inhibit ^{3}H-spiroperidol binding in the striatum (45, 54).

The TIDA neurons have some significant differences from other DA neurons. They lack an effective high-affinity DA uptake system (26); the turnover of DA in these neurons is stimulated by PRL (25) so that a shortloop negative feedback system contributes to the regulation of PRL secretion in vivo. The TIDA neurons also appear to lack autoreceptors (24) so that low doses of DA agonists do not produce further decreases in the release of DA and do not affect PRL secretion in man or laboratory animals.

The possibility of an abnormality in the TIDA neurons or pituitary DA receptors has been extensively investigated in schizophrenic patients because it would have important implications for the DA hypothesis of schizophrenia. For example, a shift to the left in the dose-response curve of the ability of DA agonists such as apomorphine or bromocriptine to decrease serum PRL levels in drug-free schizophrenics as compared to controls would suggest DA receptor supersensitivity in the schizophrenic patient's pituitary glands. A smaller increase in serum PRL levels following administration of a low dose of a neuroleptic would also be consistent with increased release of DA from the TIDA neurons, supersensitivity of pituitary DA receptors, decreased metabolism of DA, or some other mechanism which might account for excessive dopaminergic antagonism of the neuroleptic-induced increase in PRL secretion.

Basal Serum PRL

Basal serum PRL levels have been studied in unmedicated acute and chronic schizophrenic patients by many investigators and found to be within normal limits in nearly all subjects (8, 35, 53, 54, 56, 57, 76). A small proportion of subjects in some studies have elevated basal serum PRL levels (53, 36) but this may be due to stress, failure to allow sufficient time, which may be as long as two months, for the effect of long-acting neuroleptics to terminate, or the persistence of the sleep-related increase in PRL secretion after awakening. We have recently obtained evidence that single or even multiple basal serum samples obtained by venipuncture at 0800 hrs may produce misleading data about basal PRL secretion. The correlation coefficients for PRL levels in the mean of three samples obtained at 15 min intervals between 0900 and 1000 hrs on each of two days were 0.98 and 0.86 in 19 schizophrenic patients and 20 normal controls, respectively ($p < .001$). The correlation coefficient for PRL levels in two basal blood samples obtained via direct venipuncture on consecutive days from 28 unmedicated schizophrenic patients was 0.54 ($p < .01$). The correlation coefficient between the mean of three basal serum PRL determinations and the catheter serum PRL levels on one of the three days in 17 schizophrenic patients was 0.47, $p < .025$. Thus, these results indicate that the basal serum PRL levels, though providing some indication of PRL secretion, produce, when the levels are within the normal range, less reliable results than the samples obtained via catheter.

The mean serum PRL levels in new groups of normal controls and chronic schizophrenic patients (diagnosis by RDC criteria) from our laboratory are given in Table 5. The schizophrenic patients had been withdrawn from neuroleptic drugs for at least 7 days and most had been drug-free for more than a month. No significant difference between basal or catheter serum PRL levels in male and female normal controls was found. Basal PRL levels in female schizophrenic patients tended to be elevated. Basal PRL levels in male schizophrenic patients and catheter PRL levels in male and female schizophrenic patients were not significantly different from normal. There was a trend for the variance in basal serum PRL levels in the male chronic schizophrenic patients to be greater than that of the controls but this was not noted in the catheter PRL values. No evidence of decreased serum PRL levels in schizophrenic patients was obtained in this study. The apparently increased basal PRL levels in female schizophrenic patients, compared to normal controls without any difference in catheter PRL levels between the two groups, suggests that one of the factors which could increase basal serum PRL levels influenced these results. In any event, the number of female subjects is small.

We examined the correlations between basal serum PRL levels and the following variables in chronic schizophrenic patients: age, age of onset, duration of illness, presence of delusions, hallucinations, total psychotic symptoms, first rank symptoms, anxiety, total Brief Psychiatric Rating Scale scores and total Global Assessment score. None of the correlations reached statistical significance. There was a trend

TABLE 5. SERUM PRL LEVELS IN MALE AND FEMALE SCHIZOPHRENIC AND NORMAL CONTROLS

	Basal		Catheter	
Group	Males	Females	Males	Females
Normal Controls	26.7 $\pm$ 10.6 (23)	30.2 $\pm$ 13.0 (24)	27.3 $\pm$ 15.8 (23)	29.5 $\pm$ 12.6 (20)
Chronic Schizophrenics	32.9 $\pm$ 18.9 (23)	51.8 $\pm$ 20.4 (13)	26.5 $\pm$ 14.3 (22)	28.8 $\pm$ 12.7 (15)

for delusions and hallucinations to be more common in female schizophrenic patients with lower serum PRL levels.

Brambilla et al. (7) studied serum PRL levels in catheter samples obtained from chronic schizophrenic patients who had last received neuroleptic treatment at least 10 days prior to study. Serum PRL levels markedly lower than normal were found in six of the 10 patients studied before, as well as 3 and 6 days after withdrawal from a subsequent 30 day course of haloperidol treatment. This is consistent with the hypothesis of increased dopaminergic activity in the TIDA neurons or increased response to DA by pituitary DA receptors. The explanation of the low serum PRL levels in these patients will require further study. It has recently been reported that lower serum PRL levels were found in those schizophrenic patients withdrawn from medication as part of a drug-free trial who were most likely to have a worsening of their symptoms followed by a full-blown relapse (15, 46). These patients also responded best to neuroleptics when they were restarted. These results were consistent with increased TIDA as well as increased dopaminergic activity in those DA neurons which contribute to the exacerbation of psychosis.

We have obtained serum samples at 15 min intervals from 0900 to 2100 hrs from six chronic schizophrenic patients and three normal controls. No significant difference in the pattern of PRL secretion in these subjects was noted (54).

Sleep PRL Levels

There has been only one report of serum PRL levels during sleep in schizophrenic patients. We (54) found the expected increase in PRL levels beginning shortly after sleep onset with the peak at 0500-0600 hrs in two chronic schizophrenic patients treated with fluphenazine decanoate. Additional studies in drug-free and medicated patients are clearly indicated.

CSF PRL Levels

Wode-Helgodt et al. (100) reported that PRL levels in the CSF of 43 unmedicated chronic schizophrenic patients were not significantly different from that of normal controls. Similar results have been reported by Rimon et al. (73) who also found that CSF PRL levels were significantly higher in non-lobotomized patients than in those who had had a lobotomy.

Effect of L-Dopa or Apomorphine on Serum PRL Levels

The ability of apomorphine and L-dopa to suppress PRL levels in schizophrenics and normal controls has been studied by a number of investigators. The methodology of these studies has been briefly described in discussing the results of these agents on GH secretion so only the PRL findings will be summarized here. Meltzer et al. (55), Ettigi et al. (29) and Rotrosen et al. (76) found no difference in the ability of apomorphine to suppress PRL levels in schizophrenic patients and controls whereas Tamminga et al. (91) reported that apomorphine produced a lesser decrease in PRL levels in schizophrenic patients than in normals. Tamminga et al. (91) also reported a lesser decrease in PRL levels following L-dopa in schizophrenics than in normals whereas Rotrosen et al. (77) and Brambilla et al. (7) found no significant difference in the PRL decrease in the two groups.

We have now administered apomorphine, 0.75 mg subcutaneously, to 23 chronic and 11 acute schizophrenic patients, 44 other psychiatric patients and 21 normal controls. The results are given in Tables 6 and 7

TABLE 6. APOMORPHINE-INDUCED PROLACTIN AREA UNDER THE CURVE

	Area Under the Curve	
Group	Male	Female
Chronic Schizophrenics	84.34 (12)*	129.66 (11)
Acute Schizophrenics	123.46 (5)	160.09 (6)
Manics	74.12 (5)	125.06 (10)
Depressives	72.18 (5)	123.30 (3)
Controls	99.28 (7)	125.09 (11)
Others	84.39 (10)	100.95 (11)
	Baseline PRL	
Group	Male	Female
Chronic Schizophrenics	18.31 (12)	29.08 (11)
Acute Schizophrenics	26.73 (5)	36.35 (6)
Manics	15.96 (5)	27.68 (10)
Depressives	17.46 (5)	31.99 (3)
Controls	22.52 (7)	27.70 (11)
Others	19.67 (10)	24.42 (11)

*(N)

and Fig. 5. The magnitude of the PRL decrease was significantly correlated with the baseline level of PRL and sex so these factors were partialled out. No significant difference in the PRL responses in any of the groups were found although there was a tendency for the PRL response in the acute schizophrenic patients to be greater than that of the other patient groups. When the acute and chronic schizophrenic patients were divided into those whose illness had persisted for less than or more than 4 years, as was done with the GH response data, no significant difference in PRL response to apomorphine was noted. Thus, only the GH response to apomorphine differs in schizophrenic patients divided into those whose illness has persisted for less than or more than 4 years.

Effect of TRH on PRL Secretion

Brambilla et al. (12) reported that the PRL response to 500 ug of TRH i.v. was significantly greater in 20 schizophrenic patients than in 8 normal controls. The patients had been withdrawn from neuroleptic medication for 10 days in 17 cases, for 3 months in one case and for 1 year

TABLE 7. EFFECT OF DIAGNOSIS AND SEX ON APOMORPHINE-INDUCED PROLACTIN AREA UNDER THE CURVE, COVARYING OUT SERUM PROLACTIN BASELINE

Analysis of Covariance

Source of Variation	Adjusted Sums of Squares	Adjusted df	Adjusted Mean square	F	p
Groups	2807.78	5	561.56	1.73	.14
Sex	373.42	1	373.42	1.15	.29
Groups x Sex	299.86	5	59.97	.18	.97
Covariate (Baseline PRL)	99094.96	1	99094.96	304.66	.0001
Error	26996.99	83	325.26		

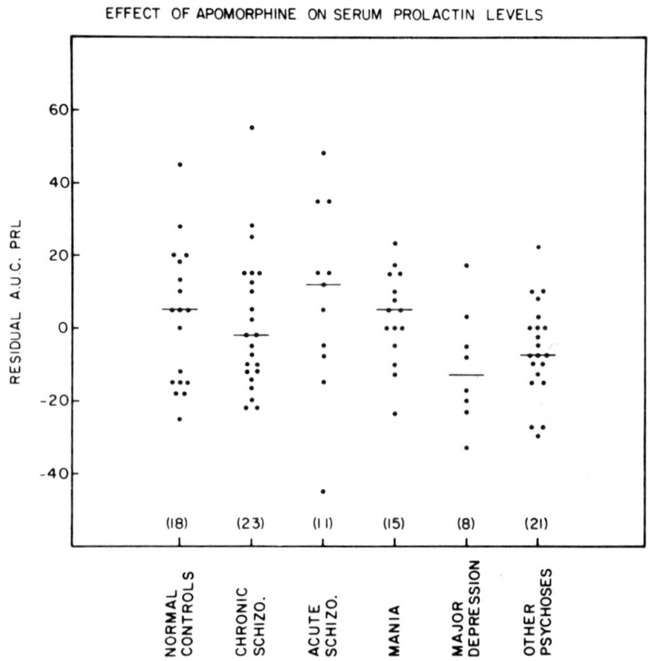

FIG. 5. Residual PRL areas under the curve (AUC) with baseline PRL and sex effect covaried out for normal controls and five groups of psychiatric patients. (N = number of subjects).

in two cases. However, Prange et al. (70) found no difference in the PRL response following TRH in 15 unmedicated chronic schizophrenic patients and 17 normal controls. There was a markedly greater response in female patients and controls than in male patients and controls. The explanation of the difference between the two studies is unclear; further investigation is warranted.

Effect of Single Dose of Neuroleptic on Serum PRL Levels

The release of DA from the TIDA neurons and the sensitivity of pituitary DA receptors are major factors which determine the magnitude of and time course of the PRL response to neuroleptic administration. Increased release of DA from the TIDA neurons or supersensitivity of DA receptors in the pituitary would be predicted to produce a smaller or shorter PRL response. This has stimulated considerable clinical investigations in schizophrenic patients. Thus, Meltzer et al. (54) found no difference in the PRL response to a 50 mg dose of chlorpromazine (CPZ) in 16 male schizophrenic patients and 6 normal controls. Gruen et al. (35) found no significant difference in the PRL response to 25 mg CPZ in 10 male normal control and 8 male schizophrenic patients.

We have now carried out a study in which 12.5 and 25 mg CPZ was given i.m. to male and female schizophrenic patients and controls (51). The controls also received saline i.m. on the third study day. Serum PRL levels were monitored prior to and after the injections in blood samples obtained via indwelling venous catheters. The results of this study will be briefly summarized here (Tables 8, 9). The PRL area under the curve was significantly corrleated with baseline PRL levels for the 12.5 mg

TABLE 8. EFFECT OF 12.5 mg CHLORPROMAZINE ON PROLACTIN AREA UNDER THE CURVE

Group	Males	Females
Schizophrenics	208 ± 110* (14)+	152 ± 66 (11)
Controls	202 ± 63 (7)	233 ± 129 (9)

*Mean ± S.D.
+(N)

dose but not for the 25 mg dose. There was no significant difference in the response to 12.5 mg or 25 mg for males and females. There was a strong trend which just missed statistical significance for the female schizophrenic patients to have a smaller response than female controls, particularly after the 12.5 mg dose ($t = 1.66$, $N = 20$, $p = 0.12$). The response to 25 mg was signigicantly greater than to 12.5 mg in both patients and controls. The PRL response to 12.5 mg CPZ was significantly greater than to saline in the controls. We found a significant negative correlation ($r = -0.46$, $N = 24$, $p = .018$) between severity of delusions rated on the SADS-C at admission and serum PRL response to CPZ 25 mg i.m. There was no significant relationship between the PRL response to either dose of CPZ and the clinical response to CPZ following treatment with 200 mg CPZ/day for 1 week and 400 mg/day for a second week. There were trends for a positive correlation between clinical response as measured by changes in BPRS rating between admission and discharge and the magnitude of the PRL response to 12.5 or 25 mg CPZ i.m. during the placebo period. No relationship between duration of illness and the magnitude of the PRL response to either dose of CPZ was noted. The PRL response to CPZ 25 mg i.m. was significantly correlated with the basal serum PRL levels at the end of the first and second treatment weeks ($r = 0.55$ and 0.64, $p < 0.05$), respectively.

These results suggest that female schizophrenic patients may have increased release of DA from the TIDA neurons, an enhanced response to DA, or, for pharmacokinetic reasons, absorb smaller amounts of CPZ than normal control females.

TABLE 9. EFFECT OF 25 mg CHLORPROMAZINE ON PROLACTIN AREA UNDER THE CURVE

Group	Males	Females
Schizophrenics	281 ± 114* (18)+	316 ± 146 (11)
Normals	337 ± 61 (7)	410 ± 288 (9)

*Mean ± S.D.
+(N)

Gonadotrophins, Gonadal Steroids and Adrenal Androgens in Schizophrenia

Gonadal Steroids: Brambilla and Penati (11) have provided a detailed review of studies through 1977 of gonadal function, gonadotrophins and sex hormone levels in schizophrenic patients. These studies will only be briefly discussed here and several recent related studies will be cited. Brooksbank et al. (14) and Tourney and Hatfield (94, 95) have reported normal levels of testosterone, androstenedione and other androgenic steroids in male schizophrenic patients. Arato et al. (2) also found normal testosterone levels in 17 chronic schizophrenic patients. However, Brambilla and Penati (11) reported markedly reduced serum testosterone levels in 92% of a group of 29 chronic schizophrenic patients. Urinary estrogen secretion was reduced in half of the 24 female schizophrenic patients studied. Urinary pregnanediol secretion was also reduced in hebephrenic and paranoid patients studied within the first two years of their psychoses. Contrary to this report, urinary 17-ketosteroids have been reported to be significantly increased compared to normal controls in schizophrenics withdrawn from neuroleptics for five days prior to study (96). The magnitude of the increase was slight and may be due to previous drug treatment. The clinical significance of the reported changes in gonadal hormone output appears modest. They could assume greater importance if they reflected neurotransmitter abnormalities in the regulation of LRH release. It is more likely they reflect the results of chronic institutionalization and drug treatment.

Adrenal Androgens

Tourney and Hatfield (94, 95) reported that institutionalized and non-institutionalized chronic schizophrenic patients had significantly decreased plasma dehydroandrosterone and dehydroepiandrosterone (DHEA) levels in comparison with acute schizophrenics and normal controls. This is one of the adrenal androgens and is secreted along with cortisol under the stimulus of ACTH. In subsequent studies from Tourney's laboratory (27, 93), DHEA and its sulfate conjugate (DHEA-SO_4), testosterone, aldosterone and cortisol were measured at 0800, 1130, 1600 and 2100 hrs in 10 chronic schizophrenic patients and 10 male controls. The patients were drug-free and had been hospitalized for at least 4 years. No differences in testosterone, aldosterone or DHEA-SO_4 levels were found over the three time periods. However, various analyses of the DHEA and cortisol data suggested that these two parameters could be used together to distinguish the schizophrenic patients and controls. The controls had higher levels of DHEA and showed a better synchronization of cortisol and DHEA levels. A linear discriminant function model using the four DHEA levels also distinguished the schizophrenic patients from the controls. This model has not bee confirmed with an independent group of patients and controls. DHEA secretions is not influenced by hyperprolactinemia (68). An ealier uncontrolled study reported improvement in "contact with reality" and willingness to engage in normal social interactions following prolonged administration of DHEA (86). Further investigation of the relevance of adrenal androgens to schizophrenia in males appears indicated.

Gonadotrophins

Brambilla et al. (9) reported that male chronic schizophrenic patients suffering from puberty-onset chronic hebephrenia had decreased plasma FSH, LH and testosterone levels. The levels found were comparable to prepubertal levels. These results were consistent with previous studies of decreased gonadal function in schizophrenics by Rey et al. (72), Suwa et al. (87) and Persky et al. (69). Johnstone et al. (36) reported mean serum FSH levels at the upper end of normal and mean serum LH levels at the lower end of normal in 16 chronic schizophrenic patients. Six of the patients had FSH levels greater than normal and 11 had LH levels slightly lower than normal. A significant positive correlation was found between FSH and poverty of speech and a significant negative correlation between FSH and delusions. Three other studies have reported normal basal levels of LH in male and female schizophrenics during or after withdrawal of chronic neuroleptic treatment (4, 23, 64). Arato et al. (2) studied serum prolactin, testosterone, FSH and LH levels in relation to sexual activity (frequency of intercourse) and potency in 17 married male schizophrenic patients treated with fluphenazine decanoate for 1-3 years. Ten of the patients had normal sexual function while 7 were impaired. There were no significant differences in prolactin or testosterone levels between the two groups. PRL levels were elevated in both groups compared to normals. Testosterone levels were within normal limits. The patients with normal sexual function had increased levels of LH whereas FSH levels were within normal limits in both groups. What relationship, if any, the elevated LH levels had to normal sexual function in the neuroleptic-treated males is not clear. The results of these studies must be viewed with caution because of the episodic nature of FSH and LH secretion and the possible effects of long-term hospitalization and previous long term neuroleptic treatment. However, in view of the evidence that DA can inhibit LH secretion in man (48), it would be of interest to pursue the possibility that the decreased LH levels in schizophrenia may reflect increased dopaminergic activity. This is currently under investigation in our laboratory.

LRH Administration

Brambilla et al. (8) administered three doses of LRH: 50, 100 or 150 μg, to schizophrenic patients and controls and found that the increase in LH and FSH levels which occurred after LRH administration was significantly greater in the schizophrenic patients than in the control group. Administration of CPZ had no effect on the test. No differences in the magnitude of the LH or FSH response to the three doses of LRH were observed. Brambilla et al. (8) considered the possibility that the excessive response to LRH in schizophrenics may be related to the greater response to LRH in prepubertal children than in adults. However, Naber et al. (64) found that the increase in LH produced by 250 μg LRH was not significantly different in schizophrenic patients chronically treated with neuroleptic drugs and normal controls.

Clomiphene Citrate Administration

Because of the evidence suggesting hypothalamic-pituitary gonadal deficiency, Brambilla et al. (13) administered clomiphene citrate, 150 mg/day, for 8 days to 16 chronic behephrenic schizophrenic patients, 10 of whom were drug-free, and to 5 normal controls. Reduced basal FSH, LH and testosterone levels were present in the patients. The LH and testosterone increases observed in the controls were entirely suppressed in both the drug-free and neuroleptic-treated patients but there was no difference in the FSH response. The lack of effect on LH and testosterone was attibuted to the inability of clomiphene to further diminish the inhibitory effect of androgens on LH release from the pituitary. Further replication of these results and, if verified, clarification of the mechanism, appears indicated.

Comment

Further studies to determine if the LH or FSH response to LRH administration and the DHEA-SO_4 diurnal rhythm and response to ACTH administration are abnormal in chronic schizophrenic patients, whether these are related to each other, or to subtype of schizophrenic such as the so-called "defect state" which is of current interest, appears warranted. In view of the extensive evidence that hyperprolactinemia can affect the secretion of LRH (78) and the possibility of its interference with gonadal function directly (see refs. 30, 74, for further discussion), it is important to keep in mind that current or past neuroleptic-induced hyperprolactinemia may be a significant cause of abnormalities in hypothalamic-pituitary gonadal function in schizophrenics.

Self-Induced Water Intoxication and the Syndrome of Inappropriate Antidiuretic Hormone Secretion

Smith and Clark (83) reviewed 18 reports of 27 cases of self-induced water intoxication in schizophrenic patients, sixteen of whom had at least temporary evidence of the syndrome of inappropriate ADH secretion (SIADH). They also added another 20 cases of their own. Normal individuals cannot induce water intoxication in themselves by maximal oral water intake but for unknown reasons some schizophrenic patients can. Patients suffering from self-induced water intoxication present with an organic psychosis and seizures superimposed on the schizophrenic psychopathology. Approximately 12 of the 47 cases reviewed by Smith and Clark (83) were not receiving neuroleptic drugs at the time of development of the syndrome. They proposed that SIADH might be caused by increased dopaminergic activity in the neural centres which regulate thirst and ADH release. They suggested that self-induced water intoxication or SIADH in neuroleptic-treated patients might, as has been postulated for tardive dyskinesia, be due to a denervation supersensitivity phenomenon in dopaminergic neurons which regulate thirst and ADH release.

Conclusions

There is little evidence to suggest an abnormality in the TIDA neurons or pituitary DA receptors in schizophrenic patients. The low basal levels of serum PRL reported by Brambilla et al. (7) in a small group of male chronic schizophrenic patients and the slightly diminished PRL response to 12.5 mg CPZ in female schizophrenics which we noted (51) suggests that some schizophrenics may have increased activity of the TIDA neurons. There are some promising suggestings of aberrant gonadotrophin secretion or response in chronic schizophrenic patients. Whether such differences are secondary to chronic neuroleptic treatment or chronic institutionalization rather than a primarily abnormality in the hypothalamo-pituitary-gonadal axis remains to be determined.

It is not the purpose of this review to comment on the integrity of the adrenal, thyroid or endorphinergic systems in schizophrenia. However, we believe it can be concluded that there is as yet no conclusive evidence of major abnormalities in the secretion of those hormones in any substantial proportion of patients diagnosed schizophrenic. This contrasts significantly with the status of the endocrine system in the major depressive disorders where there is robust evidence for state-dependent abnormalities in the hypothalamic-adrenal and hypothalamic-thyroid axis. In view of the widespread assumption that there are major functional and probably structural abnormalities in the brains of schizophrenic patients, the apparent integrity of the neuroendocrine system in most schizophrenic patients is somewhat surprising. It may be that newer methods of studying the endocrine system will yet reveal abnormalities that are related to the pathophysiology and etiology of schizophrenia in the endocrine systems reviewed here.

REFERENCES

1. Ahn, A. H., Gardner, E. and Makman, M. H. (1979): Eur. J. Pharmacol. 53:313-317.
2. Arato, H., Erdos, A. and Polgar, M. (1979): Pharmakopsychiatry 12:426-431.
3. Beg, A. A., Varma, V. A., Dash, R. J. (1979): Am. J. Psychiatry 136:914-917.
4. Beumont, P., Jr., Corker, C. S., Friesen, H. G., Kolakowska, T., Mandlebrote, B. M., Marshall, J., Murray, M.A.F. and Wiles, D. H. (1974): Brit. J. Psychiatry 124:420-430.
5. Bird, E. D., Spokes, E. G. and Iversen, L. J. (1978): Science 204:93-94.
6. Blumberg, J. B., Taylor, R. E., Sulser, F. (1975): J. Pharm. Pharmac. 27:126-128.
7. Brambilla, F., Bellodi, L., Negri, F., Smeraldi, E. and Malagoli, G. (1979): Psychoneuroendocrinology 4;329-339.
8. Brambilla, F., Guastalla, A., Guerrini, A., Rovere, C., Legnani, P., Sarno, M. and Riggi, F. (1976): Acta Psychiat. Scand. 54:275-286.
9. Brambilla, F., Guerrini, A., Riggi, F. and Ricciardi, J. (1974): Dis. Nerv. Sys. 362-367.
10. Brambilla, F., Guerrini, A., Rovere, C., Guastalla, A., Riggi, F., and Recchia, M. (1975): Neuropsychobiology 1:267-276.
11. Brambilla, F. and Penati, G. (1978): In: Perspectives in Endocrine Psychobiology, edited by F. Brambilla, P. K. Bridges, E. Endioczi, and G. Heuser, pp.309-422. J. Wiley and Sons, London.
12. Brambilla, F., Rovere, C., Guestalla, A., Guerrini, A. and Riggi, F. (1976): Acta Psychiat. Scand. 54:131-145.
13. Brambilla, F., Rovere, C., Guastalla, A., Guerrini, A., Riggi, F. and Burbati, G. (1977): Acta Psychiat. Scand. 56:399-406.
14. Brooksbank, B. W., MacSweeney, D., Johnson, A. L., Cunningham, A. E., Wilson, D. A. and Coppen, A. (1970): Brit. J. Psychiatry 117: 412-420.
15. Brown, W. A. and Laughren, T. (1981): Am. J. Psychiatry 138:237-239.
16. Bucht, G., Gottfries, C. G., Roos, B. -E. and Winblad, B. (1979): In: Biology-Psychiatry Today, edited by J. Obiols, C. Ballus, E. Gonzalez Monclus, and J. Piyols, pp.381-388. Elsevier/North Holland Biomedical Press.
17. Caron, M. G., Raymond, Beaulieu, M., Raymond, V., Gagne, B., Drouin, J., Lefkowitz, R. J. and Labrie, F. (1978): J. Biol. Chem. 253:2244-2253.
18. Chalmers, R. J., Bennie, E. H., and Johnson, R. H. (1978): Clin. Endocrinol. 8:75-79.
19. Clarenback, P., Prunkl, R., Riegler, M. and Cramer, A. (1978): Neuroscience 3:345-348.
20. Collu, A. R., Jequier, J. C., Leboeuf, G., Letarte, J. and Duchaine, J. R. (1975): J. Clin. Endocrin. Metab. 41:981-984.
21. Cronin, M. J. and Weiner, R. I. (1979): Endocrinology 104:307-312.
22. Crow, T. J., Baker, H. F., Cross, A. J., Joseph, M. H., Lofthouse, R., Longden, A., Owen, F., Riley, G. J., Glover, V. and Kelljack, W. S. (1979): Brit. J. Psychiat. 134:249-256.
23. Czernik, A. and Kleesiek, K. (1979): Nervenzat 50:527-553.

24. Demarest, K. T., Alper, R. H. and Moore, K. E. (1979): J. Neural Transmission 46:183-193.
25. Demarest, K. T. and Moore, K. E. (1979a): J. Neural Transmission 46:263-277.
26. Demarest, K. T. and Moore, K. E. (1979b): Brain Res. 171:545-551.
27. Erb, J. L., Kadane, J. B., Tourney, G., Mickelsen, R., Trader, D., Szabo, R. and Davis, V. (1981): J. Clin. Endcrinol. Metab. 52: 181-186.
28. Ettigi, P., Lal, S., Martin, J. B., Frieser, H. G. (1975): J. Clin. Endocrinol. Metab. 40:1094-1098.
29. Ettigi, P., Nair, N.P.V., Lal, S., Cervantes, P. and Guyda, H. (1976): J. Neurol. Neurosurg. Psychiat. 39:870-876.
30. Fang, V. S., Refetoff, S. and Rosenfield, R. L. (1974): Endocrinology 95:991-998.
31. Farley, I. J., Price, K. S., McCullough, E., Deck, J. H., Hordynski, W. and Hornykiewicz, O. (1978): Science 200:456-458.
32. Friend, W. C., Brown, G. M., Jawahir, G., Lee, T. and Seeman, P. (1978): Am. J. Psychiatry 135:839-841.
33. Gil-Ad, I., Dickerman, Z., Weizman, R., Weizman, A., Tyano, S. and Laron, Z. (1981): Amer. J. Psychiatry 138:357-360.
34. Gomes, U.C.R., Shanley, B. C., Potgeiter, L. and Roux, J. T. (1980): Brit. J. Psychiat. 137:346-351.
35. Gruen, P. H., Sachar, E. J., Langer, G., Altman, N., Leifer, M., Frantz, A. and Halpern, F. S. (1978): Arch. Gen. Psychiatry 35: 108-116.
36. Johnstone, E. C., Crow, T. J. and Mashiter, K. (1977): Psychol. Med. 7:223-228.
37. Joseph, M. H., Baker, H. F., Johnstone, E. C. and Crow, T. J. (1976); Psychopharmacology 51:47-51.
38. Kebabian, J. W. and Calne, D. B. (1979): Nature 277:93-96.
39. Kleinman, J. E., Bridge, P., Karoum, P., Speciale, S., Jr., Starb, R., Zaleman, S., Gillin, J. C. and Wyatt, R. J. (1980): In: Perspectives in Schizophrenia Research, edited by C. F. Baxter and T. Melnechuk. Raven Press, New York.
40. Krulich, L. (1979): Ann. Rev. Physiol. 41:603-615.
41. Lake, C. R., Sternberg, D. E., van Kammen, D. P., Ballenger, J. C., Ziegler, M. G., Post, R. M., Kopin, T. J. and Bunney, W. E. (1980): Science 207:331-333.
42. Lal, S., Guyda, H., Bikadoroff, S. (1977): J. Clin. Endocrinol. Metab. 44:766-770.
43. Langer, G., Heinze, G., Reim, B. and Matussek, N. (1976): Arch. Gen. Psychiatry 33:1471-1475.
44. Langer, G. and Matussek, N. (1977): Psychoneuroendocrinology 2: 379-382.
45. Langer, G., Sachar, E. J., Gruen, P. H. and Halpern, F. S. (1977): Nature 266:639-640.
46. Laughren, T. P., Brown, W. A. and Williams, B. W. (1979): Am. J. Psychiatry 136:108-110.
47. MacLeod, R. M. (1975): In: Frontiers in Neuroendocrinology, edited by L. Martini and W. F. Ganong, pp.169-194. Raven Press, New York.
48. Martin, W. H., Rogol, A. D., Kaiser, D. L., Thorner, M. O. (1981): J. Clin. Endocrinol. Metab. 52:650-656.
49. Masala, A., Delitala, G., Aloqua, S. and Devilla, L. (1977): Clin. Endocrinol. 7:253-256.
50. Meltzer, H. Y., Busch, D. and Fang, V. S. Psychoneuroendocrinology (in press).

51. Meltzer, H. Y., Busch, D., So, R., Holcomb, H. and Fang, V. S. (1980a): In: Perspectives in Schizophrenia, edited by C. Baxter and T. Melnechuk, pp.149-172. Raven Press, New York.
52. Meltzer, H. Y., Busch, D., Young, M., Tricou, B. J., Nasr, S., Metz, J. and Fang, V. S. (1980b): In: progress in Psychneuroendocrinology, edited by F. Brambilla, G. Racagni and D. de Wied, pp.283-294. Elsevier/North Holland, Amsterdam.
53. Meltzer, H. Y. and Fang, V. S. (1976): Arch. Gen. Psychiatry 33: 279-286.
54. Meltzer, H. Y., Goode, R. J. and Fang, V. S. 91978): In: Psychopharmacology: A Generation of Progress, edited by M. A. Lipton, A. DiMascio, and K. F. Killiam, pp.509-530. Raven Press, New York.
55. Meltzer, H. Y., Goode, D. J., Fang, V. S., Schyve, P. and Young, M. (1976): Lancet 2:1142.
56. Meltzer, H. Y., Sachar, E. J. and Frantz, A. A. (1974): In: Neuropsychopharmacology of Monoamines and Their Regulatory Enzymes, edited by E. Usdin, pp.299-316. Raven Press, New York.
57. Meltzer, H. Y., Sachar, E. J. and Frantz, A. G. (1974): Arch. Gen. Psychiatry 31:564-569.
58. Meltzer, H. Y. and So, R. (1979): Life Sciences 25:531-536.
59. Meltzer, H. Y. and Stahl, S. (1976): Schiz. Bull. 2:19-76.
60. Motson, R. W., Glass, D. N., Smith, D. A. and Daly, J. R. 91978): Clin. Endocrinol. 8:315-326.
61. Muller, E. E., Nistico, G. and Scapagnini, U. (1977): In: Neurotransmitters and Anterior Pituitary Function, pp.249-253. Academic Press, New York.
62. Murri, L,, Cerrone, G., Muratorio, A., Isidore, A. and Rotolo, A. (1973): Rev. Pat. Nerv. Ment. 94:391-400.
63. Murri, L., Cerone, G., Periozzi, F., Mancini, G. M. and Nurzia, A. (1973): Boll. Soc. Ital. Biol. 49:1490-1495.
64. Naber, L., Ackenheil, G., Laakman, G., Fischer, H. and von Werder, K. (1980): Pharmakopsychiat. 13:325-330.
65. Nathan, R. S., Sachar, E. J., Ostrow, L., Asnis, G. M., Hallbreich, U., and Halpern, P. S. (1981): J. Clin. Endocrinol. Metab. 52: 807-809.
66. Overall, J. E. and Gorham, D. R. (1962): Psychol. Rep. 10:799-812.
67. Pandey, G. N., Garver, D. L., Tamminga, C., Ericson, S., Ali, S. I., and Davis, J. M. (1977): Amer. J. Psychiatry 134:518-522.
68. Parker, L. N., Chang, S. and Odell, W. D. (1978): Clin. Endocrinol. 81:1-5.
69. Persky, H., Zuckerman, M. and Curtis, G. (1968): J. Nerv. Met. Dis. 146:488-497.
70. Prange, A. J., Jr., Loosen, P. T., Wilson, I. C., Meltzer, H. Y. and Fang, V. S. (1979): Arch. Gen. Psychiatry 36:1086-1093.
71. Ray, K. R. and Wallis, M. (1981): Biochem. J. 194:119-128.
72. Rey, J., Nicholson-Bailey, U., and Trappi, A. (1957): Brit. Med. J. 2:843-850.
73. Rimon, R., Liica, J., Kampman, R. and Hyppa, M. (1981): Neuropsychobiology 7:87-93.
74. Rolland, R. and Corbey, R. S. (1978): Europ. J. Obstet, Gynec. Reprod. Biol. 7:337-348.
75. Rotrosen, J., Angrist, B. M., Clark, C., Gershon, S., Halpern, P. S. and Sachar, E. J. (1978): Am. J. Psychiatry 135:949-951.
76. Rotrosen, J., Angrist, B., Gershon, S., Paquin, J., Branchey, L., Oleshansky, M., Halpern, F. and Sacher, E. J. (1979): Brit. J. Psychiat. 135:444-456.

77. Rotrosen, J., Angrist, B. M., Gershon, S., Sachar, E. J. and Halpern, P. S. (1976): Psychopharmacology 51:1-7.
77b. Rotrosen, J., Angrist, B. M., Pacquire, J. et al. (1978); Psychopharmacology Bulletin 14:14-17.
78. Rubin, R. T., Poland, R. E., Sobel, J., Tower, B. B. and Odell, W.D. (1978): J. Clin. Endocrinol. Metab. 47:447-452.
79. Rubovits, R. and Klawans, H. L. (1972): Arch. Gen. Psychiatry 27: 502-507.
80. Schilkrut, R., Chandra, O., Osswald, M., Ruther, E., Baarfusser, B. and Matussek, N. (1975): Neuropsychobiology 1:70-79.
81. Schimmelbusch, W. M., Mueller, P. S., Sheps, J. (1971): Brit. J. Psychiatry 118:429-436.
82. Sherman, L., Kim, S., Benjamin, F. and Kolodny, H. D. (1971): N. J. Med. 284:72-74.
83. Smith, W. O. and Clark, M. L. (1979): Am. J. Psychiatry 137: 1053-1060.
84. Snyder, S. H., Banerjee, S. P., Yamamura, H. J. and Greenberg, D. (1974): Science 184:1243-1253.
85. Spitzer, R. L., Endicott, J. and Robins, E. (1977): Research Diagnostic Criteria, Third Edition, Biometrics Research. New York State Psychiatric Institute.
86. Strauss, E. B., Sands, D. E., Robinson, A. M., Tandall, W. J., and Stevenson, W.A.H. (1952): Brit. Med. J. 3:64.
87. Suwa, N., Yamashita, J., Ito, K., Yoshimura, Y. and Moroji, T. (1966): J. Nerv. Ment. Dis. 143:36-46.
88. Sylvalahti, E. and Pekkarinen, A. (1977): J. Neural Trans. 40: 221-226.
89. Takahashi, Y., Kipnis, D. M. and Daughaday, W. H. (1968): J. Clin. Invest. 47:2079-2090.
90. Takahashi, K., Takahashi, S., Honda, Y., Shizime, K., Trie, M., Sakuma, M. and Tsushima, T. (1967): Folia Psychiat. Neurol. Jap. 21:87-105.
91. Tamminga, C. A., Smith, R. C., Pandey, G., Frohman, L. A. and Davis, J. M. (1977): Arch. Gen. Psychiatry 36:1199-1203.
92. Taube, S. L., Kirstein, L. S., Sweeney, D. R., Heninger, G. R. and Maas, J. W. (1978): Am. J. Psychiatry 135:78-82.
93. Tourney, G. and Hatfield, H. L. M. (1973): Biological Psychiatry 6:23-36.
94. Tourney, H. L. and Hatfield, L. (1972): Arch. Gen. Psychiatry 27: 753-755.
95. Tourney, G. and Erb, J. L. (1979): Biological Psychiatry 14: 395-404.
96. Varma, V. K., Amma, M.K.P., and Ghosh, A. (1978): Ind. J. Med. Res. 67:443-452.
97. Vigneri, R., Pezzino, V., Squatrito, S., Calandia, A. and Maricchilo, M. (1974): Neuroendocrinology 14:356-361.
98. Volovka, J., Pairs, L. G. and Ehrlich, Y. H. (1979): Schiz. Bull. 5:227-250.
99. Wing, J. K., Birley, L. T., Cooper, J. E., Graham, P. and Issacs, A. D. (1967): Brit. J. Psychiatry 113:499-515.
100. Wode-Helgodt, B., Eneroth, P., Fyro, B., Gullberg, B., Sedvall, G. (1977): Acta Psychiat. Scand. 56:280-293.

Neuroendocrinology and Psychiatric Disorder,
edited by G. M. Brown, et al.
Raven Press, New York 1984.

Pharmacoendocrinology of Schizophrenia

John M. Davis, Caryn Vogel, Robert Gibbons, Ivan Pavkovic, and M. Zhang

General Considerations

In using a hormonal system to understand the effects of a given drug on transmitters, we are not necessarily simply studying the effects of a drug on a given hormone. The many interrelating systems, with multiple inputs, and multiple feedback systems make interpretation complicated (14, 17, 72, 99, 109, 140). A transmitter may, for example, govern: (1) diurnal rhythms of a given hormone; (2) sleep-related excretion of that hormone; and (3) response to challenge tests (for example, insulin-induced hypoglycemia). The same considerations apply to the response of a hormone to any pharmacologic drug with a known mechanism of action. Hence it is most useful to focus on the effects of a drug on mechanisms that to the extent possible control a specific aspect of that hormonal system. Drugs that pass or do not pass the blood brain barrier (BBB) may be an important tool in localizing the level at which a drug acts. It is important however, to recognize that a drug which does not pass the blood brain barrier can act in the median eminence, presumably on any axonic synapse, so it should not be assumed to always act on the pituitary.

The response of the pituitary may depend, in part, on feedback of peripheral hormones as well as prior exposure to the hypothalamic factors. For example, high cortisol levels result in a decreased TSH response (148, 156, 181, 194). Therefore, one might speculate that the reduced TSH response to TRH seen in depressed patients may relate to the increased cortisol seen in this condition.

Statistical Reanalysis of Data

In some of the papers we review, the authors failed to statistically analyze their data, so when data was available in tables or graphs, we performed the statistical analysis and present these results in our review.

It is not uncommon for studies to use normal values from their laboratory as a control group. One problem with this approach is that these subjects are often young and healthy. Another problem is that abnormal values are sometimes excluded from the norms. To determine the effect of this on the statistical validity of such experiments, we simulated the effect by excluding 3 high values from a simulated control group. Generating entirely random data but excluding 3 high values out of 20 patients in a control group, resulted in finding an abnormality by a two tailed t-test at the .05 level almost half of the time (two tailed 47%, one tailed 68%) (N = 20 in experimental and N = 20 in control group). This finding underlines the importance of using all data in so- called normal control groups.

Mechanism of Action of Antipsychotic Drugs

We will discuss the use of endocrine techniques to investigate the way that neuroleptic drugs may affect disease states or brain substances such as neurotransmitters. The cause of schizophrenia is unknown, but the probable mechanism by which antipsychotic drugs help schizophrenia is thought to be through blockade of dopamine receptors. There is evidence that almost all antipsychotic drugs have an antidopamine effect, which is generally that of receptor blockade. But several, such as reserpine or tetrabenazine, lower dopamine nerve activity by lowering brain dopamine levels. The observation in our laboratory that apomorphine, at a dose level that would be expected to stimulate presynaptic dopamine receptors and slow dopamine release, has an apparent antipsychotic action when administered acutely in schizophrenic patients is consistent with an antidopamine mechanism of action (41, 178, 184). The observation that pretreatment with alphamethylparatyrosine (a drug that interferes with catecholamine synthesis) reduces the dose necessary to produce an antipsychotic response is also consistent with the theory that antipsychotic response occurs as a result of mechanisms involving catecholamines.

Antipsychotic Potency and Prolactin Response

A striking correlation exists between ability of drugs to block dopamine receptors in various test systems and their clinical potency in man (43, 172, 173, 179). One of the cornerstones in our understanding of how neuroleptics help schizophrenia is the close relationship between the clinically effective dose of a drug in man and the ability of that drug to bind to dopamine receptors. In man, dopamine blockade at a pituitary level can be evaluated by measuring plasma prolactin levels. Initial studies in rats by Clemens et al. (37) showed that drugs with antipsychotic activity stimulate prolactin secretion, whereas structurally similar drugs without antipsychotic activity do not. The dopamine blocking isomer of butaclamol (+), but not its inactive form (-) increases prolactin and benefits schizophrenia (42, 198). Potency of drugs that block spiroperidol binding in the rat pituitary is correlated with effects on striatal binding (119, 121, 122), but there are some departures from the expected relationship. Langer et al. (92, 93, 94, 95) and Gruen et al. (62, 63) systematically investigated the prolactin stimulating potency of neuroleptics and compared it to the clinical effectiveness in schizophrenia, i.e. the dose necessary to treat schizophrenia as empirically derived from controlled studies. Although each subject received several (but not all) neuroleptics and the sample size was small, the dose required to elevate prolactin correlated well with the clinical antipsychotic dose. We have plotted clinical antipsychotic potency against the potency on dopamine receptors, using Seeman's data (173) and Langer's data on human prolactin simulating potency on the same graph (not shown). The curves paralleled each other, but the prolactin potency was shifted slightly to the left. The dose needed to benefit schizophrenia is higher than the dose needed to increase prolactin in man. Insofar as a hormonal response is an indicator of dopamine blockade, this data provides a link between dopamine receptor homogenates and animal test systems, such as stereotyped behaviour in rats, and dose of antipsychotic in schizophrenics. Potency in elevating prolactin in man provides an index of dopamine blockade in man which can be correlated with antipsychotic dose.

Crowley and MacDonald (46) studied the effects of thioridazine and thiothixene on prolactin. Patients received thioridazine or thiothixene in a ratio of 25 to 1 although, based on empirical data (49), a 20 to 1 conversion ratio should have been used to achieve an equal therapeutic efficacy. (However, conversion ratios are very crude calculations). Both neuroleptics produced comparable increases in prolactin. Thioridazine would produce very slightly less prolactin increase than thiothixene given equal antipsychotic dosage.

Cotes et al. (42) noted that alpha-flupenthixol and increased prolactin produced improvement in schizophrenia while beta-flupenthixol which did not produce improvement in schizophrenia, also did not produce an increase in prolactin. The alpha isomer, but not the beta isomer, is also active in blocking dopamine in animal preparations. Johnstone and coworkers (70, 71) had similar findings.

Two drugs, clozapine and melperone, are exceptional cases. Sedvall (171) found that clozapine (600 mg per day) failed to elevate prolactin and that melperone elevated prolactin slightly. In this study, melperone elevated prolactin much less than thiothixene at an equivalent antipsychotic dose. If there was a strong relationship between prolactin elevation and antipsychotic dose, then it would be expected that both melperone and thiothixene would elevate prolactin to the same degree. Clozapine did not elevate prolactin at all in plasma or CSF. Chlorpromazine was found to elevate prolactin less than equivalent thiothixene.

Sachar et al. (167), Kane, Cooper, Sachar and their coworkers (74), and Meltzer (118) reported the effect of clozapine in doses of 12.5 mg to 900 mg a day in a total of 18 subjects and found no significant increase in prolactin levels. A modest elevation was noted in a few patients given very high doses of clozapine. Lal and Nair (89, 138) observed that 200 mg of chlozapine produced a statistically significant (17%) decrease in basal serum prolactin levels in drug-free chronic schizophrenics. Parenthetically, this group found that clozapine significantly inhibited the apomorphine-induced growth hormone in drug-free chronic schizophrenics without altering baseline growth hormone.

Sulpiride is relatively more potent in elevating prolactin (45, 107, 130) than in producing antipsychotic effects even though in therapeutic doses sulpiride is clearly an effective antipsychotic agent (32, 125, 126, 154, 189). Clozapine is an effective antipsychotic agent which is not particularly potent in elevating prolactin, and incidentally, does not produce extrapyramidal side effects.

Belmaker (6) found that high doses of propranolol neither influenced prolactin nor helped schizophrenia. Elizur (54) observed that propranolol did not have an impressive effect on prolactin levels, but did improve schizophrenia. Wilson and his coworkers (200) studied basal prolactin levels and metoclopramide=stimulated prolactin levels before and after treatment with propranolol. No clinical change was noted. The basal prolactin levels and the stimulated prolactin test decreased and, the differences, though small, were significant. Hanssen (64) found that propranolol slightly decreased basal prolactin and nocturnal prolactin rise.

There is contradictory evidence as to the therapeutic efficacy of propranolol in schizophrenia. If propranolol does in fact help some schizophrenics, then the mechanism of action may be an important clue. If the finding that propranolol at these high doses fails to alter prolactin is substantiated, this would tend to rule out the dopaminergic mechanism of action of propranolol, although it is, of course, possible that propranolol could have an antidopaminergic effect through a mechanism involving receptors other than dopamine pituitary receptors.

For most neuroleptic drugs there is a fairly striking parallel between ability to block dopamine receptors as measured by prolactin elevation and antipsychotic potency in man. The exact meaning of the discrepancies may or may not be important. Poorer penetration into the brain than into the pituitary would easily explain certain discrepancies, but none of great theoretical interest. A high affinity to specific receptors in the mesolimbic system and relatively low affinities in other systems may be an important clue to mechanism of action of antipsychotics. Despite these exceptional cases, excellent correlation between the wide variety of assays of dopamine receptor blockade - direct measure of receptor binding, pituitary effects, animal behaviour, extrapyramidal side effects - to clinical dose together with other evidence is consistent with the theory that antipsychotic drugs produce their behavioral effects in schizophrenia by blocking dopamine receptors.

Endocrinology as a Tool for Investigation of Drug Effect on Transmitters

Neuroendocrine studies are particularly useful in the initial evaluation of new drugs. Endocrine tests in animals may offer important information on the effect of these drugs on transmitter substances. Similar studies in humans are also necessary, since there is always the problem of intraspecies difference. For example, many of the provocative stimuli that increase growth hormone in humans fail to do so in the rat, even though intraspecies differences are the exception rather than the rule.

Many drugs will affect multiple transmitter substances at higher dose levels. In trying to infer drug action in humans from animal studies, there is always the question of whether a given effect on a transmitter will occur at the dose given in humans. Doses in man may be substantially smaller than doses given to animals. In addition, there are considerable interspecies differences between animals and humans in amount and type of drug metabolites formed. Chronic administration of a drug in humans may yield reasonable levels of a metabolite that would not have formed an appreciable concentration in an acute animal experiment. Hence, in humans a drug might produce different actions than seen in the initial animal screening (115) because of differing doses, duration, or metabolites. Meltzer's study (123) of fluoxetine is an excellent example of the use of endocrine changes to provide evidence of the effects of drugs on transmitters. Fluoxetine has been thought to be a serotonergic drug. Meltzer's observation that it has dopminergic effects adds an important clue to the clinical pharmacology of fluoxetine.

Site of Action of Antypsychotics on Prolactin Secretion

It is likely that the most important loci for the regulation of plasma prolactin are dopminergic systems external to the BBB. Evidence in support of this is that doperidone, a drug which does not pass the BBB, elevates prolactin levels in humans (19, 28, 151). Moreover, dopamine, which does not cross the blood brain barrier, decreases plasma PRL levels (8, 98). Furthermore, administration of carbidopa, a peripheral decarboxylase inhibitor, which lowers peripheral dopamine level, produces an elevation of prolactin (15). It would seem reasonable to presume that the site at which neuroleptic drugs elevate prolactin levels would be, at least in a large part, outside the BBB. The locus is probably the dopamine receptor on the pituitary (16, 173).

Tolerance to Antipsychotic Prolactin Stimulation

Several authors have failed to find a decrease in prolactin levels after neuroleptic treatment of approximately one month (63, 114). However, these studies used neuroleptic doses that increased with time and the increase in dose would produce higher prolactin levels that might have cancelled out any decrease due to tolerance.

Mielke, Gallant, and Kessler (125) provide data that we analyzed to determine how long tolerance takes to develop. They studied six patients who received fixed doses of neuroleptics for 80 days. Our statistical analysis of their data did not reveal any trend over time in prolactin levels except that the levels on day 80 were about 43% lower than day 52. This difference did not reach statistical significance due to large variance, but it does hint that tolerance may develop after about 80 days. Sulpiride dose levels were not held constant, and in general, similar doses were used on day 80 as on day 24 or 52. Prolactin levels were not lower at day 80 than on earlier days. There was no correlation between changes in dose or prolactin levels between day 24 or day 52 and day 80, indicating that the slight increase in dose did not cancel out a decrease in prolactin level due to development of tolerance. This possibility cannot be completely ruled out unless fixed dose studies are done.

In the great majority of patients treated acutely with antipsychotic drugs, prolactin increases substantially, often by a factor of 200% or 300%. A number of investigators have measured prolactin levels in patients receiving long-term neuroletpics (Table I). One hundred and forty-seven or roughly 50% of the 291 patients studied on long-term neuroleptics have prolactin levels within the normal range (2, 9, 10, 51, 80, 82, 110, 124, 132, 133, 134, 135, 196, 199). This data provides striking evidence that tolerance occurs with long-term antipsychotic medication.

Naber and his coworkers (132, 133, 134, 135) measured baseline prolactin levels as well as the TRH-stimulated prolactin in two separate groups of chronic schizophrenic patients taking long-term neuroleptics. No males (of 35) and only 7 females (of 45) showed an elevation in baseline prolactin. However, the authors observed that there was a marked increase in prolactin following the injection of TRH in both men and women. This observation is important since one possible explanation for tolerance to prolactin increase would be that the lactotropic cells become depleted and, hence, the pituitary can no longer secrete large amounts of prolactin. The fact that TRH can elevate plasma prolactin levels indicates that there is adequate reserve of potentially releasable prolactin.

Two studies which did not include data that could be readily summarized in our table are consistent with tolerance. Martin-du-Pan et al. (110) investigated 17 chronic schizophrenic patients treated for long periods with neuroleptics. Elevation in prolactin was seen only during concomitant anticholinergic administration.

Casacchia et al. (31) studied chronic patients treated with fluphenazine decanoate (n = 5) or haloperidol (n = 6) for an interval longer than six months. Prolactin levels were slightly but not significantly elevated over controls.

Tardive Dyskinesia

Tardive Dyskinesia has been hypothesized to be due to hypersensitivity of striatal dopamine receptors, presumed to be caused by an increased number of receptor sites secondary to neuroleptic induced dopamine blockade (100). If the pituitary prolactin system functioned in an analogous way, one would expect an increase in the number of dopamine receptor sites in the pituitary after chronic neuroleptic treatment. Hence, one would expect that in tardive dyskinesia there would be lower basal prolactin levels and a greater magnitude of decrease in serum prolactin (or increase in growth hormone) following apomorphine or dopamine.

However, Friend, Brown and their coworkers (58) reported that the binding of haloperidol to rat pituitary was decreased (not increased) in rats following chronic haloperidol treatment. In our group, Tamminga et al. (185, 186) using apomorphine and dopa provocative agents to stimulate growth hormone and reduce prolactin, respectively, showed that chronic schizophrenic patients with or without tardive dyskinesia had slightly lower prolactin response than controls to dopa. Similarly, chronic schizophrenic patients with and without tardive dyskinesia had sluggish growth hormone responses to apomorphine. This data is not consistent with the up regulation that has been postulated (185, 186, 55).

It is known that when neuroleptic drugs are discontinued, tardive dyskinesia generally increases, yet prolactin has been found empirically to decrease (4, 39). Asnis and coworkers (4) studied six patients with tardive dyskinesia and found that their prolactin levels were similar to those of controls after neuroleptic withdrawal or patients later given a chlorpromazine challenge.

Cohen and Cooper (38) investigated four patients with tardive dyskinesia while they were taking neuroleptics. Three of the four had normal plasma prolactin levels and all four had somewhat limited responses to TRF. Jeste and coworkers (69) investigated 12 patients with tardive dyskinesia and 12 matched controls. In both groups eight were chronic schizophrenics and four patients had organic brain syndromes. It may be concluded that there is no demonstrated relationship of tardive dyskinesia to altered prolactin. Therefore, dopamine receptor responses in the pituitary differ from ones of the basal ganalia or the denervation hypothesis of tardive dyskinesia is incorrect.

Laughren, Brown, and Williams (97) noted that 3 of 11 patients removed from neuroleptics relapsed in a one month drug free period and those three had prolactin levels of less than 6 ng/ml while on chronic neuroleptic treatment vs. 12.2 ng/ml for the whole group. In a second study (23), those patients who had prolactin levels of less than 6 ng/ml on chronic neuroleptics relapsed faster during a 40 week drug free period (mean = 6.5 weeks) than those with higher prolactin levels (mean = 18 weeks, $p = .025$ one-tailed t-test). These fast relapsing patients also had low prolactin levels during acute neuroleptic drug treatment. This replicable finding may offer a clue for the mechanism to explain why patients who manifest low prolactin response to neuroleptics relapse rapidly following discontinuance of neuroleptics.

Chouinard and coworkers (35) studied patients for which neuroleptic drugs were discontinued and penicillin was substituted for 6 weeks. A greater decrease in prolactin levels was postively correlated with a worsening of psychosis over this time period. This finding should be tempered because of the small sample size.

Effects of Other Drugs on Prolactin

In the laboratory, drug free normal volunteers can be used as experimental subjects. However, in the clinic, if we are using prolactin as if it were an indicator of neuroleptic biological effect, it should be recognized that many patients would be on other medications which can potentially alter prolactin (116, 117). We will review evidence relevant to some, but this is by no means exhaustive (108, 124). Van Kammen and coworkers (192) found that amphetamine, 20 mg i.v., significantly raised prolactin levels in drug free schizophrenic patients. However, Janowsky et al. (68) found that a dose of methylphenidate that produced a profound behavioral activation (increased anxiety, talkativeness), failed to decrease prolactin. Janowsky and Davis both have found methylphenidate to be substantially more potent than amphetamine in worsening psychosis. This is the reverse potency of the effect of the drugs on prolactin. Agents that either raise plasma dopamine or stimulate dopamine receptors can also profoundly lower prolactin levels (86, 100, 108).

Turkington (190) reported that the tricyclic antidepressants imipramine and amitriptyline elevated prolactin levels but Meltzer (120) failed to confirm the increase. Nielsen (142) measured prolactin in depressed patients receiving nortriptyline. We calculate from their data that a small but significant elevation was produced. Nordgren and Scheele (144) found that nortriptyline did not alter either basal or TRH-stimulated prolactin in depressed patients. Widerlov et al. (195) also found neither nortriptyline or chlorimipramine to clearly alter basal or TRH-stimulated prolactin. Galenberg (59) studied 24-hour prolactin secretion in a young woman who experienced galactorrhea associated with amoxapine and found elevated 24-hour prolactins. Nomifensin, a drug which inhibits dopamine reuptake and norepinephrine reuptake, has an inhibitory effect that lowers plasma prolactin levels (60). However, its use as a test has been questioned (52).

Roccatagliata and his coworkers (158) administered trazodone to drug free patients at a dose of 200 mg i.v. and observed a very slight (17%) acute decrease in prolactin levels, but whether this decrease in prolactin is meaningful remains to be seen. Trazodone inhibits the reuptake of serotonin and also may effect beta noradrenergic systems.

Stern and his co-workers (182) observed that single oral doses of buproprion produced suppression of prolactin with an inconsistent effect on growth hormone in man. Deprenil may increase prolactin (124).

It is of interest that serotonin and its precursors can stimulate prolactin in man (75, 91, 113). Masala and his coworkers (112) report that fluoxetine had no clear effect on fasting prolactin levels, but significantly enhanced insulin-induced prolactin response. Fluoxetine was observed by Meltzer (123) to produce a dystonic reaction, Parkinsonian rigidity, and an increase in serum prolactin levels, a profile of findings which suggests that this agent either directly or indirectly may decrease dopaminergic activity in the striatum and at a pituitary level and/or tubero-infundibular level. Quipazine somewhat irregularly produces an increase in prolactin levels in normal and neurologically ill subjects (149).

Cosignani and his coworkers (44) found two serotonin antigonists, metergoline and methysergide, that decreased the prolactin response to nursing. However, metergoline and methysergide also have dopaminergic properties. They may also directly affect dopamine receptors in the pituitary lactotrophis (83). A third serotonin antagonist, cyproheptadine, has antihistaminic atropinic properties; it did not modify prolactin response to nursing (53) and had no effect on basal prolactin (141, 159) or insulin-stimulated prolactin response (141) or prolactin response to apomorphine (159). There are studies that fail to find a serotonin effect on prolactin; hence, more data is needed (57). An H_1 antagonist was reported to reduce prolactin release and an H_2 antagonist also stimulates prolactin release in man (152, 160).

Catlin and his coworkers (33) have shown that human beta-endorphin can increase prolactin. The mechanism by which endorphin produces this effect and the locus of the effect is yet to be worked out. The mechanism of prolactin interaction with the endorphin system is complex (85).

With respect to EABA related effects, Tamminga and her coworkers (183) found that muscimol elevated prolactin and growth hormone levels in patients with schizophrenia and Huntington's chorea. Nair et al. (137) found that neither Baclofen nor Sodium Valproate altered prolactin.

Mackay et al. (105), Van Kammen (192) and also Lal and Nair (89) report that lithium has little effect on prolactin levels.

Buckman and his coworkers (26) found that indomethacin had no effect on basal or perphenazine-stimulated prolactin secretion.

Since antiparkinsonian drugs are frequently given with neuroleptics, it is of interest that Lal and his coworkers (88) found that benztropine plus haloperidol produced slightly greater elevation in prolactin level than haloperidol alone in normals. Nathan et al. (141) found that atropine inhibited evening insulin induced elevation of prolactin.

Use of Plasma Prolactin Level to Monitor Central Effect of Antipsychotic Drugs

The elevation of prolactin following administration of a neuroleptic may be quantitatively related to the plasma neuroleptic level. There are substantial individual differences in plasma neuroleptic levels for patients on a constant dose. Furthermore, there is evidence that plasma neuroleptic levels may correlate with side effects or with therapeutic efficacy. In addition, it is important to measure plasma neuroleptic levels for working out the mechanisms of certain drug-drug interactions and for various other purposes. Much of the work on plasma neuroleptic levels suffers from serious methodolgic problems which should be considered briefly.

Curry, Marshall, Davis and Janowsky (47) noted wide (20 fold) individual differences in plasma levels of chlorpromazine in patients receiving comparable doses and suggested an inverted U-shaped relationship between plasma level and clinical response. Only a few valid studies on the relationship of plasma levels to clinical efficacy in which patients received a fixed dose of a neuroleptic drug have been performed, and most found results consistent with the originally proposed inverted U-shaped relationship. Unfortunately, many studies of dose response relationships have utilized variable doses adjusted by clinicians to obtain a desired effect. An inadequate response in some patients might well lead a physician to increase the dose. This would, in turn, increase the plasma level. Hence in a flexible dose design, it would be expected that high plasma levels would occur in nonresponders receiving high doses. Furthermore, some patients will respond at a higher plasma level. This design therefore removes the lower end of the therapeutic window. Similarly, side effects can cause the physician to lower a patient's dose. The correlation between plasma levels or prolactin levels and clinical response in such a flexible dose design is meaningless.

Another metholdological problem is the correlation of plasma levels of neuroleptics over time versus clinical response over time. Even in patients on a constant dose, plasma levels will steadily increase until the patient reaches steady-state. If the plasma levels are increasing, we would expect the prolactin level to increase. If a flexible dose is used, the dose increases over time. There is obviously going to be a highly artifactual correlation between these three variables.

Additional methodological limitations exist. Placebo responders will recover regardless of the plasma level, and some patients do not respond to neuroleptics at all, no matter what the dose. In such cases, one would anticipate no correlation between plasma levels and therapeutic response. Of course, the patient will improve with adequate doses of drugs until the maximal level of improvement possible for him is achieved. The degree of psychopathology remaining would reflect the patient's maximum capacity to improve with optimal doses of neuroleptics. It would not be expected that plasma levels would correlate with this because the optimal capacity is a function of an aspect of their disease not associated with drug effect. It is important to methodologically distinguish between the drug-produced improvement and the patient's maximal capacity for improvement. One may speculate that if chronically treated patients were taken off drugs until they relapsed and were then treated with low doses, the percent improvement produced by the drug compared to the percent improvement possible for that patient would be an index of a possible effect that may relate to plasma levels.

The literature on the relationship between hormones and neuroleptic treatment is apparently often contradictory. It is common to see statements saying that (1) there is a correlation between plasma prolactin levels and response to neuroleptic treatment, or (2) that there is no relationship between plasma prolactin levels and response to neuroleptic treatment, or (3) that studies on this question show mixed results. For the most part, these statements are based on studies with a methodologic flaw - not using a constant dose.

A few valid or at least partially valid studies comparing plasma levels with efficacy and side effects, will be considered. Wiles et al. (197) did a flexible dose study of patients receiving chlorpromazine. This study is flawed because the presence of side effects could have caused the clinician to use a lower dose. However, patients with extrapyramidal side effects had relatively high mean plasma chlorpromazine and prolactin levels as compared to those who did not show extra pyramidal effects. Of the five patients who had prolactin levels under 30 ng/ml and chlorpromazine below 50 ng/ml, none exhibited extrapyramidal side effects. Of the patients who had plasma levels and prolactin above these cutoff points, six out of seven had extrapyramidal side effects.

Van Putten, May, and Wilkins (193) performed a methodologically valid study on schizophrenic patients treated with a constant dose of chlorpromazine. Ten of these patients developed akinesia and 26 did not. Plasma and saliva chlorpromazine levels and plasma prolactin levels did not differentiate between the patients who did nor did not develop the side effects.

There are very few studies comparing changes of prolactin consequent to neuroleptic drug treatment with improvement that use correct methodology. Cotes et al. (42) treated patients with a fixed dose of flupenthixol and note a significant correlation of prolactin levels to total symptom changes. Wode-Helgodt (201) did a methodologically excellent study on patients treated with a fixed dose of chlorpromazine: 200, 400 or 600 mg a day. In male schizophrenics there was a positive correlation between improvement and prolactin elevation at 4 weeks. The dose was fixed and a 200 mg and 400 mg dose schedule would be considered low, shereas 600 mg would be a moderate dose. In an investigation designed to elucidate the lower end of the therapeutic window, it is appropriate to use low doses. If a combination of low fixed dose and rapid metabolism results in plasma levels that are too low to produce a therapeutic effect, then one may expect a positive correlation between clinical outcome and plasma level or its surrogate, plasma prolactin level. Studies that use a high oral dose in which most patients have at least moderate plasma levels are not adequate to discern the lower end of the therapeutic window. Sedvall (171) was unable to demonstrate a relationship between prolactin levels and clinical improvement in female patients receiving chlorpromazine, thiothixene, or melperone. Perhaps changes in estrogen levels introduced too much variability in prolactin levels.

It should be noted that prolactin levels could be more valid measure than plasma drug levels for certain purposes insofar as a central antipsychotic effect could be produced by an active metabolite not measured by a specific assay of the unchanged drug. In theory, a drug precursor could be metabolized to an active drug which will produce an antipsychotic effect. Prolactin levels reflecting the biological effect of the drug might have much more clinical relevance than the blood level of an inactive drug.

Physiological Determinants of Prolactin Secretion

Estrogen Status

Many determinants of prolactin levels may not be correlated with clinical efficacy or side effects of drugs and which may detract from the usefulness of prolactin levels in following neuroleptic therapy. A consistent finding that runs through all the studies is that women have substantially higher prolactin responses to neuroleptics than do men (25, 62, 63, 102, 114, 145). Furthermore, exogenous estrogens increase the prolactin response to neuroleptics (25) although they do not have a large effect on basal prolactin.

Goode, Meltzer, and Fant (61) observed that prolactin levels of women who developed a postpartum psychosis treated with neuroleptics were higher than a group of nonpostpartum women treated with similar doses of antipsychotics.

Since men and women have profoundly different responses to neuroleptics, it is generally not valid to intermix mena dn women for statistical study. Furthermore, prolactin response could conceivably vary throughout the menstrual cycle and certainly would be expected to vary in women taking significant external estrogens. The estrogen content of certain birth control pills may not necessarily be sufficent to produce a large effect. Judd and his coworkers (73) studied women at several points in the menstrual cycle and noticed that increasing concentrations of endogenous estrogens were associated with a relative resistance in prolactin response to dopamine infusion as well as an increase of prolactin after withdrawal of dopamine infusion. It is clear that plasma prolactin levels, like drug plasma levels, must be compared separately in men, premenopausal women, and possibly also postmenopausal women. The estrogenic status of women may be an important determinant of prolactin response to neuroleptic.

Pulsatile Release and Nonspecific Factors

Because prolactin is secreted episodically, a single sample may not be an accurate measure of prolactin secretory status. For research purposes, multiple sampling should be done. In a study where prolactin response and haloperidol levels were measured after intravenous administration of haloperidol in single dose, Ohman et al. (146) noted that serum prolactin concentrations initially oscillated, exhibiting peaks and troughs over an 80 ng/ml range at a time when the haloperidol level was fairly constant. If this oscillation is a common phenomenon, verified by future research, it reveals the limitations of a single prolactin value after an acute administration of neuroleptic as a measure of response. Changes associated with age, sex, race, body size, medical diseases, thyroid status, gonodotropic status and possibly other factors add to the difficulty in interpretation. Stress induced secretion of hormones can be a major confounding factor (27, 29, 30, 147, 157, 180). For example, the stress of blood drawing can markedly increase cortisol secretion. This is illustrated in Fig. 1, which shows the stress of second-year medical studients, who are relatively naive with respect to the pain associated with having blood drawn. In another context, Mori et al. (129) found that the prolactin elevation produced by sulpiride was enhanced when subjects consumed a low sodium diet.

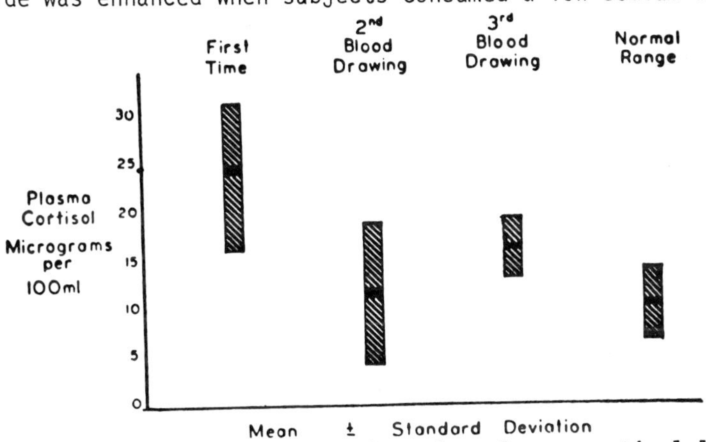

FIG. 1. The mean and standard deviations for plasma cortisol levels emphasize the significant elevation of plasma cortisol at the first blood letting. There is a slight elevation at the third blood drawing which is ascribed to the stress of approaching examinations (58).

Correlation of Prolactin Level to Antipsychotic Drug Level

Since plasma drug levels are used as an aid to dose adjustment to achieve maximal clinical benefit with minimal side effects and since prolactin levels could potentially be used for the same purposes, it is important not only to understand plasma levels but also to know how they interrelate with prolactin levels. If prolactin levels were highly correlated to plasma levels, they could be used in place of plasma levels. Many studies show a rough relationship between prolactin levels and plasma levels for a variety of drugs. Such corrleations range from values of practically 1 to values of zero, but most studies show a moderate relationship, so there is no doubt that prolactin levels in some sense are a function of drug levels (81). Rama-Rao et al. (1954) found that there was no signfiicant correlation between sulpuride concentration and prolactin. Similarly, Brown and Laughren (23) found that prolactin elevations induced by neuroleptics were not significantly correlated to their plasma levels measured by radioreceptor assay.

For a study by Linnoila and coworkers (103) on mentally defective patients treated with haloperidol, we calculated a correlation between the two variables of 0.98 for females, and for the males a correlation of 0.33. For 10 mental defectives treated with thioridazine, there was a correlation between total thioridazine and mesoridazine plasma levels and prolactin of 0.12.

In a study by Ohman, Forsman, and Larsson (146) we calculate that the increase in prolactin correlated positively with plasma level of haloperidol (men r = 0.82 and women r = .83, average correlation for 4 weeks of treatment).

Based on data presented in a graph form (128), we calculated a correlation for men of approximately 0.6 and for women of 0.5 between haloperidol and prolactin levels on day 9. We found the correlation between peak plasma butaperazine and prolactin after a single dose of drug in males and females to be 0.5 to 0.8 respectively. After several weeks steady-state butaperazine, an increment in prolactin correlated 0.2 and 0.4 for men and women (177).

In six normal men studied by Nikitopoulou and his coworkers (143), prolactin levels correlated (r = 0.28) with thioridazine plasma levels and with thioridazine metabolite plasma (r = 0.22). The unchanged thioridazine correlated with its metabolites (r = 0.53).

Rubin, Forsman, and their coworkers (162) did an extensive methodological study of several methods for assaying haloperidol and two methods for assaying prolactin. We calculate from their data that the correlation between plasma haloperidol levels measured chemically by gas chromatography and prolactin levels is 0.66. The percentage of free haloperidol level also correlated with average prolactin value, yielding r = 0.78. The results of the various other methodologies in general paralleled the findings.

Rubin and Hays (165) report cross-sectional correlations (separate correlations for each timepoint) of prolactin and haloperidol, taken roughly every 20 minutes in seven normal subjects given 0.5 mg. We averaged the individual correlations of each timepoint after the first two and found that integrated prolactin response was correlated to the integrated haloperidol concentration (r = 0.77, i.v.; r = 0.94, i.m.). Because there were sample-to-sample variations due to episodic release of prolactin, averaging of PRL values over a considerable time period would help eliminate this source of variability. Rubin and coworkers (163, 164) discuss how many samples are needed to define an endocrine response and also discuss methodology.

Hays and Rubin (65) have also compared prolactin response to TRH and prolactin response to haloperidol. The variability in prolactin response to TRH was much smaller than the variability of prolactin response to haloperidol. This suggests one cannot explain the variability in prolactin response to haloperidol by pituitary reserve. Hays and Rubin (65) suggest that different patients have different sensitivities for their pituitary dopamine receptors and hence different responses to haloperidol.

Ceiling Effect

Gruen and his coworkers (62, 63) suggested that there might be a ceiling effect to the prolactin dose-response curve. At low doses, a dose increase would result in increased response (i.e. linear portion of the dose-response curve). When a dose of antipsychotic that would produce a maximum stimulation of prolactin was given, then increasing the dose would yield no greater prolactin levels. The mean increase in prolactin above baseline at a dose of approximately 200 mg was 46 ng/ml and at a dose of 400 mg was 73 ng/ml. The increase of prolactin was 27 ng/ml when the dose was increased from about 600 mg to 800 mg; the increment was essentially negligible, namely a mean increment of 0.65 ng/ml. The evidence shows a striking ceiling effect. Linnoila et al. (103) also found a ceiling effect with thioridozine. Wilson and coworkers (199) found a dose-related mean rise in prolactin in chronic patients receiving low doses of thioridazine (low defined as 20-30- mg, medium as 40-80, and high as 80-300). Elizur et al. (54) found a ceiling effect in schizophrenics given i.v. haloperidol.

Kolakowska et al. (80) administered a 50 mg intramuscular injection of chlorpromazine to patients on clinical doses of neuroleptics. In some patients the chlorpromazine challenge was ineffective in raising prolactin. Wiles et al. (196) reported a higher prolactin response after 25.0 mg. of fluphenazine enanthate than after 12.5 mg. Therefore, prolactin responses had not peaked out at doses of prolixin of 12.5 mg per week suggesting that if there is a ceiling, it must be higher than this dose. Rama-Rao et al. (155) did not find a ceiling prolactin response to haloperidol as suggested by Gruen et al. (62, 63) but rather a linear relationship at doses of 5-40 mgs in female schizophrenics.

Effects of Antipsychotic Drugs on Growth Hormone

Sherman and his coworkers (175) reported that insulin-stimulated growth hormone levels were lower when patients were being treated with chlorpromazine growth hormone levels. Chalmers et al. (34) found similar results. Mims and coworkers (127) observed that chlorpromazine blunted the L-dopa induced rise in growth hormone. Schwimm et al. (170) found that pimozide decreased the peak of growth hormone after arginine and exercise. Collu (40) found that pimozide did not lower basal GH to a significant degree. Masala et al. (111) found pimozide administration did not lower either basal or DOPA-stimulated levels significantly.

Saldanka et al. (169) found that basal plasma growth hormone was slightly but not significantly lower in patients after chlorpromazine administration, and the increase in plasma growth hormone in response to insulin-induced hypoglycemia was somewhat blunted, but the difference was not statistically significant. Beumont et al. (9) studied patients receiving chronic neuroleptics and found that basal and insulin induced growth hormone was normal and, indeed, elevated in a few subjects.

Rotrosen and his coworkers (159) found that haloperidol blocked the growth hormone response to apomorphine. Clarenbach and his coworkers (36) found that haloperidol produced a modest and clearly not statistically significant decrease in stage 4, sleep-induced secretion of growth hormone.

Although we cannot disentangle the effects of psychiatric diagnosis from psychiatric drugs, since most schizophrenics are on antipsychotics and most non-schizophrenics are not, both the diagnosis of schizophrenia and the presence of neuroleptic medication decrease the methylphenidate induced elevation of growth hormone.

There may be methodologic problems in studying the effects of antipsychotics on basal growth hormones in that growth hormone is already at so low a level that it may be hard for any treatment to reduce it still further. Furthermore, any real drug effect must be small and it could therefore be eliminated by any random growth hormone peaks caused by stress or other nonspecific factors.

Tyson and Friesen (191) studied the response of 7 women to 25 mg chlorpromazine i.m., finding baseline plasma growth hormone levels of 4.2 ± 0.5 (mean ± sem) and a 90 minutes post-injection growth hormone of 0.7 ± 0.3. Significance cannot be assessed by paired t-test because the correlation of pre to post levels is not given.

Benjamin and his coworkers (7) reported that basal levels of GH, as well as levels after a glucose tolerance test, were distinctly lower in three patients on Thorazine than in controls and other study groups.

Not all studies found that antipsychotic drugs lower growth hormone levels. One study reported a modest increase. Cotes et al. (42) found no change after alpha-flupenthixol in 11 out of 13 subjects, and two subjects showed an increase in growth hormone.

Mielke, Gallant, and Kessler (125) investigated 16 severely-ill chronic schizophrenics receiving sulpiride. The average growth hormone level fell from a baseline of 4 ng/ml ± 1.7 (SEM) to an average of 0.93 ng/ml ± 0.28, a difference of -3.08 ± 1.7 (paired t-test, t = 1.82, (df=15), p less than 0.09 as analyzed by us).

Rubin and his coworkers (166) studied the effects of 0.25 and 0.5 mgs haloperidol i.m. in normal volunteers and found no effect on growth hormone.

Beg and coworkers (5) investigated five schizophrenic patients at baseline before drug administration, during thirteen weeks of antipsychotic drugs, and again at two weeks following drug withdrawal. They found no significant differences in either basal growth hormone excretion or maximal response to insulin-induced hypoglycemia. This group also investigated subjects on chlorpromazine in comparison to normal controls and again found no difference between either basal growth hormone levels or in maximal response to insulin stimulation.

Age can also affect hormonal response. Elderly subjects may have a lower and less consistent growth hormone response to many dopamine agonists such as dopa, apomorphine, or lergotrile (104, 168, 188). Age can alter neuroleptic plasma levels but if age also alters the hormonal response to a given plasma level, this introduces another variable which may mean that the given hormonal level may not have a 1-to-1 correlation with plasma level (18, 24).

Effects of Stimulants on GH

The growth hormone response to d-amphetamine is normal in schizophrenics (92). Parkes et al. (150) noted that 20 mg of amphetamine caused an increase in growth hormone in normal subjects. Brown and his coworkers (21) found that small oral doses of amphetamine or methylphenidate (20 mg of each) stimulate growth hormone release, amphetamine being more potent than methylphenidate. Many dopamine agonists stimulate growth hormone and interact with this system in complicated ways (1, 20, 22, 67, 87). Because dopamine is an important transmitter in growth hormone control, it should not be neglected (3, 71, 187).

Effects of Neuroleptic Drugs on LH and FSH

Although many studies show a slight decrease resulting from the acute or subacute administration of neuroleptics on LH or FSH secretion, most studies reveal that acute neuroleptics do not change LH secretion.

Collu et al. (40) studied 10 adult male volunteers for 4 days, treated with either 2 mg or 4 mg of pimozide. Plasma LH and FSH levels were slightly lower, but only LH decreased significantly after pimozide. Plasma testosterone level was virtually identical to baseline.

Rubin and his coworkers (166) found that two doses of haloperidol, 0.25 mg and 0.5 mg i.m. to 5 normal controls produced no significant changes in plasma LH or FSH.

Brambilla and coworkers (11, 12) studied chronic schizophrenics stabilized on haloperidol, finding that serum FSH, LH and testosterone fell within normal limits. Brooksbank and his coworkers (13) found no difference in the urinary excretion of androgens between controls and schizophrenic patients. All but two of the latter group were on antipsychotic medication. Cotes et al. (42) studied levels of FSH and LH and testosterone in patients treated with the active alpha isomer of flupenthixol and compared the results with those obtained using the inactive isomer as a placebo. They found little difference in these hormones between drugs. Beumont (9, 10) found normal LH levels in most premenopausal female patients on phenothiazine although several patients apparently did not have mid-cycle gonadotropin peaks and were amenorrheic. Males and postmenopausal females had normal LH. Males had slightly lower testosterone levels on phenothiazine than after the drug was withdrawn. Laughren, Browne, and Petruccia (96) studied 7 chronic schizophrenics: (1) on chronic medication, (2) during a 4 week placebo washout period, and (3) after 4 weeks of acute treatment with thioridiazine. Most testosterone levels were within the normal range. However, there was a slight but statistically significant decrease after both acute and chronic thioridazine treatment.

In a crossover experiment, normal volunteers were given either pimozide or fusaric acid at the mid-point of the menstrual cycle. These drugs significantly decreased the LH surge and very slightly or non-significantly decreased the FSH surge. Response to LH and FSH to LRH was not affected by either drug (101).

Casacchia et al. (31) found that plasma levels of gonadotropins and testosterone were normal in chronic schizophrenics complaining of decrease in libido and who had been on neuroleptics six months or more. Nathan and his coworkers (139) found that penfluridol slightly but non-significantly decreased testosterone. Czernik and Kleesiek (48) found schizophrenics on depot neuroleptics to have similar basal and LHRH-stimulated FSH and LH levels in comparison to controls.

Murray et al. (131) administered chlorpromazine (125 mg) to male sexual offenders and found plasma testosterone and LH levels to be essentially unchanged.

Magrini (106) and Martin-du-Pan et al. (110) studied schizophrenics on prolonged antipsychotic drug treatment with or without antiparkinsonian drugs and found that basal levels of estrogen and testosterone were normal as well as estrogen responses to stimulation with HCG or bormocryptine. Siris et al. (176) found that FSH and LH were slightly decreased in patients on pimozide. Testosterone levels did not change.

Arato et al. (2) found normal testosterone and FSH concentrations in all patients on long-term neuroleptics. Those patients who had sexual dysfunctions such as reduced libido and/or potency on long-term neuroleptic treatment had elevated prolactin levels (although not significantly) as well as normal serum LH levels. Sexual dysfunction was present in 17 of 27 chronic schizophrenics on long-action fluphenazine decanoate Naber (136), studying 12 male and 10 female chronic schizophrenics, found that basal LH levels or LHRH stimulated LH levels were normal, i.e., within normal limits, although an occasional patient had a low basal value. Caution in interpreting data on effects of neuroleptics on gonadotropins is indicated since prolactin can alter CNS amines such as dopmaine as well as having other effects (56, 66, 84, 153, 161).

Antipsychotic Effects on TRH and Cortisol

Neuroleptics given acutely produce no change in thyroid-stimulating hormone in most studies (174). When changes were produced, studies are equally divided as to whether the effect was an increase or a decrease. Naber, Steinbock, and Greil (136) studied 9 acute schizophrenics before and after acute treatment with antipsychotic agents. The antipsychotic drugs did not alter triiodothyronine or basal and stimulated TSH. Wode-Helgodt (202) found that treatment of schizophrenics with neuroleptics for two to four weeks did not alter TSH levels. In their study, ten normal subjects were studied after receiving two oral doses of haloperidol; the basal level of TSH was significantly increased and the stimulated TSH increase was also slightly elevated after drug (79). Lamberg et al. (90) administered a single dose of chlorpromazine (50 mg) or the same dose for 8 days and in both experiments found the treated group to have slightly lower basal and TSH stimulated TSH. Although Lamberg et al. (90) found a decreased TSH response to TRH after neuroleptic treatment, most authors found both normal baseline values as well as stimulated TSH values in patients treated with neuroleptics (48, 136).

Since prolactin can feedback on CNS systems and modify other hormones, interpretation of data should be made with caution (26).

Czernik and Kleesiek (48) as well as Beumont et al. (9) found no change in basal or insulin-stimulated cortisol between schizophrenics on neuroleptics and controls. Saldanka and coworkers (169) studied and compared the cortisol response to hypoglycemia in schizophrenics and found no difference before or after one week of 300 mg chlorpromazine. Collu et al. (40) found that 2 or 4 mg pimozide for 4 days did not alter cortisol levels.

DISCUSSION

An occasional report will state that neuroleptics produce an elevation or decrement in an endocrine parameter in a subgroup of patients. It is important to recognize that there is a significant methodological artifact that comes from small sample studies where subgroups are identified. By random variation alone, abnormal values are encountered. The endocrine system is sensitive to stress and many other extraneous factors. Patients may occasionally have a low or high value. When several patients have an abnormal value, it is certainly reasonable to investigate whether a subgroup exists, and to characterize it the investigator systematically inspects the information that he has on his group of patients to see if the group with the abnormal endocrine finding is dependable subgroup. If we take a random walk through many variables, there must always be a variable that characterizes any subsample by chance alone. We can then characterize an optimal cut-off point to maximize this difference. We have performed a computer "Monte-Carlo" simulation where many sets of random data were inspected by a computer utilizing methods to simulate this clinical process of identifying a subgroup. The computer identified abnormal values on one variable, characterized a subgroup by inspection of the variable to define a subgroup and then optimized the parameters to identify the optimal cut-off points in the process. This more or less parallels clinical research identification for subgroup differences. Starting with absolutely randomly generated data, the computer can find statistically significant differences in 50% of the experiments. Such procedure gives a great opportunity for fortuitous associations. Of course, in any empirical research the investigator properly must look for meaningful relationships, but before they become fact, the material needs to be verified by replication. For many endocrine parameters, an occasional study finds an elevation or vice-versa. It is difficult to completely rule out that many of these changes are real and occur either in certain subgroups or only under certain conditions.

There are many clinical variables that do affect endocrine results. The endocrine system is labile and affected by a wide variety of factors. When disturbed mental patients are tested, they are often in the midst of an acute episode during which they are not receiving drugs. An internal process, such as hallucinations or delusions, could produce an internal stress not evident to the investigator. It is reasonable to expect a certain amount of noise in such a labile system. Undoubtedly, the occasional high values or occasional low values might result from such factors. In my judgement, before an endocrine abnormality can be said to be proven in a serious mental disease, it must be clearly replicated by several investigators and be an effect of sufficient magnitude to stand out above the noise. In addition, we have commented above on the statistical artifacts which could magnify such chance associations. Undoubtedly, the occasional elevation or decrement reported by some investigators may be the result of such factors.

SUMMARY

There is a substantial body of evidence which indicates that antipsychotic drugs produced a marked elevation in plasma prolactin, presumably because of the dopaminergic blockade at a pituitary level. The dose-response relationship of the effect of the drug on the pituitary differ from the dose-response relationship with the antipsychotic effect in patients with psychosis. The dose-response curve is such that a lesser amount of neuroleptic is required to produce an elevation of prolactin than is required to produce an antipsychotic effect. In addition, there is an important difference in time course. The pituitary effects occur early, even within the first few hours, and are fairly stable over the months. An antipsychotic effect is noticeable in a patient given intramuscular or neuroleptic within a few hours of injection. The degree of improvement produced in schizophrenia has a different time course. Although it starts in the first few hours, the onset is rather gradual. There is a fair increase in antipsychotic effect in the first week, but the antipsychotic effect is still increasing at week 6 although it is beginning to level out. There is still improvement between week 6 and week 25. Furthermore, there is some evidence that there may be tolerance to the neuroleptic property of elevating prolactin in patients who have been on antipsychotics for many years. The data on this is not absolutely definitive but suggestive. There is also evidence that tolerance may not develop to the antipsychotic properties of the neuroleptics over great lengths of time. Patients who have been on neuroleptics for ten years are still responsive to them. The proper experiments have not been done to rule out whether there is some degree of tolerance to the antipsychotic effects over time, but within the limits of our present knowledge, there appears to be a different time course of the prolactin effect and the antipsychotic effect of neuroleptic. The antipsychotic drugs do not produce a marked effect on other endocrine parameters. They may have minor effects in certain situations and certainly variable results are found in different experiment. We review the literature here not in detail, but as an overall generalization that neuroleptics do not produce a marked effect in growth hormone, cortisol, thyroid and sexual-hormone axis.

REFERENCES

1. Angrist, B., Ain, M., Rotrosen, J., Gershon, S., Halpern, F. S. and Sachar, E. J. (1979): J. Neurol. Transmission 44:249-262.
2. Arato, M., Erdos, M. and Polgar, M. (1979): Pharmakopsychiatry 12: 426-431.
3. Arosio, M., Moriondo, P., Trauaglin, P., Ambrosi, B., Beck-Peccoz, P, Puglisi, F. C., Secchi, F. and Faglia, G. (1980): J. Clin. Endocrin. Metab. 51:454-461.
4. Asnis, G. M., Sachar, E. J., Langer, G., Halpern, F. S. and Fink, M. (1979): Psychopharmacology 66:247-250.
5. Beg, A. A., Varma, K. V. and Dash, R. J. (1979): Am. J. Psychiatry 136:914-916.
6. Belmaker, R. H., Ebstein, R. P., Dasberg, H., Levy, A., Sedvall, G. and Van Praag, H. M. (1979): Psychopharmacology 63:293-296.
7. Benjamin, F., Casper, D. J. and Kolodny, H. H. (1969): Obstetrics and Gynecology 34:34-39.
8. Besses, G. S., Burrow, G. N., Spaulding, S. M. and Donabedian, R. K. (1975): J. Clin. Endocrinol. Metab. 14:985-988.
9. Beumont, P.J.V., Corker, C. S., Friesen, H. G., Kolakowska, T., Mandelbrote, B. M., marshall, J., Murray, M.A.F. and Wiles, D. H. (1974): Br. J. Psychiatry 124:420-430.
10. Beumont, P.J.V., Gelder, M. G., Friesen, H. G., Harris, G. W., MacKinnon, P.C.B., Mandelbrote, B. M. and Wiles, D. H. (1974): Br. J. Psychiatry 124:413-419.
11. Brambilla, F. A., Guerrini, A., Guastalla, A., Rovere, C. and Riggi, F. (1975): Psychopharmacologia 44:17-22.
12. Brambilla, F., Guerrini, A., Riggi, F. and Ricardi, F. (1974): Dis. Nerv. Syst. 34:362-368.
13. Brooksbank, B.W.L., MacSweeney, D. A., Johnson, A. L., Cunningham, A. E., Wilson, D. A. and Coppen, A. (1970): Br. J. Psychiatry 117:413-420.
14. Brown, G. M., Friend, W. C. and Chambers, J. W. (1979): In: Clinical Neuroendocrinology: A Pathophysiological Approach, edited by G. Tolis, pp.47-81. Raven Press, New York.
15. Brown, G. M., Garfinkel, P. E., Warsh, J. J. and Stancer, H. C. (1976): J. Clin. Endocrin. Metab. 43:236-239.
16. Brown, G. M., Seeman, P. and Lee, T. (1976): Endocrinology 99: 1407-1410.
17. Brown, G. M. and Seggie, J. A. (1980): Psychiatrics Clinics of North America 3(1):205-221.
18. Brown, G. M., Stancer, H. C., Moldofsky, H., Harman, J. H., Murphy, J. T. and Gupta, R. N. (1978): Arch. Gen. Psychiat. 35: 1261-1264.
19. Brown, G. M., Verhaegen, H. and Van Wimersna Griedanos, T. B. (1981): Clin. Endocrinol. 3:275-282.

20. Brown, W. A. (1977): Arch. Gen. Psychiatry 34:1103-1108.
21. Brown, W. A., Corriveau, D. P. and Ebert, M. H. (1978): Psychopharmacology 58:189-195.
22. Brown, W. A., Krieger, D. J., Van Woert, M. H. and Ambani, L. M. (1974): J. Clin. Endcorinol. Metab. 38:1127-1129.
23. Brown, W. A. and Laughren, T. (1981): Am. J. Psychiatry 138: 237-239.
24. Brown, W. T., Sanberg, P. R. and McGeer, P. L. (1977): Arch. Neurology 36:452-453.
25. Buckman, M. T. and Peake, G. T. (1973): J. Clin. Endocrinol. Metab. 37:977-979.
26. Buckman, M. T., Peake, S. T. and Srivastara (1979): Horm. Metab. Res. 11:395-398.
27. Burrow, G. N., May, P. B., Apaulding, S. W. and Donabedrian, R. K. (1977): J. Clin. Endocrinol. Metab. 45:65-72.
28. Camanni, E., Genazzini, A. R., Massara, F., LaRosa, R., Cocchi, D. and Muller, E. E. (1980): Neuroendocrinology 30:206.
29. Camanni, E., LoCoco, R., Lanzar, P. and Janni, A. (1979): Acta Endocrinologica 91:609-615.
30. Camanni, E., LoCoco, R., Longo, A., Lansara, P. and Janni, A. (1980): In: Central and Peripheral Regulation of Prolactin Function, edited by R. M. MacLeod and U. Scapagnini, pp.353-356. Raven Press, New York.
31. Casacchia, M., Meco, G., Carchedi, F., DiCeglie, M., Falashi, P., Rocco, A., Pompei, P. and Frajese, G. (1979): In: Neuroendocrine Correlates in Neurology and Psychiatry, edited by E. E. Muller and A. Agnoli, pp.211-224. Elsevier Press, Amsterdam.
32. Cassano, G. B., Castrogiovanni, P., Conti, L. and Bonollo, L. (1975): Curr. Ther. Res. 17:189-201.
33. Catlin, D. H., Poland, R. E., Gorelick, D. A., Gevner, R. H., Hui, K. K., Rubin, R. T. and Choh, H. I. (1980): J. Clin. Endocrinol. Metab. 50:1021-1025.
34. Chalmers, R. J., Johnson, R. H., Keogh, H. J. and Nanda, R. N. (1978): J. Neurol. Neurosurg. Psychiat. 41:135-139.
35. Chouinard, G., Jones, B. D. and Annable, L. (1978): Am. J. Psychiatry 135;1409-1410.
36. Clarenbach, P., Prunkl, R., Riegler, M. and Cramer, A. (1978): Neuroscience 3:345-348.
37. Clemens, J. A., Smalstig, E. G. and Sawyer, B. D. (1974): Psychopharmacology 40:123-127.
38. Cohen, K. L., Cooper, R. A. and Altshule, S. (1979): New Eng. J. Med. 300:46.
39. Collu, R., Choumard, G., Jones, B. D. and Annable, L. (1978): Clin. Res. 26:840.
40. Collu, R., Jequier, J. C., Leboeuf, J. and Ducharme, J. R. (1975): J. Clin. Endocrinol. Metab. 41:981-984.
41. Corsini, G. U., DelZompo, M., Maconi, S., Chianchetti, C. and Mangoni, A. (1977): In: Symposium on Non-Striatal Dopaminergic Neurons, edited by E. Costa and G. L. Gessa, pp.645-648. Raven Press, New York.
42. Cotes, P. J., Crow, T. J., Johnstone, E. C., Bartlett, W. and Bourne, R. C. Psychological Med. 8:657-665.
43. Creese, I., Burt, D. R. and Synder, S. H. (1976): Science 194: 546.
44. Crosignani, P. G., Lambroso, G. C. Mattei, A., Caccamo, A. and

Trojsi, C. (1979): J. Clin. Endocrinol. Metab. 48:335-337.
45. Crosignani, P. G., Reschini, E., Perrachi, M., Lombroso, G. C., Mattei, A. and Caccamo, A. (1977): J. Clin. Endocrinol. Metab. 45: 841-844.
46. Crowley, T. J. and Hydinger-MacDonald, M. (1981): Arch. Gen. Psychiat. 38:668-675.
47. Curry, S. H., Marshall, J. H. L., Davis, J. M. and Janowsky, D. S. (1970): Arch. Gen. Psychiat. 22:289-296.
48. Czernik, A. and Kleesiek, K. (1979): Nervenarzt. 50:527-553.
49. Davis, J. M. (1974): J. Psychiat. Res. 11:65-69.
50. Davis, J. M., Morrill, R., Fawcett, J., Upton, U., Bondy, P. and Spirok H. (1962): J. Psychosomatic Res. 6:83-86.
51. DeRivera, J. L., Lal, S., Ettigi, P., Hontela, S., Muller, H. F. and Friesen, H. G. (1976): Clin. Endocrinol. 5:273-282.
52. Dunne, M. J., Walker, J., Cowden, E. A. and Ratcliff, J. G. (1979): Lancet 2:1243.
53. Egge, A. C., Rogol, A. D., Varma, M. M. and Blizzard, R. M. (1977): J. Clin. Endocrinol. Metab. 44:210-213.
54. Elizur, A., Segal, S., Yenet, A. and Ben-David, M. (1979): Isr. Ann. Psychiatry 17:318-327.
55. Ettigi, P., Nair, N.P.V., Lal, S., Cervantes, P. and Guyda, H. (1976): J. Neurol. Neurosurg. Psychiatry 39:870-876.
56. Evans, W. S., Rogol, A. D., MacLeod, R. M. and Thorner, M. O. (1980): J. Clin. Endocrinol. Metab. 50:103-107.
57. Ferrari, C., Caldara, R., Romuss, M., Rawpin, P., Telloli, P. and Zaatar, S. (1979): In: Neuroendocrinology: Biological and Clinical Aspects, edited by A. Poller and R. M. MacLeod, pp.299-306. Academic Press, New York.
58. Friend, W. C., Brown, G. M., Jawahir, G., Lee, T. and Seeman, P. (1978): Am. J. Psychiatry 135:839-841.
59. Gelenberg, A. S., Cooper, D. S., Doller, J. C. and Maloof, F. (1979): JAMA 242:1900-1901.
60. Gerazzani, A. R., Camanni, F., Massara, F., Picciolini, E., Cocchi, D., Belforte, L. and Muller, E. E. (1980): Acta Endocrinologica 93:139-148.
61. Goode, D. J., Meltzer, H. Y. and Fang, S. (1980): Psychoneuroendocrinology 5:345-351.
62. Gruen, P. H., Sachar, E. J., Altman, N., Langer, G., Tabrizi, M. A., and Halpern, F. S. (1978): Arch. Gen. Psychiat. 35:1222-1227.
63. Gruen, P. H., Sachar, E. J., Langer, G., Altman, N., Leifer, M., Frantz, A. and Halpern, F. S. (1978): Arch. Gen. Psychiatry 35: 108-116.
64. Hanssen, T., Heyden, T., Sundberg, L., Wetterberg, L. and Eneroth, P. (1978): Lancet 1:101-102.
65. Hays, S. E. and Rubin, R. T. (1981): Psychoneuroendocrinology 6: 45-52.
66. Huws, D. and Groom, G. V. (1977): Postgrad. Med. J. 53(suppl. 4): 175-181.
67. Janowsky, D. S., Leichner, P., Parker, D., Judd, L. L., Huey, L. and Clopton, P. (1978): Arch. Gen. Psychiatry 35:1384-1389.
68. Janowsky, D. S., Leichner, P., Parker, D., Judd, L., Huey, L. and Clopton, P. (1978): Psychopharmacology 58:43-47.
69. Jeste, D. V., Neckers, L. M., Wagner, R. L., Wise, C. D., Staub, R. A., Rogol, A., Potkin, S. G., Bridge, T. P. and Wyatt, R. J. (1981): J. Clin. Psychiatry 42:75-77.

70. Johnstone, E. C., Crow, T. J. and Mashiter, K. (1977): Psychol. Med. 7:223-231.
71. Johnstone, E. C. and Ferner, F. N. (1980): Br. J. Clin. Pharm. 10:5-21.
72. Judd, S. J., Lazarus, L. and Smythe, G. (1976): J. Clin. Endocrinol. Metab. 43:313-317.
73. Judd, S. J., Rakoff, J. S. and Yen, S.S.C. (1978): J. Clin. Endocrinol. Metab. 47:494-498.
74. Kane, J., Cooper, T., Sachar, E., Halpern, F.S. and Bailine, S. (1981): Psychopharmacology 73:184-187.
75. Kato, Y., Nakai, Y., Imura, H., Chihara, K. and Ohgo, S. (1974): J. Clin. Endocrinol. Metab. 33:873.
76. Kebabian, J. W. and Calner, D. B. (1979): Nature 277:93-96.
77. Keogh, H. J., Johnson, R. H., Nanda, R. N. and Sulaiman, W. R. (1976): J. Neurol. Neurosurg. Psychiat. 39:244-249.
78. Kirkegaard, C., Bjorum, B., Cohn, D., Faber, J., Lauridsen, U. B., and Nerup, J. (1977): Psychoneuroendocrinology 2:131-136.
79. Kirkegaard, C., Bjorum, N., Cohn, D. and Lauridsen, U. B. (1978): Arch. Gen. Psychiatry 35:1017-1021.
80. Kolakawska, T., Fraser, S., Franklin, M. and Know, I. (1981): Psychopharmacology 72:283-285.
81. Kolakowska, T., Orr, M., Gelter, M., Heggie, M., Wiles, D. and Franklin, M. (1979): Br. J. Psychiat. 135:352-359.
82. Kolakowska, T., Wiles, D. H., Gelder, M. G. and McNeilly, A. S. (1976): Psychopharmacology 49:101-107.
83. Krulick, L., McCann, S. M. and Myfield, M. D. (1981): Endocrinology 108:1115-1124.
84. Lachelin, G.C.L., LeBlanc, H. and Yen, S.S.C. (1977): J. Clin. Endocrinol. Metab. 44:728-732.
85. Lal, H., Brown, W., Drawbaugh, R., Hynes, M. and Brown, G. (1977): Life Sci. 20:101-106.
86. Lal, S., DeLaVega, C. E., Sourkes, T. L. and Friesen, H. G. (1973): J. Clin. Endocrinol. Metab. 37:719-724.
87. Lal, S., Guyda, H. and Bikadorof, F. (1977): J. Clin. Endocrinol. Metab. 44:766-780.
88. Lal, S., Mendis, T., Cervartes, P., Guyda, H. and DeRivera, J. J. (1979): Neuropsychobiology 5:327-331.
89. Lal, S. and Nair, N.P.V. (1979): In: Neuroendocrine Correlates in Neurology and Psychiatry, edited by E. E. Muller and A. Agnoli, pp.179-194. Elsevier North Holland Biomedical Press.
90. Lamberg, B. A., Linnoila, M., Fogelholm, R., Olkimora, M., Kotilainen, P. and Saarinen, P. (1977): Neuroendocrinology 24: 90-97.
91. Lancranjan, I., Wirz-Justica, A., Puhringer, W. and Del Pozp, E. (1977): J. Clin. Endocrinol. Metab. 45:588-593.
92. Langer, G. (1979): In: Neuroendocrine Correlates in Neurology and Psychiatry, edited by E. E. Muller and A. Agnoli, pp.71-88. Elsevier North Holland, Amsterdam.
93. Langer, G., Sachar, E. J., Gruen, P. H. and Halpern, F. S. (1977): Nature 266:639-640.
94. Langer, G. R., Sachar, E. J. and Halpern, F. S. (1978): Psychoneuroendocrinology 3:165-169.
95. Langer, G., Sachar, E. J., Halpern, F. S., Gruen, P. H. and Solomon, M. (1977): J. Clin. Endocrinol. Metab. 45:996-1002.
96. Laughren, T., Brown, W. and Petruccia, J. (1978): Am. J. Psychaitry

135:492-494.
97. Laughren, T. P., Brown, W. A. and Williams, B. W. (1979): Am. J. Psychiat. 131:108-110.
98. Leblanc, H., Lachelin, G.C.L., Abu-Fadil, S. and Yen, S.S.C. (1976): J. Clin. Endocrinol. Metab. 43:668.
99. Leebaw, W. F., Woolf, P. D. and Lee, L. A. (1978): J. Clin. Endocrinol. Metab. 47:480-487.
100. Lemberger, L. and Crabtree, R. E. (1979): Science 205:1151-1153.
101. Leppaluoto, J., Mannisto, P., Ranta, T. and Linnoria, M. (1976): Acta Endocrinol. 81:455-460.
102. Lindholm, H., Gullberg, B., Ohman, A. and Sedvall, G. (1978): Psychopharmacology 57:1-4.
103. Linnolia, M., Viokari, M. and Vaisanen, H. (1980): Acta Pharmacol. Toxicol. 46:1159-1160.
104. Maany, O., Frazer, A. and Mendels, J. (1975): J. Clin. Endocrinol. Metab. 40:762-763.
105. MacKay, A.V.P., Sheppard, G.P., Saha, B. K., Motley, B., Johnson, A. L. and Marsden, C. D. (1980): Psychological Medicine 10:583-587.
106. Magrini, G., Mean, F., Martin-du-Pan, R., Baumann, P. and Feiber, J. P. (1979): In: Neuroendocrinology: Biological and Clinical Aspects, edited by A. Polleri and R. M. MacLeod, pp.351-357. Academic Press, New York.
107. Mancini, A. M., Guitelman, A., Vargas, C. A., Debeljuk, L. and Aparicio, N. J. (1976): J. Clin. Endocrinol. Metab. 42:181-184.
108. Martin, J. B., Smarthji, L. and Tolis, G. (1974): J. Clin. Endocrinol. Metab. 39:180-182.
109. Martin, J. B., Reichlin, S. and Brown, G. M. (1977): Clinical Neuroendocrinology. Davis, Philadelphia.
110. Martin-du-Pan, R. and Baumann, D. (1979): Psychoneuroendocrinology 3:245-252.
111. Masala, A., Delitala, G., Alagna, S. and Devilla, L. (1977): Clinical Endocrinology 7:253-256.
112. Masala, A., Delitala, G., Devilla, L., Alagna, S. and Rovasio, P. (1979): J. Clin. Endocrinol. Metab. 49:350-352.
113. MacIndoe, J. H. and Turkington, R. W. (1973): J. Clin. Invest. 52:1972-1978.
114. Meltzer, H. Y. and Fang, V. S. (1976): Arch. Gen. Psychiatry 33: 279-286.
115. Meltzer, H. Y., Gang, V. S., Simonovich, M. and Paul, S. M. (1977): Eur. J. Pharmacol. 41:431-436.
116. Meltzer, H. Y., Fessler, R. G., Simonovich, M. and Fang, V. S. (1978): Psychopharmacology 56:255-259.
117. Meltzer, H. Y., Goode, D. J. and Fang, V. S. (1978): In: Psychopharmacology: A Generation of Progress, edited by M. A. Lipton, A. DiMascio and K. F. Killam, pp.509-529. Raven Press, New York.
118. Meltzer, H. Y., Goode, D. J., Schyve, P. M., Young, M. and Fang, V. S. (1979): Am. J. Psych. 136:1550-1555.
119. Meltzer, H. Y., Paul, S. M. and Fang, V. S. (1977): Psychopharmacology 51:181-183.
120. Meltzer, H. Y., Piyakalmala, S., Schyve, P. and Fang, V. S. (1977): Psychopharmacology 51:185-187.
121. Meltzer, H. Y., Simonovich, M., Fang, V., Piyakalamala, S. and Young, M. (1978): Life Sciences 23:605-610.
122. Meltzer, H. Y., So, R., Miller, R. J. and Fang, V. A. (1979):

Life Sciences 25:573-584.
123. Meltzer, H. Y., Young, M., Metz, J., Fang, V. S., Schyve, P. M. and Arora, R. C. (1979): J. Neurol. Transmission 45:165-175.
124. Mendlewicz, J. and Youdim, M.B.H. (1977): Lancet 48:507.
125. Mielke, D. H., Gallant, D. M. and Kessler, C. (1977): Am. J. Psychiatry 134:1371-1375.
126. Mielke, D. H., Gallant, D., Ronigen, J. J., Kessler, C. and Kessler, B. (1977): Dis. Nerv. Syst. 38:569-571.
127. Mims, R. B., Scott, C., Modebe, O. and Bethume, J. (1975): J. Clin. Endocrinol. Metab. 40:256-259.
128. Moller, H. J., Kissing, W. and Maurach, R. (1981): Pharmakopsychiatry 14:27-34.
129. Mori, M., Kobayashi, I., Ohshima, K., Marute, S., Shimomura, Y. and Fukuda, H. (1980): Acta Endocrinologica 94:25-29.
130. Muller, E. E., Stefanini, E., Camanni, F., Locatetlli, V., Massara, F., Spano, P. F. and Cocchi, D. (1979): J. Neural Transmission 46:205-214.
131. Murray, M.A.F., Bancroft, J.H.J., Anderson, D. C., Tennent, T. G. and Carr, P. J. (1975): J. Endocrinol. 67:179-188.
132. Naber, D., Ackenheil, M. and Laakmann, G. (1980): In: Advances in Biochemical Psychopharmacology, edited by F. Cattabeni, P. F. Spano, G. Racagni and E. Costa, p.24. Raven Press, New York.
133. Naber, D., Ackenheil, M., Laakmann, G., Fischer, H. and Von Werder, K. (1980): Pharmakopsychiatry 13:325-330.
134. Naber, D., Finkbeiner, C., Fischer, B., Zander, K. J. and Ackenheil, M. (1980): Neuropsychobiology 6:181-189.
135. Naber, D., Fischer, F. and Ackenheil, M. (1979): Commun. Psychopharmacol. 3:59-65.
136. Naber, D., Steinbock, H. and Greil, W. (1980): Prog. Neuropsychopharmacology 4:199-206.
137. Nair, N., Lal, S., Schwartz, G. and Thavundayil, J. X. (1980): In: Long Term Effects of Neuroleptics, edited by F. Cattabeni, P. F. Spano, G. Racagri and E. Costa. Raven Press, New York.
138. Nair, N.P.V., Lal, S., Cervantes, P., Yassa, R. and Guyda, H. (1979): Neuropsychobiology 5:136-142.
139. Nathan, R. S., Asnis, G. M., Dyrenfurth, I., Halpern, F. S., Halbreich, U., Ostrow, L. C. and Sachar, E. J. (1980): Lancet 2:94.
140. Nathan, R. S., Sachar, E. J., Ostrow, L., Asnis, G. M., Halbreich, V. and Halpern, F. S. (1981): J. Clin. Endocrinol. Metab. 52:807-809.
141. Nathan, R. S., Tabrizi, M. A., Halpern, F. S. and Sachar, E. J. (1980): J. Clin. Endocrinol. Metab. 51:90-92.
142. Nielsen, J. (1980): Neuropsychobiology 6:52-55.
143. Nikitopoulou, G., Thorner, M., Crammer, J. and Ladev, M. (1976): Clin. Pharm. Ther. 21:422-429.
144. Nordgren, L. and V. Scheele, C. (1980): Pharmacopsychiatry 14: 61-65.
145. Ohman, R. and Axelsson, R. (1978): Eur. J. Clin. Pharmacol. 14: 111-116.
146. Ohman, R., Forsman, A. and Larsson, M. (1980): Curr. Ther. Res. 27:137-143.
147. Onishi, T., Miyai, K., Izumi, K., Nakanishi, H. and Kumahara, Y. (1975): J. Clin. Endocrinol. Metab. 40:30-32.
148. Otsuki, M., Dakoda, M. and Baba, S. (1973): J. Clin. Endocrinol.

36:95-102.
149. Parati, E. A., Zanardi, P., Cocchi, D., Caraceni, T. and Muller, E. E. (1980): J. Neurol. Transmission 47:273-297.
150. Parkes, I. D., Debono, A. G. and Marsden, C. D. (1976): Lancet 1:483.
151. Pourmand, M., Rodriquez-Arnao, M., Weightman, D., Hall, R., Cook, D., Lewis, M. and Scanlon, M. (1980): Clin. Endocrinol. 12:211-215.
152. Pontiroli, A., Silva, E. and Mazzoleni, I. (1981): J. Clin. Endocrinol. Metab. 52:924-928.
153. Quigley, M. E., Judd, S. J., Gilliland, G. B. and Yen, S.S.C. (1979): J. Clin. Endocrinol. Metab. 48:718-720.
154. Rama-Rao, V. A., Bailey, J. and Coppen, A. (1981): Psychopharmacology 73:77-80.
155. Rama-Roa, V. A., Bishop, M. and Coppen, A. (1980): Am. J. Psychiatry 137:518-521.
156. Re, R. N., Kourides, I. A., Ridgway, E. C., Weintraub, B. D. and Maloof, F. (1976): J. Clin. Endocrinol. Metab. 43:338.
157. Refetoff, S., Fang, V. S., Rapoport, B. and Friesen, H. G. (1974): J. Clin. Endocrinol. Metab. 38:450-457.
158. Roccatagliata, G., De Cecco, L., Rossato, P. and Albano, C. (1979): Int. Pharmacopsychiatry 14:260-263.
159. Rotrosen, J., Angrist, B., Gershon, S., Paquin, J., Branchey, L., Oleshansky, M., Halpern, F. and Sachar, E. J. (1979): Br. J. Psychiatry 135:444-456.
160. Rowley-Jones, D. (1978): Lancet 2:635.
161. Rubin, R. T. (1980): Lancet 2:370.
162. Rubin, R. T., Forsman, A., Heykonts, J., Ohman, R., Tower, B. and Michiels, M. (1980): Arch. Gen. Psychiat. 37:1069-1074.
163. Rubin, R. T. and Forster, B. (1980): Comm. Psychopharmacol. 4(1): 41-47.
164. Rubin, R. T. and Hays, S. E. (1978): Psychopharmacology Bulletin 14:9-11.
165. Rubin, R. G. and Hays, S. E. (1979): Psychopharmacology 61:17-24.
166. Rubin, R. T., Poland, R. E., O'Connor, D., Gouin, P. R. and Tower, B. B. (1976): Psychopharmacology 47:135-140.
167. Sachar, E. J., Gruen, P. H., Altman, N., Halpern, F. S. and Frantz, A. G. (1976): In: Hormones, Behaviour and Psychopathology edited by E. J. Sachar, p.161. Raven Press, New York.
168. Sachar, E. J., Mushrush, G., Perlow, M., Weitzman, E. D. and Sassin, j. (1972): Science 178:1304.
169. Saldanha, V. F., Havard, C.W.H., Bird, R. and Gardner, R. (1972): Clin. Endocrinol. 1:173-180.
170. Schwimm, C., Schward, H., McIntosh, C., Milstrey, H. R., Wills, B. and Kobberling, J. (1976): J. Clin. Endocrinol. Metab. 43:1183-1185.
171. Sedvall, G. (1979): In: Neuroendocrine Correlates in Neurology and Psychiatry, edited by E. E. Muller and A. Agnoli, pp.195-209. Elsevier Press, Amsterdam.
172. Seeman, P., Chau-Wong, M., Tedesco, J. and Wong, K. (1975): Proc. Natl. Sci. U.S.A. 72:4376-4380.
173. Seeman, P., Lee, T., Chau-Wong, M. and Wong, K. (1976): Nature 261:717-719.
174. Sekso, M., Solter, M., Banovac, K., Vizner, B. and Petek, M. (1977): Acta Iug. Med. 31:321-332.
175. Sherman, L., Kim, S., Benjamin, F. and Kolodny, H. D. (1971):

New Eng. J. Med. 284:72-74.
176. Siris, E. S., Siris, S. G., van Kammen, D., Docherty, J. P., Alexander, P. E. and Bunney, W. E. Jr. (1980): Am. J. Psychiatry 137:211-213.
177. Smith, R. C., Tamminga, C., Crayton, J. and Davis, J. (1979): Psychopharmacology 66:29-33.
178. Smith, R. C., Tamminga, C. A. and Davis, J. M. (1977): J. Neural Transm. 40:171-176.
179. Snyder, S. H., Creese, I. and Burt, D. R. (1975): Psychopharmacol. Commun. 1:663-673.
180. Spitz, I. M., Almaliach, U., Rosen, E., Polishuk, W. and Rabinowitz, D. (1977): J. Clin. Endocrin. Metabolism 45:1173-1178.
181. Sowers, J. R., Carlson, H. E., Brautbar, N. and Hershman, J. M. (1977): J. Clin. Endocrinol. Metab. 44:237.
182. Stern, W. C., Rogers, J., Fang, V. and Meltzer, H. (1979): Life Sciences 25:1717-1724.
183. Tamminga, C. A., Neophtides, A., Chase, T. N. and Frohman, L. A. (1978): J. Clin. Endocrinol. Metab. 47:1348-1351.
184. Tamminga, C. A., Schaffer, M. H. Smith, R. C. and Davis, J. M. (1978): Science 200:567-568.
185. Tamminga, C. T., Smith, R. C., Pandey, G., Frohman, L. and Davis, J. M. (1976): Soc. for Neuroendocrinology 6:699.
186. Tamminga, C. A., Smith, R. C., Pandey, G., Frohman, L. A. and Davis, J. M. (1977): Arch. Gen. Psychiatry 34:1199-1203.
187. Terry, L. C. and Martin, J. B. (1981): Endocrinol. 108:1869-1871.
188. Thorner, M. O., Ryan, S. M., Wass, J.A.H., Jones, A., Boulloux, P., Williams, S. and Besser, G. M. (1978): J. Clin. Endocrinol. Metab. 47:372-378.
189. Toru, M., Shimazono, Y., Miyasaka, M., Kokubo, T., Mori, Y. and Nasu, T. (1972): J. Clin. Pharmacol. 12:221-229.
190. Turkington, R. W. (1972): Arch. Intern. Med. 130:349-354.
191. Tyson, J. E. and Friesen, H. G. (1973): Am. J. Obstet. and Gynecol. 116:377-387.
192. Van Kammen, D. P., Docherty, J. P., Marder, S. P., Siris, S. G. and Bunney, W. E., Jr. (1978): Life Sciences 23:1487-1492.
193. Van Putten, T., May, P. and Wilkins, J. (1980): Am. J. Psychiatry 137:1446-1448.
194. Vissen, T. S. and Lambert, S.W.J. (1981): Acta Endocrinologica 96:480-483.
195. Widerlov, E., Wide, L. and Sjostrom, R. (1979): Acta Psychiat. Scand. 58:449-456.
196. Wiles, D., Franklin, M., Dencker, S. J., Johansson, R., Lundi, L. and Malm, U. : 71:131-136.
197. Wiles, D. H., Kolakowska, T., McNeilly, A. S., Mandelbrote, B. M. and Gelder, M. G. (1976): Psychol. Med. 6:407-415.
198. Willoughby, J. O., Brazeau, P. and Martin, J. B. (1977): Endocrinology 101:1298-1303.
199. Wilson, R. G., Hamilton, J. R., Boyd, W. D., Forrest, A.P.M., Cole, E. N., Boyns, A. R. and Griffiths, K. (1973): Br. J. Psychiatry 127:71-74.
200. Wilson, J. D., King, D. J. and Sheridan, B. (1979): Clin. Pharmacol. 7:313.
201. Wode-Helgodt, B., Borg, S., Fyro, B. and Sedvall, G. (1978): Acta Psychiat. Scand. 58:149-173.
202. Wode-Helgodt, B., Eneroth, P., Fyro, B., Gullberg, B. and Sedvall, G. (1977): Acta Psychiat. Scand. 56:280-293.

Neuroendocrinology and Psychiatric Disorder, edited by G. M. Brown, et al. Raven Press, New York 1984.

Is Prolactin a Marker for Brain Dopamine Function?

Michael O. Thorner and William S. Evans

Prolactin secretion from the anterior pituitary is under predominantly inhibitory hypothalamic control (14). The catecholamine dopamine is now considered to be the major, if not the sole, physiologic hypothalamic prolactin inhibiting factor (31). Dopamine is synthesized by the tuberoinfundibular dopaminergic neurons (TIDA) which have their cell bodies in the arcuate and periventricular nuclei of the medial basal hypothalamus with terminals ending on the hypothalamic-hypophyseal portal capillaries at the median eminence. Dopamine secreted by these neurons is transported by the portal system to the anterior pituitary where the neurotransmitter binds to plasma membrane dopamine receptors on the lactotroph, activating as yet undefined mechanisms which tonically inhibit prolactin release (18). Thus, serum prolactin levels reflect in an inverse manner both the tone of this dopamine pathway and the sensitivity of the dopamine receptor on the lactotroph. Prolactin release increases as the effective dopamine concentration reaching the pituitary is reduced. Such a reduction occurs following administration of various drugs which act as dopamine receptor blockers (the butyrophenones and phenothiazines), as catecholamine depleting agents (reserpine), as false neurotransmitters (alpha-methyl dopa) and also may accompany processes in which the dopamine delivery system is physically disrupted (hypothalamic or pituitary disease, pituitary stalk section) (57). Prolactin secretion may be directly stimulated by various substances including estrogen and thyrotropin-releasing hormone (TRH). Estrogen clearly has a physiologic role since prolactin secretion is greater in women than in men, and is also increased in normal situations where circulating estrogen concentrations are elevated such as pregnancy. The role of TRH in the control of prolactin secretion is unclear at the present time. There is a dissociation in the secretion of prolactin and TSH (16); during sleep serum prolactin levels rise without a parallel increase in serum TSH. Furthermore, during suckling there is a rise in prolactin secretion which is not accompanied by any change in TSH secretion. Recently, extremely low concentrations of vasoactive intestinal peptide (VIP) have been shown to directly stimulate prolactin release in rats (25); the physiological significance of this observation is uncertain.

In order to be able to evaluate data on prolactin secretion in schizophrenia it is important to recall the patterns of prolactin secretion in normal subjects. There are marked changes in circulating prolactin levels from fetal life to old age (Figure 1). In the fetus up to 25 weeks of gestation serum prolactin levels are slightly higher than in normal adults. From 25 weeks until birth fetal serum prolactin levels rise progressively and may exceed 500 ng/ml. After birth there is a fall over the first week to between 50 and 80 ng/ml and by six weeks serum prolactin has reached prepubertal levels of 15 ng/ml. Such levels are maintained until the time of puberty when a small rise in prolactin levels (measured between 1000-1130 h) occurs at stage 2 (i.e. the breast bud stage) of breast development in girls (56). Serum prolactin levels in girls after menarche are higher than before puberty and exceed values seen in boys and men although there is overlap in the ranges.

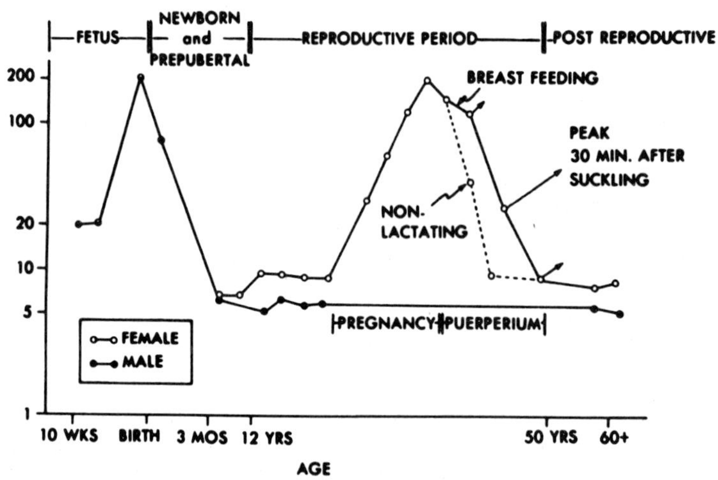

FIG. 1. Average serum prolactin levels at various periods of life in human male (●) and female (O) subjects. The length of the arrows in females who are breast-feeding is intended to indicate the magnitude of the increase in serum prolactin after each episode of suckling (reproduced from ref. 15 with permission).

During pregnancy prolactin levels rise with the highest values occurring during the third trimester. Following delivery prolactin levels fall and are normal at two weeks if lactation does not take place. However, if breast feeding occurs basal prolactin levels remain elevated and, with suckling, rise yet higher over 30 minutes, then falling gradually until the next feed. While breast feeding continues, the basal prolactin levels remain elevated above those seen in non-pregnant women. As supplemental food is introduced to the infant and as suckling episodes diminish in frequency, serum prolactin falls (38).

Concentrations of circulating prolactin do not remain constant throughout a 24 hour period. Serum levels rise shortly after the onset of sleep (by 50-100%) and then fall towards morning. That this rise is related to sleep rather than time of day has been demonstrated by shifts in prolactin release which occur simultaneously under conditions of acute day/night sleep reversal (44, 47). Such sleep-associated prolactin secretion can be suppressed by hypercortisolism (both exogenous and from Cushing's syndrome) (9, 27) and is lost in subjects with pathologic hyperprolactinemia. Of interest is a recent report (24) suggesting that prolactin concentrations in the cerebrospinal fluid (CSF) of the rhesus monkey appear entrained with such sleep-associated rises in serum prolactin; i.e., during normal sleep-awake cycles, peak CSF prolactin levels occurred between 0200 h and 0500 h with minimum values being found at 1500 h. That CSF prolactin values tend to parallel serum values has been shown in normal and MtTW15 tumor bearing rats and in humans with both intra and supra-sellar tumors (29). The source of such prolactin and the manner in which the hormone enters the CSF remain unclear; thus, the significance of studies on CSF prolactin levels in psychiatric patients are difficult to evaluate.

Although a prolactin surge occurs in temporal association with the LH surge during the afternoon of proestrus in rats, no such change in prolactin secretion has been documented during the midcycle phase of the menstrual cycle in women (37). Enhanced release of prolactin is seen, however, in response to various forms of emotional and physical states and may occur in women during stimulation of the breast by sexual partner and during sexual intercourse (43).

With the above in mind it becomes obvious that consideration must be given to the time of day, the sex, and the developmental state of the subject when measuring serum prolactin. Recently Moult and colleagues (41) examined the question of randomly obtained serum prolactin levels as compared to those collected during multiple sampling. When a forearm vein was cannulated between 0830-0930 hours and samples withdrawn every 15 minutes for two hours (the first taken 45 minutes after cannulation), the initial prolactin concentration (i.e. at 45 minutes) was elevated in 74% of the subjects. Values progressively fell over the two hour sampling period in 38% and 44% of those with initially elevated values fell into the normal range. Furthermore, when the mean of the last three samples taken during this period (defined as the basal or "unstressed" prolactin level) was compared to the mean of several randomly obtained prolactin levels, basal concentrations were found to be 27% lower than random concentrations. Thus, when an accurate representation of the circulating prolactin level is required, attention must be paid not only to the variables noted above but also to the manner in which the prolactin is drawn. We currently utilize methodology similar to that described above. A heparin-lock cannula is inserted between 0700-0800 h and, after one hour, samples are withdrawn at 20 minute intervals on at least three occasions. The mean of these samples is taken as the basal prolactin level. All measurements of serum prolactin during and after a given treatment regimen are obtained in the same manner. Although the studies performed in psychiatric patients have rarely been performed in this manner, prolactin levels have only occasionally been reported to be abnormal.

In Vivo and In Vitro Studies of the Control of Prolactin Secretion

MacLeod and Lehmeyer (34) using static incubations of rat anterior hemipituitaries demonstrated that catecholamines were capable of inhibiting prolactin release. Compared to norpinephrine, dopamine was significantly more potent in suppressing prolactin secretion.

Physiological studies involving measurement of dopamine in the portal blood of rats by Neill and colleagues confirmed a complex but definite inhibitory role of the catecholamine in both tonic and dynamic prolactin release by the pituitary (11, 12, 18, 46). Pharmacological studies demonstrated that the ergot alkaloids are capable of inhibiting and the neuroleptics (e.g. haloperidol) stimulating prolactin release (Figure 2). Such effects appear to be mediated by interaction of these agents with dopamine receptors located on the lactotroph. The subject of dopamine receptors in the anterior pituitary has recently been reviewed by Cronin (10). Both agonist and antagonist binding to dopamine receptors of the anterior pituitary have been satisfactorily defined by several groups. The potency with which a variety of dopaminergic drugs compete for the binding sites correlates well with the ability of these drugs of affect prolactin release *in vitro*. Furthermore, binding sites of the dopamine antagonist haloperidol have been visualized on the plasmalemma of

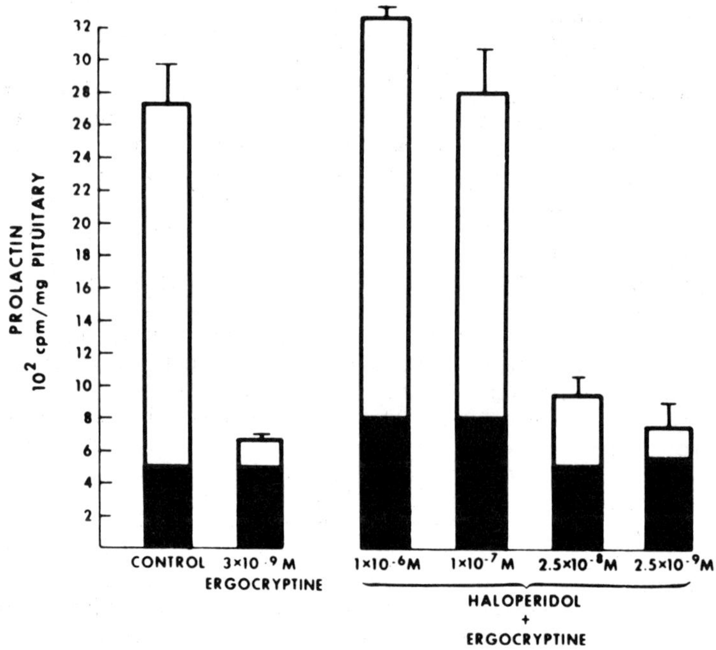

FIG. 2. Blockade of the ergocryptine-mediated inhibition of prolactin release by haloperidol. 3 x 10^{-9} M ergocryptine was incubated alone and in the presence of varying concentrations of haloperidol in flasks containing four hemipituitary glands; three flasks per group (reproduced from ref. 32 with permission).

lactotrophs with an immunocytochemical technique. Although the identity of the second messenger for the dopamine receptor remains controversial, there is good evidence that it may involve the inhibition of calcium influx or adenylate cyclase (infra vide).

When the pituitary is isolated from hypothalamic influences prolactin release becomes maximal. The stimulus for this secretion appears to be intrinsic to the cell and is poorly understood. The observation of action potentials in anterior pituitary cells (10% of cells) (52, 53) has led to the suggestion that these spikes, which have the characteristics of slow calcium spikes - i.e. being dependent on extracellular calcium rather than sodium ions - may participate in stimulus secretion coupling of prolactin. This observation may be of particular significance since two factors which affect prolactin release, TRH and dopamine, are known to stimulate and inhibit spiking, respectively (52, 53). Although the concept of stimulus secretion coupling has been addressed in studies of many secretory systems, including some cells of the anterior pituitary, its application to studies of the control of prolactin release by the lactotroph curiously has been largely neglected. We recently have performed studies investigating the effects on prolactin release of some factors which have been shown to alter stimulus secretion coupling and/or spiking of anterior pituitary cells.

Our studies were performed using rat anterior pituitary cells in a perifusion column (30, 62). This is a simple and very sensitive method for examining the dynamics of control of pituitary hormone secretion and

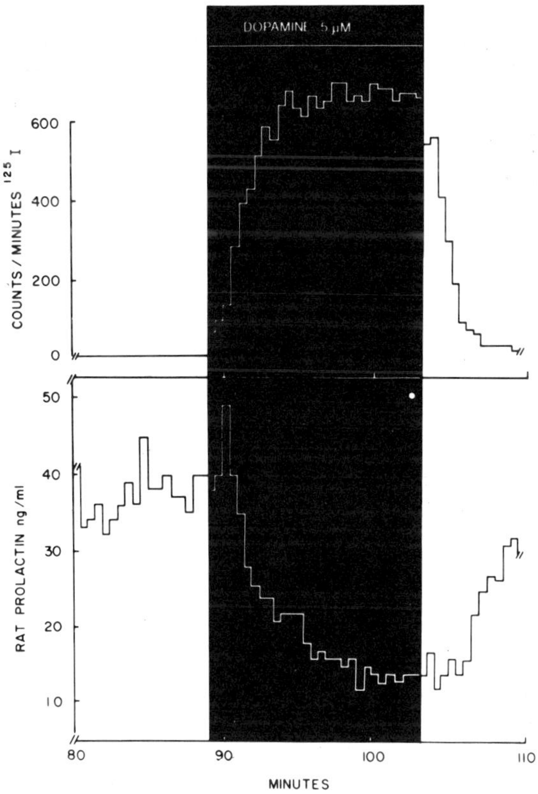

FIG. 3. The rapid onset and recovery from a 15 minute dose of 5 M dopamine on the release of prolactin from pituitary cell column. Upper panel: counts per minute ^{125}I-luteinizing hormone used as indicator for dopamine concentration in 0.5-minute fractions of eluate from pituitary cell column. Lower panel: concentration of rat prolactin in eluate from column (reproduced from ref. 51 with permission).

is admirably suited for the investigation of such questions. Using this technique we have been able to follow the dynamics of prolactin release from isolated cells at minute to minute intervals. As shown in Figure 3 an inhibitory effect of dopamine was observed within three minutes after the commencement of perifusion of the cells with the catecholamines, but three minutes before peak dopamine levels were achieved. By the time that peak dopamine levels occurred, prolactin levels were already suppressed to 45% of baseline and only a further 20% suppression was observed five minutes later. Three minutes following the withdrawal of dopamine prolactin was still maximally inhibited but one minute later prolactin levels had doubled and 2.5 minutes later still prolactin levels had recovered to 80% of those observed before exposure to dopamine. From these results it is clear that the inhibitory effects of dopamine are rapid and are just as rapidly reversible. Although the effects of dopamine on action potentials occur within seconds, the effects observed here appear to be slower; this apparent discrepancy probably reflects the limitations of our _in vitro_ system and may well have no physiological significance.

The mechanism by which dopamine inhibits prolactin secretion is poorly understood. We have presented evidence to suggest that calcium rather than cyclic AMP is the physiological intracellular regulator of prolactin release (54). Other groups, however, have suggested that in the pituitary dopamine may indeed affect intracellular cyclic AMP by inhibiting adenylate cyclase (17); this activity would be in contrast to the brain where dopamine appears to stimulate adenylate cyclase (26). Irrespective of whether or not calcium is the second messenger, it is clear that the withdrawal of calcium from the medium bathing pituitary cells leads to a rapid inhibition of prolactin release. Addition of calcium leads to recovery of prolactin secretion. Similarly, ions or drugs which block calcium channels (e.g. verapamil and D-600, the methoxy derivative of verapamil) all inhibit basal prolactin secretion in vitro. Thus, there is little doubt that in order to sustain basal prolactin secretion extracellular calcium is required. In contrast basal secretion of other anterior pituitary hormones is unaffected by these manipulations although stimulated secretion is inhibited. Sodium channels appear to be unimportant in the control of prolactin secretion.

When cells were exposed over four hours to calcium free medium prolactin release was inhibited. After 2.5 hours of exposure of the cells to calcium-free medium a supramaximal dose of dopamine (5 μM) had no effect on prolactin release, suggesting that the release process was already maximally inhibited. On re-exposure of the cell to physiological concentrations of extracellular calcium there was a massive release of prolactin and the cells once more were sensitive to dopamine. Both manganese (2 mM) and D-600 (1 μM) were effective in inhibiting spontaneous prolactin release. However, following withdrawal of manganese prolactin secretion recovered immediately while the effect of D-600 was prolonged. Takahara and colleagues also showed that the calcium channel blocking agent, nefedepine, inhibited spontaneous prolactin release in vitro (51).

The hypothesis that tonic prolactin secretion is maintained by influx of extracellular calcium and that dopamine inhibits this process is supported by some experiments performed by our laboratory using the calcium ionophores which enhance calcium transport across membranes. The ionophore A23187 had no effect at doses of 1 nM to 10 μM on tonic prolactin secretion in the presence of 2.5 mM calcium. However, it overcame in a dose-dependent fashion the inhibitory effects of dopamine.

Irrespective of whether dopamine affects cyclic AMP stimulation in the lactotroph, the administration of compounds which stimulate adenylate cyclase, (e.g. prostaglandin E_1 or chloratoxin) is able to alter the release of cyclic AMP from cells but these treatments do not affect either basal prolactin secretion or the inhibition of prolactin secretion by dopamine. Thus we believe that cyclic AMP is probably unimportant in the physiologic regulation of prolactin secretion; calcium appears more important. However, effects of cyclic AMP on prolactin synthesis (rather than release) may be significant (36).

From the point of view of the discussion of prolactin as a marker of TIDA activity and other brain dopamine function, the effects of estrogen on prolactin secretion are of only minor significance. For the sake of completeness it needs to be stressed that estrogens do play an extremely important role in the regulation of physiological prolactin production. Pituitary glands from female rats contain several fold more prolactin than is found in glands from male rats. Gonadectomy decreases pituitary prolactin content and biosynthetic capacity, both of which are restored by the administration of estrogens (33). Specific estrogen receptors which have been identified in pituitary tissue are directly stimulatory for the generation of messenger RNA which then codes for prolactin synthesis (49, 50, 61). Estrogen administration increases the circulating concentration of prolactin, but the primary action of the steroid is on the synthesis of prolactin. The stimulatory effect of estradiol on prolactin secretion may be mediated through modulation of the inhibitory action of dopamine. There is little doubt that dopamine mediated inhibition of prolactin secretion is decreased in pituitary glands following treatment with estradiol (28, 32). Evidence is accumulating that the binding of ^{3}H estradiol to pituitary receptors is decreased following the administration of ergot alkaloids (dopamine agonists) and may represent a mechanism through which the monoaminergic and estrogenic systems interact to regulate prolactin synthesis and release (42). Furthermore, estradiol may have an indirect action in stimulating prolactin secretion by affecting the turnover of hypothalamic dopamine; decreased dopamine release into the portal capillaries diminishes tonic inhibition of prolactin secretion (13)(Figure 4). Parenthetically, the enhanced secretory reserve induced by estrogen is manifest clinically by the greater response of prolactin to neuroleptics and other stimuli, such as estrogen, in women than in men.

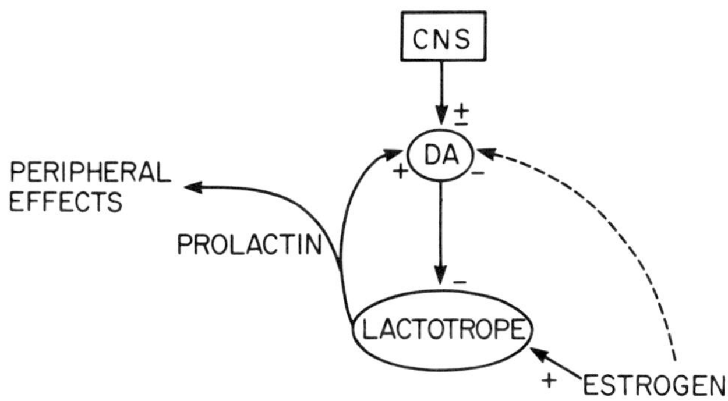

FIG. 4. Schematic representation of the interrelationships between the lactotrope dopamine and estrogen in the control of prolactin secretion (reproduced from ref. 52 with permission).

Prolactin as a Marker for Brain Dopamine Function

Although many questions remain unanswered, much progress has been made in elucidating the mechanisms responsible for the control of prolactin secretion. Can such knowledge help bring about a better understanding of neurologic and psychiatric disorders in which aberrant brain dopamine metabolism is involved? Recently, this possibility has received much investigative attention. For some time it has been evident that the fundamental abnormality in Parkinson's disease centers around a deficiency of nigrostriatal dopamine (4, 21). Conversely, a situation of excessive dopaminergic tone in the striatum has been hypothesized as an etiologic factor in Huntington's disease (21, 22). However, of prime interest to this discussion is the possibility that schizophrenia may be associated with abnormalities in brain dopamine metabolism. Much of this conjecture is based on the fact that administration of the neuroleptics, which are potent dopamine receptor blockers, often leads to definite improvement in symptoms in the schizophrenic patient (5, 19, 20; see chapter 2 by Davis and colleagues). It would be reasonable to speculate that, since several neuropsychiatric disorders appear to involve abnormal brain dopamine pathways, then prolactin secretion, which is a good marker of TIDA activity, might be useful in the diagnosis and monitoring of such disease states. The issues surrounding this thesis, however, are complex. It must be recalled that there are at least four functionally separate central dopaminergic systems: (1) the nigrostriatal in which cell bodies in the pars compacta of the substantia nigra have axons which terminate in the caudate and putamen of the corpus striatum; (2) the mesolimbic which arises from the central tegmental area in the region of the interpeduncular nucleus and innervate the limbic forebrain structures (nucleus accumbens, paraolfactory, prefrontal and septal areas); (3) the mesocortical ascending tract originating in the same mesencephalic region with axons to the frontal, cingulate, and the entorhinal cortex; and (4) the tuberoinfundibular dopaminergic neurons (TIDA) whose characteristics have been described above. Dopamine is the primary neurotransmitter in each of these systems and, for the TIDA, prolactin is an excellent indicator of dopaminergic activity. Unfortunately, there is no known readily accessible marker for dopaminergic activity in the nigrostriatal, mesolimbic and mesocortical systems. The question of vital importance is obvious: can there be a functional problem entirely isolated to one of the dopaminergic systems or will such a problem in any one of the pathways be reflected in the others? If the latter were true, then abnormalities of the higher dopaminergic systems might well be documented by changes in the TIDA as represented by aberrations in prolactin secretion. Examination of the various pathways immediately suggests definite physiological differences. Firstly, in the nigrostriatum, there is good evidence for the presence of both pre- and post-synaptic dopamine receptors (59). Conversely, studies have failed to document the presence of pre-synaptic dopamine receptors in the TIDA in the median eminence (6). Secondly, following acute administration of the dopamine receptor blocking drug thioproperazine, the nigrostriatal pathway appears much more sensitive to activation of dopamine synthesis than either the mesocortical or mesolimbic tracts (23). Thirdly, treatment on a chronic basis with neuroleptics results in a situation of tolerance in the nigrostriatal system which is not seen in the mesolimbic, mesocortical, or TIDA pathways (2, 23, 60). Fourthly, the concentration of dihydroxyphenylacetic acid (DOPAC) which is a primary product of dopamine metabolism is significantly less in the TIDA than in the other dopaminergic systems (58). Fifthly, both electrophysical (3) and biochemical (40) studies have shown that the function of the nigrostriatal and mesocortical systems increases following administration of dopamine receptor antagonists and decreases after dopamine receptor agonists; similar studies on the TIDA have shown no such responses, thus suggesting that this system is not controlled by a short-loop dopaminergic feedback system. Moreover, the TIDA is responsive to changes in prolactin concentration, a situation not observed in the limbic system. The effect of prolactin on the nigrostriatum is controversial (1, 35, 45).

The specific evidence concerning prolactin secretion in schizophrenia has been extensively reviewed in chapters 1 and 2 by Meltzer and Davis. Most studies have found no definite abnormality of basal prolactin secretion in schizophrenic subjects. Furthermore, it should be recalled that, while institution of therapy with the neuroleptics is followed within minutes or hours by elevated serum prolactin levels, the antipsychotic effects may require weeks to become manifest (39). Similarly, discontinuation of some of these drugs is followed by normalization of serum prolactin within two to three days; during this time no deterioration in the psychiatric status occurs (39). Finally, extremely effective antipsychotic drugs are in use which do not elevate serum prolactin levels (20, 48). From the discussions by Meltzer and Davis, it is clear that, with few exceptions, all drugs used in the treatment of psychosis have dopamine antagonist properties which are manifest by stimulation of prolactin secretion. A perhaps paradoxical finding is that during chronic neuroleptic treatment, serum prolactin levels are most elevated at the initiation of therapy but over the subsequent months or years may fall. The explanation for this phenomenon is unclear. It is conceivable that prolactin secretion is controlled by a variety of stimulatory and inhibitory factors of which dopamine is only one. Chronic elevation of serum prolactin might result in modulation of such non-dopaminergic factors, resulting in lowered prolactin concentrations. Another possibility relates to the concept of receptor supersensitivity. Cheung and Weiner (7) examined the effect of lesioning the medial basal hypothalamus of rats on prolactin release. As would be expected, disruption of the tonic hypothalamic inhibitory influence led to increased prolactin release when measured at one and 14 days after surgery. The dopamine agonist apomorphine diminished serum prolactin when administered on day 1 but had a much greater inhibitory effect on the day 14 animals. Similar results were obtained in a later study by the same group (8). Medial hypothalamus-lesioned rats were sacrificed at one and 14 days; pituitary cells were exposed to dopamine and apomorphine using a static incubation technique. Dopamine (10^{-8} M) and apomorphine (5×10^{-8} M) both exerted a significantly greater degree of inhibition of the day 14 animals as opposed to the day 1 animals. These results were interpreted as consistent with an increased sensitivity of dopamine receptors on the prolactin secreting lactotroph. In patients, chronic treatment with dopamine receptor antagonists might be expected to result in a similar situation of supersensitivity. If such were the case, enhanced tuberoinfundibular dopamine turnover (resulting from elevation of serum prolactin) might result in dopamine concentrations at the lactotroph sufficient to overcome partially the receptor blockade effect of the neuroleptic by acting on supersensitive receptors, receptors, resulting in some, but not complete lowering of serum prolactin. It must be emphasized that this mechanism, although tenable, is without clinical documentation.

CONCLUSIONS

The current evidence would thus seem to argue that the various dopaminergic pathways in the central nervous system are functionally independent; i.e., an abnormality in one may well not be reflected in the activity of another. A neurologic or psychiatric disorder stemming from a dysfunction in one dopaminergic pathway would not, of necessity, be expected to be associated with definite abnormalities in another, particularly since feedback mechanisms are different. The fact that prolactin secretion appears normal in schizophrenia, suggesting intact TIDA function, neither proves nor discounts the possibility of deranged function in one or more of the higher dopaminergic systems. Hopefully, future research efforts will result in markers for the striatal and limbic systems in a manner similar to that of prolactin for the TIDA; such markers will prove invaluable in correlating clinical manifestations of various neuro-psychiatric disorders with biochemical and/or physiological disturbances within the brain. For now, however, while measurement of serum prolactin may be useful in monitoring compliance of those patients taking antipsychotics with dopamine antagonist properties, levels of the hormone do not appear to be useful discriminators of higher dopaminergic dysfunction.

REFERENCES

1. Annunziato, L. (1979): Neuroendocrinology 29:66-76.
2. Bowers, M. B. and Rozitis, A. (1974): J. Pharm. Pharmacol. 26: 743-745.
3. Bunney, B. S., Walters, J. R., Roth, R. H. and Aghajanian, G. K. (1973): J. Pharmacol. Exp. Ther. 185:560-571.
4. Calne, D. B. (1977): Ann. Neurol. 1:111-119.
5. Carlsson, A. (1978): Am. J. Psychiatry 135:164-173.
6. Chen, H. T. personal communication.
7. Cheung, C. Y., Weiner, R. I. (1976): Endocrinology 99:914-917.
8. Cheung, C. Y., Weiner, R. I. (1978): Endocrinology 102:1614-1620.
9. Copinschi, G., L'Hermite, M., Leclercq, R., Golstein, J., Vanhaelst, L., Virasoro, E. and Robyn, C. (1975): J. Clin. Endocrinol. Metab. 40:442-449.
10. Cronin, M. J. (1981): In: Neuroendocrine Perspectives, Vol. 1, edited by E. E. Muller and R. M. MacLeod. Elsevier/North Holland, Amsterdam (in press).
11. de Greef, W. J. and Neill, J. D. (1979): Endocrinology 105:1093-1099.
12. de Greef, W. J., Plotsky, P. M., Neill, J. D. (1981): Neuroendocrinology 32:229-233.
13. Eikenburg, D. C., Ravitz, A. J., Gudelsky, G. A. and Moore, K. E. (1977): J. Neural Transm. 40:235-244.
14. Everett, J. W. (1954): Endocrinology 54:685-690.
15. Friesen, H. G. (1978): Ann. R. Coll. Phys. Surg. Canada 11:275-281.
16. Gautvick, K. M., Tashjian, A. H., Jr., Kourides, I. A., Weintraub, B. D., Graeber, C. T., Maloof, F., Suzuki, K. and Zuckerman, J. E. (1974): N. Engl. J. Med. 290:1162-1165.
17. Giannattasio, G., DeFerrari, M. E., Spada, A. (1981): Life Sci. 28:1605-1612.
18. Gibbs, D. M. and Neill, J. D. (1978): Endocrinology 102:1895-1900.
19. Gruen, P. H. (1978): Med. Clin. North Am. 62:409-424.
20. Gruen, P. H., Sachar, E. J., Langer, G., Altman, N., Leifer, M., Frantz, A. and Halpern, F. S. (1978): Arch. Gen. Psych. 35:108-116.
21. Hornykiewicz, O. (1977): Adv. Exp. Med. Biol. 90:1-20.
22. Hornykiewicz, O. (1979): In: Advances in Neurology, Vol. 23, edited by T. N. Chase, N. S. Wexler and A. Barbeau, pp.679-686. Raven Press, New York.
23. Julou, L., Scatton, B. and Glowinski, J. (1977): Adv. Biochem. Psychopharmacol. 16:617-624.
24. Kalin, N. H., Insel, T. R., Cohen, R. M., Risch, S. C. and Murphy, D. L. (1981): J. Clin. Endocrinol. Metab. 52:857-858.
25. Kato, Y., Iwasaki, J., Abe, H., Yanaihara, N., Imura, H. (1978): Endocrinology 103:554-558.
26. Kebabian, J. W., Petzold, G. L., Greengard, P. (1972): Proc. Natl. Acad. Sci. USA 69:2145-2149.
27. Krieger, D. T., Howanitz, P. J., and Frantz, A. G. (1976): J. Clin. Endocrinol. Metab. 42:260-272.

28. Labrie, F., Ferland, 1., Dipaolo, T. and Veilleux, R. (1981): In: Central and Peripheral Regulation of Prolactin Function, edited by R. M. MacLeod and U. Scapagnini, pp.99-115. Raven Press, New York.
29. Login, I. S. and MacLeod, R. M. (1977): Brain Res. 132:477-483.
30. Lowry, P. J. (1974): J. Endocrinol. 62:163-164.
31. MacLeod, R. M. (1976): In: Frontiers in Neuroendocrinology, Vol. 4, edited by L. Martini and W. F. Ganong, pp.169-194. Raven Press, New York.
32. MacLeod, R. M. and Lamberts, S. W. J. (1979): In: Neuroendocrine Correlates in Neurology and Psychiatry, edited by E. E. Muller and A. Agnoli, pp.89-101. Elsevier/North Holland, Amsterdam.
33. MacLeod, R. M. and Lehmeyer, J. E. (1971): In: Lactogenic Hormone, edited by G. E. Wolstenholme and J. Knight, pp.53-82. Churchill/ Livingstone, London.
34. MacLeod, R. M. and Lehmeyer, J. E. (1974): Endocrinology 94: 1077-1085.
35. MacLeod, R. M. and Login, I. S. (1977): Adv. Biochem. Psychopharmacol. 16:147-157.
36. Maurer, R. A. (1981): 63rd Annual Meeting of the Endocrine Society, Abstract #38.
37. McNeilly, A. S. and Chard, T. (1974): Clin. Endocrinol. 3:105-112.
38. McNeilly, A. S., Howie, P. W. and Houston, M. J. (1980): In: Research Frontiers in Fertility Regulation, edited by G. I. Zatuchni, M. H. Labbok and J. J. Sciarra, pp.102-116. Harper and Row, New York.
39. Meltzer, H. Y. and Fang, V. S. (1976): Arch. Gen. Psych. 33: 279-286.
40. Moore, K. E. and Wuerthele, S. M. (1979): In: Progress in Neurobiology, edited by G. A. Kerkut and J. W. Phillis, pp.325-359. Pergamon Press, New York.
41. Moult, P.J.A., Dacie, J. E., Rees, L. H. and Besser, G. M. (1981): Clin. Endocrinol. 14:387-394.
42. Nagy, I., Valdenegro, C. A., Login, I. S., Snyder, F. A. and MacLeod, R. M. (1979): In: 1st International Congress on Hormones and Cancer, Rome, edited by S. Iacobelli, pp.193-207. Raven Press, New York.
43. Noel, G. L., Suh, H. K. and Frantz, A. G. (1974): J. Clin. Endocrinol. Metab. 38:413-423.
44. Parker, D. C., Rossman, L. G. and Vanderlaan, E. F. (1973): J. Clin. Endocrinol. Metab. 36:1119-1124.
45. Perkins, N. A., Westfall, T. C., Paul, C. V., MacLeod, R. M. and Rogol, A. D. (1979): Brain Res. 160:431-444.
46. Plotsky, P. M., de Freef, W. J. and Neill, J. D. (1979): The Endocrine Society, 61st Annual Meeting, abstract #449.
47. Sassin, J. F., Frantz, A. G., Kapen, S. and Weitzman, E. D. (1973): J. Clin. Endocrinol. Metab. 37:436-440.
48. Sedvall, G. (1979): In: Neuroendocrine Correlates in Neurology and Psychiatry, Developments in Neurology, Vol. 2, edited by E. E. Muller and A. Agnoli, pp.195-209.
49. Seo, H., Refetoff, S., Martino, E., Vassart, G. and Brocas, H. (1979): Endocrinology 104:1083-1090.
50. Shupnik, M. A., Baxter, L. A., French, L. R. and Gorski, J. (1979): Endocrinology 104:729-735.
51. Takahara, J., Yunoki, S., Yamane, Y., Yamauchi, J., Yakushiji, W.

Kageyama, N., Fujino, K. and Ofuji, T. (1979): Proc. Soc. Exp. Biol. Med. 162:31-33.
52. Taraskevich, P. S. and Douglas, W. W. (1977): Proc. Natl. Acad. Sci. USA 74:4064-4067.
53. Taraskevich, P. S. and Douglas, W. W. (1978): Nature 276:832-834.
54. Thorner, M. O., Hackett, J. T., Murad, F. and MacLeod, R. M. (1980): Neuroendocrinology 31:390-402.
55. Thorner, M. O. and MacLeod, R. M. (1980): In: Progress in Reproductive Biology, Vol. 6, edited by P. O. Hubinont, pp.1-23. Karger, Basel.
56. Thorner, M. O., Round, J., Jones, A., Fahmy, D., Groom, G. V., Butcher, S. and Thompson, K. (1977): Clin. Endocrinol. 7:463-468.
57. Turkington, R. W., Underwood, L. E. and Van Wyk, J. J. (1971): N. Engl. J. Med. 285:707-710.
58. Umezu, K. and Moore, K. E. (1979): J. Pharmacol. Exp. Ther. 208: 49-56.
59. Usdin, E., Kopin, I. J. and Barchas, J., editors (1979): In: Catecholamines: Basic and Clinical Frontiers, pp.387-604. Pergamon Press, New York.
60. van Praag, H. M. (1977): Br. J. Psychiatry 130:463-474.
61. Vician, L., Shupnik, M. A. and Gorski, J. (1979): Endocrinology 104:736-743.
62. Yeo, T., Thorner, M. O., Jones, A., Lowry, P. J. and Besser, G. M. (1979): Clin. Endocrinol. 10:123-130.

Neuroendocrinology and Psychiatric Disorder,
edited by G. M. Brown, et al.
Raven Press, New York 1984.

Evaluation of Neuropharmacologic Strategies in Schizophrenia

Lawrence A. Frohman

The hypothesis underlying the studies which have been reviewed in chapters 1 and 2 by Drs. Meltzer and Davis is that the use of neuropharmacologic probes which modify the secretion of anterior pituitary hormones may have value in detecting abnormalities of tuberoinfundibular-pituitary function which reflect similar abnormalities in the mesolimbic system. This concept has been referred to as the "pituitary window hypothesis" (Figure 1). There are several implications in studies preformed to test this hypothesis. First, knowledge of specific neurotransmitter effects on anterior pituitary hormones must be available and second, a direct effect of the neurotransmitter on pituitary hormone secretion would greatly facilitate interpretation of the results. The recognized role of dopamine as a prolactin-inhibiting factor fulfills this criteria. However, for the other anterior pituitary hormones, there are intermediary hypothalamic releasing and inhibiting factors, making interpretation a bit more complex. In addition, the hypothesis implies that the neurotransmitter abnormality which might be uncovered is generalized or, at least, that a similar defect is present in the hypothalamus and in the mesolimbic system.

A very large number of studies have been performed and extensively reviewed. In particular, the excellent reviews by Drs. Meltzer and Davis have already addressed several of the critical problems in this area. The nature of neurotransmitter abnormality which has served as the focus for most of the studies is based on the original observation that the primary action of all neuroleptic drugs which are effective in the treatment of patients with schizophrenia is that of dopamine receptor antagonism. From this has emerged the concept of an increase in dopaminergic tone as the pathogenic basis for schizophrenia. If one then assumes a similar increase of dopaminergic tone to be present in the hypothalamus, the list of alterations in pituitary function which might be expected are indicated in Table 1.

A number of general difficulties are encountered in attempting to compare the various published studies. In many, the age, sex, and relationship to the menstrual cycle have not been adequately controlled nor sufficient data provided in the reports. All of the pituitary hormones are affected by these factors, and in particular, growth hormone (GH), LH, FSH and prolactin secretion are markedly influenced by ovarian and testicular hormones. GH secretion is also influenced by the nutritional status with altered responses being observed in patients with protein calorie malnutrition, anorexia nervosa, and obesity. Another major difficulty relates to the underlying disease of the patient and to aspects of treatment. In many of the reports, the diagnostic criteria for schizophrenia has been variable and furthermore, the possible existence of numerous subgroups with clinically indistinguishable manifestations provides an alternative explanation for the heterogeneity of

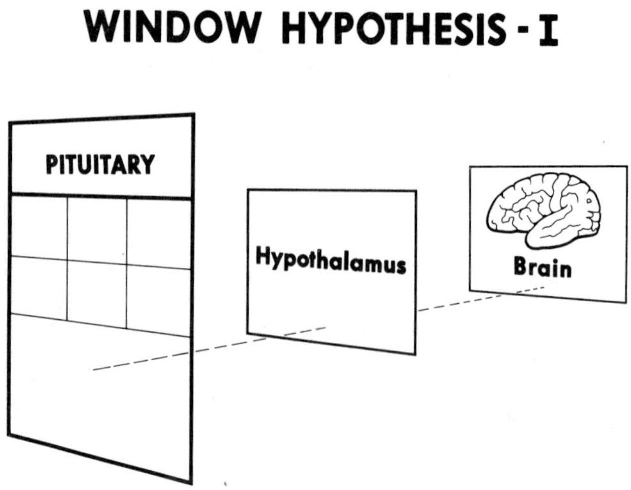

FIG. 1. The pituitary as a window to the brain - original hypothesis.

responses observed. Lastly, many of the patients have been studied during drug therapy or after varying periods of drug withdrawal. It remains to be determined whether the effects of the drug on hypothalamic-pituitary function persist for shorter or longer periods of time than those on behaviour.

With the exception of the studies focusing on prolactin, already evaluated by Dr. Thorner (chapter 3), the vast majority of reports in the literature relate to growth hormone secretion. These have focused on dopamine agonists such as apomorphine, which serve as a probe of the dopamine receptor, dopaminergic precursors such as L-dopa, which reflect both the processes of precursor uptake and decarboxylation as well as receptor activity, and other stimuli of GH secretion, which may involve dopaminergic or noradrenergic neurotransmission such as insulin hypoglycemia. Most of the studies have not revealed any differences in the GH responses to the various stimuli between schizophrenic and normal subjects while a few have shown a decrease in responses with increased duration of disease. It has been noted that similar decreases have been

TABLE 1. NEUROENDOCRINE CONSEQUENCES OF INCREASED HYPOTHALAMIC DOPAMINERGIC TONE

PROLACTIN	↓
GH	↑
LH (FSH)	↓ (↑)
ACTH	– (↓)
TSH	↓
ADH	?

TABLE 2. NEUROTRANSMITTER CONTROL OF SOMATOSTATIN

DOPAMINE	+
NOREPINEPHRINE	(?) +
ACETYLCHOLINE	−
ENDORPHINS/ ENKEPHALINS	−
NEUROTENSIN	+

observed in affective disorders and are thus not specific for schizophrenia. Tamminga et al. (1) studied chronic schizophrenics after long-term neuroleptic therapy with and without symptoms of tardive dyskinesia. In both groups the GH responses were normal or diminished in comparison with healthy controls. Thus, both in schizophrenics where an increased dopaminergic tone has been hypothesized and in tardive dyskinesia where nigrostriatal dopaminergic hypersensitivity occurs, no evidence of an enhanced response to dopaminergic agents could be demonstrated in evaluating the hypothalamic-pituitary axis. An occasional patient exhibited a normal or slightly supranormal response which could be due to individual variation or could reflect the heterogeneous population under study.

A complexity in the interpretation of manipulations of the dopaminergic pathways in the hypothalamus relates to the fact that there are two hypothalamic factors which control GH secretion: a GH-releasing factor, the structure of which has recently been reported, and a GH-inhibiting factor (somatostatin). The neurotransmitter control of somatostatin has been shown to involve a number of neurotransmitters, including dopamine (Table 2). Since somatostatin secretion is stimulated by dopamine (2), a similar stimulatory effect of this neurotransmitter on GH-releasing factor may also be present in order to account for the net stimulatory effect of dopamine on GH release. In addition, other compensatory mechanisms involving the other neurotransmitters which control somatostatin secretion may very well be altered in an attempt to compensate for the excessive stimulation by dopamine, should it be present.

The actions of somatostatin are not specific for GH secretion and include an equally potent inhibiting effect on basal and TRH-stimulated TSH secretion. Thus, were somatostatin secretion to be increased in patients with schizophrenia and to cause the occasionally observed decrease in GH responses, it would be expected that a decrease in basal or stimulated TSH secretion would also be observed. However, all of the studies on TSH secretion in patients with schizophrenia have indicated responses indistinguishable from normal controls.

In normal subjects, TRH stimulates TSH and prolactin but not GH secretion. However, GH responses to TRH have been observed in a number of conditions, most notably acromegaly, anorexia nervosa, depression, chronic renal failure, and protein malnutrition. The responses in acromegaly occur rapidly, i.e. within 15 minutes (3), and have been attributed to the presence of TRH receptors on the neoplastic somatotrophs. In anorexia nervosa, in contrast, the response is considerably delayed, peaking at 45-90 minutes (4). The mechanism of this response is unknown but its slow onset is incompatible with an effect on the pituitary considering the very rapid half-life (a few minutes) of TRH in circulation and is more consistent with a yet to be defined effect within the CNS. The responses to TRH and also to LHRH occasionally observed in patients with schizophrenia are similarly delayed (5) and are presumably a CNS-mediated effect. The neurotransmitter mechanism involved is still unknown.

The secretion of gonadotropins in patients with schizophrenia has been extensively studied, primarily by Brambilla and her associates (see chapter 1 by Dr. Meltzer), and the results have not provided any consistent pattern of change. There is a suggestion of a decrease in basal levels of LH and an increase in the response to LHRH. The extent to which these findings may be associated with acute stress responses or to neuroleptic drug therapy has not been entirely clarified. Since most neuroleptics stimulate the release of prolactin secretion and hyperprolactinemia can lead to altered gonadotropin regulation, the disturbances may, in part, be related to the use of these agents. Despite these effects, female patients who have recovered from acute schizophrenic episodes and who are on chronic neuroleptic therapy marry at an expected frequency and appear to have a nearly normal fertility (personal communication, D. Offer). Amenorrhea is not a recognized problem among these individuals. Consequently, it appears that gonadotropin secretion is maintained reasonably well despite the psychopathology.

ACTH secretion is generally normal in patients with schizophrenia with the exception of reports which relate to patients in the acute stages of their illness, where stress is a major factor. Vasopressin secretion also appears to be normal in schizophrenics though it has been reported that forced fluid intake can lead to water intoxication, a phenomenon not observed in normals. There is evidence for dopaminergic innervation of the posterior pituitary and suggestive evidence exists for dopaminergic regulation of vasopressin secretion. These factors do not, however, imply an abnormality of dopaminergic regulation of this hormone in schizophrenia.

It is, therefore, necessary to look for evidence that neurotransmitter function in individual brain regions is area specific and that disorders associated with changes in neurotransmitter levels are restricted to localized brain regions. Both phenomena are supported by several lines of evidence. Extensive studies of dopamine receptors, particularly involving the semi-rigid tetrahydronaphthaline enantiomers have demonstrated differences between renal, pituitary and striatal dopamine receptors (6, 7) as shown in Figure 2. Such differences not only suggest the possibility of separate and unrelated function but also raise the prospect of the development of tissue specific dopamine agonists.

In reports from a number of laboratories, there is evidence for separate mechanisms of control of somatostatin in various neural and extraneural brain regions. Norepinephrine stimulates somatostatin secretion in the cortex but not in the hypothalamus (8), dopamine stimulates somatostatin in the hypothalamus (2) but not in the stomach (9), and 2-deoxy-glucose stimulates somatostatin secretion in the hypothalamus but not in the cortex (10). GH stimulates hypothalamic somatostatin secretion (11) but the release of somatostatin into cerebrospinal fluid is inhibited by GH (12). Thus, evidence is accumulating that the control of secretion of neurotransmitters and neuropeptides may be site specific.

Recent studies summarized in Table 3 have also indicated alterations in the concentration of neurotransmitters and neuropeptides in specific brain regions associated with the CNS diseases (13). It would, there-

SYSTEM DEPENDENT DOPAMINE AGONIST POTENCY

RENAL VASODILITATION	RAT STRIATAL C-AMP	NEURONAL FIRING INHIBITION HELIX ASPERSA	^{3}H-DOPAMINE DISPLACEMENT CALF STRIATUM	INHIBITION RAT PROLACTIN RELEASE
DOPAMINE	DOPAMINE	DOPAMINE	ALPHA ROTAMER	BETA ROTAMER
BETA ROTAMER	BETA ROTAMER	BETA ROTAMER	DOPAMINE	DOPAMINE
ALPHA ROTAMER (partial)	ALPHA ROTAMER (partial)	ALPHA ROTAMER (inactive)	BETA ROTAMER	ALPHA ROTAMER

FIG. 2. Differences in potency exhibited by dopamine and the alpha and beta rotamers of the semirigid tetrahydronaphthalene analogs in various tissues. The potencies are listed in decreasing order and suggest differences in the nature of the dopamine receptor in these tissues.

fore, not be surprising that functional disturbances could also be site specific. Of particular interest is the observation that somatostatin levels are increased in the caudate, putamen and globus pallidus in patients with Huntington's disease (14). Inasmuch as GH responses to dopaminergic stimuli are increased in this disorder, the presence of increased concentrations of somatostatin in the hypothalamus would not be expected to occur.

In summary, even if the pituitary window hypothesis is valid, it appears that the markers currently being examined are too remote from the CNS regions of interest, i.e., we need to measure releasing and/or inhibiting factors rather than pituitary hormones. However, it is not clear at which sites this can be accomplished in human subjects. Blood levels of somatostatin and TRH and of CSF somatostatin appear not to reflect hypothalamic secretion. More than one releasing and/or inhibiting factor is involved in the control of individual pituitary hormones and the control of individual releasing factors involves

TABLE 3. LOCALIZED NEUROTRANSMITTER ALTERATIONS

DISORDER	NEUROTRANSMITTER	SITE
Parkinson's Disease	Dopamine ↓	Basal ganglia
Huntington's Disease	GABA ↓	Putamen, caudate
	Substance P ↓	Putamen, globus pallidus
	Somatostatin ↑	Caudate, putamen globus pallidus
	Cholecystokinin ↓	> Basal ganglia
	Met-enkephalin ↓	
Alzheimer's Disease	Somatostatin ↓	Hippocampus, cortex

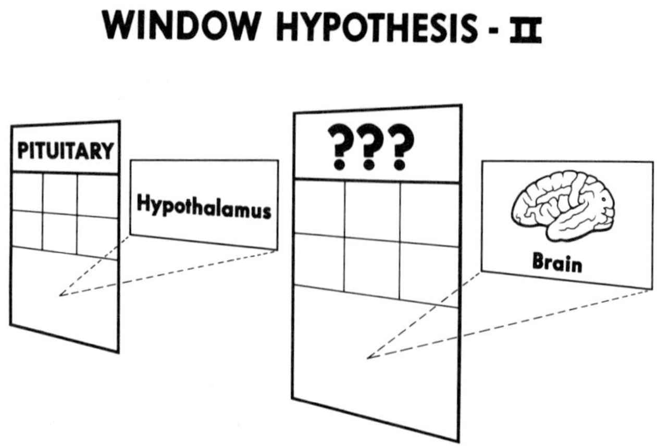

FIG. 3. Proposed modification of the pituitary window hypothesis.

multiple neurotransmitters, opening the possibility of compensatory changes. Finally, target organ hormone and metabolic substrate feedback from extra-CNS sites will also modify releasing factor and pituitary hormone secretion and may obscure any changes due to primary CNS dysfunction.

An alternate view (Figure 3) is that pituitary hormone measurements may provide an adequate reflection of hypothalamic function but another window must be obtained to observe the mesolimbic region. Most of the currently available information would tend to support this hypothesis. Consequently, while neuroendocrine studies may provide important new information concerning hypothalamic-pituitary alterations in schizophrenic patients, it does not appear likely that they will be fruitful avenues to study the neurochemical disturbances involved in the pathogenesis of schizophrenia.

REFERENCES

1. Tamminga, C. A., Smith, R. C., Pandey, G., Frohman, L. A. and Davis, J. M. (1977): Arch. Gen. Psychiat. 34:1199.
2. Maeda, K. and Frohman, L. A. (1980): Endocrinology 106:1837.
3. Irie, M. and Tsushima, T. (1972): J. Clin. Endocrinol. Metab. 35: 97.
4. Maeda, K., Kato, Y., Yamaguchi, N., Chihara, K., Ohgo, S., Iwasaki, Y., Yamamoto, Y., Moridera, K., Kuromaru, S. and Imura, H. (1976): Acta Endocrinol. 81:1.
5. Gil-Ad, I., Dickerman, Z., Weizman, R., Weizman, A., Tyano, S. and Laron, Z. (1981): Am. J. Psychiatry 138:357.
6. Rick, J., Szabo, M., Payne, P., Kovathana, N., Cannon, J. G. and Frohman, L. A. (1979): Endocrinology 102:1234.
7. Goldberg, L. I., Volkman, P. H., Kohli, J. D. and Kotake, A. N. (1977): In: Advances in Biochemical Pharmacology, Vol. 16, edited by E. Costa and G. Gessa, p.251. Raven Press, New York.
8. Bennett, G. W., Edwardson, J. A., de Cotte, D. M., Berelowitz, M., Pimstone, B. L. and Kronheim, S. (1979): J. Neurochem. 32:1127.
9. Goto, Y., Berelowitz, M. and Frohman, L. A. (1981): Am. J. Physiol. 240:E274.

10. Berelowitz, M., Dudlak, D. and Frohman, L. A. (1982): J. Clin. Invest. 69:1293.
11. Berelowitz, M., Firestone, S. and Frohman, L. A. (1981): Endocrinology 109:714.
12. Berelowitz, M., Perlow, M. J. and Frohman, L. A. (1982): Brain Res. 241:355.
13. Kreiger, D. T. and Martin, J. B. (1981): New Engl. J. Med. 304: 876.
14. Cooper, P. E., Aronin, N., Bird, E. D., Leeman, S. E. and Martin, J. B. (1981): Neurology 31:64.

Neuroendocrinology and Psychiatric Disorder,
edited by G. M. Brown, et al.
Raven Press, New York 1984.

Prolactin Secretion and Dopaminergic Neurons: An Evaluation of Neuropharmacologic Strategies

K.E. Moore and K.T. Demarest

Many psychopharmacologists believed that some of the symptoms of schizophrenia result from the overactivity of certain dopamine (DA) neuronal systems in the brain. This "DA hypothesis of schizophrenia" is primarily derived from pharmacological evidence; namely, that symptoms of this disease are ameliorated by the administration of DA receptor blocking drugs (neuroleptics) (21). These drugs presumably act by reducing the actions of hyperactive DA neurons somewhere in the brain. The precise site of the antipsychotic actions of neuroleptics is unknown, but it is generally believed to be in limbic and/or cortical regions of the forebrain. Thus, neuroleptics appear to reduce schizophrenic symptomatology as a result of their ability to alter the transmission process at the terminals of mesolimbic-cortical neurons by blocking postsynaptic DA receptor sites (38). By implication it is suspected, but not proven, that mesolimbic-cortical DA neurons are overly active in the schizophrenic brain. Considering the close functional relationship between limbic and striatal brain regions (e.g. see 12), the hypothesis that schizophrenia involves the exclusive disruption of the mesolimbic-cortical DA neuronal system may be unrealistically restrictive (11).

The activity of mesolimbic-cortical DA neurons has been estimated in animals by measuring the rates of synthesis, metabolism and turnover of DA in brain regions (e.g. nucleus accumbens, olfactory tubercle, frontal cortex) which contain terminals of these neurons. Similar studies cannot be performed in schizophrenic patients although DA neuronal activity in the central nervous system has been estimated from measurements of metabolites of this neurotransmitter in lumbar cerebrospinal fluid. Unfortunately, these metabolites probably do not represent DA released from mesolimbic-cortical neurons, but rather from nigrostriatal neurons which terminate in the striatum adjacent to the lateral cerebral ventricles, or from DA neurons which terminate in the spinal cord.

Tuberoinfundibular DA neurons located in the mediobasal hypothalamus influence the secretion of certain hormones from the anterior pituitary (40), and the activity of these neurons has been estimated _in vivo_ from the concentrations of hormones, particularly prolactin, in the serum. The question to be considered in this report is: "Can serum prolactin concentrations, as an index of tuberoinfundibular DA neurons, be employed as a marker for other DA neurons in the brain, particularly those in the mesolimbic-cortical system which may be involved in the symptoms of schizophrenia?" Evidence will be presented that different DA neurons in the central nervous system subserve different functions and, in turn, are regulated by different mechanisms (25, 30). These differences are such that extrapolations from one DA neuronal system to another must be done with caution.

DISTRIBUTION AND FUNCTION OF DA NEURONS IN THE BRAIN

The distribution and functions of DA neurons has been recently reviewed (31). The pattern of distribution of these neurons in the rat brain, as revealed by histofluorescent techniques, is depicted in Figure 1. Nigrostriatal neurons, which originate in pars compacta of substantia nigra and project to the striatum (caudate-putamen), appear to participate in the regulation of postural reflexes and in the initiation of motor movements. The mesolimbic-cortical neurons, which also originate in substantia nigra and just medial to this region in the ventral mesencephalon, project to various limbic and cortical regions in the forebrain. These neurons appear to participate in fundamental psychic processes such as alertness, initiative and thought organization. Together these ascending DA neurons constitute the mesotelencephalic system (4); most of what we know about DA neurons has been learned from experimental studies on this system.

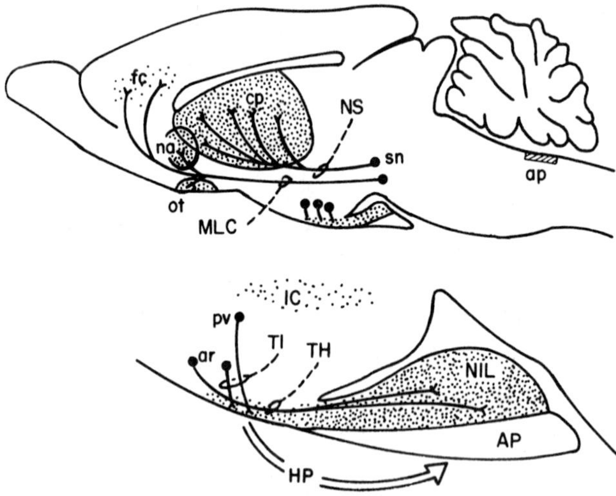

FIG. 1. Distribution of dopaminergic neuronal systems in the rat brain. The lower figure is an enlargement of the mediobasal hypothalamus and the pituitary. Abbreviations: ap, area postrema; ar, arcuate nucleus; cp, caudate putamen (striatum); fc, frontal cortex; na, nucleus accumbens; ot, olfactory tubercle; pv, periventricular nucleus; sn, substantia nigra; AP, anterior pituitary; NIL, neurointermediate lobe (posterior pituitary); HP, hypophyseal portal system. Dopaminergic neuronal systems; mesotelencephalic (composed of NS, nigrostriatal and MLC, mesolimbic-cortical); IC, incertohypothalamic; TH, tuberohypophysial; TI, tuberoinfundibular.

Several groups of DA perikarya are located within the hypothalamus. Of these the tuberoinfundibular DA system will be featured in the present discussion. The cell bodies of these neurons are located in the arcuate and periventricular nuclei. They project to either the lateral aspect of the median eminence, where they appear to contact luteinizing hormone releasing hormone (LHRH) containing neurons, and to the external layer of the median eminence, where they terminate near the pericapillary spaces of the primary plexus of the hypophysial portal system. DA released from the latter neurons is carried in the blood to the anterior pituitary where it reacts with receptors located on lactotrophs. Activation of these receptors inhibits the release of prolactin. This hormone is under tonic inhibitory control of tuberoinfundibular neurons so that disruption of this system by blocking synthesis (α-methyltyrosine) or storage (reserpine) of DA in the nerve terminal, or by blocking the actions of DA at anterior pituitary receptors (neuroleptics) causes serum concentrations of prolactin to increase. DA agonists (e.g. bromocriptine) mimic the actions of DA at pituitary receptors and thereby cause serum concentrations of prolactin to decrease.

Much less is known about other hypothalamic DA neurons. Cell bodies of tuberohypophysial DA neurons are also located in the arcuate nucleus; their axons project to the neurointermediate lobe of the pituitary. Little is known about the functions of these neurons, but they appear to be activated by water deprivation or salt loading (1). Several groups of DA neurons comprise the incertohypothalamic DA neuronal system. Those in the caudal region of the hypothalamus appear to project to the spinal cord (5), while the distribution of axons from perikarya in the rostral hypothalamus is unknown, as is their function.

PROLACTIN AND TUBEROINFUNDIBULAR DA NEURONS

Tuberoinfundibular DA neurons play an important role in regulating the release of prolactin, luteinizing hormone (LH), and possibly growth hormone (GH) from the anterior pituitary (28, 40). These neurons have attracted the interests of psychoneuroendocrinologists because serum concentrations of prolactin can be measured in a relatively easy and non-invasive manner in order to study their activity and receptor sites in man and animals. For example, this system provides an excellent model for investigating the dopaminergic properties of drugs - DA agonists reduce and DA antagonists increase serum concentrations of prolactin. Furthermore, there is a good correlation between the antipsychotic and prolactin-elevating properties of neuroleptics (6, 16). Rubin and Hays (37) have prepared an excellent review on the applications of neuroleptic-induced changes in serum concentrations of prolactin, and have discussed critically the limitations of these applications.

It has been proposed that neuroleptic-induced changes in tuberoinfundibular DA neuronal activity, as evidenced by alterations in serum prolactin concentrations, may parallel changes in other DA neurons and their receptors (19) and thereby serve as a "window to the brain" (Davis et al., chapter 2). Although serum prolactin concentrations are often assumed to reflect tuberoinfundibular DA neuronal activity, it must be remembered that the secretion of this hormone is also regulated by other mechanisms. For example, putative 'prolactin releasing factors' may play a role in controlling prolactin secretion in different physiological (e.g., stress, lactation) and pathological states (40). Thus, although the concentration of prolactin is a useful index of neuroleptic antagonism at DA receptors in the anterior pituitary (22, 37) it does not always reflect tuberoinfundibular DA neuronal activity. Furthermore, tuberoinfundibular neuronal activity does not usually reflect activity of other DA neurons, including those in the mesolimbic-cortical system implicated in schizophrenia. It is becoming increasingly clear that there are important differences among the various DA neuro s. There appear to be no consistent differences in serum prolactin concentrations in schizophrenic patients and appropriate normal controls (Meltzer et al. chapter 1). Because of differences in DA neurons, however, one cannot conclude that the functioning of mesolimbic-cortical DA neurons are _not_ abnormal in the schizophrenic brain. Some of the differences in properties of different DA neurons are described below.

NIGROSTRIATAL AND MESOLIMBIC-CORTICAL DA NEURONS

It has been suggested that from an anatomical point of view the ascending DA neurons should be classified as a single unit - the mesotelencephalic DA system (4). From a functional, pharmacological and biochemical standpoint, however, it is frequently useful to consider the mesolimbic-cortical and nigrostriatal DA neuronal systems as separate entities. DA terminals in limbic regions appear to be important for the neuropharmacological actions of some central stimulants. For example 6-hydroxydopamine-induced lesions limited to terminals of the mesolimbic-neurons in nucleus accumbens block the locomotor stimulant and self-administration properties of indirect-acting DA agonists such as d-amphetamine and cocaine (15, 18, 35). Injections of neuroleptics selectively into nucleus accumbens also block locomotor stimulant actions of d-amphetamine (32).

Many drugs have similar neurochemical effects in terminal regions of nigrostriatal and mesolimbic-cortical DA neurons. Monoamine oxidase inhibitors increase the concentration and reduce the rate of synthesis of DA while reserpine causes just the opposite effects in all forebrain regions (8). Acute administration of neuroleptics increase and DA agonists decrease the rate of DA synthesis and turnover to a similar degree in all forebrain regions (29).

There are, however, subtle but important differences in some of the characteristics of mesolimbic-cortical and nigrostriatal DA neurons, particularly in their response to pharmacological manipulations. Many of these differences undoubtedly relate to neuronal circuitry; there are differences in feedback loops and the afferent and efferent neuronal connections of the two systems (7, 12). There are also striking differences in the sensitivity of presynaptic receptors to DA agonists, with receptors on the terminals of mesolimbic neurons being 5-10 times more sensitive to apomorphine than are those on terminals of nigrostriatal neurons (36). It may be possible to exploit this difference if selective presynaptic DA agonists can be developed. Such drugs might be expected to preferentially inhibit synthesis and possibly release of DA from mesolimbic DA neurons (see below). d-Amphetamine causes a marked increase in the _in vivo_ rate of DA synthesis in terminals of nigrostriatal neurons, _but has_ essentially no effect in terminals of mesolimbic neurons in nucleus accumbens and olfactory tubercle (17). In addition, nigrostriatal and mesolimbic DA neuronal systems respond differently to chronic administration of neuroleptics; tolerance develops more rapidly to neuroleptic-induced biochemical changes in DA neurons terminating in the striatum than in mesolimbic regions (13).

TUBEROINFUNDIBULAR AND MESOTELENCEPHALIC DA NEURONS

Differences between properties of tuberoinfundibular neurons and those DA neurons which comprise the ascending mesolimbic-cortical and nigrostriatal systems are more pronounced than are the differences between the latter two neuronal systems. Detailed studies of tuberoinfundibular DA neurons had to wait the development of techniques which were sensitive enough to quantify the activity of these neurons. Technical problems have limited electrophysiological studies, but a variety of histochemical and biochemical techniques have permitted the estimations of rates of synthesis and turnover of DA in the median eminence of the rat; these studies have been recently reviewed (28). The properties which distinguish tuberoinfundibular neurons from other DA neurons in the mammalian brain, and thus make their responses to drugs different, are outlined below. Some of these differences are depicted schematically in Figure 2.

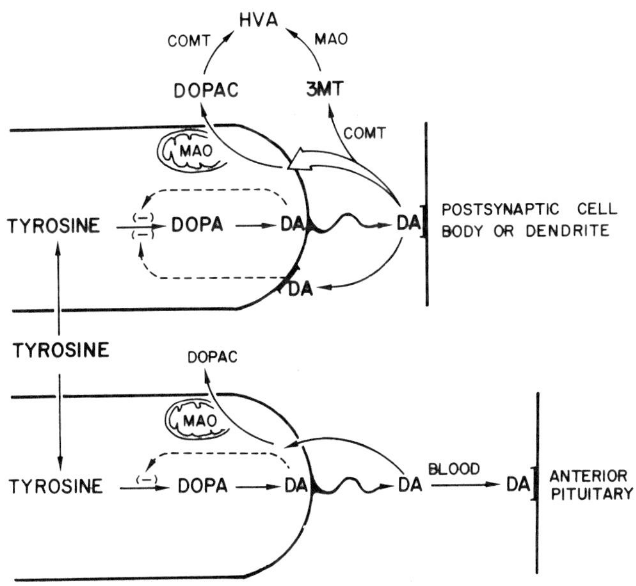

FIG. 2. Schematic diagram of (a) mesotelencephalic and (b) tuberoinfundibular dopaminergic nerve terminals. COMT, catechol-o-methyltransferase; D, dopamine; DOPAC, 3,4-dihydroxyphenylacetic acid; HVA, homovanillic acid; MAO, monoamine oxidase; 3MT, 3-methoxytryramine.

In the terminals of mesotelencephalic neurons (Figure 2, top) DA is synthesized in two steps beginning with the hydroxylation of tyrosine to form DOPA. This process is catalyzed by tyrosine hydroxylase, the rate-limiting enzyme in the synthetic process. DOPA in turn, is decarboxylated to DA by an ubiquitous enzyme, aromatic L-amino acid decarboxylase. The synthesized DA can then be stored in synaptic vesicles, or released in response to nerve action potentials. The released DA is then free to activate postsynaptic receptors, some of which may be linked to adenylate cyclase. In the synaptic cleft DA is also free to interact with presynaptic or 'autoreceptors'. Activation of these receptors inhibits the synthesis of DA; it may also inhibit release, but this has not been proven conclusively (see discussion by Raiteri et al. (33)). DA is removed from the synaptic cleft by a high affinity amine uptake system which transports DA back into the presynaptic terminal where the amine can be oxidatively deaminated by intraneuronal monoamine oxidase to form dihydroxyphenylacetic acid (DOPAC). This metabolite can be further metabolized by o-methylation to form homovanillic acid (HVA).

The activity of mesotelencephalic DA neurons in rats has been estimated biochemically by measuring: 1) the concentration of DA metabolites in brain tissue or CSF (increased metabolites reflect increased neuronal activity), 2) the rate of DA synthesis (accumulation of DOPA after the administration of a decarboxylase inhibitor), and 3) the rate of disappearance of DA following inhibition of synthesis with the tyrosine hydroxylase inhibitor, α-methyltyrosine. The latter two techniques have also been employed in studies on tuberoinfundibular neuronal systems. In addition, the activity of tuberoinfundibular DA neurons has been estimated by quantifying the amount of DA in hypophysial portal blood (3, 10) and in the anterior pituitary (2).

The DA synthetic processes are basically the same in tuberoinfundibular and mesotelencephalic DA neurons. There are, however, major differences in biochemical dynamics of other processes; these are depicted schematically in Figure 2 (bottom). DA is released from tuberoinfundibular neurons, not into a synaptic cleft (at least in the medial part of the median eminence), but rather into the blood where it is transported to and activates receptors on cells in the anterior pituitary. On the basis of the structural requirements for DA agonists and antagonists the characteristics of DA receptors is essentially the same in the forebrain and the anterior pituitary. That is, at present there are no drugs which selectively block 'specific' DA receptors in the brain. On the other hand, the coupling of DA receptors to adenylate cyclase appears to be quite different, with DA stimulating the enzyme in forebrain regions and either having no effect (14) or inhibiting (9) the enzyme in the anterior pituitary.

Tuberoinfundibular DA neurons lack a high affinity amine uptake system which plays an important role in the dynamics of other catecholaminergic neurons. The lack of this uptake system in tuberoinfundibular neurons has important pharmacological considerations. First, these neurons are resistant to destruction by 6-hydroxydopamine, which gains access and thereby accumulates to toxic levels in other catecholaminergic neurons. Secondly, the concentraiton of DOPAC in the median eminence is relatively low in the median eminence and does not change in parallel with other biochemical indices of tuberoinfundibular neuronal activity (39). That is, in mesotelencephalic DA neurons the released DA is recaptured by the neuronal terminal and is converted to DOPAC so that the concentration of this metabolite reflects DA neuronal activity. A similar effect does not occur in tuberoinfundibular neurons because the DA is quickly removed from the terminal regions by the blood, and the neuron lacks a mechanism for recapturing the released amine.

Drugs such as d-amphetamine, methylphenidate and cocaine, which exert behavioural effects by blocking DA uptake into mesotelencephalic DA neuronal terminals (23) have little effect on tuberoinfundibular neurons since they have no transport mechanism with which to interact. Consequently, the potent "indirect" DA agonists have only a modest ability, if any, to reduce the secretion of prolactin in animals (34) and in man (19). Furthermore, d-amphetamine does not alter the rate of DA synthesis in terminals of tuberoinfundibular neurons as it does in mesotelencephalic neurons (17).

Another unique characteristic of tuberoinfundibular DA neurons is their lack of an acute response to the administration of DA agonists or antagonists; these drugs decrease and increase, respectively, the activity of other DA neurons. These compensatory responses appear to be mediated via long neuronal feedback loops and/or 'short-loop' feedback mechanisms which are controlled by putative autoreceptors (30). Since most tuberoinfundibular DA neurons do not appear to make synaptic contact with other neurons, they obviously cannot be regulated by neuronal feedback loops, and their lack of response to dopaminergic drugs suggests that they also lack autoreceptors. This has been confirmed by direct experimentation. Drugs such as γ-butyrolactone and baclofen, by reducing impulse traffic in DA neurons thereby reducing the release of DA and activation of the inhibitory autoreceptors, increase the rate of synthesis of DA in forebrain regions. This effect can be reversed in a dose-dependent manner by DA agonists acting on presynaptic receptors. These effects do not occur in the median eminence (24).

On the other hand, tuberoinfundibular DA neurons are unique in that they are selectively stimulated by prolactin. Systemic or intracerebroventricular injections of this hormone, or endocrinological (estrogens) or pharmacological (neuroleptics) manipulations which increase serum concentrations of prolactin will also increase tuberoinfundibular DA neuronal activity after a latent period of several hours (26). By this sluggish hormonal-neuronal feedback mechanism prolactin regulates its own release. Tuberoinfundibular neurons are unique among other DA neurons in that they are not directly regulated by DA receptor-mediated mechanisms, but rather by the very hormone that they control. Thus, although the functions of all DA neurons are disrupted by the DA receptor blocking actions of neuroleptics, tuberoinfundibular neurons have properties that are unique. In turn, the major ascending DA neurons have properties that are not shared by tuberoinfundibular neurons. It is unreasonable to expect, therefore, that the activities of the latter neurons, as estimated by serum concentrations of prolactin, can adequately serve as a "marker" for other DA neurons. This is clearly seen when the temporal relationship of neuroleptic drug actions are determined in the clinic (20). The serum concentration of prolactin increases shortly after a neuroleptic is administered and is maintained at elevated levels as long as the drug is administered; serum prolactin concentrations fall to control values shortly after neuroleptic administration ceases. On the other hand, the antipsychotic effect of neuroleptics becomes manifest only after days of treatment, and relapses often do not occur until several weeks after treatment stops. Clearly, there is a dissociation between the time course of action of neuroleptics as antipsychotics (mesolimbic-cortical system) and on prolactin secretion (tuberoinfundibular system).

In summary, many unique properties of tuberoinfundibular DA neurons have been known for some time. Nevertheless, investigators have persisted in their efforts to examine these neurons because of the potentially important information that might be obtained from their study in schizophrenic patients (or in patients with other mental disorders). Reports that there are no major differences between the prolactin responses (tuberoinfundibular neuronal activity?) in schizophrenic and normal controls (Meltzer et al. chapter 1) probably have little bearing on the possible role that dysfunctions of the mesolimbic-cortical DA neuronal system play in schizophrenic symptomatology. Nevertheless, further studies on the effects of psychoactive drugs on serum concentrations of selected pituitary hormones in humans, and basic research into the properties of tuberoinfundibular DA neurons in animals will eventually assist investigators to better understand the central control of pituitary hormone release mechanisms, and in the basic neurobiology of important DA neuronal systems in the brain.

Specific Antagonists of Mesolimbic-Cortical DA Neurons

It would be highly advantageous to have antipsychotic drugs which are devoid of extrapyramidal and endocrinological side effects. Theoretically such compounds might interact with the mesolimbic-cortical DA neurons. To date, most clinically available neuroleptics appear to block DA receptors in the anterior pituitary and in different parts of the brain with equal effectiveness, although those in the anterior pituitary are relatively more sensitive. It is possible that some unique characteristics of DA receptors at terminals of the mesolimbic-cortical neurons will be discovered which would make them selectively sensitive to pharmacological blockade. Alternatively, it may be possible to synthesize compounds with selective presynaptic receptor agonist properties which would be specific for shutting down synthesis and possibly release of DA from mesolimbic-cortical neurons, and not from nigrostriatal neurons. These compounds would be expected to have antipsychotic properties with minimal extrapyramidal side effects. This is not outside the realm of possibility since, at least in the rat, putative DA autoreceptors on mesolimbic-cortical neurons appear to be more sensitive to DA agonists than are those on nigrostriatal neurons (36). Such a presynaptic DA agonist would probably lack endocrine side effects mediated by changes in tuberoinfundibular nerve activity since these neurons appear to lack autoreceptors (8). It may also be possible to selectively disrupt neuronal circuits that have input to or output from the mesolimbic-cortical DA neurons. Basic information on the chemical characteristics of neurons which comprise these afferent and efferent connections are needed to facilitate this research. New animal screening methods would, therefore, have to be developed to search for these compounds. The DA receptor properties of currently available neuroleptics can be readily detected from their ability to increase serum concentrations of prolactin. Drugs which interact specifically with mesolimbic-cortical neurons should be without effect on the 'prolactin test'.

Tuberohypophysial DA Neurons

Until recently tuberohypophysial DA neurons have been largely ignored. The properties of these neurons, which are anatomically related to those in the tuberoinfundibular system, are markedly different from those in the latter system. For example, they are not stimulated by increased in serum concentrations of prolactin (27). On the other hand, tuberohypophysial DA neurons resemble the major ascending DA neurons in that their activity can be acutely altered by the administration of DA agonists and antagonists (8). The functions of these neurons are unknown, but since they are selectively activated by dehydration or NaCl loading (1), they may play a role in the regulation of antidiuretic hormone (ADH) release from the posterior pituitary. More experimental studies on this relatively neglected DA neuronal system are needed, but it is interesting to speculate that dysfunction of these neurons could possibly play a role in the bizarre syndrome of inappropriate ADH secretion and self-induced water intoxication in schizophrenic patients (see Meltzer et al. chapter 1).

ACKNOWLEDGEMENTS

Many experiments reported in this review were supported by USPHS Grant NS 9174. The assistance of Diane Hummel in the preparation of this manuscript is gratefully acknowledged.

REFERENCES

1. Alper, R. H. and Moore, K. E. (1980): Neuroendocrinology 31: 112-115.
2. Apud, J., Cocchi, D., Iuliano, E., Casaneuva, F., Müller, E.E. and Racagni, G. (1980): Brain Res. 186:226-231.
3. Ben-Jonathan, N., Oliver, C., Weiner, H. J., Mical, R. S. and Porter, J. C. (1977): Endocrinology 100:452-458.
4. Björklund, A. and Lindvall, O. (1978): In: Limbic Mechanisms, edited by K. D. Livingston and O. Hornykiewicz, pp.307-331. Plenum Press, New York.
5. Björklund, A. and Skaerberg, G. (1980): Brain Res. 177:170-176.
6. Clemens, J. A., Smalstig, E. B. and Sawyer, B. D. (1974): Psychopharmacology 40:123-127.
7. Costa, E. (1977): Adv. Biochem. Psychopharm. 16:557-563.
8. Demarest, K. T. and Moore, K. E. (1979): J. Neural. Transmission 46:263-277.
9. Giannattasio, G., Elisabetta de Ferrari, M. and Spada, A. (1981): Life Sci. 28:1605-1612.
10. Gibbs, D. M. and Neill, J. B. (19780: Endocrinology 102:1895-1900.
11. Hornykiewicz, O. (1978): Neuroscience 3:773-783.
12. Jones, D. L., Mogensen, G. J. and Wu, M. (1981): Neuropharmacology 20:29-37.
13. Julou, L., Scatton, B. and Glowinski, J. (1977): Adv. Biochem. Psychopharmacol. 16:617-624.
14. Kebabian, J. W. and Calne, D. B. (1979): Nature 277:93-96.
15. Kelly, P. H. and Iversen, S. D. (1976): Europ. J. Pharmacol. 40: 45-56.
16. Langer, G., Sachar, E. J., Gruen, P. H. and Halpern, F. S. (1977): Nature 266:636-640.
17. Lyness, W. H., Demarest, K. T. and Moore, K. E. (1980): Neuropharmacology 19:883-889.
18. Lyness, W. H., Friedle, N. M. and Moore, K. E. (1979): Pharmacol. Biochem. Behav. 11:553-556.
19. Meltzer, H. Y. (1980): Psychiatric Clinics of North America 3:277-298.
20. Meltzer, H. Y. and Fang, V. (1976): Arch. Gen. Psychiat. 33: 279-286.
21. Meltzer, H. Y. and Stahl, S. M. (1976): Schizophrenic Bull. 2: 19-76.
22. Merali, Z. and Lapierre, Y. D. (1981): Int. J. Ment. Health 9: 140-161.
23. Moore, K. E. (1978): In: Handbook of Psychopharmacology, Vol. 11, edited by L. L. Iversen and S. H. Snyder, pp.41-98. Plenum, New York.
24. Moore, K. E. and Demarest, K. T. (1980): Brain Res. Bull. 5(Suppl. 2):531-536.
25. Moore, K. E. and Demarest, K. T. (1982): In: Frontiers in Neuroendocrinology, Vol. 7, edited by W. F. Ganong and L. Martini, pp.161-190. Raven Press, New York.
26. Moore, K. E., Demarest, K. T. and Johnston, C. A. (1980): Fed. Proc. 39:2912-2916.
27. Moore, K. E., Demarest, K. T. and Johnston, C. A. (1980): In: Progress in Psychoneuroendocrinology, edited by F. Brambilla, G. Racagni and D. DeWied, pp.359-366. Elsevier/North Holland,

Amsterdam.
28. Moore, K. E. and Johnston, C. A. (1981): In: Neuroendocrine Perspectives, Vol. 1, edited by E. E. Müller and R. M. MacLeod, pp.23-68. Elsevier/North Holland, Amsterdam.
29. Moore, K. E. and Kelly, P. H. (1978): In: Psychopharmacology: A Generation of Progress, edited by M. A. Lipton, A. DiMascio and K. F. Killam, pp.221-234. Raven Press, New York.
30. Moore, K. E. and Wuerthele, S. M. (1979): Progress in Neurobiology 13:325-359.
31. Moore, R. Y. and Bloom, F. E. (1978): Ann. Rev. Neurosci. 1:129-169.
32. Pijnenburg, A.J.J., Honig, W.M.M. and Van Rossum, J. M. (1975): Psychopharmacologia 41:87-95.
33. Raiteri, M., Cervoni, A. M., de Carmige, R. and Levi, G. (1978): Nature 274:706-707.
34. Ravitz, A. J. and Moore, K. E. (1977): Life Sci. 21:267-272.
35. Roberts, D.C.S., Corcoran, M. E. and Fibiger, H. C. (1977): Pharmacol. Biochem. Behav. 6:615-620.
36. Roth, R. H. and Nowycky, M. C. (1977): Adv. Biochem. Psychopharmacol. 16:465-470.
37. Rubin, R. T. and Hays, S. E. (1980): Psychoneuroendocrinology 5: 121-137.
38. Stevens, J. R. (1973): Arch. Gen. Psychiat. 29:177-189.
39. Umezu, K. and Moore, K. E. (1979): J. Pharmacol. Exp. Ther. 208: 49-56.
40. Weiner, R. I. and Ganong, W. F. (1978): Physiol. Rev. 58:905-976.

6

Neuroendocrinology and Psychiatric Disorder,
edited by G. M. Brown, et al.
Raven Press, New York 1984.

Discussion: Schizophrenia

O. Hornykiewicz

Opening this panel discussion, I would like to make a few remarks relevant to questions raised by the speakers and discussants, all of whom have very aptly covered the quite difficult topic of neuroendocrine involvement in schizophrenia.

Specificially, I would like to reflect on two vital questions already alluded to by most of the speakers. The first question relates to whether it is possible to extrapolate from the neuroendocrine changes controlled by neurotransmitter receptors, such as the pituitary dopamine receptors, to the state of activity of dopamine receptors elsewhere in the brain. The consensus seems to be that this is a most difficult research strategy, and I would like to elaborate a little on an example that has already been mentioned by several speakers, namely Parkinson's disease. For Parkinson's disease, we have a fairly good idea what happens to the dopamine receptors in the nigrostriatal and mesolimbic dopamine systems. In both of these areas, dopamine concentrations decrease and the receptors, at least in nondopa-treated patients, become supersensitive to dopamine. There are several studies available on the levels of growth hormone and prolactin in nondopa-treated and dopa-treated Parkinson's patients. Although the results of these studies are somewhat variable, the majority suggests that basal levels of growth hormone and prolactin are within the normal range in Parkinson's patients. Also, the effect of L-dopa has been tested on these parameters and although again there are somewhat contradictory reports involving in most cases relatively few patients, on the whole the plasma growth hormone and prolactin responses seemed to be adequate. What is most important, Galea-Debono and colleagues (J. Neurol. Neurosurg. Psychiat. 40, 162-167, 1977) showed that the growth hormone response did not depend on whether the Parkinsonians responded well to L-dopa (responders) or not at all (non-responders); whether they were L-dopa "swingers"; or whether they were in their first year of L-dopa treatment or in their second to fifth treatment year. In all these subgroups of Parkinson's patients the growth hormone response was, for all practical purposes, the same, and the attained plasma levels of L-dopa did not influence the patient's growth hormone response. In other words, in this study, there was no correlation between the growth hormone response to L-dopa and the level of receptor sensitivity in the nigrostriatal and mesolimbic dopamine systems. Similarly, in a study comparing, in a comparatively small group of Parkinson patients, the therapeutic response to L-dopa with L-dopa's effect on prolactin levels (Rondot et al., Adv. Neurol. 24, 511-520, 1979), it was found that despite a good response to L-dopa, the prolactin response was quite variable, being in some patients normal, while in others there was a paradoxical or bimodal response. The L-dopa plasma levels were not significantly different for any of the patients. These results again emphasize the fact that there seems to be no correlation whatever between the sensitivity of the pituitary dopamine system to L-dopa and the dopamine receptors in the forebrain as determined by the therapeutic responsiveness to Ldopa treatment.

What can we conclude from these observations? Obviously, that if we knew nothing about the state of the dopamine receptors in the forebrain of Parkinson's patients, from neuroendocrinological data alone we would not be able to conclude that the dopamine receptors in the nigrostriatal and mesolimbic systems are, as a matter of fact, in a state of increased sensitivity. This very clearly illustrates the problems involved in this type of research strategy.

The second question I would like to raise concerns the antipsychotic mechanism of action of neuroleptics. It has been mentioned by several speakers, especially by Dr. Moore, that the most popular hypothesis postulates that the antischizophrenic effect of neuroleptics is related to the blockade of dopamine receptors in the mesolimbic, mesostriatal and mesocortical dopamine systems. I find it difficult to accept this hypothesis without reservations, especially when the effects of chronic neuroleptic administration are considered. As mentioned by Dr. Moore, chronic treatment with neuroleptics, in animals at least, produces a biochemical tolerance, and this tolerance seems to develop in all the forebrain dopamine systems, differences between the various dopamine systems being only related to time and possibly dosage. Along with the development of a biochemical tolerance to neuroleptics, there also develops a corresponding behavioural tolerance and, most importantly, supersensitivity of the forebrain dopamine receptors, that is to say increase in number of brain dopamine receptors.

The dopamine receptor supersensitivity, which develops in the forebrain of animals, also seem to develop in schizophrenic patients receiving chronic neuroleptic treatment. This is indicated by the development, in such patients, of tardive dyskinesias and what has been called withdrawal psychosis; the latter represents an acute exacerbation of the psychotic state, in some cases during neuroleptic medication, or when the dose of the antipsychotic drug is lowered or withdrawn (Chouinard and Jones, Am. J. Psychiat. 137, 16-21, 1980). These two phenomena, tardive dyskinesias and withdrawal psychosis, strongly suggest that in the schizophrenic brain, like in the laboratory animals, chronic neuroleptic treatment results in development of a supersensitivity of brain dopamine receptors, affecting, inter alia, also those dopamine regions of the brain that are specifically related to the antipsychotic effect of neuroleptic drugs. In this connection, it is interesting to note that, although chronic administration of neuroleptics in non-psychotic patients produces, in about 10 per cent of cases, tardive dyskinesias (either on withdrawal of the neuroleptic or during treatment) in none of these nonpsychotic patients have psychotic symptoms been observed to develop, neither during treatment nor upon withdrawal of the neuroleptic (C. D. Marsden, personal communication). (Similar observations have also been recorded by Chouinard and Jones, Am. J. Psychiat. 137, 16-21, 1980, in a group of manic patients on chronic neuroleptics).

How are we to interpret all these observations? In my view, there are two conclusions that may be drawn from these observations. Firstly - and this is something we have always known - procedures which increase brain dopamine activity seem to be associated with exacerbation of schizophrenic symptoms. Secondly, and most significantly, dopamine supersensitivity by itself is not sufficient to produce schizophrenic symptomatology or, more generally, psychosis. In other words, this means that whatever the mechanisms of antipsychotic effects may be, neuroleptics may influence secondary biochemical phenomena, and not the primary biochemical disturbance in schizophrenia.

I assume that the following discussion could be divided into two parts - the relevance of neuroendocrine functions as predictors of response in schizophrenia; and the relevance of these findings to the mechanism of action of antipsychotic drugs in general. May I now ask Dr. Carroll to moderate the discussion.

B. J. Carroll

I would ask this morning's speakers to respond to the points Dr. Hornykiewicz has raised.

Dr. H. Y. Meltzer

Regarding Dr. Hornykiewicz's criticism of the dopamine hypothesis, there is some evidence that tolerance does not develop in the frontal cortical regions in schizophrenics. I refer to the paper by Bacopoulos and colleagues (Science 205, 1405-1407, 1979) in which they measured homovanillic acid levels in postmortem brain specimens from schizophrenics with and without chronic neuroleptic treatment. They found persistently elevated dopamine metabolites in the forebrains of chronically treated patients, whereas tolerance was demonstrated in the striatal regions. On the other hand, we have pointed out a number of times that a distinction must be made between the time course of dopamine receptor blockade, as indicated by the prolactin system (and that is one of its big uses) and the antipsychotic effect. Dopamine receptor blockade, as we have heard many times, takes place within a matter of hours, or even minutes, following neuroleptic administration in man, but the drug's antipsychotic effect can take from days to weeks to months to develop. Similarly, when neuroleptic treatment is stopped, we have shown that dopamine receptor blockade is over within a matter of days but psychotic relapse may take weeks to months to occur. And we have also pointed out, in consideration of this, that the reduction of dopaminergic activity may in fact be leading to some other biochemical processes with a long half-life, that are in fact the relevant factors in antipsychotic effect or the onset of psychosis when the drug is stopped.

With regard to other points, a great deal has been said about dopamine receptors in the pituitary, and I have shown in a number of animal studies that there are differences between these and the limbic and striatal dopamine receptors. But there seem to be more similarities between the limbic and striatal dopamine receptors and the dopamine receptor in the hypothalamus that mediates dopaminergic stimulation of growth hormone release. As for the effect of neuroleptics on this dopamine receptor, the best work is that of Lal and Nair (In: Neuroendocrine Correlates in Neurology and Psychiatry, Muller and Agnoli, eds. 1979. Elsevier, Amsterdam, p.179) who have shown that clozapine dramatically blocks apomorphine-induced increase in growth hormone, whereas it has no effect on prolactin. And so I think that this particular receptor, which no one has done binding studies with or has ever localized, is one that deserves more attention.

Regarding Dr. Moore's idea for a receptor agonist that would produce an antipsychotic effect without endocrinological side effects, we have just published a study using a selective dopamine autoreceptor agonist in the striatal region; we found it to be tremendously potent as an *in vivo* inhibitor of rat prolactin secretion.

B. Carroll: Thank you. I am going to take the Chairman's prerogative for a few minutes and speculate as to where this field will be going in the future. We have heard several presentations from the basic endocrinologists, telling psychiatrists in the audience two things: 1) neuroendocrine systems are extraordinarily complex, and 2) we may well be 'barking up the wrong tree' if we think we are going to obtain fundamental information about schizophrenia or even about antipsychotic drug action, by the neuroendocrine window strategy. We have not heard from the psychiatric proponents why they started the neuroendocrine research approach to schizophrenia in the first place.

In principle, there are two reasons. Perhaps one can generalize from one dopamine system in the brain to another, and therefore use the tuberoinfundibular dopamine system as a model for the mesolimbic. But I believe that much of what we have just heard puts that simple idea to rest. The second reason for a neuroendocrine approach to schizophrenia might be that the pathophysiology of the disease resides in the same centers that regulate neuroendocrine function - that is, that schizophrenia is in a sense a limbic system disorder. Perhaps someone should spell this out, because many feel that this is probably not a limbic system disorder and certainly not in the same sense as affective illness. The most prominent endocrine changes in schizophrenia do indeed occur in schizoaffective disorders but not in simple schizophrenia and not in the burned out residual state.

What I am really asking is whether there is any logic in continuing with neuroendocrine studies in schizophrenia, as a way to understand the illness? Of course, it is still worth pursuing for pragmatic reasons, to help us understand the mechanism of action of new antipsychotic drugs and help in their development. The panelists should try to focus on these fundamental issues.

Dr. Meltzer: Prolactin and growth hormone secretion can indeed provide a window on the hypothalamus. I also think that by developing drugs which would not elevate serum prolactin but would inhibit apomorphine-induced growth hormone secretion, it would at last be possible to test in man for antipsychotic drugs that will inhibit mesolimbic and mesocortical dopaminergic receptors with minimal effect on the nigrostriatal system. Even in terms of negative observations, it has been extremely useful, to this point, to have established that pituitary dopamine receptors appear to be reasonably normal and not supersensitive in schizophrenic patients.

Dr. E. Müller

It appears from this discussion that the determination of growth hormone seems to give a clearer index of what is going on in the CNS. But I think that the basic question is to know how we influence the catecholamine neurotransmission when we affect the release of growth hormone? In other words, when we give drugs like apomorphine or clonidine to humans and measure the increase in growth hormone release, are we stimulating the receptors, as we think, or are we on the contrary, toning down the activity of the catecholaminergic system by the very low doses of the drugs administered? I am not certain of this. We simply need to know the answer to this question before extrapolating to other brain catecholamine systems, e.g. the mesolimbic system. We were one of the first to start such studies in normal human subjects, but I think that we need to investigate this further. The second point I would like to make is about indirectly acting dopamine agonists. This type of drug seems very promising as a probe of CNS as well as tuberoinfundibular dopamine activity and its disorders (e.g. prolactinoma). It is my opinion that in future research the administration of drugs of the amphetamine and methylphenidate type will prove a useful tool for the investigation of both CNS and anterior pituitary sensitivity to dopaminergic stimulation.

Dr. A. Prange

I think that constrictions on the endocrine window theory apply just as long as we remain strictly 'aminocentric' in our conception of mental illness. For example, Dr. Frohman has pointed out the difficulties of making step-by-step inferences - from the periphery, through the pituitary to the hypothalamus, and to the rest of the brain. For the sake of argument at least, we can avoid the necessity of one step if we grant that some of those hypothalamic hypophyseal hormones themselves have behavioural effects, and act as neuromodulators or even neurotransmitters. In this case, we need not exclusively concern ourselves with making the final inference from there to classical transmitter systems.

In addition, some of the things that we measure in the periphery - that is to say, the trophic hormones - may even get 'upstairs' through retrograde circulation to the hypothalamus, and as our compatriot David DeWied and others believe, have behavioural properties of their own. One does not have to limit oneself to the hypothalamic substances to think about behavioural effects, and it is, after all, the behavioural disorders that we are concerned with here.

Finally, to the periphery. It is a closed system, after all, with many of the secretions of the target glands having access to the brain. Now, we have always asked, what do they do to the amine systems? But I believe they have behavioural effects as well - or at least in a very complex way through the amine systems. Many of the markers we like to think of as peripheral, have central consequences of their own. If we adopt this point of view, then I think the 'window' strategy is much less constrictive than it seemed to be at the end of this morning's session.

Uriel Halbreich

When Dr. Moore compared the dopaminergic tuberoinfundibular system to other dopaminergic systems, he did not mention the role of the cholinergic system in the tuberoinfundibular prolactin regulation. We recently published a study in which we gave haloperidol and haloperidol plus benztropine mesylate. When the latter was given by itself, it had no influence on prolactin. However, when the two drugs were given together, there was a delay in the prolactin response. When more benztropine was given, the delay was longer. So I believe the situation is not as clear as presented and that there probably is some cholinergic contribution to the regulation of prolactin.

K. Moore

May I respond to the comment made by Dr. Halbreich? I did not really try to cover all the ways by which the tuberoinfundibular nerves are regulated. The point I tried to make is that prolactin is not exclusively a measure of tuberoinfundibular nerve activity. And there are a number of other systems - the cholinergic system, for instance. Dr. Muller has focused on the GABA system, and Dr. Meltzer and others have looked at the 5-HT systems. I was just trying to highlight the tuberoinfundibular nerves per se, as they relate to other dopamine mechanisms. But clearly, and as Dr. Frohman points out, there is a lot of interaction that is not completely understood. And this is very interesting, with the neuronal role in the mesolimbic system clearly different from that in the nigrostriatal system, and in turn different from that in the tuberoinfundibular system. Perhaps the object is not to work on drugs that interfere with dopamine nerve terminals, but to look at their afferent inputs and to modify the system in this way.

John Sutton

I would like to comment on a topic brought up earlier by John Davis - namely, sex differences in pituitary hormone responses. I am not referring to male/female differences which are well known to all, but to the fact that differences between the two phases of the menstrual cycle in a simple hormonal response can be just as great. Looking at the response of growth hormone to exercise in females in relation to the cycle variation, we have shown that the response during the luteal phase is much greater than during the follicular phase. This cycle - related difference in response has now been shown not only for growth hormone but also for the catecholamines epinephrine and norepinephrine. I would like to plead that not only should we be aware of male/female differences, but that even subtle modulations or minor changes in the ovarian hormones may well change the pituitary's response to simple physiological changes, such as sleep and exercise.

S. Reichlin

I was very pleased to conclude from Dr. Meltzer's remarks that the endocrine regulatory system in schizophrenia is really quite robust and that perhaps a lesson can be drawn from how well it performs, rather than how sick it is. But my specific question is, what further psychoneuroendocrine studies are indicated at this time? If you had a magic wand, what studies would you want to see next?

Dr. Meltzer: My first answer to Dr. Reichlin's question is that we need more of the same. The results look good as grouped, but hidden within them are individuals who are aberrant. Dr. Brambilla reported the group of patientw with very diminished prolactin; let us follow these up. Maybe these are the people who confirm the notion that increased tuberoinfundibular dopaminergic activity reflects increased mesolimbic dopaminergic activity.

These are some of the issues that have been skimmed over - that there is an early-onset hebephrenic group, as distinct from paranoid schizophrenia, and that these patients can be characterized by early or late onset and an aberrant growth hormone response to TRH - which, granted, is not specific, but why should it occur in schizophrenia, as well as in anorexia nervosa and acromegaly? Aberrant gonadotropin response to gonadotropin releasing hormone and to clomiphene have been particularly demonstrated by Dr. Brambilla. This has been done with small samples and needs to be extended to others. There has been very little done to combine strategies by stimulating with TRH and then trying a dose-response antagonism with L-dopa or apomorphine. That may clarify supersensitivity. Dr. Frohman has pointed out this model to be of particular advantage.

The biggest problem in schizophrenia, as opposed to the affective disorders, is that of heterogeneity. The only answer is to be patient and look at large samples, using this as a kind of screening device to better define populations that will in turn be subjected to other hypotheses - other kinds of testing extending from the original findings. Here, the neuroendocrine window is just one of a number of ways to begin the process of subtyping schizophrenics.

Dr. Rose

Herb (Meltzer), I hate to give you a hard time, because you have worked very hard and 'toiled long in the vineyards'. We have talked about the problems of looking through the wrong end of the telescope. Ed Sachar, and I guess others, postulated maybe a decade ago the concept of a window on the hypothalamus; it looks as if we have a dark glass in one window, and in the other window it is even darker, in terms of the affective disorders. But it seems that there is a message, although there are a number of things going against it. There has been a lack of consistency, and your slides clearly show this. While you gave us the overview, the trends were hard to disern. And, as has been pointed out from the large picture point of view, the basic neuroendocrinologists have told us that these systems are not that parallel. There are some parallels, but there are also some obvious discrepancies. There is also a third problem related to the amine story, with chronic drug metabolites persisting in there, firmly attached to the amine receptor.

Some of the data you presented earlier were on chronic patients, with the patients only recently off drug in terms of weeks or months, after having been on it for 5 to 10 years. This indeed further darkens the window, and I wonder if this lack of consistency of either specificity or sensitivity of endocrine findings, using provocative or basal levels, in addition to the problems of chronic neuroleptic administration in some of the subgroups, raises serious questions as to whether we are ever going to find a marker or at least parallelism between symptoms and endocrine abnormalities. This is one of the things that have emerged from our discussion and I don't think we should bury it, but it looks as if it already has 'one foot in the grave'.

Dr. M. Thorner

The points that Dr. Meltzer made are very well taken. However, I am not certain that the investigation of hormonal changes without a basic hypothesis to test, will necessarily bring more fruitful data, because of the tremendous variations we have seen in hormonal values. It is difficult enough to study normal subjects, and the basic questions you posed at the beginning have perhaps been answered, but I am not terribly optimistic that you are going to be able to distinguish different subgroups on the basis of these data. I think that perhaps a more fruitful approach would be to study the tremendous dissociation of clinical effects and hormonal change, as for the drug cloapine. Taking this approach is much more likely to produce fundamental basic knowledge than looking for hormonal changes which have proved very disappointing up to now.

Dr. R. Rubin

I would like to make a brief methodological comment. We have heard about the need to refine diagnostic subcategories of schizophrenia, in terms of differential hormone response. John Davis mentioned the importance of taking more than a single blood sample for more accurate integration of these hormone concentrations. I would simply like to comment on the problem of shifting baselines and, as an illustration, to refer back to Herb Meltzer's first slide. There is no question concerning the growth hormone response to apomorphine. But if you look at the prolactin responses, you see that in the 20 minutes prior to administrtion of apomorphine the prolactin levels were declining. Now we really don't know how much further they might have declined before stabilizing. Certainly, venipuncture is a known stimulus to prolactin increase. Now, one might conclude from these data that apomorphine arrested an otherwise normal decline of prolactin. On the other hand, some investigators, such as Rotrosen in some of his work, had a declining baseline and, simply averaging the values, came out with a rather high level. Prolactin levels continued to decrease after apomorphine. There was no difference in the slope, but it was concluded that apomorphine suppressed prolactin. So, I think that if you do not have a stable baseline, you cannot conclude certain things from your data, and I would simply like to plead for an extended sampling period in order to get the better baseline.

O. Hornykiewicz

To conclude this discussion, I simply cannot help feeling a little unhappy when the point is so strongly stressed that because there may be so many different subgroups of schizophrenics, we have to do more of the same in order to possibly find out something of significance. After all, we should not forget that a substantial number of schizophrenics do benefit, at least temporarily, from neuroleptic medication; to me, this suggests that they have something basic in common - unless we assume that what the neuroleptics influence is totally unrelated to the psychotic process. Dr. Meltzer quoted the potentially important report of Bacopoulos et al. (Science 205, 1405-1407, 1979) suggesting that in schizophrenic patients long-term neuroleptics do not produce tolerance, and by implication dopamine supersensitivity, specifically in the mesocortical dopamine neuron system. However, in this respect we first need answers to two basic questions: Firstly - what is the role of cortical dopamine in psychotic behaviour? So far, I do not see an answer to this question. Secondly - in which neuronal elements of the cortex is the dopamine metabolite homovanillic acid localized? Analyses of the human cortex, dissected into discrete areas according to the Brodmann map, disclosed only trace amounts of dopamine, except for Brodmann area 25, which was not analyzed by Bacopoulos et al. (own unpublished observations). Therefore, it seems quite possible that the cortical homovanillic acid found elevated in neuroleptic-treated schizophrenics was contained not at all in dopamine neurons but e.g. in noradrenaline neurons (where dopamine functions as an intermediate in the biosynthesis of noradrenaline).

My final point is related to the question of withdrawal psychosis which I already mentioned in my introductory remarks. It is crucial to realize that this phenomenon is not just the well-known observation that patients relapse weeks or months after withdrawal of the neuroleptic; the patients in question become worse either immediately after withdrawal of the neuroleptic or while receiving neuroleptic medication, thus requiring a substantial increase in dose in order to maintain the therapeutic response. This type of withdrawal response has been defined by Chouinard and Jones (Am. J. Psychiat. 137, 16-21, 1980) as representing a dopamine supersensitivity psychosis, that is psychosis due to development of brain dopamine supersensitivity as a consequence of chronic neuroleptic medication. The occurrence of this neuroleptic-induced dopamine supersensitivity psychosis clearly indicates that during chronic neuroleptic medication supersensitivity, and by implication tolerance, to dopamine develops also in those areas of the human brain related to the anti-psychotic effects of neuroleptics. There is no question in my mind that these and similar crucial points must seriously be considered before we can rationally discuss the value of the dopamine hypothesis of schizophrenia.

B. Carroll: Thank you. This morning's session has brought certain issues into clearer focus. There are two opinions: One is to 'not throw the baby out with the bath water' and the other is that 'maybe we are simply following the Willie Sutton principle and studying neuro-endocrinal function because that is where the money is'. I hope we can, as a result of this morning's discussion, move towards better-defined study protocols.

Neuroendocrinology and Psychiatric Disorder,
edited by G. M. Brown, et al.
Raven Press, New York 1984.

Overview of Endocrinology of Stress

Robert M. Rose

In Mason's now classic review of psychoendocrine research on the pituitary-adrenal cortical system (64), published in 1968, he noted that in the previous twenty years there had been approximately 200 publications in this area. Since that time there has been an increase of greater than an order of magnitude in the number of publications relating to changes in various endocrine systems, including corticoids, growth hormones, prolactin, catecholamines and gonadal steroids in response to a wide variety of stressful stimuli. The relevant literature is very large and growing. Many investigators utilize maximally stressful stimuli such as exposure to inescapable shock to probe the dynamics of various physiological systems responsive to stress including neurotransmitter-endocrine interactions, while others study how individuals differ in their response to less overwhelming though clearly distressing life events. Investigation of responses to the wide variety of stressful stimuli studied (including all relevant physiological and psychological work) represents a significant portion of biomedical research as has been pointed out in a forthcoming publication from the Institute of Medicine entitled "Research on Stress in Health and Disease" (34). Even if we restrict our attention to research into endocrine responses to stress, the field is too vast to encompass in a single review all relevant endocrine systems and all classes of stressful stimuli. This review therefore, will attempt to summarize only selected areas in the endocrinology of stress.

Early stress research in animals emphasized that responses of the organism to a wide variety of stimuli were non-specific. These included studies of the adrenal responses to a variety of physical stressors (108) such as exposure to heat, cold, exercise and so forth. Early research with human subjects paralleled animal research by studying adrenal responses, initially by measurement of blood eosinophils, to the physical stress of rowing or exercise. In 1975, Mason (68) pointed out that much of early research into stress, especially that involving exposure of animals to a variety of physical stimuli, shared one important characteristic. One of the primary qualities of the stressful experience was the exposure of the animal to a novel, strange or unfamiliar environment. Thus, the common thread that may have explained these animals' responses was the psychological relevance of the stimulus rather than the particular physical stressors to which they were exposed. In subsequent research, Mason (68) was able to document that exposure of animals to a variety of different physical stimuli including heat, cold and reduction of caloric intake, was not necessarily associated with activation of the adrenal cortical system, especially when it was done in such a way that the animal could not readily detect changes in the environment, i.e. no sudden changes, being fed on schedule with non-nutrative food pellets, etc. We will, therefore, restrict most of our attention to the relevant psychoendocrine literature and not attempt to summarize endocrine responses to various physical stresses independent of any psychologically stressing aspects.

Investigators also began to appreciate the significance of individual differences in the responses of human subjects when confronted with potentially challenging or threatening stimuli. Further research which will be described in greater detail in this review focussed on how individuals can avoid being stressed when exposed to threatening environmental situations; a concept later labelled under the general rubric of "coping responses". In other words, we became much more aware of the importance of how individuals perceived a given event in determining how stressful it was for them rather than attending, as we had earlier, to the characteristics of the situation or environmental task. This review will concentrate on describing research on how individuals respond endocrinologically to a wide variety of life events. We will also review studies which have attempted to investigate how individuals differ in their response to a given life situation, such as entering basic combat training in the Army, and note the psychological assessments that have been made in an attempt to predict how individuals differ in their endocrine response to altered environmental situations. We will also briefly discuss endocrine responses seen in psychiatric illness but primarily from the perspective of the psychological stress they evoke rather than a review of the specific endocrine abnormalities associated with psychiatric illness.

The psychoendocrine literature is most complete with respect to studies involving measurement of adrenal cortical responses initially as a class of metabolites (plasma or urinary 17-hydroxycorticosteroids, 17-OHCS) and more recently by the direct measurement of cortisol itself. Over the last decade, there have been an increasing number of studies measuring other hormones which are now well known to be responsive to stressful stimuli. These include plasma growth hormone, prolactin and testosterone. There is also a significant literature measuring urinary catecholamines (epinephrine and norepinephrine), but there are relatively few studies describing individual differences in plasma catecholamine responses to potentially stressful situations. Because cortisol measurements have been used most extensively to investigate individual differences in response, the review will focus primarily on those studies measuring adrenal cortical responses. However, those studies measuring other endocrine products which clarify how individuals respond differently to psychologically stressful events will also be noted and reviewed.

This review will also attempt to clarify how most of our understanding of endocrine responses relates to exposure to acutely stressful events and that in the vast majority of cases there is a rapid loss of endocrine responsivity to the initially provocative stimulus or life event, probably reflecting adaptation. This conclusion raises serious questions about the utility of studying most endocrine systems to assess differential risk for future illness that can be a consequence of exposure to various stressful conditions. Some examples of studies which reported a dissociation between endocrine responses and illness will be noted.

There has been growing interest recently in how endocrine responses to a variety of stimuli are modified by circadian variation. The review of these studies suggest an important mechanism for the difficulties individuals experience in adapting to shift work, jet travel, where our usual periodicity is disrupted. Finally, although scanty, there is exciting new evidence demonstrating the conditionability of endocrine responses, providing a potential framework for understanding response set, possibly related to risk for future illness.

A word about definition is necessary before we continue. Unfortunately, stress is used to encompass several different ideas, often in the same report. The title of this chapter, as is typical of so many papers in the field, speaks of responses to stress. This implies that the stress is outside and the individual is responding to something which is exterior to himself. Upon reflection this is clearly not true yet this habit continues and although some authors have attempted to change this and speak more precisely, it has not changed in general usage. Selye referred to the nature of the provocative event as a "stressor", as being placed in the cold was a stressor or taking an examination was a stressor. Other workers have chosen to describe the nature of the environmental or physical stimuli as the stress, and the response of the individual as strain, employing an engineering analogy. Other writers have elected to use the word stress as referring to the response of the person as being "under stress". _Stress_ therefore is used as describing a characteristic of the environment, the response of the individual, or the _interaction_ of an individual's perception of environment and his response, such that a particular situation is _stressful_ for him. Since all of these are used and at time even interchangeable, the reader must be patient and tolerant. Some workers have suggested we discard the word "stress" or concept of stress, but it tends to remain in common parlance and hence we will succumb and use it ourselves, hopefully specifying its meaning in context.

Responses To Life Events

The response capability of the individual begins early in life. Anders et al. (4) found that plasma cortisol in normal human infants showed marked increases after crying as compared to when the infants were lying quietly. The cortisol differences between crying and quiet wakefulness or REM sleep were not greater in children one to five weeks of age compared to those five to fifteen weeks of age, and they concluded that the endocrine correlates of arousal are probably present in humans as early as one week of age. Cathro et al. (24) compared normal infants with those who were born with an Rh incompatibility or with asphyxia before or during birth and found that the infants with a stormier post-natal course showed higher levels of cortisol. Gutai et al. (44) however did not find differences comparing normal infants with those who had a stressful post-natal course, such as with respiratory distress syndrome. However, studies which compare individuals to themselves, usually provide better data on the relevance of psychological state to endocrine functions than cross-sectioned studies.

Many studies report that increased cortisol secretion is associated with surgery; more recently it has been shown (50) that this increase is due not only to changes in metabolism but also to an increased secretion of cortisol to a maximum level. Normal feedback inhibition does not occur presumably due to increased corticotrophin releasing factor (CRF). Other workers have found that individuals anticipating surgery may show as great an increase as that occurring during surgery, thereby emphasizing the importance of psychological perception. Czeisler et al. (28) measured plasma cortisol every 20 minutes over 24 hours in patients on the day prior to elective coronary artery bypass surgery. When patients underwent preoperative surgical preparation, (scrubbing the chest) they showed very large increases in plasma cortisol, even at midnight when cortisol secretion is normally very low. In some patients this increase was even larger than that associated with the normal rise during sleep prior to awakening (122). Thus, anticipation of the surgical event itself was a very provocative stimulus.

Numerous studies have documented that anticipation of examinations provokes adrenal secretion (64). Attempts to correlate the rise in cortisol with the degree of emotionality exhibited by the subjects, (as determined by a variety of psychological tests) have not been consistent (10).

Admission to a hospital has been noted to be generally very provocative of cortisol secretion (64). An interesting exception to this finding is a report by Woodman et al. who studied cortisol and catecholamine responses in prisoners admitted to a maximum security hospital (128). These individuals were tested not only following admission but during exposure to a variety of potentially unpleasant stimuli such as mental arithmetic under pressure. A significant number of subjects were endocrinologically unresponsive to admission or the potentially stressful mental arithmetic. They noted that these unresponsive individuals showed "many psychopathic behaviour patterns". This was not a predictive study but it is clearly in the same direction as other studies which emphasize the potential impact of any potentially stressful event is dependent on the perception of the individual who is exposed to this situation.

Several investigators have noted that prolonged exercise, especially exhausting exercise, leads to an increase in cortisol secretion as well as a number of other stress labile hormones (110, 111). This was noted in individuals exposed to exhausting exercise (45) (73% of maximum O_2 uptake) both before and after training. Thus, this level of exercise is clearly a significant physiologic stimulus given the work done. Cortisol, growth hormone and catecholamines interact synergistically to mobilize blood glucose. Similarly, cortisol has been found to be significantly elevated following a marathon by trained runners (77). Mason et al. (67) also found that individuals anticipating exhausting exercise showed very significant rises in cortisol as well as other stress labelled hormones, levels comparable to that seen during the actual conduct of the physical task.

From these studies, as well as many not specifically cited, it is apparent that individuals show a significant adrenal cortical activation when exposed to important changes in their environment. Not only just anticipation of surgery, or examination, or exercise can be provocative of cortisol secretion, but also the response to moving when that is very important or distressing. Kral et al. (53) studied aged men and women who had to be relocated. They found that especially psychiatrically impaired men showed a significant increase in plasma cortisol following their relocation.

The reader may be struck with the ubiquity of situations which can provoke significant endocrine responses. However, the studies summarized so far have focussed on group differences and although many mention that there were individuals who were not observed to respond, systematic efforts were not undertaken to investigate or predict why some individuals failed to show significant endocrine responses.

Individual Differences In Responses To Potentially Stressful Events

A clue to one of the more relevant variables that may explain how individuals adapt, comes from earlier animal studies. In subjecting rhesus monkeys to the task of avoiding electric shock by pressing a lever over a 72 hour period, Mason et al. (65) found that the animals showed the most brisk cortisol responses during their first or second 72 hour experience. By the time the animals experienced their third or fourth three day shock avoidance, cortisol responses were no longer elevated compared to baseline, and in some animals were even below normal. Animals quickly adapted to the stressful nature of this stimulus and there was no longer an evidence of adrenal cortical arousal. One might generalize from these studies that endocrine responses undergo rapid extinction upon re-exposure to the stimulus. A similar finding was observed in measuring plasma corticosterone and pituitary changes in rats following prolonged exposure to stress. Pollard et al. (83) found that after 20 days of exposure to shock avoidance animals failed to show any rise in corticosterone; the intense secretory activity observed in the cells of the adrenohypothesis that secrete ACTH was no longer observed after 20 days and corticotrope activity returned to control levels. These findings are especially relevant to Selye's hypothesis that after prolonged exposure to stress there is a stage of pituitary or adrenal insufficiency, referred to as "stage of exhaustion". This observation of a lack of pituitary activation following prolonged exposure strongly supports the argument that animals adapt to most stressful stimuli except extreme situations such as observed in some captured monkeys exposed to repeated, novel and intense manipulations (75).

Many workers have become impressed with the fact that individuals adapt or accommodate to most stressful stimuli upon being re-exposed to them and thus they lose their stressful quality. Upon reflection it is apparent that most stressful psychological stimuli that have been shown to be provocative of a variety of endocrine responses, are acute or novel in nature and that upon re-exposure endocrine responses extinguish reflecting adaptation.

A recent study of parachute jumpers (117) provides support for these conclusions. First-time parachutists show a very large increase in cortisol and other stress labile hormones such as growth hormone or prolactin on their first jump, and by subsequent jumps most individuals fail to show any increase in hormonal levels following the jump. Experienced parachutists show a brief anticipatory response in cortisol levels which return to baseline levels before the jump actually occurs. There is some psychological anticipation of the event, however, it is highly damped as the individual becomes accommodated to the task.

The studies in animals and men documenting the rapid adaptation of endocrine responses to re-exposure suggest a strategy that might be followed in attempting to understand why certain individuals fail to show endocrine response when exposed initially to potentially stressful psychological stimuli. The internal dialogue might go something like, "I've seen this before" or "The consequences of this are not very important to me". How individuals arrive at that state seems to vary very widely and is not of primary importance in determining whether or not he or she demonstrates an endocrine response upon being confronted or challenged by a potentially stressful event. The task facing the investigator wishing to predict how individuals respond to potentially stressful psychological events is to assess the presence and effectiveness of various attitudes or defenses (coping styles) that individuals may employ upon being confronted or challenged with a particular task or event. This has proved to be an elusive task, but there are a number of studies in which investigators have successfully predicted individual differences in endocrine response. In 1964 Wolff and colleagues (126, 127) studied the parents of children dying of leukemia. These parents lived on a ward at NIMH and were studied by a team of investigators while they were responding to exacerbations and remissions in their child's struggle with leukemia, which during this period of time usually ended in death. The investigators were able to predict the parents' level of urinary cortisol metabolites (17-OHCS) during this difficult period. They focussed on the defenses of the parents and the effectiveness of these defenses. It is of note that some parents were extremely demonstrative and even hysterical in their discussion of their child's illness, while other individuals were much quieter and seemed to "suffer in silence". These workers pointed out that hysterical behaviour could also serve as a defense against the distress of perceiving the child's death, as indicated by the relatively normal levels of corticosteroid excretion among women who demonstrated this behaviour. Other individuals were deeply disturbed, although they were reluctant to verbalize their feelings and were correctly judged to be very distressed by the illness and death of their child. This classic study also pointed out that individuals could cope by denying the illness and only when this denial was challenged was there evidence of psychological stress and increased 17-OHCS excretion. Some individuals are observed to have very high levels of 17-OHCS on the day in which they had an interview with the psychiatrist or, for example, were forced to spend the day sitting and talking with their child which they had previously been able to avoid. This study emphasized that what was most relevant was not the type of defense or whether or not it was psychologically healthy or effective, but whether or not it was successfully utilized by the individual to protect himself from feelings of being stressed, as measured by the level of adrenal cortical activation.

In an attempt to replicate this finding in another population, my colleagues and I (88, 82) studied young men during their first month of basic combat training in the Army. Urinary 17-OHCS were used as an index of adrenal cortical activation. We were able to successfully predict individuals' average level of 17-OHCS during the first four weeks of basic training. Similar to Wolff et al. we found that what individuals told us about how distressed or disturbed they were by being in the Army was not necessarily a very good indication of their actual level of psychological arousal and by itself not predictive of endocrine response. Some individuals complained loudly, but were really not very disturbed or stressed by basic training, while other individuals were much quieter and we only gained some appreciation of the degree of their distress by reports of their behaviour from medical corpsmen who lived with the men and met with us regularly to discuss the recruits. Assessment of their psychological maturation was not particularly helpful in predicting their endocrine response, but what was most important and relevant was the degree to which they were able to isolate or protect themselves by any means possible from the demands of basic training and their being severely threatened or humiliated by it.

The crucial importance of the individuals' perception of potentially stressful events as the major variable in determining their adrenal cortical responses is exemplified by two studies that were done during the Vietnam War. One group (Bourne et al.) studied a group of men in the Special Forces who had intercepted a message that their isolated camp was to be attacked by the Viet Cong in a few days (12). Urine samples from the men in the camp both before and during the expected attack as well as several days following were collected. The attack did not occur but there was significant differences in urinary 17-OHCS excretion observed among the men. Most of the Special Forces' enlisted personnel were eager and enthusiastic about the impending attack and spent much of their time in task-oriented activities, such as bringing in extra ammunition and fortifying their defenses. Their behaviour and attitude was in sharp contrast to the captain and radio operator, who spent much of their time communicating with the Commanding Officer in battalion headquarters. The captain was under considerable pressure to perform well. Both the radio operator and the captain showed sharp increases in their urinary 17-OHCS levels on the day of the expected attack compared to levels on the days preceding and following this day. Although this was not a predictive study, one would conclude from these observations that the captain and radio operator were significantly stressed by the events, consistent with the nature of their contact with superior officers. This was in contrast with the enlisted men who engaged in positively viewed activities, i.e. the opportunity to engage the enemy, relief from the boredom and lack of productive activity as they perceived their status prior to this anticipated event.

Another study by Bourne et al. involved the measurement of the urinary 17-OHCS in helicopter medics who were involved in medical evacuation flights (11). The striking finding was that urinary 17-OHCS levels on days in which the medics flew were not significantly different from days that they stayed on the base. One might have expected that when they were flying and facing the real danger of being shot down there would be increased stress, as reflected by elevated urinary steroid excretion. Bourne noted that different men employed different ways of dealing with the potential threat of being shot down including obsessional defenses, and intensification of their religious beliefs. It was striking that all of these individuals who were involved in a more chronic stress activity showed complete adaptation to their medical evacuation missions, as judged by their excretion of urinary corticosteroids.

Analagous observations have been made in animals. As noted previously, when monkeys are subjected to 72 hour shock avoidance (65) they show no elevation of adrenal cortical activation after the first few episodes and when chronically exposed they show even lower levels than baseline. Social variables among animals have also been shown to be relevant in determining their response to stress. When dominant and aggressive rhesus monkeys were subjected to shock avoidance they showed a very brisk increase in adrenal cortical activity (62). However, several monkeys who were much more submissive and less aggressive failed to show any increase of adrenal cortical activity when subjected to shock avoidance. One of these monkeys was studied in order to determine the adequacy of his pituitary and adrenal reserves. There was a brisk rise in urinary 17-OHCS following ACTH as well as following metyropone, which tests pituitary ACTH reserve. Thus the lack of response in this animal was not related to any adrenal or pituitary insufficiency, but rather to the particular task not being stressful for that animal. One might speculate that for subordinate and submissive animals, avoidance of negative punishment is not as novel or as potentially stressful an event as it is for a dominant male or "alpha" male to engage in frequent responses to avoid punishment. A parallel observation, although anecdotal, was observed in one of the helicopter medics (11). One of the men who had very low adrenal steroid excretion was in a fight and sustained a laceration to his scalp which subsequently became infected and required medication. During this time, concurrent with the laceration becoming infected, he had a very large increase in urinary 17-OHCS reflecting the intact responsiveness of his pituitary adrenal cortical system to this external physical stress, and indicating that his previous low level of steroid excretion was psychological in origin and not due to an unresponsive or refractory pituitary or adrenal gland.

Katz and collaborators (49) were able to predict adrenal cortical levels as measured by cortisol secretion rate in patients who underwent breast tumor biopsy for determination of potential malignancy. They found that those women who employed defenses such as isolation and denial, often had the lowest cortisol secretion rate prior to the biopsy compared to those women who were overly distressed and worried about the biopsy and its implications. This study is perhaps a most telling example of what seems to matter most, from a psychoendocrine standpoint, is the effectiveness of the defense in protecting the individual from being acutely distressed or aroused rather than its psychological adaptive value. That is to say, many of the women who had low cortisol levels in anticipation of the biopsy had waited a dangerously long period of time before seeking medical attention and thus endangered their lives. From this perspective, their coping defenses were maladaptive. However, from the context of preventing or protecting them from being stressed or aroused, these defenses were successful.

More recently children's cortisol responses to hospitalization for elective surgery have been studied (51). Cortisol production rates while the children were still at home and had just learned they had to come into the hospital in two weeks did not correlate with individual cortisol levels obtained the day after admission to the hospital. Children were interviewed and given Rorschach tests. Those children who were observed to be less distressed and who showed less rigid, more flexible psychological coping styles, were correctly predicted to have lower cortisol production rates ($r = 49$, $p < .02$) in response to hospitalization. In this study the cortisol level reflects adaptation to the process of hospitalization, and there is a greater parallel between the efficacy of the coping style in protecting against distress associated with psychoendocrine response and its utility in helping the child adjust psychologically to the hospital.

From these studies we can conclude that individuals differ significantly with respect to their perceptions of various life events. Even events which appear to be stressful to everyone such as an impending breast tumor biopsy or a physical operation, are viewed very differently by individuals. That is to say, individuals differ significantly in the degree to which they screen themselves from the realization or impact of a distressing life event. Sometimes there are negative psychological consequences to the extent that the ability to confront an unpleasant event and to seek appropriate help early, such as tumor biopsy and subsequent operation, may be impaired by the very mechanisms that prevent distress. Another way of saying this is that it is not always adaptive to avoid acute stress.

Responses To Chronic Stress

Despite its large theoretical importance, there are relatively few studies describing endocrine responses to chronic stress. As noted earlier, studies with experimental animals indicate that adaptation occurs relatively rapidly, in three to six weeks in animals that are exposed to a variety of stressful stimuli. Investigators have noted that chronically stressed animals, however, are different from naive controls. Sakellaris (104) found that chronically stressful rats have more rapid endocrine responses to other novel stimuli than do unexposed controls, even though they fail to show any adrenocortical responses to the original stressor after repeated re-exposure.

There is relatively little data available in human subjects. Burchfield (18), in a recent review, postulated that most potentially stressful life events occur on a chronic intermittent basis for human subjects. She hypothesized that after experience, individuals develop an anticipatory response which is reflected both in endocrine and autonomic arousal but then when actually exposed to the stressful event, show no changes compared to baseline. This anticipatory response has not been studied endocrinologically in human subjects. Fenz (37) described an anticipatory response in experienced parachutists using heart rate as the dependent measure and noted that experienced parachutists showed a rise prior to the event as contrasted to novice jumpers who continued to show elevation throughout the course of the parachute jump. Whether there are significant endocrine anticipatory responses upon re-exposure to a familiar but once stressful event has yet to be documented in human studies.

The relatively few studies in human subjects measuring chronic adrenocortical responses parallel those in animals. Namely, there is very little change from the unstimulated state. In a study of paramedics and firefighters, Dutton et al. (33) found that when he compared the urinary corticoids for either group there was no substantial change in levels comparing days worked and days off. The firefighters had an opposite response with higher corticoids on the days off. Timio et al. (114, 115) reported on the urinary secretion of adrenaline, noradrenaline and urinary corticoids in two groups of workers while on the job. One group were employees in a confectionery factory who usually worked on a piece work basis while others were on salary working on an assembly line. Both groups showed increased levels of catecholamines and urinary steroids when they were paid on a piece work basis. This was true even for the confectionery workers who were accustomed to this type of employment, in that they showed a drop in levels when their pay for the four days was guaranteed by salary. Sheetmetal workers showed a rise in their urinary corticoids and epinephrine when their pay was changed to a piece work basis. These results were replicated when these same groups of workers were studied six months later. This study not only shows that a novel situation such as change of basis of pay at work can be stressful, but it also shows there may be a chronic increase in levels in individuals whose pay is directly proportional to the amount of output, i.e. piece work.

Most studies of individuals engaged in difficult tasks to which they have been exposed for some time, however, fail to demonstrate any significant endocrine responses in these subjects. Experienced pilots studied during strenuous flight failed to show elevations of growth hormone or prolactin, compared to the significant responses of novice pilots (81). Studies of experienced truck drivers working for 11 hours on four consecutive days (26) failed to show significantly higher cortisol on the driving days compared to non-driving days, not dissimilar from an earlier study of helicopter medics in Vietnam.

Measures of plasma cortisol in air traffic controllers while they are actually working planes failed to reveal a very close relationship between the magnitude of work performed and levels of plasma cortisol. When men were studied as their own control, there was a slight increase in plasma cortisol when workload increased for some subjects (97). Other variables such as mood at work, attitude towards the job, however, did contribute significantly to predicting when increased work was provocative of increased plasma cortisol secretion. These later studies along with other investigations strongly support the concept that individuals adapt to chronic work stress although there were men whose cortisol did show a consistent rise when workload increased. It is interesting to know these men were among the most competent as judged by their peers and also showed rather high investment in their work.

Another study on the relationship between cortisol and everyday stresses such as white collar work was reported by Caplan et al. (20). They studied high level NASA administrators and scientists and compared plasma cortisol measured at two times in the day with individual's reports of workload and job strain. Among those reporting higher workload, they found a significantly lower cortisol level in the morning while those with lower amounts of reported workload showed the usual diurnal drop of cortisol during the day. One interpretation is that those with greater workload showed a suppression of cortisol in response to the work. However, frequent samples were not drawn, and the exact nature of the shift in diurnal curve cannot be interpreted. However, these results do suggest that rather than seeing a persistent elevation of cortisol during chronic exposure to a potentially stressful stimulus, certain individuals may actually suppress below baseline, a result which has been reported by Mason for monkeys (65).

A study by Curtis et al. (27) provides additional evidence for the lack of adrenal cortical activation during confrontation with a chronically stressful stimulus. He studied phobic patients during the course of their treatment when they were confronted with the phobic object (flooding *in vivo*). Despite the very large increases in anxiety measured by self ratings or as observed by the investigators, plasma cortisol failed to show any increase during the flooding sessions. The session started at 7.00 at night which is a time of rather low cortisol but individuals, if sufficiently distressed by a novel stimulus such as being prepared for surgery, (Czeisler et al.) (28) are capable of showing a profound increase in plasma cortisol. The lack of response during the same time patients were behaviourally very aroused indicates the possibility of suppression and/or adaptation to a chronically distressing stimulus, i.e. phobic object, which in some ways parallels the results obtained in individuals exposed to chronic work stress.

One interesting exception to the usually rapid adaptation shown by cortisol following a repeated exposure to initially provocative stimuli was described by Weiss et al. (121). They subjected rats to a single inescapable shock or repeatedly forced them to swim in cold water daily for several minutes over a two week period. Those animals who had repeated exposure to shock showed adaptation as manifested by failure to show elevated corticoid levels following the final day of exposure to shock. However, animals exposed to chronic swimming experiences failed to adapt and showed elevated corticosterone following the final day of either another swimming experience similar to that after being subjected for the first time to an inescapable shock. This is an unusual study, without much precedent in the literature, and may reflect a special difficulty these animals have in adapting to swimming, although this remains unclear.

However, most studies in animals and man report that adaptation to chronic stress occurs rather rapidly and that reexposure to a familiar stimulus which was initially distressing, fails to lead to adrenocortical activation. In contrast, studies of adrenomedullary activity as measured by epinephrine and norepinephrine excretion suggest that adaptation may not occur as rapidly as would appear from studies of adrenocortical function.

Chronic Stress and Illness

In some of the theoretical literature on stress and illness, the authors have hypothesized that after exposure to chronically stressful stimuli or life events individuals tend to develop an illness or, to put it more precisely, are at an increased risk for developing illness. It has been postulated that one possible mechanism accounting for this increased predisposition is chronic alteration of endocrine activity. This concept evolved from studies of the way in which a large variety of potentially stressful stimuli produce significant changes in a variety of endocrine systems. However, as noted above, man and animal do not demonstrate altered endocrine activity following repeated exposure to stressful stimuli. If altered endocrine state does represent a pathogenic mechanism involved in becoming ill following exposure to repeated stressful life events, then one must document such altered endocrine responses in those exposed to chronic and not just acute stressful stimuli. Most studies fail to find continued alterations of endocrine activity in chronically exposed animals or humans.

Exposure to acutely stressful stimuli leads to reduced protein synthesis in rat brain, a result which could have adverse developmental sequelae. Kuhn and co-workers (57) studied the effects of maternal deprivation in rat pups. Animals that had been separated from their mothers at one week of age showed a decline in immuno-reactive growth hormone which was reversed when the animals were returned to their mother. This change in growth hormone was not accompanied by changes in corticosterone or prolactin but did parallel the decrease in ornithine decarboxylase (ODC) which is a crucial enzyme in the brain catalyzing protein synthesis.

Several studies have been reported that show pathological sequelae following repeated exposure to stressful stimuli although little adrenocortical change has occurred. Natelson et al. (76) reported the development of acute gastroduodenal mucosal lesions, lasting for up to one week, in monkeys exposed to shock avoidance experiments. This stress was particularly severe because level presses, which allowed the animals to avoid shock in an experiment lasting for ten to eleven weeks was reprogrammed to cause shocks at the end of the study. The gastroduodenal lesions, albeit short-lived, occur without significant parallel elevation of urinary 17-OHCS excretion.

Siegel et al. (109) exposed lambs to active shock avoidance during neonatal development, consisting of fifteen sessions over ages four to nine weeks, each session consisting of eight two-second period of shock. Both the experimental animals and the age-matched controls were then studied at eight months of age in active shock avoidance study lasting ten days. Both the experimental neonatally stressed animals and their age-matched controls showed significant elevations in plasma corticosteroid levels immediately following each avoidance session, no differences being observed between the two groups. This occurred despite the fact that the control animals for whom the avoidance was a novel experience lost significant body weight during the training period while the neonatally stressed animals did not show such weight loss. It is of interest that the previous stressful experience resulted in a form of "protection" from weight loss, and the authors concluded that this neonatal stressful experience did not appear to have a maladaptive effect even in light of the fact that both groups of animals showed similar arousal response as measured by plasma corticoids. Thus the experimental animals, when later re-exposed to shock avoidance, did not show any differences from controls in endocrine response, although they had a differential response in terms of weight loss. One thus concludes that one would have to look elsewhere outside the adrenocortical system or another non-endocrine mediator, to assess the relevant physiological variable to explain the differential weight loss in the experimental animals.

In summary, exposure to chronically stressful stimuli or environments, associated with an increased risk for future illness, has not been shown to be associated with long lasting differences in adrenocortical responsivity. Data involving the response of other endocrine systems to chronic stimuli are generally not available. This raises serious questions about alterations in endocrine responses functioning as the underlying mechanism leading to the development of illness. One possible exception to this may be the influence of diurnal rhythms in endocrine response, to be reviewed later.

Endocrine Function in Psychiatric Patients

In a series of studies Sachar and co-workers demonstrated that some schizophrenic patients and some patients with major depressive illness have increased levels of cortisol secretion and increased levels of urinary catecholamines. In schizophrenics elevated urinary 17-OHCS were seen early during acute psychotic turmoil and fell during the course of the illness when the patients developed a delusional system which was interpreted as having a "protective" effect (100, 102). In the depressed patients with elevated cortisol production rates values fell after recovery (103, 101).

We now believe that there are probably two different mechanisms associated with the elevations of cortisol in these patients. In schizophrenic patients, elevated cortisol has been interpreted as an indicator of the amount of stress being experienced, whereas changes in depression reflect a central pathogenetic abnormality. Elevated cortisol secretion in schizophrenic patients is suppressed by dexamethazone while many depressed patients do not suppress with dexamethasone. As is described in significantly more detail in another chapter in this volume, the hypercortisolemia seen in depression has now been found by Sachar (101), Carroll (22) and other workers not to reflect the stress of the illness but rather is central to the disorder, probably reflecting altered levels of neurotransmitters in other parts of the brain as well as in the tuberoinfundibular area of the hypothalamus. The hypercortisolemia and lack of suppression by dexamethasone probably reflects a basic biological defect in some depressed patients, more prevalent in those with the endogenous sub-type.

Some patients studied by Sachar (98, 99) showed an increase in cortisol when they came to confront painful issues central to their distress during the course of therapy. Although this work has not recently been replicated, a change in cortisol may reflect the change in inner distress which they experience during the course of therapy. These findings parallel those reporting how individuals differ in response to externally distressing events.

Catecholamines

Systematic investigation of catecholamine response to emotionally provocative situations extends back to Cannon's time. His now classic research leading to the fight-or-flight hypothesis (19) clearly implicates epinephrine and norepinephrine secretion as sensitive to a wide variety of emotional stimuli. Catecholamines are involved in many important control systems including the regulation of blood pressure, heart rate, cardiac output, shunting of blood from the viscera to brain and muscle and mobilization of blood glucose. It has been known for many years that increases in catecholamines secondary to emotional stress, not only is related to blood pressure regulation but indeed may serve a crucial role in the pathophysiology of a number of illnesses, especially hypertension, cardiac arrhythmias and onset of pulmonary edema. Nevertheless, research in the psychoendocrinology of epinephrine and norepinephrine has lagged considerably behind research in the control of cortisol secretion.

This lag can be attributed mainly to difficulties in the measurement of catecholamines. Although we have achieved considerable consensus about a variety of methods to measure cortisol secretion, in which measurement of plasma levels correlates highly with isotope dilution studies, no such consensus exists in relation to the measurement of catecholamines.

Earlier studies concentrated on measuring urinary catecholamines by fluorometric techniques. These are extremely difficult technically and investigators were frequently plagued by high blanks and lack of reproducibility because of contaminating fluorescent substances. Epinephrine was differentiated from norepinephrine by subtracting one set of absorption curves from another and interfering substances would effect this correction. An example of these difficulties can be seen in reviewing the literature on the norepinephrine response to standing from a supine position. Earlier results indicated a five to ten percent increase of norepinephrine while more specific methods such as using radio-enzymatic techniques which employed the methylation of noradrenalin to form epinephrine by the enzyme PNMT (phenylethanolamine-n-methyltransferase) indicate a two-fold increase (60). Using the more specific radio-enzymatic technique indicates that resting plasma levels in the supine males are approximately 250 picograms per ml. which is considerably lower than data provided by most fluorometric techniques (36, 38). Even greater difficulty is involved in measuring plasma epinephrine. The best methods using radio-enzymatic techniques reveal a resting plasma level of approximately 40 picograms per ml., but this is at the low end of the sensitivity of the method such that a very great deal of variability is involved. Consequently, even today it is very difficult to measure reliably the basal levels of norepinephrine and epinephrine from which one can calculate the increase secondary to a variety of provocative stimuli (36). Reports of basal state levels of catecholamines in the nanogram per ml. range are very suspect.

Earlier results were also confused by the fact that different individuals show different rates of metabolism of injected norepinephrine (38). Although metabolic clearance of norepinephrine is relatively constant in given individuals, there is considerable variation among individuals. This means that urinary techniques which compare groups of individuals with varying stimuli may yield confusing results, unless the same subjects are studied in each situation.

I have digressed to discuss these technical issues because they raise serious questions about the previous results, especially when authors characterize some situations as clearly provocative of only epinephrine and not norepinephrine and vice versa.

A wide variety of situations have been shown to increase urinary catecholamine levels. These include exposure to examinations, watching distressing motion pictures, being forced to perform mental arithmetic, physical exercise, sleep deprivation and gravitational stress (66, 39). Earlier studies, similar to those in the cortisol literature, did not differentiate between individuals, even though it was apparent that significant individual differences were observed, given the variances in group mean values. Whether these relate to the differences in arousal or relate to problems in methodology are not clear.

Earlier work by Ax (5) and Funkenstein (40) suggested that certain individuals were norepinephrine responders (designated by them as "anger out") and other epinephrine responders ("anger in"). There is now serious question as to whether or not this conclusion is valid, because of methodological issues raised above as well as the fact that their data have not been replicated using more sophisticated radioenzymatic techniques.

Mason and colleagues found using fluorometric techniques that exposure of rhesus monkeys to noxious stimuli with unpredictability and uncertainty, blood epinephrine and norepinephrine were found to increase (66). However, they reported that when the stimulus was merely noxious and repetitive or stereotyped, epinephrine did not increase and norepinephrine alone was elevated. This conclusion is analogous to that reported by Frankenhaeuser (39) who found that conditions characterized by novelty, anticipation and unpredictability were associated with rises in fluorometrically measured epinephrine in the urine. When the subjects appear to gain control over the situation and move from a state of helplessness to mastery, epinephrine fell. Norepinephrine secretion appeared more related to whether or not the situation was atention-demanding or there was vigilance or increased effort associated with the task. Whether or not these differences which discriminate between epinephrine and norepinephrine, as suggested by these groups of workers, will hold when specific and sensitive plasma techniques are employed rather than fluorometric techniques in plasma or urine, is yet to be demonstrated. However, recent work reported by Dimsdale and Moss (30), utilizing the more sensitive and reliable plasma radioenzymatic assay technique, tend to support the concept that uncertainty plus vigilance are associated with increased catecholamine secretion, particularly that of epinephrine. They found that medical house officers experienced a significant elevation in plasma epinephrine levels three minutes following the start of their grand rounds presentation, which for most subjects remained elevated at about the mid-point or fifteen minutes.

It does appear that catecholamine secretion is responsive to a variety of psychologically distressing events in a manner similar to that for cortisol secretion. However, the psychoendocrinology of catecholamine secretion differs in some ways from that of cortisol (46). Catecholamine responses do not extinguish upon re-exposure to stressful stimuli as rapidly as do those of cortisol. Experienced parachutists continued to show increased catecholamine excretion when other endocrine responses extinguish when expert status is gained (117). Repeated immobilization stress in rats causes repeated adrenal norepinephrine increase (59); the authors of one report postulated that the adaptation of the adrenal medulla to repeated stress is characterized by enhanced ability to replace released catecholamines more rapidly rather than diminished release after repetition of the stress. These data are analogous with the findings reported by Henry and co-workers (47) who studied mice housed in an intercommunicating box system that led to repeated aggressive confrontations as one mouse had to back up to permit passage of another animal. They reported that more dominant animals, who forced more confrontations by moving around more, not only showed increases in blood pressure but elevated adrenal epinephrine norepinephrine were observed in these groups. They also found that tyrosine hydroxylase, the rate-limiting enzyme for norepinephrine synthesis, as well as PMNT, (catalyzing the conversion of norepinephrine to epinephrine) was significantly increased in these animals. Thus, the chronic social stimulation secondary to repeated aggressive confrontations between these male mice, was associated with increased levels and increased capacity for synthesis of both epinephrine and norepinphrine. These studies may serve as a model for the appearance of hypertension in individuals who are exposed continually to a potentially stressful environment, such as has been observed in air traffic controllers (95).

Another difference between secretory patterns of catecholamines and cortisol, is the difference in response to pleasant as well as unpleasant emotions (61, 71). Both catecholamines and cortisol have been shown to fall following relaxing or non-stimulating movies (64, 66, 39), and both hormone systems are actuated after viewing distressing, shocking or emotionally provocative movies. However, there is evidence that catecholamines may also increase in intensely pleasurable situations under conditions unassociated with cortisol secretion. Patkai (80) reported that catecholamine secretion increased during a game playing session which was described by the subjects in positive terms as pleasantly arousing. Weideking and colleagues (124) reported that plasma norepinephrine measured by sensitive and reliable radio-enzymatic techniques showed significant increases associated with sexual arousal and sexual intercourse. It is not clear whether these increases in norepinephrine secretion are related more to the arousal or vigilance aspects of these stimuli, or other aspects of pleasurable emotions, but there is an absence of parallel reports in the literature documenting the increase in cortisol secretion with positively arousing or stimulating situations.

One further difference in catecholamine and cortisol responses is related to predictive studies. There have been a few studies attempting to predict which individuals in a given situation would respond with either epinephrine or noepinephrine upon being exposed to the stimulus or environment. Thus, the relevance of differences in coping maneuvers of defensive styles that has characterized many studies in research in the adrenal cortical system have not yet been paralleled in the study of peripheral noradrenergic or adrenal-medullary endocrinology.

In summary, interest in catecholamines predates that for cortisol and is most important because of the very widespread and potent effects catecholamines have physiologically. However, research in this area has been hampered by several factors. Perhaps the most telling relates to the technical difficulties in measuring catecholamines either in urine or in plasma. Current methods, however, promise a higher degree of sensitivity and specificity, although to date this has been demonstrated more clearly for plasma norepinephrine than for plasma epinephrine. Therefore, it has been difficult to draw very firm conclusions regarding the exact qualities of potentially stimulating events on catecholamine secretion. Nevertheless, the bulk of the literature, taken as a whole, does suggest that catecholamine responses to stimuli adapt more slowly than that for cortisol, that attention or vigilance may continue to provoke increased norepinephrine secretion and thus, stressful stimuli on a chronic basis may be more stimulating of catecholamine secretion than that for cortisol. The nature of individual differences in response in catecholamine physiology have yet to be investigated and which differences between stimuli that lead to norepinephrine and nor epinephrine secretion are still unclear.

Growth Hormone

In many ways growth hormone responds in a similar manner to that observed for cortisol and the catecholamines. Growth hormone is responsive to a wide variety of stressful stimuli (43, 70). Elevations of growth hormone have been reported following surgery (78, 105), physical exercise (106), watching stressful movies (58), stressful interviews (2), both written and oral examinations (112), venepuncture (93) and taking psychological tests (73).

As noted in a recent review by Brown et al. (15), growth hormone is not usually as responsive as ACTH-cortisol. In most studies of stress which report both cortisol and growth hormone responses in humans, there are more subjects who show an elevation of cortisol than of growth hormone. The measurement of growth hormone responses to a variety of psychological stimuli, however, is complicated by the nature of its secretion. Growth hormone is secreted episodically in very large bursts which rapidly fall toward baseline (15, 93). This episodic secretion appears to be the usual mode of growth hormone secretion as well as that in response to specific stimuli. Growth hormone may rise from an almost undetectable baseline to a large peak and fall within an hour. Investigators who have studied growth hormone with frequent repeat samples often report that on control days there are episodes of secretion of growth hormone as well as that observed during the experimental day (15, 16). This greatly complicates the interpretation of growth hormone responses to specific emotional stimuli.

Also analogous to the observations made for cortisol and catecholamines, the anticipation of exercise, seeing a movie, or taking a test, can lead to even larger increases in growth hormone than that observed during the test itself.

Most investigators resport that cortisol and growth hormone responses to both physical and psychological stimuli can be dissociated. It is most likely that separate mechanisms control growth hormone and cortisol secretion (15, 87). Growth hormone secretion is influenced by both hypothalamic growth hormone releasing factor as well as somatostatin (growth hormone release inhibiting factor). The regulation of growth hormone secretion is complex. It has been shown that growth hormone is responsive to a number of different physiologic stimuli, blood levels of glucose and various aminoacids as well as stage of sleep. However, it has been demonstrated that the release of growth hormone to psychological stimuli is mediated by mechanisms that do not involve changes in plasma glucose (17) as many studies have shown the growth hormone responses to psychological stimuli occur without changes in blood glucose levels.

The dissociation between cortisol and growth hormone response may be related to stimulus intensity. Subjects who show growth hormone responses also show significant cortisol responses although the converse is not true, indicating perhaps that a more intense stimulus is needed to provoke release growth hormone than cortisol (93). However, Brown and Heniger suggested another explanation than stimulus intensity to explain differences between growth hormone and cortisol responses. They found that growth hormone responses were more prominent in subjects with greater field independence (17), but this has not yet been replicated.

Another dimension which may discriminate between those who are growth hormone responders from those who are not was reported by Green and associates (42) who observed patients undergoing cardiac catheterization. Subjects who were judged to be "anxious but engaged" during the catheterization showed cortisol responses, but those who were anxious and did not engage with others showed growth hormone responses in addition to cortisol. These results were in part replicated by Kurokawa and colleagues in observing growth hormone responses to gastroscopy (58). Subjects who were judged to be anxious and engaged during the procedure showed elevated free fatty acid levels but no growth hormone responses, while those judged to be anxious and not engaged showed elevations in both free fatty acids and growth hormone.

Another study reported by Abplanalp and co-workers (2) also provides information about the association between psychological state, cortisol and growth hormone secretion. They studied 21 healthy women through one menstrual cycle with repeated endocrine assays for cortisol and growth hormone. The subjects' endocrine response to stressful interviews was investigated. Those women who reported a significant increase in state anxiety following the interview showed significant increases in cortisol or growth hormone. Eleven out of 21 women had a rise in cortisol and of these, only six showed parallel increases in growth hormone. Of the eight growth hormone responders, only two did not have increases in cortisol, suggesting that growth hormone responses rarely occur in the absence of cortisol and seem to require more intense stimulation. Those subjects responding with both elevated growth hormone and cortisol had the largest increases in state anxiety following the interview. No relationship was found between trait anxiety and endocrine response or propensity to respond during different phases of the cycle.

One clear exception to the conclusion that growth hormone elevation rarely occurs in the absence of the increases in cortisol is a study reported by Miyabo and colleagues (73). They studied both neurotic and normal subjects during a mirror drawing test. Although the non-neurotic subjects showed cortisol responses, elevations in growth hormone were found only in the neurotic subjects, with no consistent elevations in control subjects. In addition, they found that among the neurotic group growth hormone responses were inversely correlated with cortisol ($R = -0.84$). This report of a rise in growth hormone without a rise in cortisol in this subset of patients is a unique observation, which requires replication and is not readily explained.

Another type of psychological stress that appears to have a significant influence on growth hormone secretion has been reported in those children who were found to have significantly reduced height for their chronological age and described initially by Powell and co-workers in

1967 as psychosocial dwarfism (85). Endocrine studies of these patients indicated a reduced pituitary-adrenocortical response to metyrapone as well as low or absent growth hormone response to hypoglycemia. Upon readmission to the hospital, the patients exhibited a very rapid catch-up in growth. At this same time significant improvements were seen in the endocrine abnormalities, with a return to normal growth hormone responses to insulin hypoglycemia. In addition, Powell and co-workers in 1973 reported that these children also showed an absence of growth hormone secretion that usually is observed during slow wave sleep (86). There is some controversy about this as Krieger and associates have suggested the endocrine findings were related to malnutrition (55, 56). However, their subjects were different and selected in terms of retardation of language and psychomotor development rather than on the basis of growth retardation.

In summary, growth hormone is clearly a stress labile hormone which seems to require a somewhat higher threshold of stimulus intensity before increases are seen. Research in this field may be confused by the abrupt episodic nature of growth hormone secretion as well as by the fact that a variety of physiological stimuli seem to influence growth hormone secretion. Nevertheless, studies of growth hormone secretions indicate that differences in coping style (anxious engaged versus non-engaged), may provide an explanation of why some subjects may show a response. It is also possible that the differences in being engaged or not may function as moderating or diminishing the intensity or level of stress experienced by the subjects and that stimulus intensity may be the most parsimonious explanation of why growth hormone is or is not secreted along with cortisol.

Prolactin

There are now numerous studies documenting the response of prolactin to stressful stimuli (14, 79). Prolactin clearly rises during surgery (79, 129). It has also been reported to increase associated with other procedures such as gastroscopy, proctoscopy and pelvic examination (52). The fact that women may respond to gynecological examination with an increase in prolactin may lead to a mis-diagnosis of hyperprolactinemia and to inappropriate treatment with bromocriptine (52).

There are relatively few studies of prolactin response to psychologically disturbing stimuli. Although this hormone has been reported to rise during parachute jumping or after induction of motion sickness (35) it has not been observed to increase following venepuncture. Similar to the observation that cortisol responses may be dissociated from growth hormone responses, prolactin responses may also be dissociated from those of cortisol (84) and growth hormone (74). Although there is insufficient evidence at this time to be certain, it does appear as if prolactin, similar to growth hormone, requires a more intensely disturbing or provocative stimulus compared to that leading to an increase in cortisol or catecholamine levels. It is not yet known whether there are particular psychological stimuli which are specifically provocative of prolactin secretion which are not at the same time associated with increased cortisol, catecholamine or growth hormone secretion. In other words, are there either certain psychologically stressful situations which are only associated with prolactin secretion?

Similar to growth hormone, prolactin is also secreted in response to other nonstressful stimuli. Prolactin is normally secreted in nursing women following stimulation of the nipple and is intimately involved in the production of milk (113). Stimulation of the nipple or areola in non-lactating is also associated with prolactin secretion in some manner (14).

The significance of prolactin secretion, secondary to psychologically social stimuli, is not clear. Initially prolactin was believed to be only related to stimulation of breast tissue following childbirth and secretion of milk, but it is now becoming increasingly clear that it has much more widespread effects in the body. It has been shown to have significant influences on androgen metabolism, osmoregulation, as well as influencing other metabolic events in the body (116). However, its exact role in homeostasis and its significant elevation in response to stress is as yet unclear.

Testosterone

In contrast to responses of cortisol, catecholamines, growth hormone and prolactin, testosterone levels fall following exposure to stressful stimuli. Initially observed in the rat following ether anesthesia (6), the fall in testosterone has been reported in monkeys and man as a result of exposure to a variety of different stimuli (90, 89). Surgery has been reported by several investigators to induce a fall in testosterone (25, 23, 69). The underlying mechanism however, remains unclear. LH or FSH levels have not been observed to parallel the fall in testosterone (23). As LH has been reported to fall following surgery in the rat, or suppressed by social subordination in the monkey (13), the absence of such a fall in LH in man is hard to explain. It has been suggested that the drop in testosterone during surgery may be secondary to increased corticoids acting either to suppress LH release by the pituitary or LH action on the testis (31). However, if the latter mechanism is correct, there should be a rebound increase in LH, secondary to the diminished negative feedback of falling testosterone. As this has not been observed, the mechanism leading to suppression of testosterone remains unclear.

Psychological stimuli have also been reported to lead to an inhibition in testosterone secretion. One of the earliest reports attempting to assess androgen responses to predominately psychological stress was our study which compared the secretion of metabolites of testosterone (androsterone, etiocholanolone and testosterone) in men during their first month of basic combat training in the army (90). In addition, we also studied a small group of men in Vietnam under threat of attack whose change in cortisol excretion was discussed above (89). Both the men in training and in Vietnam showed significantly lower levels of urinary metabolites of testosterone possibly reflecting inhibition of testosterone secretion.

We also studied plasma testosterone levels in 18 young men in army officer candidate school which provides a more direct measure of testicular secretion (54). Plasma testosterone levels were significantly lower during the earlier, more stressful part of the course as contrasted with each man's levels immediately prior to completion of the training course. Physical activity levels were approximately the same during the fourth week of training when the men's testosterone were determined and during the comparison 21st week. These results provided evidence that psychological stress can suppress levels of circulating plasma testosterone, using individuals as their own controls as well as comparing men with other groups. These results were replicated by Aakvaag et al. (1) who studied plasma testosterone and testosterone binding globulin in men during a rigorous five day combat training mission. The individuals studied experienced a significant fall in testosterone, associated with a rise in testosterone binding globulin. These changes lead to an even greater fall in free rather than total testosterone and hence a marked decrease in hormone available to the tissues.

These observations in men documenting an inhibition of testosterone secretion during exposure to psychological stress is analagous with several different observations in rhesus monkeys living in social groups. Rose et al. (91) showed that male rhesus monkeys who were defeated in social encounters experienced a significant inhibition of plasma testosterone which lasted for many weeks which isolated them from the group. This inhibition did not appear to be related to inability of the pituitary or testis to respond as several males showed a very brisk and significant increase in plasma testosterone upon being reintroduced to a group of sexually receptive females. It has been shown in this study and others that females may serve during the breeding season as a positive stimulus to increase plasma testosterone among male monkeys (7, 8). This study was replicated in another group of aimals who were defeated but this time as a group when their social group was displaced by another more dominant group (92). Animals in the defeated group also showed falls in plasma testosterone levels without any confounding influence of physical injury.

There is also preliminary evidence to indicate that plasma testosterone can rise during potentially stressful situations. Monkeys who were victorious following aggressive encounters showed a brief increase in plasma testosterone in contrast to the fall associated with defeat in the subordinate males (8, 9). Analogous observations in humans have not been done.

Stress has been shown to influence the onset of puberty in the male rhesus monkey (94). Males who experience significant physical trauma in their third year fail to show the characteristic rise in testosterone that occurs during the breeding season when they are three, but did so the following year. In addition, juvenile males who lived in groups with a significant number of older adult males had lower testosterone levels than late juveniles living with fewer older males (94).

Ward has shown prenatal stress in pregnant rats leads to more feminine behaviour in male offspring, with lower levels of male copulatory behaviour and higher rates of female lordotic responding (118), which persists even after treatment with testosterone (119). She has recently shown that this altered behaviour is mediated by a fall in testosterone in the fetal male rats, secondary to the immobilization stress of their mothers (120). Although there are no analogous studies in humans, these reports raise interesting questions about the interaction between stress, androgen secretion and male behaviour at adolescence or later in life.

Other Endocrine Systems

There are a number of reports involving the responses of other endocrine systems to psychological stress. These include thyroid hormone, insulin, aldosterone, as well as many of the more recently described peptides including beta endorphin, the enkephlins and possibly others such as substance P. With the advances in neuroendocrinology, we have learned that the brain exercises some control over most endocrine systems. However, the literature on effects of psychological stress on these hormone systems is not sufficiently developed, especially in human subjects to warrant review. However, as we have observed with other endocrine systems such as prolactin, growth hormone and others, there is little doubt that these other hormone systems will be found to be significantly influenced by a variety of psychological events as methods for their measurement become more widespread and systematic study proceeds.

Diurnal Variations and Endocrine Responsivity

It is now well established that hypothalamic pituitary systems in man are closely linked to the 24 hour sleep-wake cycle (123). This is related to sleep but acutely can be dissociated from sleep. There is now abundant evidence for diurnal cycles in the secretion of cortisol, testosterone, growth hormone, prolactin and probably catecholamines. The peak of the diurnal cycle appears to represent the sum of a number of rapidly repeating pulsatile secretory episodes, while the trough reflects very few widely spaced secretory episodes. For cortisol these intense, frequent secretory bursts which determine the diurnal peak start approximately three to four hours prior to awakening and last until shortly after awakening. During the day, there is a variable, intermittent number of secretory episodes, while the trough of the diurnal curve reflects a period of minimal cortisol secretion, usually beginning close to the sleep onset and lasting for the first few hours of sleep.

Kaneko and co-workers (48) have recently reported studies in the cortisol system that suggest that these diurnal differences are not only a reflection of a differential rate of corticotropin-releasing factor (CRF) secretion by the hypothalmus, but also are determined by considerable amplification of these differences by both the pituitary and the adrenal. Thus, they found that the pituitary is more responsive in that part of the day which corresponds to peak secretory activity to a given level of CRF, which in turn leads to a two-fold amplication of peak versus trough differences in ACTH levels stimulated by a smaller change in CRF secretion. Furthermore, the adrenal also is differentially receptive to ACTH stimulation during that part of the day that corresponds to peak secretory activity, so that a given amount of ACTH leads to a significantly larger increase in cortisol secretion during this time. Combining the amplification of both the pituitary secretion of ACTH to CRF stimulation and the adrenal secretion of cortisol following ACTH stimulation, one finds a six to eight-fold amplification comparing peak to trough differences in the much smaller differences in the amount of CRF secreted during the diurnal cycle. Therefore, changes in diurnal variation appear to be both the product of differential neurosecretory activity from the nervous system during the circadian cycle, amplified by increased responsiveness in both the pituitary and adrenal cells.

The combination of both central and peripheral differences in responsiveness during the 24 hour cycle may account for the difficulty that individuals have in adapting their endocrine secretion when they change their sleep-wake cycle.

Akerstedt (9) has reported on a number of laboratory and field studies of altered sleep-wake patterns and circadian rhythms in the sympathoadrenalmedullary system, as measured by urinary secretion of epinephrine and norepinephrine. These studies, along with that of other investigators, have concluded that it is very difficult for individuals to adapt to the changes that are imposed by shift work. Individuals who work consistently at night but do not rotate shifts do not seem to have the difficulties of those who experience shift changes either rapidly such as one a week or even more slowly varying patterns once a month (125).

Thus, Akerstedt et al. (3) reported that individuals who shift regularly once a week between working at day and working at night failed to show appropriate changes in diurnal excretion of adrenaline or noradrenaline. The peak secretion that occurs during daytime working hours did not shift to occur at night when they worked at night, but instead persisted during the day when they were sleeping. They similarly found that individuals who shifted only once a month also had serious difficulties. Even by the third week of night work, they still failed to show the appropriate alteration in adrenaline excretion so that the trough occurred during sleep.

Recently, in a very careful study involving repeated measurements of cortisol secretion throughout the 24 hour period while individuals were studied in a sleep lab, but had flown from Brussels, Belgium to Chicago, Illinois, Desir and collaborators studied the effects of jet lag (29). They found that approximately three to four weeks following the individuals' westward flight from Europe to Chicago, the subjects did develop some evidence of local time appropriate peak (acrophase) secretion but failed to show minimum cortisol secretion before and following sleep onset. Thus, subsequent to the seven hour time shift involved in flying westward, individuals were still secreting large amounts of corticosteroids during a period of time in which the adrenal activity is usually quiescent. It was interesting to note that almost immediately, however, upon their return home following the 30 day stay in the west, individuals' endocrine pattern reverted towards normal and within the ten days was very similar to that prior to their trip, suggesting that the systems involved seem to "remember" their original condition. Return to normal sleep activity patterns was much more evident on their return back to their native environment.

Most studies of endocrine responsivity to stressful stimuli have not involved assessments altering the diurnal pattern and seeing how endocrine response might change (see also Chapter 12). There are, however, a number of studies which have shown that exposure to stressful stimuli at the normal peak of diurnal activity as opposed to trough leads to a significant increased endocrine activity. Thus, Seggie and Brown who studied corticosterone, prolactin and growth hormone (107) found that there was generally a higher level of endocrine activity when animals were subjected to stress at the normal crest of the diurnal curve compared to the trough. Duration of the elevation was more influenced than was the absolute peak response level. Other investigators (32) have found that the percentage increase of cortisol activity is greater at the trough but that is because the level is lower and the absolute increase in levels of cortisol is equal in crest and trough. In other words, expressed another way, it seems as if endocrine response to stressful stimuli compared to basal secretion became elevated throughout the entire day and that levels are higher both at the peak and the trough, thus the circadian pattern is maintained. These results are analogous to those reported by Akerstedt (3) who followed adrenaline secretion during 72 hours of a performance of a vigilance task. Adrenaline excretion following response to the stressful stimuli showed equal absolute increases when these occurred during the peak as opposed to the trough of normal adrenaline circadian curve. There are no studies to my knowledge of the differential response to a variety of stressful stimuli, of individuals whose sleep-wake cycle has been shifted by measures such as jet travel or shift work. This might be a fruitful area for inquiry to explain why individuals report such intense discomfort and difficulty in adapting to shift work or jet lag following air travel. There is significant indirect evidence to suggest that frequent changes in the sleep-wake cycle may be a significant stress of itself and the imposition of exposure to other additional stressful stimuli may produce physiological changes that are particularly maladaptive, but this has yet to be studied.

Conditioned Endocrine Responses

This review has summarized some of the evidence documenting the sensitivity and responsiveness of various endocrine systems to wide varieties of environmental stimuli. Despite this, there is relatively little data relating to the conditionability of endocrine systems to stimuli, despite the very significant evidence for conditioned learning in the autonomic nervous system (72).

Levine and Coover (63) showed that rats having very limited access to food and water showed elevated corticosteroid levels immediately prior to feeding and drinking, which fell dramatically within five minutes after they began. This fall after feeding could be interrupted if the animals received water alone or an empty drinking tube. They interpreted their findings of rapid suppression in the pituitary adrenal system to reflect conditioning to stimuli associated with prior reinforcement.

A recent report by Graham and Desjardins (41) provided the first evidence for classical conditioning of LH and testosterone secretion in the rat. Males were exposed daily to a neutral stimulus, methyl salicylate vapors, immediately followed by access to a sexually receptive female for fourteen trials. On the fifteenth trial they were exposed to the methylsalicylate by itself and were found to show a significant increase in both testosterone and LH identical to males who only had access to a receptive female for fifteen days. This study provides direct evidence for the conditionability of the pituitary-gonadal system, which may account for the observation that the anticipation of sexual activity in men can be a provocative stimulus for increased testosterone secretion (17). It may also provide a theoretical basis for potentially altered response to stressful stimuli in those with appropriate past experiences.

Summary

The earliest studies of stress response have emphasized the wealth of endocrine responses to a wide variety of stressful stimuli. Early markers minimized the importance of the novel, strange or unfamiliar qualities of the stressful experience and the psychological relevance of the stimulus focussing primarily on the characteristics of one particular stressor. Early research overlooked the importance of individual differences in response to stressful life events neglecting the impact of differences in the extent to which individuals could screen themselves from the impact of a distressing life situation.

Despite its theoretical importance, there are relatively few studies describing endocrine responses to chronic stress. Most studies now find that in both animals and man there is rapid adaptation to chronic stress and re-exposure to a familiar stimulus which is once distressing fails to lead to adrenocortical activation. There is some exception to this in that secretion of epinephrine/norepinephrine may relate not only to the degree to which the stimulus is distressing but also to its demanding attention or requiring continued vigilance.

Despite the theoretical importance that altered endocrine activity may contribute to the risk of illness that follows exposure to chronic stress, little evidence is available to support this conclusion especially regarding adrenocortical responses where most data are available. There are several negative studies which report a dissociation between repeated exposure to stressful stimuli, physiological changes and elevated endocrine responsiveness.

More recent studies involving diurnal variation in endocrine responsivity suggest that this may be a very important parameter to evaluate. Individuals have considerable difficulty in adapting to rapid changes in their sleep-wake cycle with respect to the circadian variation of both cortisol and catecholamines. It is possible that interaction between altered sleep-wake cycle with the concomitant inappropriate endocrine secretion combined with exposure to stressful stimuli may be particularly maladaptive although this is yet to be systematically investigated. There is also recent evidence that documents the conditionability of the endocrine system which provides a further avenue for investigation of how endocrine responses to stress may effect long term health.

REFERENCES

1. Aakvaag, A., Bentdal, O., Quigstad, K., Walstad, P., Ronningen, H., Fonnum, F. (1978): Int. J. Androl. 1:22-31.
2. Abplanalp, J. M., Livingston, L., Rose, R. M., Sandwisch, D. (1977): Psychosom. Med. 39(3):158-177.
3. Akerstedt, T. (1979): Acta Physiol. Scand. Suppl. 469.
4. Anders, T. F., Sachar, E. J., Kream, J., Roffwarg, H. P., Hellman, L. (1970): Pediatrics 46(4):532-537.
5. Ax, A. (1953): Psychosom. Med. 15:433.
6. Bardin, C. W., Peterson, R. E. (1967): Endocrinology 80:38-44.
7. Bernstein, I. S., Rose, R. M., Gordon, T. P. (1977): Anim. Behav. 25:609-614.
8. Berstein, I. S., Gordon, T. P., Rose, R. M. (1978): Behav. Biol. 24:400-404.
9. Bernstein, I. S., Rose, R. M., Gordon, T. P., Grady, C. L. (1979): Aggressive Behav. 5:329-339.
10. Bloch, S., Brackenridge, C. J. (1972): J. Psychosom. Res. 16:25-33.
11. Bourne, P. G., Rose, R. M., Mason, J. W. (1967): Arch. Gen. Psych. 17:104-110.
12. Bourne, P. G., Rose, R. M., Mason, J. W. (1968): Arch. Gen. Psych. 19:135-140.
13. Bowman, L. A., Dilley, S. R., Keverne, E. B. (1978): Nature 275: 56-57.
14. Boyd, A. E. III, Reichlin, S. (1978): Psychoneuroendocrinology 3: 113-130.
15. Brown, G. M., Seggie, J. A., Chambers, J. W., Ettigi, P. G. (1978): Psychoneuroendocrinology 3:131-153.
16. Brown, W. A., Henninger, G. (1975): Am. J. Psych. 132(11):1172-1176.
17. Brown, W. A., Henninger, G. (1976): Psychosom. Med. 38(2):145-147.
18. Burchfield, S. R. (1980): Psychosom. Med. (in press).
19. Cannon, W. B. (1929): In: Bodily changes in Pain, Hunger, Fear and

Rage, C. T. Branford Co., Boston.
20. Caplan, R. D., Cobb, S., French, J.R.P. (1979): J. Psychosom. Res. 23:181-192.
21. Carroll, B. J. (1976): Psychosom. Med. 38:106-121.
22. Carroll, B. J. (1978): In: Psychopharmacology: A Generation of Progress, edited by M. A. Lipton, A. DiMasco and K. F. Killam, p.487. Raven Press, New York.
23. Carstensen, H., Amer, I., Wide, L., Amer, B. (1973): J. Steroid Biochem. 4:605-611.
24. Cathro, D. M., Forsyth, C. C., Cameron, J. (1969): Arch. Dis. Childh. 44:88-95.
25. Charters, A. C., Odell, W. D., Thompson, J. C. (1969): J. Clin. Endocrinol. Metab. 29:63-71.
26. Cullen, J., Fuller, R., Dolphin, C. (1979): Psychoneuroendocrinology 4:107-115.
27. Curtis, G., Buxton, M., Lippman, D., Nesse, R., Wright, J. (1976): Biol. Psych. 11(1):101-107.
28. Czeisler, C. A., Moore Ede, M. C., Regestein, Q. R., Kisch, E. S., Fang, V. S., Ehrlich, E. N. (1976): J. Clin. Endocrinol. Metab. 42(2):273-283.
29. Desir, D., Cauter, E. V., Fang, V. (1981): J. Clin. Endocrinol. Metab. 52:628-641.
30. Dimsdale, J. E., Moss, J. (1980): Psychosom. Med. 42(5):493-497.
31. Doerr, P., Pirke, K. M. (1975): Abst. 10th Acta Endocrinologica Congress, suppl.199:228.
32. Dunn, J., Scheving, L., Millet, P. (1980): Am. J. Physiol. 223(2): 402-406.
33. Dutton, L. M., Smolensky, M. H., Leach, C. S., Lorimor, R., Hsi, B. P. (1978): J. Occ. Med. 20(2):111-115.
34. Eliot, G. (1981): Nat. Acad. Sci. Instit. Med. (in press).
35. Eversmann, T., Gottsmann, M., Uhlich, E., von Wender, K., Scriba, P. C. (1978): Aviation, Space Environ. Med. 53-57.
36. Falke, H. E., Kirkenhager, W. H. (1978): In: Circulating Catecholamines and Blood Pressure, edited by W. H. Birkenhager, H. E. Falker. University Park Press, Baltimore, Maryland.
37. Fenz, W. D. (1975): In: Stress and Anxiety, edited by I. G. Sarason C. D. Spielberger, Hemisphere, Wiley Press, New York.
38. FitzGerald, G. A., Hossmann, V., Hamilton, C. A., Reid, J. L., Davies, D. S., Dollery, C. T. (1979): Clin. Pharmac. Therap. 26(6): 669-675.
39. Frankenhaueser, M. (1975): In: Emotions - Their Parameters and Measurement, edited by L. Levi. Raven Press, New York.
40. Funkenstein, D. H. (1955): Sci. Amer. 74:192-193.
41. Graham, J. M. Desjardins, C. (1980): Science 210:1039-1041.
42. Greene, W. A., Conron, G., Schlach, D. S., Schreiner, B. F. (1970): Psychosom. Med. 32(6):599-614.
43. Greenwood, F. C., Landon, J. (1966): Nature 210:540-541.
44. Gutai, J., George, R., Koeff, S., Bacon, G. E. (1972): J. Ped. 81(4):719-725.
45. Hartley, I. H., Mason, J. W., Hogan, R. P., Jones, L. G., Kotchen, T. A., Mougey, E. H., Wherry, F. E., Pennington, L. I., Ricketts, P. T. (1972): J. Appl. Physiol. 33(5):607-610.
46. Hennessy, J. W., Levine, S. (1979): Prog. Psychobiol. Physiol. Psychol. 8:133-178.
47. Henry, J. P., Stephens, P. M., Axelrod, J., Mueller, R. A. (1971):

Psychosom. Med. 33(3):227-237.
48. Kaneko, M., Kiroshige, T., Shinsako, J., Dallman, M. F. (1980): Am. J. Physiol. 239(3):R309-R316.
49. Katz, J. L., Weiner, H., Gallagher, T. F., Hellman, L. (1970): Arch. Gen. Psych. 23:131-142.
50. Kehlet, H., Binder, C. (1973): J. Clin. Endocrinol. Metab. 36(2): 330-333.
51. Knight, R. B., Atkins, A., Eagle, C. J., Evans, N., Finkelstein, J. W., Fukushima, D., Katz, J., Weiner, H. (1979): Psychosom. Med. 41(1):40-49.
52. Koninckx, P. (1978): Lancet:273.
53. Kral, V. A., Grad, B., Berenson, J. (1968): Canad. Psychiat. Assn. J. 13(3):201-209.
54. Kreuz, L. E., Rose, R. M., Jennings, J. R. (1972): Arch. Gen. Psych. 26:479-482.
55. Krieger, I. (1973): In: Endocrine Aspects of Malnutrition, Marasmus Kwashiorkor and Psychosocial Deprivation, edited by L. I. Gardner and P. Amacher, pp.129-162. Kroc Foundation, California.
56. Krieger, I., Good, M. H. (1970): Am. J. Dis. Child. 120:95-102.
57. Kuhn, C. M., Butler, S. R., Schanberg, S. M. (1978): Science 201: 1034-1036.
58. Kurokawa, N., Suematsu, H., Tamai, H., Esaki, M., Aoki, H., Ikemi, Y. (1977): J. Psychosom. Res. 21:231-235.
59. Kvetnansky, R., Mikulaj, L. (1970): Endocrinology 87:738-743.
60. Lake, C. R., Zeigler, M. G., Kopin, I. J. (1976): Life Sci. 18: 1315-1326.
61. Lamprecht, F., Eichelman, B., Thoa, N. B., Williams, R. B., Kopin, I; J; (1972): Sci. 177:1214-1215.
62. Levine, M. D., Gordon, T. P., Rose, R. M. (1969): In: Stress: Physical and Behavioural Interactions, Proceedings of Second INternational Congresso fPrimatology, Vol. 1, pp.204-210. Karger, Basel/New York.
63. Levine, S., Coover, G. D. (1976): Physiol. Behav. 17:35-37.
64. Mason, J. W. (1968): Psychsom. Med. 30:576-607.
65. Mason, J. W., Brady, J. V., Tolliver, G. A. (1968): Psychosom. Med. 30:608-630.
66. Mason, J. W. (1968): Psychosom. Med. 30:631-653.
67. Mason, J. W., Hartley, L. H., Kotchen, T. A., Mougey, E. H., Ricketts, P. T., Jones, L. G. (1973): Psychosom. Med. 35(5): 406-414.
68. Mason, J. W. (1975): J. Human Stress 1(1):6-12.
69. Matsumoto, K., Takeyasu, K., Mizutani, S. (1970): Acta Endocrino. 65:11-17.
70. Meyer, V., Knobil, E. (1967): Endocrinology 80:163-171.
71. Mikulaj, L., Kvetnansky, R., Murgas, K. (1976): In: Catecholamines and Stress, edited by E. Usdin. Pergamon Press, Oxford.
72. Miller, N. E. (1969): Science 163:434-445.
73. Miyabo, S., Hisada, T., Asato, T., Mizushima, N., Ueno, K. (1975): J. Clin. Endocrinol. Metab. 42(6):1158-1162.
74. Miyabo, S., Asato, T., Mizushima, N. (1977): J. Clin. Endocrinol. Metab. 44(5):947-951.
75. Nagle, J. P., Cammock, E. E., Nyhus, L. M., Harkins, H. N. (1965): J. Appl. Physiol. 20:131-133.
76. Natelson, B. H., Dubois, A., Sodetz, F. J. (1977): Dig. Dis. 22(10):888-897.

77. Newmark, S. R., Himathongkam, T., Martin, R. P., Cooper, K. H., Rose, L. I. (1976): J. Clin. Endocrinol. Metab. 42(2):393-394.
78. Newsom, H. H., Rose, J. C. (1971): J. Clin. Endocrinol. Metab. 33:481-487.
79. Noel, G. L., Suh, H. K., Stone, J. G., Frantz, A. G. (1972): J. Clin. Endocrinol. Metab. 35(6):840-851.
80. Patkai, P. (1970): Rep. Psychol. Lab., no. 294, Univ. Stockholm.
81. Pinter, E. J., Tolis, G., Guyda, H., Katsarkas, A. (1979): Psychoneuroendocrinology 4:79-82.
82. Poe, R. O., Rose, R. M., Mason, J. W. (1970): Psychosom. Med. 32(4):369-378.
83. Pollard, I., Bassett, J. R., Cairnscross, K. D. (1976): Neuroendocrinology 21:312-330.
84. Popp, M. B., Srivastava, L. S., Knowles, H. C. (1977): Surg. Gyn. & Obst. 145:517-524.
85. Powell, G. F., Brasel, J. A., Raiti, S., Blizzard, R. M. (1967): New Eng. J. Med. 276:1279-1283.
86. Powell, G. F., Hopwood, N. J., Barratt, E. S. (1973): J. Clin. Endocrinol. Metab. 37:674-679.
87. Reichlin, S.: In: Textbook of Endocrinology, edited by R. Williams. Saunders Co., New York (in press).
88. Rose, R. M., Poe, R. O., Maston, J. W. (1968): Arch. Int. Med. 121:406-413.
89. Rose, R. M. (1969): Psychosom. Med. 31(5):405-417.
90. Rose, R. M., Bourne, P. G., Poe, R. O., Mougey, E. H., Collins, D. R., Mason, J. W. (1969): Psychosom. Med. 31(5):418-436.
91. Rose, R. M., Gordon, T. P., Bernstein, I. S. (1972): Science 178: 643-645.
92. Rose, R. M., Bernstein, I. S., Gordon, T. P. (1975): Psychosom. Med. 37(1):50-61.
93. Rose, R. M., Hurst, M. W. (1975): J. Human Stress 1(1):22-36.
94. Rose, R. M., Bernstein, I. S., Gordon, T. P., Lindsley, J. G. (1978): Psychosom. Med. 40(1):60-70.
95. Rose, R. M., Hurst, M. W., Kreger, B. E. (1978): Psychosom. Med. 40(1):86.
96. Rose, R. M. (1978): In: Psychopharmacology: A Generation of Progress, edited by M. A. Lipton, A. DiMascio and K. F. Killam. Raven Press, New York.
97. Rose, R. M., Hall, R. P., Hurst, M., Jenkins, D.: (submitted).
98. Sachar, E. J., Harmatz, J., Bergen, H., Cohler, J. (1966): Arch. Gen. Psych. 15:310-319.
99. Sachar, E. J., Mackenzie, J. M., Binstock, W. A., Mack, J. E. (1967): Arch. Gen. Psych. 16:461-470.
100. Sachar, E. J. (1970): Prog. in Brain Res. 32:316-324.
101. Sachar, E. J., Hellman, L., Roffwarg, H. P., Halpern, F. S., Fukushima, D. K., Gallagher, T. F. (1973): Arch. Gen. Psych. 28: 19-24.
102. Sachar, E. J., Kanter, S. S., Buie, D., Engle, R., Mehlman, R. (1970): Am. J. Psych. 126(8):1067-1078.
103. Sachar, E. J., Hellman, L., Fukushima, D. K., Gallagher, T. F. (1970): Arch. Gen. Psych. 23:289-298.
104. Sakellaris, P. C., Vernikos-Danellis, J. (1975): Endocrinology 97:597-602.
105. Salter, C., Fluck, D. C., Stimmler, L. (1972): The Lancet.
106. Schalch, D. S. (1967): J. Lab. Clin. Med. 69(2):256-269.

107. Seggie, J. A., Brown, G. M. (1975): Canad. J. Physiol. Pharmacol. 53:629-637.
108. Selye, H. (1950): In: Stress: The Physiology and Pathology of Exposure to Stress. Acta Inc., Med. Publ., Montreal.
109. Siegel, B. J., Moberg, G. P. (1980): Hormones and Behavior 14: 136-145.
110. Sutton, J. R., Young, J. D., Lazarus, L., Hickie, J. B., Maksvytis, J. (1969): Australian Ann. Med. 18(69):84-90.
111. Sutton, J. R. (1978): Med. Sci. Sports 10(1):1-6.
112. Syvalahti, E., Lammintausta, R., Pekkarinen, A. (1976): Acta Pharmacol. Et Toxicol. 38:344-352.
113. Thorner, M. O. (1977): Clinics Endocrinol. Metab. 6(1):201-222.
114. Timio, M., Gentili, S. (1976): Brit. J. Prev. Soc. Med. 30: 262-265.
115. Timio, M., Pede, S., Gentili, S. (1977): G. Ital. Cardio. 7: 1080-1087.
116. Tyson, J. E., Pinto, H. (1978): Clinics Obst. Gyn. 5(2):411-434.
117. Ursin, H., Baade, E., Levine, S. (1978): In: Psychobiology of Stress. Academic Press, New York.
118. Ward, I. L. (1972): Science 175:82-84.
119. Ward, I. L. (1977): J. Comp. Physiol. Psychol. 91(3):465-471.
120. Ward, I. L., Weisz, J. (1980): Science 207:328-329.
121. Weizz, J. M., Glazer, H. I., Phovecky, L. A., Brick, J., Miller, N. E. (1975): Psychosom. Med. 37(6):522-534.
122. Weitzman, E. D., Fukushima, D., Nogeire, C., Roffwarg, H., Gallagher, T. F., Hellman, L. (1971): J. Clin. Endocrinol. Metab.
123. Weitzman, E. D., Boyer, R. M., Kapen, S., Hellman, L. (1975): Rec. Prog. in Hormone Res. 31:399-446.
124. Wiedeking, C., Lake, C. R., Ziegler, M. (1977): Psychosom. Med. 39(2):143-148.
125. Winget, C. M., Hughes, L., LaDou, J. (1978): J. Occ. Med. 20(3): 204-210.
126. Wolff, C. T., Friedman, S. B., Hofer, M. A., Mason, J. W. (1964): Psychosom. Med. 26:576.
127. Wolff, C. T., Hofer, M. A., Mason, J. W. (1964): Psychosom. Med. 26:592.
128. Woodman, D. D., Hinton, J. W., O'Neill, M. T. (1978): J. Psychosom. Res. 22:133-136.
129. Yokota, H., Kawashima, Y., Hashimoto, S., Manabe, H., Onishi, T., Aono, T., Matsumoto, K. (1977): J. Surg. Res. 23:196-200.

Neuroendocrinology and Psychiatric Disorder,
edited by G. M. Brown, et al.
Raven Press, New York 1984.

Classification and Description of Stress

Holger Ursin and Robert C.C. Murison

(In Chapter 7) Rose demonstrates clearly that the endocrine system is very reactive to environmental and psychological factors, and, also to "stress". However, in order to clarify what the psychoneuroendocrinology of "stress" really is about it is necessary to first define and second to demonstrate the validity of the concept of stress. In our opinion, this is a more important issue than the reliability of hormone measurements. We also believe it futile to understand the brain mechanisms that affect the hormone levels without understanding the psychological functions that are involved. Recent progress in basic behaviour research seems to reveal fairly consistent and comprehensible principles.

The stress concept Selye described in his 1936 paper (27) was very dramatic. A non-specific response appeared after "diverse nocuous agents" such as exposure to cold, to surgical injury, spinal shock, muscular exercise and intoxication. The thymus, spleen, liver, and lymph glands decreased in size, fat tissue disappeared, body temperature fell, pleural and peritoneal transudate occurred, and gastric ulcers appeared. This picture differs markedly from the present day concept of stress research in which commuters, trade union members and air traffic controllers have their complaints validated against the level of corticosteroid derivatives secreted in their urine. While Selye (28) himself states that absence of stress only occurs after death, present reforms aim at eliminating "stress" from the work environment. This paradoxical situation reveals that we do not have any clear and generally accepted definition of stress and this problem is not solved by improving the methods for hormone detection. It may also be difficult to identify brain mechanisms for a phenomenon until we know precisely what phenomenon it is that we are studying.

A major problem with the term "stress" is the attribution power it has acquired in popular language. A variety of diseases are "explained" as due to "stress", and the self-evident remedy is to abolish stress. On the other hand, stress is also supposed to be an asset: it helps performance (9), it is actively sought by sensation seekers, and may have a training effect (see ref. 30 for further discussion). Further confusion arises from the fact that the term is partly used about the stimulus situation , and partly about the response. It may either be used as a noun for a state of activation and sense of time pressure or it may be a verb (I stress you, you stress me). To be stressed may be flattering, or a sign of incompetence.

A large part of the popularity of the term seems due to the acceptability of the idea that anything you do not like is bad for your health. If so, it is simply your duty to avoid it. This is within the tradition of the general and sweeping health definition of the World Health Organization. If health is a total state of well being, any "stress" that interferes with this well-being is not healthy. Within this latter definition it is not necesary that the state produces any known somatic disease. As a source of interference with life qualities and well-being it is a "non-health-producing" agent anyway.

To be valid for psychoneuroendocrine research the stress concept used must encompass as much of the popular use of the word as possible. However, it should also cover some physiological and medical reality. In the following we will identify the somatic process, the stimuli that leads to this state, and why it is of interest at all.

The Stress Response: Activation

Selye made it clear that we are dealing with a general and non-specific process. The relevant stimuli must converge on one process, which then diverges to a variety of (or perhaps all) somatic processes. Both Selye and Cannon used the term "general alarm reaction", but described only parts of the somatic response we now acknowledge to occur. The general activation theory based on the brain stem system described by Moruzzi and Magoun (21) is a complete system, which satisfies all the demands of such a model. This brain stem system receives input from peripheral as well as central sources, then produces EEG activation as well as muscular changes, behavioural changes and general changes in the autonomic system (see Figure 1) as well as the endocrine system, as is evident from Rose's paper (Chapter 7).

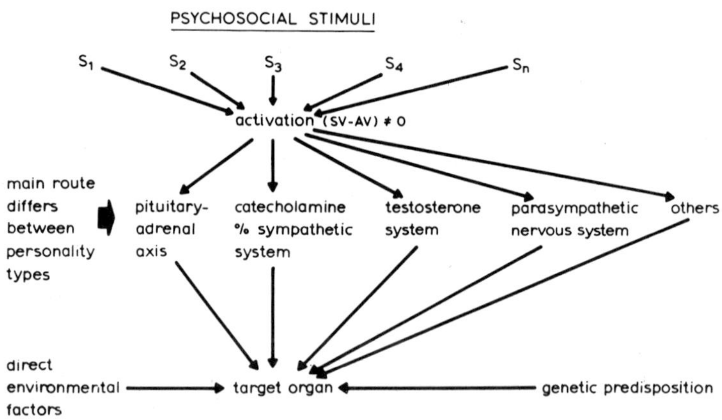

FIG. 1. The convergent paths between stimuli and the psychosomatic target organ via the activation system.

The use of the term activation rather than stress clarifies which somatic process we are dealing with. It also makes it clear when the response occurs, why it is so common, and why people seek it. The concept is reasonably simple to convey to the general public, and it has no erroneous attribution properties in the layman's language. This process is adaptive in that it will not produce pathology under normal circumstances, and it is not an atavistic "stone age" response which kills us as a punishment for our unnatural ways of life.

This is our basic position for evaluation of the validity and reliability of the measurements discussed by Rose. We regard them all as indicators of activation. The reason why so many indicators can be used for one process follows simply from activation theory. We deal with a general, unspecific response. The simplest operational definition of stress therefore, is that it is the process which produces a change in your favourite physiological parameter. It is reasonable to base the decision of indicator on reliability, convenience and economy. However, confusion and debate could be avoided if one realizes that, whatever measure selected, it is still only one of the possible indicators, and not necessarily the most interesting from a pathogenic point of view.

One additional point is that for multivariate studies some of the endocrine responses form distributions so skewed that they are not well suited for any type of correlation studies. This is true, for instance, for growth hormone with its great proportion of zero responders (34). Testosterone seems to have a bimodal response pattern, a shortlasting rise which is resistant to coping, and a pronounced decrease, which is subjected to the coping effect (see later) (6).

The Stress Stimuli (Stressors)

The word "stress" is also used to describe stimuli producing activation. Selye used the term stressor for the stimulus. In physical technology stress is used for the stimulus, strain for the "response". For instance, the law of elasticity states that strain = K . stress. The analogue model has been suggested for psychological stress (8), but most researchers seem more impressed by the lack of any linearity in the relationship between the stimuli and the stress response. Since the brain is built as network rather than a straightforward reflex automaton there is very little hope that we will be able to identify simple and general rules for "stressors", or that we will be able to measure them in simple physical terms.

We have no arguments with Rose on the characterization of the stimuli that qualifies as "stressors", but we would like to expand his discussion of working life realities since it is important for the validity argument. We find it necessary to discriminate between physical and psychological loads. The physical work load is relatively simple to measure reliably, but is not very valid for present day work or "stress" related diseases. Machines do the heavy physical work, but the "stress" remains, or may be even worse than before. The strain must depend on other types of load. Psychological loads consist partly of information loads and, partly of the load produced by emotional factors (29). The emotional load may be quantified by scaling subjective reporting, or by measuring the activation level (32). Information load does not cost energy and does not lead to activation in itself. When "stress" is reported due to high emotional factors, like worries about not being able to solve the problem. Since emotions require at least some information on capacity, performance may deteriorate further (14), which again may give rise to more emotional activation.

TABLE 1. CLASSIFICATION OF LOADS

Load	Physical	Work
		Environmental, Pollution
	Psychological	Information
		Emotion

The validity of the stress concept hinges on the possible relationship to psychosomatic disease. There is a remarkable agreement between studies in animals and in humans in what the essential psychological parameters are for the development of somatic pathology. Lack of control, poor or missing response feedback or lack of information on performance combined with high work load have been identified as pathogenetic factors both in rat ulceration studies (20) and in studies involving health and welfare issues for industrial workers (12, 17).

The Good Stress: The Adaptive Meaning of Activation

Cannon saw the activation response or the "alarm reaction", as clearly adaptive. It helps the organism to deal with acute, physical danger and demonstrates the "wisdom of the body". Later researchers (4) have been more concerned with the "stupidity" of these responses, which are supposedly inappropriate to the human condition in civilization. This rests on the possibly erroneous assumption that primitive man was mainly concerned with active and overt behaviour like flight and fight. Even in the animal world, however, inactive responses such as freezing and defensive postures are frequent and important aspects of the behavioural repertoire. Strong activation has definite unpleasant aspects to it. This has adaptive value since it motivates or "drives" the individual into finding a solution to a dangerous situation. The activation also aids the individual in acquiring this particular type of solution (9) even if there is a danger of overactivation and overload. Since it is in our power to dampen this response chemically, and since the experience of this state has negative elements, it is important to acquire a proper understanding of the state to avoid misuse of drugs and misinterpretation of the activation response.

Stress Dampening Mechanisms

When a solution has been found to a threatening situation, and the organism has learned that the solution is working, there is no need for a continued high activation level. Accordingly, activation decreases even if objectively the situation remains unchanged. This has been demonstrated for endocrine and autonomic variables in rats in avoidance tasks (1, 5) and in humans in parachute training (31). We refer to this as "coping" rather than "adaptation" (see Rose for further discussion). We prefer coping since "adapt" is used either as a passive process in sensory systems, or to express an attribution idea that explains any biological phenomenon by its existence: since it exists it must have survival value. Coping implies that brains are able to find solutions to problems, and, also that brains learn that a solution works. More formally, we assume that the subject develops a "positive response outcome expectancy" (3, 26).

Humans may also meet threats by perceptual distortions of the threatening stimulus (11). These mechanisms may be measured by paper and pencil tests, by evaluation of clinical interviews or a tachistoscopic method described by Kragh (18). The price for this activation dampening is that the situation is perceived less accurately and this activation dampening is that the situation is perceived less accurately and this may interfere with finding a proper solution. A high defense score on the Kragh test is correlated with poor performance in Swedish air force pilots and Danish attach divers (18), Norwegian parachutist trainees (31) and Norwegian divers (33). The defense mechanisms, therefore, differ from coping as defined here. It may be necessary for an individual to use defense, but coping is to be preferred.

Phasic and Tonic Activation

It is important to note that even in coping individuals some indicators of activation persist. This suggests that we have at least two different mechanism of activation, one subject to the coping effect, one that is not. Most of the physiological parameters studied in the parachutist trainees by Ursin, Baade and Levine (31) showed a marked fall with progressive training. This happened for the plasma levels of cortisol, testosterone, growth hormone, free fatty acids and blood glucose, and for the urine levels of catecholamines. However, heart rate and the difference between pre and post levels for epinephrine did not show this decrease. Also, there was some suggestion that a slight increase in testosterone could be part of this last mechanism. Ursin, Baade and Levine suggested that the two activation mechanisms could be referred to as "phasic" and "tonic" activation (Table 2). Phasic activation is the short lasting, fast acting activation observed in heart-rate and the long-lasting and slow activation characteristic of cortisol and the other hormonal changes. Phasic activation is not altered by at least the limited repeated experience given to the parachutist trainees. Similar physiological changes, at least for heart rate have been observed in personnel with very long training (2).

TABLE 2. CLASSIFICATION OF STRESS

Type of Activation	Phasic	Tonic
Duration	Short	Long
Phenomenology	Eustress	Distress
Effect	Training	Straining
Endocrine system	Epinephrine	Norepinephrine
	Testosterone	Testosterone
	Rise	Fall
		Cortisol
		Growth Hormone
Blood Changes		Blood glucose
		Free fatty acids
Circulation	Additional heart rate	Blood pressure
Effect of coping	Moderate, or none	Pronounced

The recognition of these two types of activation is essential for the discussion of the endocrine changes that occur during "stress". Increased testosterone and epinephrine do not necessarily indicate any danger of pathology. Quite to the contrary, the cardiovascular changes, for instance, may simply be a desirable training phenomenon.

Specific Activation - Specific Conflicts

The search for a separate "stress hormone" or the "best" indicator (see Rose) is a part of a general search for a specific activation pattern for specific conflicts or stress stimuli. We do not believe that this is worth searching for. One theoretical reason for this search was the psychodynamic hypothesis for the relationship between the environment and somatic disease. This position rests on the assumption that specific conflicts produce specific somatic disease. There is, to our knowledge, no empirical basis for these assumptions, in spite of a vast literature and a widespread use of the concept in psychosomatic medicine. Personality change in people with a serious disease should be considered secondary to the disease until it has been proven that this is not the case. Attributions to dynamic principles based on small and retrospective material still flourish. Hopefully, the "crisis" in stress research (35) may bring an end to this. The attributions accepted by the patient and the doctor in such a closed two-person feed-back system may be useful from a therapeutic point of view. However, therapeutic effectiveness does not elucidate or prove the operating mechanisms.

Conflict- or emotion- specific activation patterns have never been demonstrated. Lacey (19) concluded that only individual profiles existed, although a certain degree of response specificity existed within each individual. The individual variance produced by learning and by the dual innervation principle (sympathetic and parasympathetic nerves) is considerable. More consistency across individuals may appear in the studies of endocrine responses.

However, when endocrine responses are subjected to multivariate analyses, a fairly consistent picture of factor patterns emerges across studies. Rose did not refer to these studies, but he has contributed significantly to this area. The first such study analysed circulating hormone levels in 46 men undergoing basic military training (25). They found 5 factors; two factors related to androgens and estrogens, one catecholamine-factor, one cortisol-factor, and one factor related to thyroid-function. The suprarenal cortical activity was most consistently correlated with the effectiveness of the defense or coping operations, a finding which seems to be consistent with later research. Low epinephrine levels were associated with the ability to express anger openly. Persky, Zuckerman and Curtis (23) analyzed 54 male subjects, 29 mental patients and 25 hospital employees, with a battery of psychological tests and measurements of endocrine activity. Adrenocortical activity predicted anxiety and depression, whilst follicle stimulating hormone, luteinizing hormone, and thyrotopic activity related to affect expression factor. In a recent study of hormones in 71 parachutist trainees, and in 44 trainees in a longitudinal study, Ellertsen, Johnsen and Ursin (7) identified three consistent independent endocrine factors. Again, a catecholamine factor and cortisol factor were found, and in addition a testosterone-free fatty acid factor. We have reproduced these results in several unpublished Norwegian and American studies.

Both Rose et al. and Ellertsen et al. found the cortisol factor to related to high defense. In the Ellertsen material defense was measured by the Kragh test (18). As discussed previously, this test predicts low performance in parachute jumps, as well as in other performance tests. Correlations between the cortisol level and performance was consistently negative in our parachutist study. The largest negative correlations were found for tests with time pressure.

There are also interesting relationships between the catecholamine factor and psychological dimensions. The catecholamine factor related significantly to performance in intellectual tests and to performance in airborne parachutist jumps (7), and in single variable studies as well as multiple-factor studies by Frankenhaueser and her group (10). There is obvious similarity between the catecholamine responders and what has been referred to as type A behaviour (15), both for their psychological and their physiological constitution. Glass (13) has shown higher autonomic reactivity in the type A individuals, and this has been related to their susceptibility to cardiovascular disease. Special training programmes have been developed to produce other types of behaviour. This may rely on a misunderstanding of the data. If the present thinking is right, this personality type has a good chance to be able to cope with the environment. The high psychophysiological reactivity in coping individuals, or people with high ego strength (24), or in persons with high degree of internal control on the Rotter scale (16) should not be a source of undue concern and worry. Repeated short-lasting activations are not likely to produce any pathology, at least if proper rest periods are interspersed. However, sustained activation occurring in the non-coping subject, or in rats sensitized by preshock treatments have inreased susceptibility to gastric ulceration (22). Further research of this type is necessary to prove the validity of the concept of stress inducing psychosomatic disease. This approach appears more profitable than further improved methods for determination of even more hormones.

Conclusion

Classification and description of stress requires a consistent and meaningful definition of what the physiological process is. All the physiological changes accompanying stress may be summarized as "activation", a normal response in normal individuals which prepares the body and the brain to meet the challenges of everyday life. Strain may occur in the organism by activation, but the organism should not be compared with a passive machine system. There are also training properties in biological systems. Activation may be related to pathology in two ways; normal short lasting activation may be too great a load for a diseased organ, but should have only a training effect for normal healthy tissue. Sustained, long lasting activation without proper rest periods may produce somatic changes either alone or by interactions with other pathogenic agents.

The psychological conditions which produce sustained activation are to a large degree identified. Activation, and therefore the endocrine response, depends on the individual perception of the stimulus stimuation, the available responses and previous experience with stimuli and responses. When properly defined, the stress concept is useful and valid in psychoneuroendocrine research, and this research is itself important for understanding important processes involved in somatic and psychiatric health and disease issues.

REFERENCES

1. Berger, D. F., Starzec, J. J. and Mason, E. B. (1981): Physiol. Psychol. 9:81-86.
2. Blix, A. S., Stromme, S. B. and Ursin, H. (1974): Aerospace Med. 45:1219-1222.
3. Bolles, R. C. (1972): Psychol. Rev. 79:394-409.
4. Charvat, J., Dell, P. and Folkow, B. (1964): Cardiologia 44:124-141.

5. Coover, G. D., Ursin, H. and Levine, S. (1973): J. Comp. Physiol. Psychol. 82:170-174.
6. Davidson, J. M., Smith, E. R. and Levine, S. (1978): In: Psychobiology of Stress: A Study of Coping Men, edited by H. Ursin, E. Baade and S. Levine. Academic Press, New York.
7. Ellertsen, B., Johnsen, T. B. and Ursin, H. (1978): In: Psychobiology of Stress. A Study of Coping Men, edited by H. Ursin, E. Baade and S. Levine, pp.105-122. Academic Press, New York.
8. Eysenck, H. J. (1975): In: Stress and Anxiety, Vol. 2, edited by I. G. Sarason and C. D. Spielberger, pp.81-116. Hemisphere, New York.
9. Frankenhaeuser, M. (1976): In: Emotions. Their Parameters and Measurement, edited by L. Levi, pp.209-234. Raven Press, New York.
10. Frankenhaeuser, M. (1980): In: Coping and Health, edited by S. Levine and H. Ursin. Plenum Press, New York.
11. Freud, A. (1937): The Ego and the Mechanisms of Defense. Hogarth Press, London.
12. Gardell, B. (1977): Int. J. Psychol. 12:125-134.
13. Glass, D. C. (1977): Am. Sci. 65:177-187.
14. Hamilton, V. (1975): In: Stress and Anxiety, Vol. 2, edited by I. G. Sarason and C. D. Spielberger. Hemisphere (Wiley), Washington DC.
15. Jenkins, C. D. (1976): N. Eng. J. Med. 294:1033-1038.
16. Houston, B. K. (1972): J. Pers. Soc. Psychol. 21:249-255.
17. Karasek, R. A., Jr. (1979): Adm. Sci. Q. 24:285-308.
18. Kragh, U. (1960): J. Appl. Psychol. 44:303-309.
19. Lacey, I. J. (1967): In: Psychological Stress: Issues in Research, edited by M. H. Appley and R. Trumbull, pp.14-42. Appleton-Century-Crofts, New York.
20. Miller, N. E. (1980): In: Coping and Health, edited by S. Levine and H. Ursin. Plenum Press, New York.
21. Moruzzi, G. and Magoun, H. W. (1949): EEG and Clin. Nevrophysiol. 1:455-473.
22. Murison, R. and Isaksen, E. (1980): IRCS Med. Sci. 8:888-889.
23. Persky, H., Zuckerman, M. and Curtis, G. C. (1968): J. Nerv. Ment. Dis. 146:488.
24. Roessler, R. (1973): Psychophysiology 10:315-327.
25. Rose, R. M., Poe, R. O. and Mason, J. W. (1967): Psychosomatic Medicine 29:544.
26. Seligman, M.E.P. and Johnston, S.C.A. (1973): In: Contemporary Approaches to Conditioning and Learning, edited by F. T. McGruigan and D. B. Lumsden. V. H. Winston, Washington.
27. Selye, H. (1936): Nature 138:32.
28. Selye, H. (1974): Stress without Distress. Hodder & Stoughton, London.
29. Sheridan, T. and Stassen, H. (1979): In: Mental Workload, edited by N. Moray, pp.219-233. Plenum Press, New York.
30. Ursin, H. (1978): In: Psychobiology of Stress. A Study of Coping Men, edited by H. Ursin, E. Baade and S. Levine. Academic Press, New York.
31. Ursin, H., Baade, E. and Levine, S., editors (1978): Psychobiology of Stress. A Study of Coping Men. Academic Press, New York.
32. Ursin, H. and Ursin, R. (1979): In: Mental Workload, edited by N. Moray, pp.349-365. Plenum Press, New York.
33. Vaernes, R. J. (1981): Scand. J. Psychol. (in press).

34. Weitzman, E. D. and Ursin, H. (1978): In: Psychobiology of Stress. A Study of Coping Men, edited by H. Ursin, E. Baade and S. Levine. Academic Press, New York.
35. Wolf, S., Almy, T. P., Bachrach, W. H., Spiro, H. M., Sturdevant, R. A. and Weiner, H. (1979): J. Human Stress 5:27-37.

Neuroendocrinology and Psychiatric Disorder,
edited by G. M. Brown, et al.
Raven Press, New York 1984.

Neurotransmitter Mechanisms Underlying Stress Responses

William F. Ganong

Stimuli which we lump together under the term stress produce a variety of endocrine responses (10, 32). These responses, which are mediated for the most part via the pituitary gland, often include increased secretion of ACTH, and consequently of adrenal glucocorticoids. The secretion of β-LPH is also increased, since in large part it is released by exocytosis with ACTH from the same secretory granules (17). The function of circulating β-LPH is unknown, although it may be involved in the regulation of aldosterone secretion (26). Hypotension, shock, and some other stressful stimuli increase the secretion of vasopressin. Some but by no means all stressful stimuli also increase the secretion of growth hormone, and gonadotropin secretion is sometimes reduced. The secretion of the adrenal medullary hormones is often increased, as is the secretion of renin from the kidneys (10). However, the endocrine responses to stress are not stereotyped, and the response pattern varies with the stimulus. This variability deserves emphasis. Indeed, it is techniically correct to say that there is no "general stress response", only specific stress responses to specific stressful stimuli. However, many of the responses, particularly the pituitary-adrenocortical responses, are common to a large number of stressful stimuli, and because of this commonality, it is appropriate to talk of stress responses in the general snese. The important point, it seems to me, is to avoid the logical fallacy of reasoning from the general to the specific. For example, one sometimes hears the argument that stress increases ACTH secretion, and that a particular stimulus is a stress, so the particular stimulus must increase ACTH secretion. This may or may not be true, but the matter can only be settled by measuring the ACTH response to the stimulus.

In this essay, the regulation of anterior pituitary secretion is discussed and the role of neurotransmitters in the process is analyzed, using ACTH as an example.

REGULATION OF ANTERIOR PITUITARY SECRETION BY FEEDBACK AND NEURAL INPUT

The secretion of the anterior pituitary gland is regulated in part by feedback of target organ hormones directly on the pituitary, but the primary regulation is via hypophysiotropic hormones. In all probability, these hormones are all synthesized by neurons in the hypothalamus and secreted into the portal-hypophysial vessels. The seven generally accepted hypophysiotropic hormones are listed in Figure 1. The discharge of the hormone-secreting neurons is regulated in some instances by feedback of hormones on the hypothalamus, but it is also regulated by impulses in neural pathways that converge on the hypothalamus from many other parts of the brain (11). ACTH is a good example. The resting output of this pituitary hormone is stabilized by the negative feedback effect of cortisol on the anterior pituitary (Figure 2), while converging neural pathways provide an emergency override by which stress via corticotropin releasing hormone (CRH) can produce prompt increases in ACTH secretion. A similar diagram can be drawn for the secretion of TSH, with thyroid hormones exerting a negative feedback effect on the anterior pituitary, and for the gonadotropic hormones, with negative feedback being exerted in this case on the hypothalamus as well as the anterior pituitary. In the case of the gonadotropins, there is the added feature of positive feedback producing the ovulatory surge of LH secretion. Prolactin and growth hormone are each regulated by two hypophysiotropic hormones, one excitatory and one inhibitory (Figure 1).

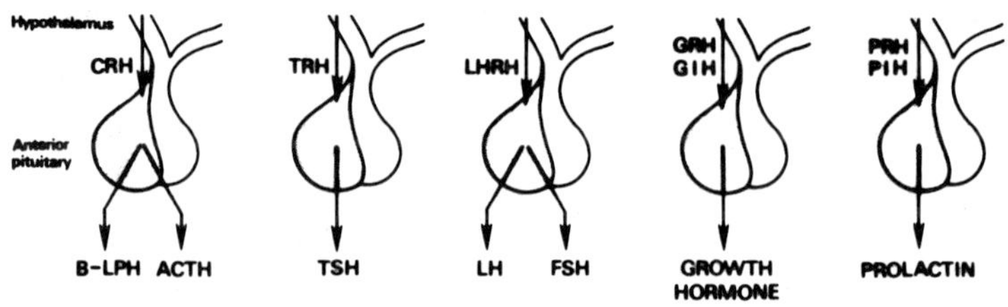

FIG. 1. Hypothalamic hypophysiotropic hormones. CRH, corticotropin releasing hormone; TRH, thyrotropin releasing hormone; LHRH, luteinizing hormone releasing hormone; GRH, growth hormone releasing hormone; GIH, somatostatin; PRH, prolactin releasing hormone; PIH, prolactin inhibiting hormone. From (11).

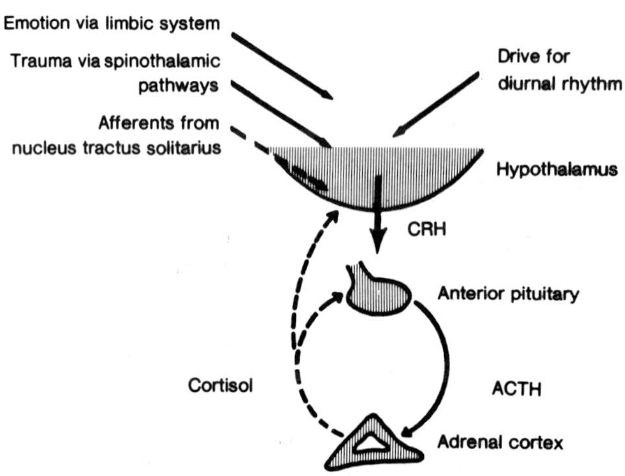

FIG. 2. Control of ACTH secretion. The solid arrows indicate stimulation and the dashed arrows indicate inhibition. From (11).

Therefore, converging stimuli can effect the secretion of each of these pituitary hormones by altering the secretion of its excitatory or the inhibitory hypophysiotropic hormone. The secretion of growth hormone, for example, can be increased by increasing the secretion of growth hormone releasing hormone or by decreasing the secretion of somatostatin. There is evidence for negative feedback effects of prolactin and growth hormone on their own secretion, and in the case of prolactin, the feedback effect is brought about by increasing the secretion of the prolactin inhibiting hormone (1).

The important point in the present context is that multiple neural inputs converge on the hypothalamic neurons that secrete hypophysiotropic hormones. Since these inputs come from many different parts of the brain and are undoubtedly of varying complexity, it is not surprising that a large number of synaptic transmitters affect the secretion of hypophysiotropic hormones. Much attention has been focussed on the role of the amine neurotransmitters, probably because of our detailed knowledge of the anatomy of the aminergic systems in the brain (Figure 3) and the many pharmacological agents that can be used to modify central aminergic transmission. However, other neurotransmitters are already known to have pronounced effects on the secretion of anterior pituitary hormones (8, 19), and it seems likely that when all the pathways and transmitters have finally been mapped, there will be respresentatives of all classes of transmitters in the neural pathways regulating anterior pituitary secretion.

ACTH

ACTH provides a good example of the role of amines and other neurotransmitters in the regulation of anterior pituitary secretion. The possible sites of action of neurotransmitters in the regulation of ACTH are summarized in Figure 4. The transmitters could, of course, be secreted at the endings of the converging neurons on the somas of the CRH-secreting neurons, or secreted some distance away in multineuron chains that end on the CRH-secreting neurons. They could also be secreted in the median eminence and act to modify the release of CRH from the endings of the putative CRH-secreting neurons, or they could be secreted directly into the portal vessels and act directly on the anterior pituitary.

A direct effect of neurotransmitters transported by the portal vessels to the pituitary seem unlikely in most instances; at one time or another, the various monoamines and acetylcholine have been tested on incubated pituitaries and generally found to be without an effect on ACTH release (41). One possible exception is norepinephrine in the rat. Norepinephrine has been reported to stimulate release of ACTH from dispersed rat pituitary cells, and the effect appears to be mediated by an α-andrenergic receptor (14, 37). A direct excitatory effect of norepinephrine on the pituitary is consistent with the observation that systemic administration of catecholamines in rats increases ACTH secretion. Indeed, the late C.N.H. Long developed a theory that the ACTH response to all stresses was due to an increase in circulating catecholamines secreted from the adrenal medulla (24). Howver, systemically administered catecholamines do not increase ACTH secretion in dogs or humans (4). The inhibitory effect of centrally released norepinephrine on ACTH secretion is discussed below. Parenthetically, however, it is worth noting that some of the difficulty demonstrating inhibition of ACTH secretion by centrally released catecholamines in rats as opposed to dogs could be due to a central inhibitory effect on CRH secretion being masked in the former species by the direct excitatory effect of catecholamines on ACTH secreting cells.

The possibility that the release of CRH and other hypophysiotropic hormones in the median eminence is modified by neurons that make axonal contacts with the terminals of the hypophysiotropic neurons has been

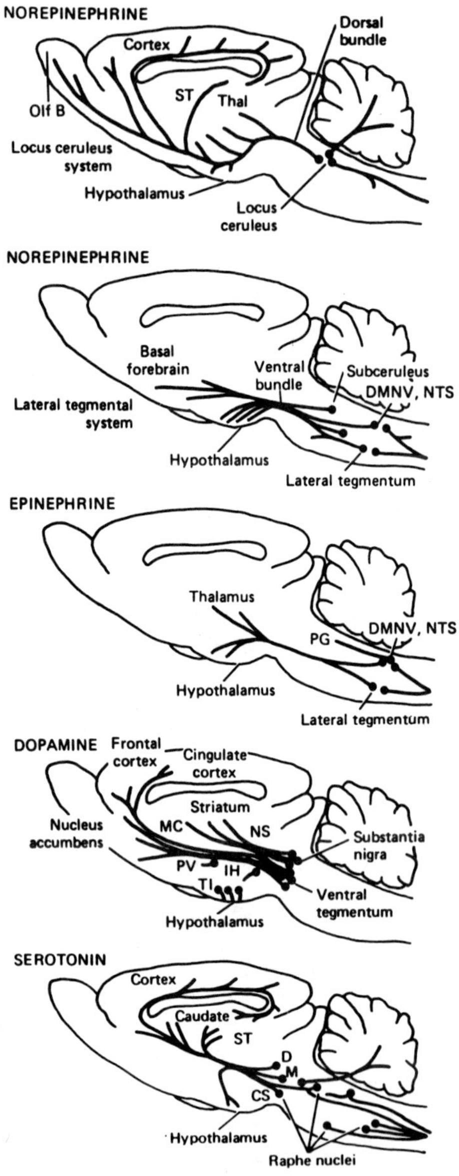

FIG. 3. Aminergic pathways in rat brain. The pathways in humans are similar. The 2 principal noradrenergic systems (locus ceruleus and lateral tegmental) are shown separately. Olf B, olfactory bulb; Thal, thalamus; ST, stria terminalis; DMNV, dorsal motor nucleus of vagus; NTS, nucleus of tractus solitarius; PG, periaqueductal gray; NS, nigrostriatal system; MC, mesocortical system; PV, periventricular system; MC, mesocortical system; PV, periventricular system; IH, incertohypothalamic system; TI, tuberoinfundibular system; D, M, and CS, dorsal, medial, and central superior raphe nuclei. From (11).

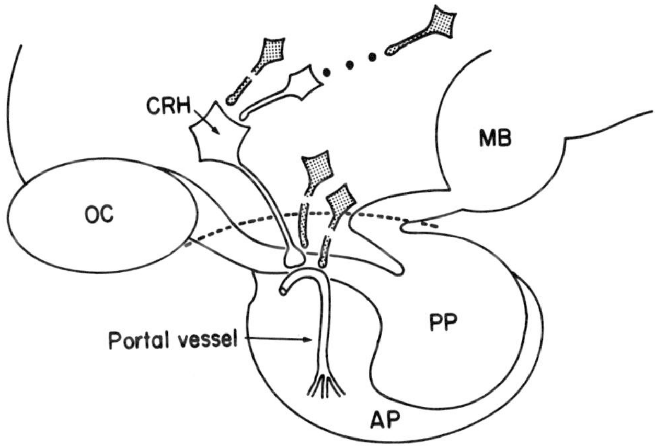

FIG. 4. Possible sites of action of neurotransmitters on ACTH secretion. The shaded neurons are postulated to secrete a particular transmitter (see text). The dashed line represents the blood-brain barrier. CRH, putative neuron secreting CRH; OC, optic chiasm; MB, mammillary body; AP, anterior pituitary; PP, posterior pituitary. From (7).

extensively discussed. One problem is that axoaxonal endings have not been identified morphologically in the median eminence of mammals (8, 41). However, monoamines may diffuse in brain extracellular fluid and act on neurons some distance away without morphologically defined subsynaptic specialization, and paracrine communication of this type has been postulated to occur in the case of serotonin in the median eminence (2). Fortunately, there is a pharmacological means for distinguishing between axoaxonal effects in the median eminence and more central actions of neurotransmitters. The median eminence is "outside the blood brain barrier" (29) and neurotransmitters acting in this location are effective upon systemic administration, whereas neurotransmitters that normally act centrally "inside the blood brain barrier" are only effective when they are injected or released within the central nervous system.

It is difficult to determine whether a given neurotransmitter that is only effective upon central release or administration is acting directly on CRH secreting neurons or in chains of converging neurons many synapses away. Indeed, there is even some debate about whether all the CRH neurons are intrahypothalamic in location (20, 27, 42). However, it is possible to narrow down the locus of action of neurotransmitters in the brain by appropriately controlled local injection experiments and by testing the effects of appropriate drugs after sectioning neural connections to the hypothalamus (hypothalamic "deafferentiation").

An additional problem in the case of ACTH is the possibility that neural effects are mediated via vasopressin. Vasopressin has appreciable CRH activity (15). Vasopressin-containing neurons of the paraventricular nucleus project to the median eminence, and there is vasopressin in portal hypophyseal blood (35). The vasopressin and neurophysin content of the median eminence are affected by adrenalectomy and steroid treatment. A number of investigators have argued that "CRH" is actually made up of two or more interacting factors, one of which is vasopressin

(15). Evidence for involvement of vasopressin in the regulation of ACTH secretion includes the observation by several investigators (although not by all) that ACTH responses to stressful stimuli are subnormal in Brattleboro rats that are congenitally unable to synthesize vasopressin. An example is the response to angiotensin II. When administered intraventricularly, this peptide stimulates the secretion of vasopressin and ACTH in normal rats. In Brattleboro rats in which there is no vasopressin response, the ACTH response to angiotensin II is present but reduced (12). Therefore, in considering the effect of neurotransmitters on ACTH secretion, one must consider not only the pathways converging on the CRH-secreting neurons, but pathways affecting the secretion of vasopressin as well.

NORADRENERGIC INHIBITION

What are the transmitters involved in the regulation of ACTH secretion? For some years, my associates and I have been developing evidence that at least in dogs, central release of norepinephrine inhibits ACTH secretion. Most of our data have been published, and have been discussed in several reviews (5, 7, 8, 9, 30), so they are only summarized here. Inhibition is produced by central administration of norepinephrine but not by intravenous administration. Therefore, the site of action of norepinephrine is inside the blood brain barrier, and not at the level of the pituitary or median eminence. Inhibition is also produced by L-dopa and by catecholamine-releasing drugs. In the context of the present symposium, it should be noted that ACTH secretion in dogs is inhibited by amphetamine and methamphetamine. We first reported inhibition by methamphetamine in 1967 (25), but we have recently conducted other experiments using amphetamine in pentobarbital anesthetized dogs in doses ranging from 15 to 250 g/kg. The results are preliminary, but there was inhibition of ACTH secretion as measured by corticoid output at all but the largest intravenous dose tested (W. F. Ganong, A. T. Boryczka and R. L. Shackelford, unpublished observations).

The receptors involved in the inhibitory effects of norepinephrine appear to be α_2 receptors because centrally administered clonidine, norepinephrine, and epinephrine inhibit ACTH secretion, whereas equal doses of phenylephrine and methoxamine do not (10). Clonidine has predominantly α_2 activity, norepinephrine and epinephrine have both α_2 and α_1 activity, and phenylephrine and methoxamine have predominantly α_1 activity (21, 23). The clonidine response is blocked by phenooxybenzamine when this α-adrenergic blocking drug is administered into the third ventricle but not when it is administered into the fourth ventricle (6), indicating that the receptors are in the diencephalon or its environs. Phenoxybenzamine blocks α_1 and α_2 receptors, whereas prazosine, which is a more selective α_1 blocking drug, has no effect on the clonidine response (R. Stith and W. F. Ganong, unpublished observations).

Are the receptors mediating catecholamine inhibition pre- or postsynaptic? There are postsynaptic α_1, α_2, β_1 and β_2 adrenergic receptors in the brain, but there are also presynaptic α_2 receptors on noradrenergic neurons that inhibit norepinephrine release (22, 23). Norepinephrine could be acting on α_1, β_1 or β_2 postsynaptic receptors to increase CRH secretion, and exogenously administered norepinephrine could act predominantly at presynaptic loci to reduce this excitatory influence. We have approached this problem in two ways. In one experiment, we administered α-methyl-p-tyrosine to reduce catecholamine synthesis, and then tested the effect of clonidine on ACTH secretion 20-24 hours later. This dose of α-methyl-p-tryosine administered on the same time schedule had previously been shown to reduce the inhibitory effect of L-Dopa on ACTH secretion (39). However, it had no effect on the inhibition of adrenal venous corticoid output produced by intravenous clonidine (Figure 5; M. Karteszi and W. F. Ganong, unpublished observations). In another experiment, we destroyed noradrenergic endings in the hypothalamus by administering 6-hydroxydopamine into the third ventricle and then tested the inhibitory effect of intravenous clonidine. Once again, the response was normal (8, 36). Therefore, receptors involved in the regulation of CRH secretion do not appear to be presynaptic α_2 receptors on the endings of noradrenergic neurons.

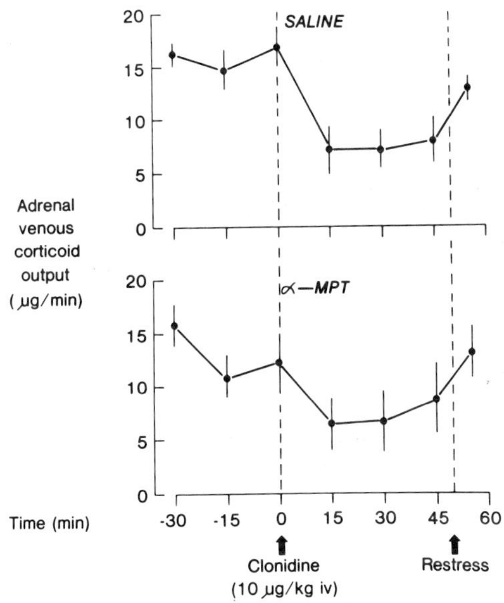

FIG. 5. Lack of effect of pretreatment with α-methyl-p-tyrosine on the corticoid response to clonidine, 10 μg/kg intravenously. Data from unpublished experiments of M. Karteszi and W. F. Ganong.

Another possibility is that there are inhibitory presynaptic α-adrenergic receptors on the endings of noradrenergic neurons that secrete neurotransmitters that stimulate CRH secretion. There is evidence, for example, for the presence of presynaptic cholinergic receptors on cholinergic neurons, for the presence of presynaptic cholinergic receptors on cholinergic neurons, and acetylcholine acts on noradrenergic neurons to modify their secretion (22, 23). Norepinephrine might act on acetylcholine secretion, and acetylcholine has been reported to stimulate ACTH release in some species (16, 19). This type of presynaptic activity of norepinephrine is not ruled out by either the α-methyl-p-tyrosine experiment or the 6-hydroxydopamine experiment.

Data on conscious as well as pentobarbital anesthetized dogs indicate that central release of norepinephrine inhibits ACTH secretion. Holland and associates (18) in our laboratory found that in conscious dogs, L-Dopa increased rather than decreased plasma corticoids. However, the stimulatory effect was converted to inhibition by pretreatment with the dopamine receptor blocking drug pimozide. Thus, it appears that there is a dopaminergic pathway that stimulated ACTH secretion in conscious dogs, and the stimulatory effect obscures the noradrenergic inhibition unless it is blocked by pimozide or pentobarbital anesthesia. The dopaminergic stimulation appears to be central, since it is unaffected by carbidopa, a drug which inhibits the formation of dopamine peripherally but does not cross the blood-brain barrier.

What is the physiological role of noradrenergic inhibition? An interesting possibility is that it mediates the inhibition of ACTH secretion produced by stimulation of the arterial baroreceptors. A decrease in blood pressure is known to increase ACTH secretion, and a pathway that inhibits ACTH secretion passes from the brain stem to the hypothalamus (31, 40). It is known that noradrenergic neurons project from in or near the nucleus of the tractus solitarius, the site of termination of baroreceptor afferents, to the hypothalamus (28), and noradrenergic inhibition could be mediated by these fibres.

POSSIBLE EXCITATORY MEDIATORS

What excitatory mediator or mediators bring about increased CRH secretion in response to stressful stimuli? The increase cannot be explained by a decrease in norepinephrine secretion because stress causes increased rather than decreased norepinephrine turnover in the brain (41), and the catecholamine-depleting drugs α-methyl-p-tyrosine and 6-hydroxydopamine do not cause a rise in resting ACTH secretion. The excitatory effect of dopamine in conscious dogs is mentioned above.

The possibility the acetylcholine is an excitatory mediator in rats is supported by in vivo and in vitro experiments (19). We were unable to reduce ACTH secretion in surgically stressed dogs by intraventricular administration of atropine and pentolinium (5), but this might be explained by species differences or failure to get the right amount of drug to the right part of the brain.

Another possible excitatory mediator is histamine. This agent increased ACTH secretion when administered intraventricularly in dogs, and so did the H_1-receptor agonist 2-methylhistamine (33). However, administration of the H_1-receptor blocking drug mepyramine in a dose that blocked the stimulatory effect of intraventricular histamine failed to lower plasma corticoids or ACTH in stressed dogs. Stimulation of H_2 receptors in the brain decreased rather than increased ACTH secretion, but the significance of this decrease is unknown.

Is serotonin an excitatory mediator? In dogs, serotonin and related drugs which increase or decrease the activity of serotonin receptors failed to affect ACTH secretion in any consistent or clearcut way (41). In rats, serotonin depletion produced by p-chlorophenylalanine (PCPA) converted the normal circadian pattern of plasma corticoid secretion into a flat curve that was higher in the morning and lower in the evening than normal corticoid values (34). However, serotonin agonists and drugs which increase the availability of extracellular serotonin stimulate ACTH secretion in this species (3). In the course of experiments on serotonergic control of renin secretion, we have also observed increased plasma corticoids upon administration of the serotonin releasing drug p-chloroamphetamine (PCA) and the serotonin agonist quipazine (38). The PCA response appears to be due to serotonin because it is blocked by administration of PCPA, and it is due to ACTH because it is blocked by hypophysectomy and mediobasal hypothalamic lesions (38; M. Karteszi, L. Van de Kar and W. F. Ganong, unpublished observations). These in vivo findings correlate with the in vitro observation that serotonin added to hypothalamic tissue in organ culture causes release of increased amounts of CRH (19). However, the exact role of serotonin in the ACTH response to various stresses in the rat has not been determined.

A third possibility is agiotensin II. This peptide stimulates ACTH secretion when administered intraventricularly, and immunocytochemical experiments have demonstrated the presence of angiotensin II-like immunoreactivity in neurons in the hypothalamus, including the median eminence (13). However, we were unable to block the response to surgical stress in dogs by injection of the angiotensin II antagonist saralasin into the third ventricle (8). The experiment needs to be repeated with more than one dose of intraventricular saralasin, but so far the data do not support the conclusion that angiotensin II is an excitatory mediator in the neural networks converging on the CRH-secreting neurons.

Many other neurotransmitters could be excitatory or inhibitory mediators involved in the regulation of ACTH secretion. However, extensive additional research is needed before a detailed picture of the exact pathways and neurotransmitters involved in the regulation of ACTH can be presented.

CONCLUSIONS

Stressful stimuli increase the secretion of some hormones and decrease the secretion of others. However, there is no uniform response, and the pattern of response varies with different stimuli.

Many stresses alter the secretion of the anterior pituitary gland by changing the rate of secretion of the various hypophysiotropic hormones secreted in the hypothalamus, and the secretion of these latter hormones is in large part under neural control. Consequently, it is not surprising that neurotransmitters have pronounced effects on anterior pituitary secretion.

ACTH is a good example of the operation of neural and feedback mechanisms in the regulation of the secretion of an anterior pituitary hormone. Resting secretion of this hormone is stabilized by the negative feedback effect of cortisol at the level of the pituitary, while neural pathways that converge on the hypothalamus provide via CRH an emergency override by which ACTH secretion can be increased to meet emergency situations. In these neural pathways, norepinephrine appears to exert an inhibitory effect. Excitation is produced by histamine and angiotensin II, and in rats but possibly not in other species, by serotonin and acetylcholine. However, the functional and morphological mapping of the excitatory pathways is incomplete and the nature of the primary excitatory mediator or mediators remains unknown.

ACKNOWLEDGEMENT

Research in the author's laboratory, including previously unpublished experiments reported in this review, is supported by USPHS Grant AM06704 and the Kroc Foundation.

REFERENCES

1. Annunziato, L. (1979): Neuroendocrinology 29:66-75.

2. Descarries, L., Watkins, K. C. and Lapierre, Y. (1977): Brain Res. 133:197-222.
3. Fuller, R. W. (1981): Neuroendocrinology 32:118-127.
4. Ganong, W. F. (1963): In: Advances in Neuroendocrinology, edited by A. V. Nalbandov, pp.92-149. Illinois Press, Urbana, Illinois.
5. Ganong, W. F. (1974): In: The Neurosciences: Third Study Program, edited by F. O. Schmitt and F. G. Worden, pp.549-563. The MIT Press, Cambridge, Mass.
6. Ganong, W. F. (1977): Fed. Proc. 36:1771-1775.
7. Ganong, W. F. (1977): Ann. N.Y. Acad. Sci. 297:509-517.
8. Ganong, W. F. (1980): Fed. Proc. 39:2923-2930.
9. Ganong, W. F. (1980): In: Catecholamines and Stress: Recent Advances, edited by E. Usdin, R. Kvetnansky and I. J. Kopin, pp.115-124. Elsevier North-Holland, New York.
10. Ganong, W. F. (1981): In: Advances in Physiological Sciences, Vol. 26, edited by Zs. Biro, A.G.B. Kovach, J. J. Spitzer and H. B. Stoner. Pergamon Press, Oxford.
11. Ganong, W. F. (1983): Review of Medical Physiology, 11th ed. Lange Medical Publications, Los Altos, California.
12. Ganong, W. F., Zimmerman, E. A., Hoffman, D. L., Keil, L. C., Shinsako, J. and Reid, I. A. (1981): Endocrinology 108:272A (abstract).
13. Ganten, D., Fuxe, K., Phillips, M. I., Mann, J.F.E. and Ganten, U. (1978): In: Frontiers in Neuroendocrinology, Vol. 5, edited by W. F. Ganong, and L. Martini, pp.61-99. Raven Press, New York.
14. Giguere, V., Cote, J. and Labrie, F. (1981): Endocrinology (in press).
15. Gillies, G. and Lowry, P. (1979): Nature 278:463-464.
16. Hedge, G. A. and DeWeid, D. (1971): Endocrinology 88:257-259.
17. Herbert, E., Roberts, J., Phillips, M., Allen, R., Hinman, M., Budarf, M., Policastro, P. and Ross, P. (1980): In: Frontiers in Neuroendocrinology, Vol. 6, edited by L. Martini and W. F. Ganong, pp.67-101. Raven Press, New York.
18. Holland, F. J., Richards, G. E., Kaplan, S. L., Ganong, W. F. and Grumbach, M. M. (1978): Endocrinology 102:1452-1457.
19. Jones, M. T., Hillhouse, E. and Burden, J. 91976): In: Frontiers in Neuroendocrinology, Vol. 4, edited by L. Martini and W. F. Ganong, pp.195-226. Raven Press, New York.
20. Krieger, D. T., Liotta, A. and Brownstein, M. J. (1977): Endocrinology 100:227-237.
21. Kobinger, W. (1978): Rev. Physiol. Biochem. Pharmacol. 81:40-100.
22. Langer, S. Z. (1977): Br. J. Pharmacol. 60:481-497.
23. Langer, S. Z. (1979): In: Catecholamines: Basic and Clinical Frontiers, edited by E. Usdin, I. J. Kopin and J. Barchas, pp. 387-398. Pergamon Press, New York.
24. Long, C.N.H. (1952): Recent Progress in Hormone Research 7:75-105.
25. Lorenzen, L. C. and Ganong, W. F. (1967): Endocrinology 80:889-892.
26. Matsuoka, H., Mulrow, P. J. and Li, C. H. (1980): Science 209: 307-308.
27. Palkovits, M. (1979): Neuroendocrinology 29:140-147.
28. Palkovits, M. and Zaborszky, L. (1977): Prog. Brain Res. 47:9-34.
29. Rappaport, S. I. (1976): Blood Brain Barrier in Physiology and Medicine. Raven Press, New York.
30. Rose, J. C. and Ganong, W. F. (1980): In: Perspectives in Clinical Endocrinology, edited by W. B. Essman, pp.1-46. Spectrum Publica-

tions, Holliswood, New York.
31. Rose, J. C., Goldsmith, P. C., Holland, F. J., Kaplan, S. L. and Ganong, W. F. (1976): Neuroendocrinology 22:352-362.
32. Rose, R. M. (1980): Advances in Psychoneuroendocrinology, Psychiatric Clinics of North America 3:251-276.
33. Rudolph, C., Richards, G. E., Kaplan, S. and Ganong, W. F. (1979): Neuroendocrinology 29:169-177.
34. Scapagnini, U., Moberg, G. P., Van Loon, G. R., de Groot, J. and Ganong, W. F. (1971): Neuroendocrinology 7:90-96.
35. Stillman, M. A., Recht, L. D., Rosario, S. L., Self, S. M., Robinson, A. C. and Zimmerman, E. A. (1977): Endocrinology 101: 42-49.
36. Stith, R. D., van de Kar, L. D., Kaplan, S. and Ganong, W. F. (1980): Fed. Proc. 39:488.
37. Vale, W. and Rivier, C. (1977): Fed. Proc. 36:2094-2099.
38. Van de Kar, L. D., Wilkinson, C. W., Brownfield, M. S., Skrobik, Y. and Ganong, W. F. (1981): Neuroscience Abstracts (in press).
39. Van Loon, G. R. and Ganong, W. F. (1969): The Physiologist 12: 381 (abstract).
40. Ward, D. G. and Gann, D. S. (1976): Endocrinology 99:1213-1219.
41. Weiner, R. I. and Ganong, W. F. (1978): Physiological Reviews 58: 905-976.
42. Yasuda, N. and Greer, M. A. (1977): Neuroendocrinology 22:48-56.

Neuroendocrinology and Psychiatric Disorder, edited by G. M. Brown, et al.
Raven Press, New York 1984.

Discussion: Stress

Seymour Levine

The mission which was entrusted to the discussion chairman was to summarize and edit the discussion and to highlight the critical points which emerged in the remarks which emanated both from the panel and from the audience. The issues could be divided into two major categories, which are: Definition and Function.

DEFINITION

The problems of defining stress have plagued workers within the field for as long as anyone can recall. There has never been a conference on stress which has not attempted to wrestle with definitional problems. This conference was no exception. Each of the papers attempted to deal with definitional problems; some utilized other words such as "activation", others attempted to categorize stress. As usual, no complete resolution was found. Some of the commentary objected to the notion of categorizing stress and it was stated (Levine) that, "I believe that with some kind of ingenuity, and a clearer perspective in examining the stimuli associated with stressful phenomena, that we could come up with a reasonable set of parameters which could effectively predict when an organism would show the biological response which is associated with those events which we classify as stress".

Perhaps one of the key issues which emerged from the papers concerned the difficulties of categorizing stress. An attempt to categorize stress in terms of its biological responses fails to account for the variety of stimuli which may elicit one or another of the endocrine responses which have been associated as indicative of stress. This issue was highlighted by the discussion which surrounded the effects of orgasm on prolactin. Thus, it was stated (Ganong) that, "Men do not have a prolactin rise when they have an orgasm. Women have a prolactin rise if they do, but no prolactin rise if they do not. The reason for emphasizing this point is not just to correct the record, but because, it seems to me, we are falling into the same old semantic trap of defining stress by the hormonal response. Just because prolactin rises, does not make the stimulus stressful. The same situation exists with other hormones such as ACTH".

What appears to be clear, both in the papers and the discussion, was that to define stress in terms of its response was both inappropriate and inadequate and that there are specific endocrine responses which may be associated with specific classes of stimuli and it may not be possible to come up with a "generalized" stress hormone. Ganong stated, "I would like to defend my statement that for each specific stimulus there is a specific response, if we have the wits to trace the pathway and understand it. Dr. Ursin and I are not in that much disagreement. The arguement is somewhat semantic, in that the pathways are so complex, they can be modified in a variety of ways and at a variety of locations. I cannot agree with the implications that we will never be able to understand the psychological complexities, or otherwise I would not be a neuroscientist". Clearly the dilemma of definition has not been put to rest as a consequence of either the papers or the discussion. It is still with us and will continue to plague us.

FUNCTION

The major bulk of the discussion dealt essentially with the functional consequences of endocrine changes that are associated with stressful events. Two major points of view were represented. Those dealing predominantly with the normal function of hormones, and in particular pituitary-adrenal hormones; and those dealing with the pathological sequelae which may be related to endocrine changes during stress.

These issues were best stated early in the discussion. Reichlin commented, "...perhaps endocrine responses are only important in telling us how the brain works. I would like to propose that the stress response, or the endocrine response to stress, is perhaps the same instrument to the psychoneuroendocrinologist. This is one way of telling us how the brain works in adaptation... The second point is the common notion that stress causes disease, which appears to be a residue of the Selye tradition. This is, perhaps pernicious. And I really think it is necessary to determine to what extent this has actually been proved. For example, has stress, however defined, caused organic destruction of tissue? I believe both of these questions are important."

Levine, in his opening remarks, made essentially the same points when he argued that with all adulation for Hans Selye, he left us with a horrible legacy: the legacy that equated stress and disease - and with a set of interwoven nuances with little or no data, which investigators have persistently pursued with little or no success. To some extent this has detracted from what I think may be the more important and interesting aspects of the activation of the pituitary-adrenal system, that it relates to perfectly normal functions. Most of us who study stress are not really interested in disease, but are interested in how the brain operates. We are concerned with how it processes information.

One of the major issues that has plagued behavioural scientists has been the issue of determining or infering "state".... Thus, the organism's distress, its emotions, its affect, have all been implied generally through some behavioural measurement. It does appear, however, that it may be possible to determine 'state' more effectively through some physiological response - either autonomic or endocrine.

These two issues, the issue of the interpretation of endocrine responses as a method of infering some aspect of CNS operation and the issue of pathophysiology caused by stress did become a major focus of the discussion. Ursin elaborated on the relationship between stress and disease. He stated that stress (or as he called it, 'activation') "does affect a lot of organs and may cause disease. If you have a diseased organ and add activation it is easy to document that this may cause functional disorders. A man with a bleeding ulcer, subjected to strong activation, will get worse and the most obvious clinical therapy is to decrease the activation. If one looks at the treatment of acute myocardial infarction, much of the management is directed towards reducing activation.

However, that is not the issue. If we are looking for maladaptation in the Selye tradition, the question is whether activation can produce disease in healthy individuals. I think the answer is yes, but I have to know what kind of activation and in whom, and more about the situation. Because most of the data are based on human studies, I think we are left with correlational evidence. Correlation studies are, and always will be, correlation studies, and will not tell us much about causation. In order to establish causation, we need animal models and I think it is in this interaction between animal models that we will eventually find the answer. Based on animal studies, I think we can now show that sustained activation will indeed produce organic disease. It has been shown for ulcers and for hypertension, and it has also been shown for mild myocardial infarction."

Rose continued with this theme by stating, "I agree with Dr. Ursin that most of the data about the relation of stress and illness in man is epidemiological and correlational, and it is risk data. As the result of stimulation by Selye, a whole host of workers have documented many hormonal changes resulting from stressful stimuli, but most of these have never been shown to be important in human illness and probably never will be. An examination of the stress literature would lead to the conclusion that physical disease, psychological illnesses and psychiatric illnesses are related with increased predisposition. Individuals who are chronically exposed to difficult life events or a succession of problems have not been found to have abnormal systems, but they are certainly different from individuals not so exposed. We cannot get a handle on that mediator.

One of the problems with the stress literature is that most of the animal work is short term and employs stressful stimuli that do not allow for individual differences in response.

The data that Dr. Ursin referred to are mainly those of acute ulceration. Weiss published an interesting study in 1975. In that study one group of animals was repeatedly shocked, and then on the last day of shocks, they were studied with regard to both corticosterone levels and brain norepinephrine. They were compared with animals receiving only one shock. The animals which had received repeated shocks - 14 or 15 times over a number of days, had decreased corticosterone and brain norepinephrine.

They then took another group of rats and forced them to take repeated 3 minute swims in cold water. They found that the animals which had repeated swims and then either an acute episode of swim or shock were very different. They showed no adaptation at all, with elevated corticosterone and brain norepinephrine levels."

Rose's conclusion was that, for most of the stress literature, very few individuals have looked at repeated experiences to see if the animals become physically ill.

In contrast to the positions taken by Rose and other discussants such as Ganong with regards to support of basic studies on animals, Carroll stated that he felt it was possible to induce real tissue lesions with stress and psychological stimuli. However, he stated, "I would like to make a plea for many more human studies on neurotransmitter pharmacology of hormone regulation. Work in dogs and rats is good, but it does suffer from the problems of species difference, and suffers in many cases from the interfering effects of anesthetics and difficulty in precisely controlling the subjective and psychological effects of the agents used to test brain function. Thus, we have made a beginning at mapping out some of the neurotransmitters involved in human ACTH regulation. Sachar and Halbreich have studied amphetamines and have shown, not a suppression but a stimulation of cortisol secretion. It may be possible, therefore, to take dexamethasone-suppressed humans (normal subjects) and demonstrate escape from dexamethasone suppression with physostigmine and L-dopa infusions. This is an approach that should be followed up by basic clinical endocrinologists, as well as psychoendocrinologists, so that we can develop a data base more applicable to human situations, rather than relying only on preclinical literature."

However, this view was not uniformly shared by all the discussants, and Rose commented, "I am still struggling with Dr. Reichlin's first question, whether hormones can be used to study adaptation? One of the most interesting themes to come out of the last decade of psychoneuroendocrine research is how hard it is to predict individual differences. Previously, I discussed a study on breast cancer, which was done with parents whose children were dying of leukemia. Although the study was reasonably conducted, we found it very difficult to look at an individual and say 'this person is adapting very well' and 'this one is not'.

We do need better animal models. Control and predictability are two of the crucial variables that determine whether or not an animal will respond, but it is much more complicated in humans, and yet we do find differences. Most of the time, people adapt quite well and turn off hormonal systems rather quickly, and this usually parallels their subjective response. Nonetheless, the prediction of response from a psychological, observational point of view is still very difficult."

Further discussions concerning psychoneuroendocrine functions illustrated an interesting controversy which was brough up by Dr. Michael Thorner when he stated, "in nature, when an animal is made sick, it is not carried to an emergency room, which is a highly abnormal situation. Here, we induce all sorts of responses which we then treat, while perhaps kidding ourselves that we are helping the patient. In fact, we actually produce the disease and then treat the disease we produce."

This question raises the old issue of whether stress or activation is representative of either the wisdom of the body as Cannon has stated, or its stupidity, as Hamburg as stated (Ursin), "The notion that psychoneuroendocrine responses are maladaptive in contemporary society was discussed and from at least one point of view, the argument was made that you have to make a distinction between man as we have in society and man that is natural. However, it is not true that, in primitive societies or in animals, strong activation necessarily leads to reactive behaviour which may be maladaptive from a societal point of view. There is a freezing response or a sitting response, that while seemingly inhibited, can be associated with a very high degree of activation - I do not believe that these responses necessarily lead to pathology. However, if this state is maintained for too long, pathology can result because it now becomes a non-adaptive response. An adaptive response is one that is part of the homeostatic regulation but cannot be endured for too long without pathology occurring."

Elkes, commenting on this issue, stated, "I'm gland the question came up, because, in a sense, it was one of the gaps in the discussion thus far. Hamburg, if I remember correctly, wrote a paper entitled 'Ancient Man of the 20th Century', in which he questioned whether we are using our adaptive capacities to the utmost. We have missed in this discussion the whole area of pain, as well as its paradox - low arousal states, which can be used for the study of responsiveness and altered responsiveness.

I think the study of low arousal states particularly, where deliberately induced and cultivated in subjects trained not only to perform but to report, can be very rewarding. This involves the use of continuing monitoring techniques, in experimental or daily life conditions. While correlational studies give one certain clusters of information, the single-subject study intensively carried out and minutely monitored for subjective information, taking into consideration environmental contingencies and incorporating deliberately induced experiments, can be much more rewarding."

Vigersky, also commenting on the same issue, said "Perhaps we can use the analogy of differences between bioactivity and immunoactivity. What we are really talking about, in terms of a stress response, is whether it is really healthy for the animal or the individual. It seems that we have yet to fine-tune what this biological response it. We have not fine-tuned it in terms of specificity and sensitivity - the same kinds of criteria we use for all immunological and hormonal responses to changes. On the one side we question whether or not these activation responses mean anything to the organism, in terms of protection or in terms of risk. But the concepts of protection, risk and detrimental effects have not been quantified in the same way as we quantify other things and therefore, we are left with somewhat nebulous parameters."

It is very clear that the discussion did not result in closure with regards to answers to these questions. The questions are certainly pertinent in terms of our conceptual framework and the approaches to research within the stress area. Ultimately, this was summed up by Dr. Elkes in his final statements in which he stated, "I have a distinct feeling of deja-vu. Thirty years ago, in the early days of psychopharmacology, we discussed exactly the same things when people found that the same drug, in the same dose and in the same animal would produce very different effects, according to the social circumstances attendant for that particular medication. The field then began to change and we used drugs as tools to lead us to the source, namely, the way the brain does it without chemical prostheses. And things began to change again. It seems to me that in this discussion, particularly the closing parts of it, the relationship between appropriate and inappropriate adaptation is crucial to the question. Simple it ain't, monistic it ain't, and linear it ain't. We are talking about a stochastic model, with very complex phase relationships - phenomena which have a certain rhythmicity of their own, based on feed-back mechanisms and considerable overlap. But what I am really trying to sense is the role of the analysis of stimulation and interpretation of the stimulus for a particular organism in a particular situation. This brings us right back to some of the principles enunciated here several times, in particular to the interpretive features of cognitive function in man. There are costs of denial and benefits for denial. There are benefits for awareness, which is the opposite to denial, and there are benefits to suppression. And I think that studies of these attitudinal parameters, in relationship to precise hormonal responses, are something we should begin to explore, to lead us from the melee of disease orientation to a much more, shall we say, normal function and health-oriented approach.

We already have in place fairly good science for pathology and disease. To my mind, we know next to nothing about normal function and health, or the science of health. As Levine keeps on pleading, let's look at how those of us who manage, and let us look at the way an individual manages in different situations, using the methods presently available. Under these circumstances, things begin to look much more possible."

The author of this summary will take the prerogative of concluding with a statement he made in the discussion, "Earlier, Rose made a point that seems to have been lost in all of this discussion, namely that it is not so much the nature of activation that is important but how individuals appear to deal with it that counts. To put this another way, one must be impressed with the way you can bombard an animal or a human and find that he is quite capable of functioning, and maintaining fairly high levels of performance. We talk about reduced arousal states, but there are industries in this world based on the creation of arousal. Just go to Las Vegas or to any amusement park. We talk about stress as a fact of life, but coping is also a predominant fact of life, and we tend to survive infinitely better because we have developed exquisite capacities to cope. Evolutionary processes have also participated in developing coping mechanisms and social animals tend to use social groups as a way of dealing effectively with stressful stimuli.

I feel that stress has become our contemporary buzz word, and although clearly there are limits and optimum levels of various stimuli to which organisms can effectively deal with I, for one, would not like to live in a world without stress."

Neuroendocrinology and Psychiatric Disorder,
edited by G. M. Brown, et al.
Raven Press, New York 1984.

Pituitary-Adrenocortical and Pituitary-Gonadal Function in Affective Disorder

Robert T. Rubin and Russell E. Poland

Major psychiatric illnesses have several biologic components - genetic, neurophysiological, neurochemical and neuroendocrine. The elucidation of the biologic correlates of psychiatric illnesses should aid in understanding their etiologies and should provide new information for differential diagnosis and prediction of treatment response. Affective disorders, in particular depression, have been the focus of psychiatric investigations because depression is a prominent illness - its lifetime incidence in the United States is 5-8%; it is the only psychiatric illness that has a significant, and often preventable, mortality; major depressive illness often recurs episodically so that patients may be at risk for much of their lives; and certain affective disorders often respond to somatic therapies, including antidepressants of several classes, antimanic agents such as lithium, and electroconvulsive treatment. The search for biologic markers in depressive illness, as clinical aids to diagnosis and prediction of treatment response, thus has a special importance.

Depressive illness encompasses a heterogeneous group of disorders that have dissimilar symptoms and response to treatment. While many individuals suffer self-limited dpressions, often precipitated by some identifiable major life stress, there is one type of depression that is characterized by a specific cluster of symptoms, a prolonged course, often a family history of similar illness, and generally a responsiveness only to somatic therapies (antidepressant medication or electroconvulsive treatment - ECT). This type of depression, called endogenous (38) or endogenomorphic (40) depression, also may follow an identifiable precipitating stress. However, the characteristic symptoms and the requirement for somatic therapy are the chief factors that allow us to characterize such a depression as endogenous. The signs and symptoms of endogenous or endogenomorphic depression have been codified in the Research Diagnostic Criteria (78) and in the DSM-III of the American Psychiatric Association (3); they include anhedonia (inability to experience pleasure), lack of energy, fatigability, reduced sexual drive, anorexia, weight loss, sleep disturbance (especially early morning awakening), depression worse in the morning, self-reproach, excessive guilt, psychomotor agitation or retardation, lack of reactivity to the environment, etc. Delusions or hallucinations (often of a depressive, somatic nature) also may be present, giving an additional psychotic dimension to the illness.

Severe endogenous depression not infrequently is accompanied by abnormalities in the secretion patterns of certain of the anterior pituitary steroid hormones (13, 21, 56, 59, 60, 62). This paper will review the published data on endocrine changes in the hypothalamo-pituitary-adrenocortical and gonadal axes in endogenous depression, with particular emphasis on the chronoendocrine aspects of these changes, including their relationships to the sleep-wake cycle. The focus will be on depression, because in bipolar (manic-depressive) patients the neuroendocrine abnormalities evident in the depressive phase of their illness often are not evident in the manic phase (14).

I. Chronoendocrinology of Normal Subjects

In humans most hormones are secreted episodically; several have prominent circadian rhythms; and some of these rhythms are linked to the sleep-wake cycle (4, 8, 24, 41, 43, 53, 58, 54, 61, 70, 81). ACTH secretion follows a prominent circadian rhythm, as does its target hormone cortisol, lowest blood levels of both hormones occurring in the early hours of the sleep period and then rapidly increasing in the later few hours of sleep to reach a maximum about the time of awakening (42). Once established, this rhythm appears to have considerable inertia, persisting when sleep is forced into a three-hour ultradian cycle and taking several weeks to readjust when the sleep-wake cycle is reversed. The individual secretory episodes of ACTH and cortisol do not correlate well with REM sleep episodes, but they do occur most frequently during the hours when REM sleep is maximal.

The gonadotropins, LH and FSH, show very little circadian rhythm in adult humans, in contrast to their higher plasma levels during sleep in pubertal subjects. The individual secretory episodes of LH are prominent and are randomly distributed throughout both day and night. FSH also is secreted episodically throughout the 24 hour period, apparently independently from LH. Circulating FSH levels are generally more stable than those of LH. In some women the midcycle ovulatory surge of LH may begin in the latter hours of sleep or at the time of awakening.

Testosterone also is secreted episodically and has a circadian rhythm, with highest levels occurring in the last hour or so of sleep. The circadian rhythm of testosterone accounts for about 20% of the total variance in its circulating levels throughout the day and night. The similarity of the testosterone circadian rhythm to that of prolactin, with testosterone following prolactin by 60 to 90 minutes, has led to the hypothesis that prolactin may play a role in the nocturnal increase of testosterone. However, manipulation of nocturnal prolactin levels by drugs (36) or by sleep-wake reversal (49) has little immediate effect on testosterone, so the relationship between prolactin and testosterone remains uncertain.

II. Sleep Architecture in Endogenous Depression

Electrophysiologic studies of sleep have shown that depression is almost always accompanied by alterations in sleep staging, including increased sleep discontinuity (disruption of sleep architecture), reduced slow-wave sleep (SWS), shortened rapid eye movement (REM) latency (the interval from the onset of sleep until the onset of the first REM period), and increased REM activity (the sum of eye movement scores during REM sleep) (45). The most prominent finding in depression is the decrease in REM latency. In normal subjects, the first REM period occurs 70 to 90 minutes after sleep onset, while in depressed patients the first REM period occurs in about half that time (31, 46). A positive correlation has been found between the severity of depression and the shortening of REM sleep latency (77). These changes in sleep stage patterns occurring in endogenously depressed patients are not a transient phenomenon; they can persist for weeks in untreated patients and for months in patients who do not respond to treatment (23, 44).

Based upon sleep electrophysiology, endogenously depressed patients can be differentiated easily from normal control subjects. Of greater clinical importance is whether endogenously depressed patients can be discriminated from other psychiatric patients, such as those with secondary depressions, schizophrenia, alcoholism, or drug addiction, and from patients with other medical disorders without psychiatric symptoms. While thorough sleep electrophysiology studies for all these groups of patients have not yet been performed, recent studies indicate that endogenously depressed patients do have unique sleep abnormalities that distinguish them from some of the other patient populations. While a detailed discussion of these abnormalities is beyond the scope of this review, they may be useful, in addition to neuroendocrine testing, as aids to differential diagnosis and prediction of treatment response (cf. 59). The importance of long term longitudinal studies of rhythm disturbances have been emphasized by Rusak (chapter 21).

III. ACTH and Cortisol Rhythms in Depression

As noted earlier, circulating ACTH and cortisol have a prominent circadian variation, with lowest levels occurring in the first few hours of sleep and peak levels occurring in the morning around the time of awakening (42). Because of the impetus given to psychoendocrine research by Selye's formulation of the general adaptation syndrome (74), and because colorimetric blood and urine corticosteroid measurement techniques were available 25 years ago, early endocrine studies of depression focused on this endocrine axis (45, 57). Many studies showed that adrenal cortical activity was increased in depressed as compared with manic or normal individuals, as reflected by elevated blood, urine and CSF cortisol concentrations. Some investigators believe that the subjectively experienced anxiety and dysphoria of the depressed patient results in an adrenal cortical stress response according to the Selye model (66), while others postulate that both the depressed affect and the increased corticosteroid secretion could be secondary to an underlying disturbance of brain function (12, 57).

Studies of the circadian pattern of corticosteroid secretion and its response to pharmacologic suppression support the latter hypothesis, namely that a CNS mechanism more fundamental than subjectively felt anxiety appears to underlie the increased corticosteroid production in endogenous depression, because increased adrenal cortical activity occurs in apathetic as well as in anxious depressives, and it occurs throughout the entire 24 hours, especially during the sleep period (16, 63, 68). Figure 1 portrays mean half-hourly serum cortisol concentrations for 15 primary endogenous depressives (six men, nine women) and eight normal age, sex, race and menstrual status-matched control subjects studied by our research group (63). Half-hourly blood sampling gives an indication of the episodically fluctuating levels of cortisol in serum. The patients had higher serum cortisol levels during most of the night and day, the difference being particularly evident between 2400 and 0300, when the mean cortisol level of the depressed patients was twice that of the control subjects. In our study the amplitude of the circadian cortisol rhythm was not blunted in the patients when compared to the controls, in contrast to the data of Sachar (67), in which the amplitude of the mean circadian cortisol rhythm in seven unipolar depressives was about half that in 54 normal controls. The circadian increase in cortisol appeared to begin several hours earlier in our patients (about midnight) compared to the control subjects (about 0300). This phase advance in cortisol secretion may be related to the circadian advance in the sleep-wake cycle (early morning awakening) that many endogenously depressed patients experience. It is of interest that following successful treatment of depressed patients, both their sleep architecture and their cortisol secretory patterns usually return to normal.

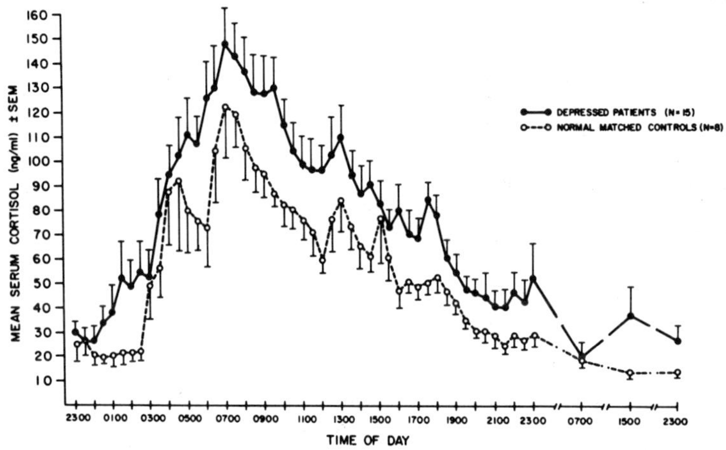

FIG. 1. Mean half-hourly serum cortisol concentrations, ± S.E.M., for 15 primary endogenous depressives and 8 normal control subjects matched to the patients on age, sex, race, and menstrual status. Immediately after the 2300 sample on the second night was drawn, dexamethasone (1 mg p.o.) was given, and samples were taken every eight hours thereafter for another 24 hours. Figure reproduced from Rubin et al. (63).

A specific indicator of the hyperactivity of the ACTH/cortisol axis in depression is the early escape of these hormones from dexamethasone (DEX) suppression. DEX (1.0 or 2.0 mg p.o.) given at midnight normally suppresses ACTH and cortisol for a full 24 hours. However, endogenously depressed patients often show an early increase in serum cortisol, between 16 and 24 hours post-DEX. Both the normal controls and the depressed patients shown in Figure 1 were given DEX (1.0 mg p.o.) at 2300 on the second night, and serum cortisol was measured every eight hours for the next 24 hours. The control subjects suppressed normally, whereas the depressed patients showed a typical pattern of cortisol escape at 16 and 24 hours post-DEX. The DEX suppression test has about 95% specificity for endogenous depression (few false positives in non-endogenously depressed patients and other types of psychiatric disorders), but its sensitivity is only 60 to 70% (30 to 40% false negatives in definitely endogenous depressives) (19). While most investigators have confirmed these percentages (15), some have found both a lower specificity and a lower sensitivity (34, 75) and have suggested that cortisol escape may correlate better with the severity of depressive symptomatology than with the diagnosis of endogenous subtype *per se*. Nevertheless, it is generally agreed that the DEX suppression test has a high construct validity, in that it is more frequently positive in diagnostically definitely endogenous compared to probably endogenous depressives and in suicidal compared to non-suicidal depressives; it normalizes with a switch from depression to mania; and it normalizes gradually with treatment (16, 19). Figure 2 depicts typical DEX suppression responses during illness and recovery in a 49 year old agitated, unipolar depressed woman with a strong family history of depression (16). The first test (2 April) was carried out three days after hospital admission, and the second (9 April) was carried out a week later, when the patient was receiving placebo medication. High midnight pre-DEX plasma cortisols and obvious cortisol escape from DEX suppression characterized the first two tests. The patient then was treated with antidepressant medication and over the next five weeks her DEX suppression tests gradually normalized as her illness remitted. At the time of her last DEX test, which showed a complete 24 hour cortisol suppression, her pre-DEX mignight cortisol level had decreased to the normal range.

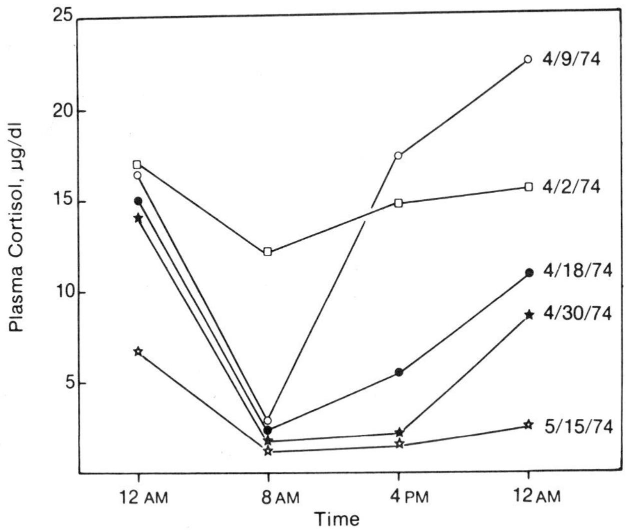

FIG. 2. Serial dexamethasone (DEX) suppression tests in a 49 year old depressed woman before (2 and 9 April, 1974) and during antidepressant drug treatment. DEX (1.0 mg p.o.) was given immediately after the first midnight plasma cortisol sample was drawn. The initial early cortisol escape from DEX suppression gradually converted to a normal, full 24 hour suppression with symptomatic improvement. Figure reproduced, with permission, from Carroll et al. (16). Copyright 1976 by the American Medical Association.

The cortisol escape from DEX suppression in depressed patients does not appear to be a result of altered pharmacokinetics of DEX metabolism (17, 63), and thus it most likely reflects enhanced limbic-hypothalamic driving of the pituitary-adrenal cortical axis. Nocturnal hypersecretion of cortisol (Figure 1) and cortisol escape from DEX suppression (Figures 1 and 2) generally occur together in endogenously depressed patients, raising the question of whether a single nocturnal blood sample for cortisol might serve the same purpose as a DEX suppression test. Carroll et al. (19) compared the sensitivity and specificity of an elevated 2330 pre-DEX plasma cortisol value with those of a positive DEX suppression test in 173 hospitalized patients. While the sensitivities of both measures were the same (65%), the specificity of an elevated 2330 plasma cortisol (55%) was much less than that of the DEX test (94%); i.e., an elevated nocturnal cortisol occurred in 45% of non-endogenously depressed patients. Papakostas et al. (51) have reported similar findings. Thus, from a diagnostic standpoint, the DEX suppression test appears to be the better of the two measures of cortisol hypersecretion.

A positive DEX suppression test also appears to be associated with certain familial types of depression. Winokur et al. (82) subdivided primary unipolar depressive illness into three groups based on family history data: pure depressive disease (history of depression but not of mania, alcoholism, or sociopathy in a first-degree relative), sporadic depressive disease (no psychiatric illness history in any first-degree relative), and depression spectrum disease (history of alcoholism, sociopathy, or both in a first-degree relative). Schlesser et al. (72) performed DEX suppression tests on 221 depressed patients, subdivided as shown in Figure 3, and on 109 control subjects. Figure 3 indicates the specificity of the DEX test for primary depression - only those patients showed abnormal tests. Similar findings have been reported by several other groups of investigators (15). Bipolar depressed patients as a group had a higher incidence of abnormal tests (85%) than did unipolar depressed patients (45%); this latter percentage also is similar to those found in several other studies (15). When the primary unipolar depressives were subdivided according to the classification of Winokur et al. (82), 76% of the familial pure depressives showed cortisol non-suppression, compared to 44% of the non-familial sporadic depressives and only 7% of the depression spectrum disease patients (those with alcoholism and/or sociopathy in a first-degree relative). These data are provocative in that they suggest a possible genetic influence on at least one neuroendocrine aspect of depression - the DEX suppression test. The data are even more intriguing in that Schlesser et al. (72) measured cortisol in only a single 0800 blood sample, taken 9 hours after DEX administration at 2300. As indicated by Figure 2, the 16 and 24 hour post-DEX blood samples often yield a much better sensitivity for cortisol escape (19). Using the full 3 x 8 hour sampling schedule, other investigators have found a considerably higher incidence of abnormal DEX tests in patients with depression spectrum disease (5/6 patients by Carroll et al. (18), 4/11 patients by Hwu et al. (35), 4/12 patients by Schlesser et al. (73) themselves, and 5/10 patients by Rubin et al. (unpublished observations)). Further attempts to resolve this question need to be undertaken.

Some investigators are attempting to use the DEX test as an aid to the choice of treatment for endogenously depressed patients and in the prediction of treatment response. Brown et al. (10) found that in a small series of patients (N = 19), those with positive DEX tests (N = 8) tended to have a better treatment response to imipramine or desipramine than to amitriptyline or clomipramine. The converse was true for the cortisol suppressors (N = 11). These investigators postulated that patients with a positive DEX test had a norepinephrine-deficiency type of depression (norepinephrine normally inhibits the hypothalamo-pituitary-adrenocortical axis) and should have responded best to drugs like imipramine or desipramine, which are strong norepinephrine reuptake inhibitors, whereas patients who showed normal cortisol suppression had a serotonin-deficiency type of depression and thus would have responded best to predominantly serotonin reuptake inhibitors like amitriptyline or clomipramine. While the initial data of Brown et al. (10) support this hypothesis, the differences in change scores among their groups were not clear-cut (11). Additional support has been provided by Cobbin et al.

(22), who found in a small number of patients (N = 14) that an abnormal DEX test predicted a poor clinical response to the antidepressant mianserin, a serotonin reuptake inhibitor, whereas normal cortisol suppression following DEX predicted a good clinical response to this drug. In this regard, Carroll et al. (20) found that depressed patients with abnormal DEX tests had normal CSF 5-HIAA concentrations, and those with normal DEX tests had low CSF 5-HIAA. Again, more extensive replication studies are needed.

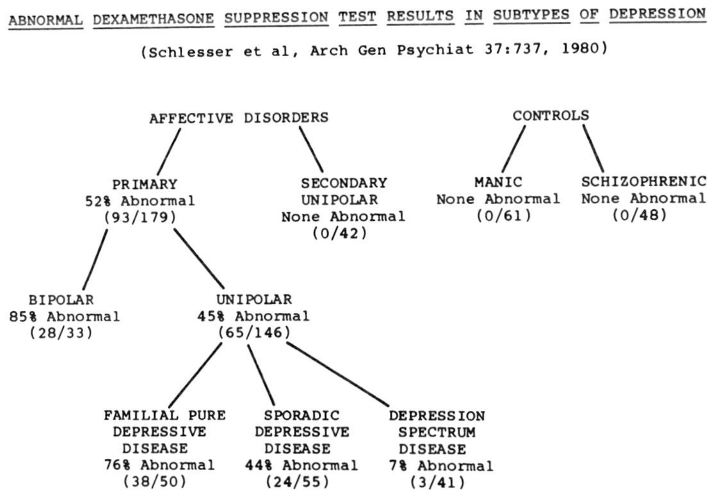

FIG. 3. Differential incidences of abnormal dexamethasone suppression tests in subtypes of depression. Dexamethasone (1.0 mg p.o.) was given as 2300, and serum cortisol was determined at 0800. The criterion for an abnormal test was cortisol > 50 ng/ml. Figure adapted from Schlesser et al. (73).

As mentioned, the DEX suppression test generally normalizes with successful treatment of the depressive episode, whether the treatment is by medication (16) or electroconvulsive therapy (1, 27). In two small series of patients (N = 8 and N = 14, respectively), Goldberg (32) and Greden et al. (33) found that patients who do not normalize their DEX tests after treatment are at higher risk for early relapse than those patients who do show a normal cortisol suppression after treatment. Here, too, further studies should be undertaken to verify the utility of the DEX test as a treatment prognosticator.

In summary, then, the DEX suppression test, as an index of hyperactivity of the hypothalamo-pituitary-adrenocortical axis in endogenous depression, appears to have the requisite sensitivity and specificity to be of high predictive value as an ancillary laboratory test in the diagnosis of endogenous depression, but only after clinical criteria have been used to narrow and focus the differential diagnosis. In this regard it appears to be better than simply the measurement of nocturnal cortisol hypersecretion, because it is more specific. Both cortisol hypersecretion and an abnormal DEX test appear to occur independently from another neuroendocrine abnormality seen in some endogenous depressives, namely a blunted TSH response to TRH (30, 39). Thus, the DEX test ultimately may be utilized best as part of a battery of diagnostic laboratory studies. Whether or not the DEX test will be a reliable predictor of the type of antidepressant medication needed for treatment and/or the potential for early relapse after treatment is discontinued remains to be determined in future investigations.

IV. Gonadotropin and Gonadal Steroid Rhythms in Depression

As noted earlier, in normal adults the gonadotropins (LH and FSH) are secreted episodically, with no apparent circadian rhythms, while testosterone has a circadian rhythm of modest amplitude, higher circulating levels occurring at night (37, 52). The gonadal steroid hormones (testosterone and the estrogens) have been implicated in the modulations of sexual and perhaps even aggressive behaviour in adulthood (9, 64, 71). Since, as noted above, decreased energy in general and decreased sexual drive in particular are part of the symptom cluster of endogenous depression, the secretion patterns of the pituitary gonadotropins and their peripheral target hormones, the gonadal steroids, may have particular relevance in this illness (55).

Only a few studies of LH and FSH patterns in depression have been reported, and their results differ. Benkert (6) measured plasma LH concentrations serially in seven unipolar endogenously depressed men and five bipolar manic men. One depressed and one manic patient had abnormally high, spiking levels, which fell to the normal range following treatment and recovery from the affective illness episode. Neither FSH nor testosterone were measured. Ettigi et al. (29) measured plasma LH concentrations prior to and following gonadotropin releasing hormone (LHRH) (100 ug i.v.) in five primary unipolar depressed men, four men with depression secondary to neuroses or sociopathy, and six normal age-matched male control subjects. Based on the single pre-LHRH injection sample, the mean baseline plasma LH levels among the three groups of subjects were not significantly different. However, Figure 2 in this paper (29) suggests that the primary depressed patients had a mean baseline LH level about half that of the secondary depressed patients and perhaps lower than the mean LH level of the normal control subjects as well. The primary depressed patients and the normal controls had apparently equivalent mean LH responses to the LHRH infusion, whereas the four patients with secondary depression had a mean LH response signficantly (about 100%) higher than those of the five patients with primary depression or the six normal controls. Testosterone also was measured in this study (28), as discussed below. Altman et al. (2) measured plasma LH concentrations serially in 12 primary, unipolar, postmenopausal depressed women and in 13 normal age-matched postmenopausal controls. The mean plasma LH concentration of the depressed women was about 30% less than that of the matched control group, a statistically signfiicant difference. Neither FSH nor gonadal steroids was determined in these women.

We recently reported a preliminary study of plasma LH and FSH concentrations measured in nine primary endogenously depressed men, eight unipolar and one bipolar, and in six age- and race-matched normal male control subjects (65). The sampling times were the same as shown in Figure 1. Average levels of both gonadotropins were 15 to 30% lower in the depressed men than in the controls both at night (2300 to 0700) and during the day (0730 to 1500). However, this was a statistically non-significant difference, in part due to the small sample size. At 1500, LHRH (100 ug i.v.) was administered. The mean LH increases following LHRH in the patients and controls were equivalent, whereas the mean post-LHRH FSH increase in the patients was about half that of the controls. We also measured testosterone in these patients, as detailed below.

These few reports of plasma gonadotropin concentrations suggest reduced diurnal and nocturnal circulating LH, and perhaps FSH, levels in depressed patients compared to matched control subjects. This difference is evident in those studies (2, 65) that utilized serial blood sampling over time to obtain an integrated measure of normally rapidly fluctuating LH levels as a result of episodic hormone secretion. Replication studies are needed to confirm or refute these findings.

There have been similarly few reported studies of gonadal steroid regulation in depression. Sachar et al. (69) measured plasma testosterone concentrations at 0800 in five bipolar and 10 unipolar depressed men during illness and again shortly after recovery. The mean pre-treatment plasma testosterone level in the patients was not significantly different from their mean post-treatment level, and both were within the range of values for normal men in the investigators' laboratory. There was a weak, non-significant correlation between the degree of loss of libido and testosterone levels (+ .41) (our calculation of rank-order correlation). Gonadotropin levels were not measured in these patients. Vogel et al. (80) determined plasma testosterone at 0900 in 27 primary, unipolar depressed men and in 13 age-matched normal male volunteers. Both total and free mean testosterone levels were significantly (about 30%) lower in the patients than in the controls. In contrast, in a subset of 15 depressives and 12 controls, the mean plasma estradiol level was significantly (about 50%) higher in the patients than in the control subjects. Unfortunately, gonadotropin levels were not measured to complement the extensive gonadal steroid data.

Ettigi and Brown (28) measured testosterone, as well as LH (29), in their primary and secondary depressed men (N = 5 and 4, respectively) and normal control subejcts (N = 6). The table in this paper (28) suggests that both the primary and the secondary depressed patients had reduced basal plasma testosterone concentrations, by 22 and 36% respectively, compared to the control subjects. These differences, however, were not statistically significant, perhaps owing to the small sample sizes.

In our aforementioned study of LH and FSH (65), we also measured plasma testosterone in the half-hourly nocturnal and diurnal samples taken from the nine primary endogenously depressed men and six matched controls. The mean plasma testosterone concentrations both at night and during the day were about 20% lower in the patients than in the controls. This finding of reduced circulating testosterone in depressed men accorded with the same finding in the study of Vogel et al. (80); however, the smaller sample size as well as the smaller magnitude of the hormone difference obviated statistical significance in our study (65).

Vogel et al. (80) also measured plasma estradiol and testosterone concentrations at 0900 twice weekly in 22 primary, unipolar premenopausal depressed women and in 10 normal age-matched premenopausal controls. The weekly mean plasma estradiol concentrations in the depressed women were significantly (60 to 80%) higher than those in the control group. The weekly mean plasma testosterone concentrations in the patients similarly were significantly (90 to 180%) higher than those in the control group. Because of decreased testosterone binding to plasma protein in the depressed women, their mean free testosterone level was 300% higher than that of the control subjects. Gonadotropins were not measured in these women.

These few reports of plasma gonadal steroid concentrations suggest that circulating testosterone levels are reduced by 20 to 30%, both at night and during the day in depressed men compared to matched controls. However, the one study of testosterone before and shortly after treatment showed no difference (69), raising the question of whether reduced circulating testosterone in depressed men is a state-dependent phenomenon. There are no other data available at present ot corroborate the findings of Vogel et al. (80) of increased circulating estradiol in depressed men and of increased circulating estradiol, and testosterone as well, in depressed women.

Taken together, these data on hypothalamo-pituitary-gonadal function in endogenously depressed patients suggest a dysfunction of this endocrine axis, as reflected by reduced circulating levels of LH, testosterone, and possibly FSH, and increased circulating levels of estradiol, in depressed men, and reduced LH, but increased estradiol and testosterone, in depressed women. As both gonadotropins and gonadal steroids were measured in the same blood samples in only a few studies, the findings become even more tenuous. Clearly, more detailed and comprehensive replication studies must be performed.

Assuming a consistent 20 to 30% reduction in circulating LH and testosterone concentrations in depressed men, what might be the psychohormonal importance of these findings? It was mentioned earlier that decreased energy in general and sexual drive in particular are part of the symptom cluster of endogenous depression (40, 78), and that the gonadal steroid hormones have CNS effects that include the modulation of sexual and perhaps aggressive behaviour in adulthood (9, 64, 71). There are ample data to indicate that hypogonadal men (those with serum testosterone concentrations 2 ng/ml) have restoration of both libido and ability to perform sexually when given testosterone replacement therapy (5, 9, 64, 71, 76), which is apparently a true pharmacological CNS effect of this androgen (26). Conversely, reduction of testosterone levels by 20% to 50% by antiandrogen treatment in patients with "deviant hypersexuality", has resulted in profound reductions of sexual drive and fantasies as well as of the deviant behaviour (7, 25, 48, 50, 79). On the other hand, there are no consistent relationships between circulating testosterone and level of sexual activity in endocrinologically and psychiatrically normal men (9, 64, 71). Thus the psychohormonal importance of reduced LH and testosterone in depressed men (assuming the preliminary endocrine findings can be replicated) is another area which future studies will need to address.

V. Discussion

This review suggests that disturbances in the secretion patterns of at least two endocrine axes are concomitants of the syndrome of endogenous depression. Because the same putative CNS neurotransmitters appear to be involved both in the modulation of affects and in the regulation of the hypothalamic releasing and inhibiting factors, it is tempting to suggest that a common CNS neurotransmitter dysfunction underlies both the depressive state and the altered endocrine dynamics. Reduced norepinephrine neurotransmission has been the prime candidate in this regard (21, 56, 60), but hypothesizing this defect has been considerably easier than demonstrating it. While attractive, and of considerable heuristic value, the catecholamine deficiency hypothesis of depression is not yet supported by sufficient evidence.

In summary, several changes in hormone dynamics occur in patients with endogenous depression. This review has focused on the hypersecretion and blunted circadian rhythms of ACTH and cortisol, the early cortisol escape from dexamethasone suppression, and the reduced secretion of LH and perhaps also of testosterone in male depressives. Some of these hormone changes may prove useful as aids in the differential diagnosis of the endogenous subtype of major depression and in the prediction of treatment response. Both the affect disturbance and the endocrine changes may be sequelae of common CNS amine neurotransmitter dysfunctions, but this attractive hypothesis remains to be verified.

REFERENCES

1. Albala, A. A. and Greden, J. F. (1980): Am. J. Psychiat. 137: 383.
2. Altman, N., Sachar, E. J., Gruen, P. H., Halpern, F. S. and Eto, S. (1975): Psychosom. Med. 37:274-276.
3. American Psychiatric Association (1980): Diagnostic and Statistical Manual of Mental Disorders, 3rd edition. Washington, D.C.
4. Aschoff, J. (1979): In: Endocrine Rhythms, edited by D. T. Krieger, pp.1-61. Raven Press, New York.
5. Bancroft, J. and Skakkebaek, N. E. (1979): In: Sex, Hormones and Behaviour, Ciba Foundation Symposium 62, pp.209-226. Excerpta Medica, Amsterdam.
6. Benkert, O. (1975): Prog. Brain Res. 42:25-36.
7. Blumer, D. and Migeon, C. (1975): J. Nerv. Ment. Dis. 160:127-137.
8. Boyar, R. M. (1978): In: The Hypothalamus, edited by S. Reichlin, R. J. Baldessarini and J. B. Martin, pp.373-386. Raven Press, New York.
9. Brown, W. A. (1980): Int. J. Ment. Health 9:45-66.
10. Brown, W. A., Haier, R. J. and Qualls, C. B. (1980): Lancet i: 928-929.
11. Brown, W. A. and Qualls, C. B. (1981): Psychiat. Res. 4:115-128.
12. Carroll, B. J. (1976): Psychosom. Med. 38:106-121.
13. Carroll, B. J. (1978): In: Psychopharmacology: A Generation of Progress, edited by M. A. Lipton, A. DiMascio and K. F. Killam, pp.487-497. Raven Press, New York.
14. Carroll, B. J. (1979): In: Manic Illness, edited by B. Shopsin, pp.163-176. Raven Press, New York.
15. Carroll, B. J. (1981): Br. J. Psychiat. (in press).
16. Carroll, B. J., Curtis, G. C. and Mendels, J. (1976): Arch. Gen. Psychiat. 33:1039-1044.
17. Carroll, B. J., Schroeder, K., Mukhopadhyay, S., Greden, J. F., Feinberg, M., Ritchie, J. and Tarika, J. (1980): J. Clin. Endocrinol. Metab. 51:433-437.
18. Carroll, B. J., Greden, J. F., Feinberg, M., James, N. McI., Haskett, R. F., Steiner, M. and Tarika, J. (1980): Psychiat. Res. 2:251-258
19. Carroll, B. J., Feinbreg, M., Greden, J. F., Tarika, J., Albala, A. A., Haskett, R. F., James, N. McI., Kronfol, Z., Lohr, N., Steiner, M., de Vigne, J. P. and Young, E. (1981): Arch. Gen. Psychiat. 38: 15-22.
20. Carroll, B. J., Greden, J. F. and Feinberg, M. (1981): In: Recent Advances in Neuropsychopharmacology, edited by B. Angrist, et al., pp.307-313. Pergamon Press, Oxford.
21. Checkley, S. A. (1980): Psychol. Med. 10:35-53.
22. Cobbin, D. M., Cairncross, K. D., Jurd, S., Veltman, D. G. and Pohlen, G. H. (1981): Neuroendocrinology Lett. (in press).

23. Coble, P.A., Kupfer, D. J., Spiker, D. G., Neil, J. F. and McPartland, R. J. (1979): J. Affect. Disorders 1:131-138.
24. Copinschi, G., L'Hermite, M., Golstein, J., Leclercq, R., Desir, D., Vanhaelst, L., Virasoro, E., Robyn, C. and Van Cauter, E. (1978): In: Progress in Prolactin Physiology and Pathology, edited by C. Robyn and M. Harter, pp.165-172. Elsevier, Amsterdam.
25. Cooper, A. J., Ismail, A.A.A., Phanjoo, A. L. and Love, D. L. (1972): Brit. J. Psychiat. 120:59-63.
26. Davidson, J. M., Camargo, C.A. and Smith, E. R. (1979): J. Clin. Endocrinol. Metab. 48:955-958.
27. Dysken, M. W., Pandey, G. N., Chang, S. S., Hicks, R. and Davis, J. M. (1979): Am. J. Psychiat. 136:1328-1329.
28. Ettigi, P. G. and Brown, G. M. (1979): In: Neuroendocrine Correlates in Neurology and Psychiatry, edited by E. E. Muller and A. Agnoli, pp.225-238. Elsevier/North Holland, Amsterdam.
29. Ettigi, P. G., Brown, G. M. and Seggie, J. A. (1979): Psychosom. Med. 41:203-208.
30. Extein, I., Pottash, A.L.C. and Gold, M.S. (1981): Psychiat. Res. 4:49-53.
31. Gillin, J. C., Duncan, W., Pettigrew, K. D., Frankel, B. L. and Synder, F. (1979): Arch. Gen. Psychiat. 36:85-89.
32. Goldberg, I. K. (1980): Lancet i:376.
33. Greden, J. F., Albala, A. A , Haskett, R. F., James, N. McI., Goodman, L., Steiner, M. and Carroll, B. J. (1980): Biol. Psychiat. 15:449-458.
34. Holsboer, F., Bender, W., Benkert, O., Klein, H. E. and Schmaus, M. (1980): Lancet ii:706.
35. Hwu, H. -G., Rudorfer, M. V., and Clayton, P. J. (1981): Arch. Gen. Psychiat. 38:363.
36. Jacobs, L. S., Mendelson, W. B., Rubin, R. T. and Bauman, J. E. (1978): J. Clin. Endocrinol. Metab. 46:561-566.
37. Judd, H. L. (1979): In: Endocrine Rhythms, edited by D. T. Krieger, pp.299-324. Raven Press, New York.
38. Kendell, R. E. (1976): Brit. J. Psychiat. 129:15-28.
39. Kirkegaard, C. and Carroll, B. J. (1980): Psychiat. Res. 3:253-264.
40. Klein, D. F. (1974): Arch. Gen. Psychiat. 31:447-454.
41. Krieger, D. T., editor (1979): In: Endocrine Rhythms (Comprehensive Endocrinology, Vol. 1). Raven Press, New York.
42. Krieger, D. T. (1979): In: Endocrine Rhythms, edited by D. T. Krieger, pp.123-142. Raven Press, New York.
43. Krieger, D. T. and Aschoff, J. (1979): In: Endocrinology, Vol. 3, edited by L. J. DeGroot, G. F. Cahill, W. D. Odell, L. Martini, D. H. Nelson, J. T. Potts, E. Steinberger, and A. Winegrad, pp. 2079-2109. Grune and Stratton, New York.
44. Kupfer, D. J. (1976): Biol. Psychiat. 11:159-174.
45. Kupfer, D. J. (1977): In: Animal Models in Psychiatry and Neurology, edited by I. Hanin and E. Usdin, pp.181-188. Pergamon, Oxford.
46. Kupfer, D. J., Foster, F. G., Coble, P., McPartland, R. J. and Ulrich, R. F. (1978): Am. J. Psychiat. 135:69-74.
47. Mason, J. W. (1968): Psychosom. Med. 30:576-607.
48. Meyer, W. J., Walker, P. A., Wiedeking, C., Money, J., Kowarski, A. A., Migeon, C. J. and Borgaonkar, D. (1977): Fertil. Steril. 28:1072-1076.
49. Miyatake, A., Morimoto, Y., Oishi, T., Hanasaki, N., Sugita, Y.,

Iijima, S., Teshima, Y., Hishikawa, Y. and Yamamura, Y. (1980): J. Clin. Endocrinol. Metab. 51:1365-1371.
50. Money, J., Wiedeking, C., Walker, P., Migeon, C., Meyer, W. and Borgaonkar, D. (1975): Psychoneuroendocrinology 1:165-178.
51. Papakostas, Y., Fink, M., Lee, J., Irwin, P. and Johnson, L. (1981): Psychiat. Res. 4:55-64.
52. Rebar, R. W. and Yen, S.S.C. (1979): In: Endocrine Rhythms, edited by D. T. Krieger, pp.259-298. Raven Press, New York.
53. Rubin, R. T. (1975): In: Hormones, Homeostasis, and the Brain, Prog. Brain Res. Vol. 42, edited by W. H. Gispen, Tj. B. van Wimersma Greidanus, B. Bohus and D. deWied, pp.73-80. Elsevier, Amsterdam.
54. Rubin, R. T. (1980): In: Physiology in Sleep, edited by J. Orem and C. D. Barnes, pp.181-201. Academic Press, New York.
55. Rubin, R. T. (1981): Int. J. Ment. Health 10(2-3):43-59.
56. Rubin, R. T. and Kendler, K. S. (1977): In: Depression: Clinical Biological and Psychological Perspectives, edited by G. Usdin, pp.122-138. Brunner/Mazel, New York.
57. Rubin, R. T. and Mandell, A. J. (1966): Am. J. Psychiat. 123: 387-400.
58. Rubin, R. T. and Poland, R. E. (1976): Psychoneuroendocrinology 1: 281-290.
59. Rubin, R. T. and Poland, R. E. (1981): In: Neuroendocrine Perspectives, Vol. 1, edited by R. M. MacLeod and E. E. Müller, pp.305-337. Elsevier/North Holland, Amsterdam.
60. Rubin, R. T., Gouin, P. R. and Poland, R. E. (1973): In: Psychiatry Proceedings of the V World Congress of Psychiatry, edited by R. de la Fuente and M. N. Weisman, pp.1036-1039. Excerpta Medica, Amsterdam.
61. Rubin, R. T., Poland, R. E., Rubin, L. E. and Gouin, P. R. (1974): Life Sci. 14:1041-1052.
62. Rubin, R. T., Poland, R. E. and Hays, S. E. (1979): In: Biological Psychiatry Today, edited by J. Obiols, C. Ballus, E. Gonzalez Monclus and J. Pujol, pp.684-688. Elsevier/North Holland, Amsterdam.
63. Rubin, R. T., Poland, R. E., Blodgett, A.L.N., Winston, R. A., Forster, B. and Carroll, B. J. (1980): In: Progress in Psychoneuroendocrinology, edited by F. Brambilla, G. Racagni, and D. deWied, pp.223-234. Elsevier/North Holland, Amsterdam.
64. Rubin, R. T., Reinisch, J. R. and Haskett, R. F. (1981): Science 211:1318-1324.
65. Rubin, R. T., Poland, R. E., Tower, B. B., Hart, P. J., Blodgett, A. L.N. and Forster, B. (1981): In: Steroid Hormone Regulation of the Brain, edited by K. Fuxe, J. -A. Gustafsson, and L. Wetterberg. pp.387-396. Pergamon, Oxford.
66. Sachar, E. J., Hellman, L., Fukushima, D. K. and Gallagher, T. F. (1970): Arch. Gen. Psychiat. 23:289-298.
67. Sachar, E. J. (1975): In: Topics in Psychoendocrinology, edited by E. J. Sachar, pp.135-156. Grune and Stratton, New York.
68. Sachar, E. J., Hellman, L., Roffwarg, H. P., Halpern, F. S., Fukushima, D. K. and Gallagher, T. F. (1973): Arch. Gen. Psychiat. 28:19-24.
69. Sachar, E. J., Halpern, F., Rosenfeld, R. S., Gallagher, T. F. and Hellman, L. (1973): Arch. Gen. Psychiat. 28:15-18.
70. Sassin, J. F. (1977): In: Neurobiology of Sleep and Memory, edited by R. R. Drucker-Colin and J. L. McGaugh, pp.361-372. Academic

Press, New York.

71. Schiavi, R. C. and White, D. (1976): J. Sex. Marital Ther. 2: 214-228.
72. Schlesser, M. A., Winokur, G. and Sherman, B. M. (1980): Arch. Gen. Psychiat. 37:737-743.
73. Schlesser, M. A., Winokur, G. and Sherman, B. A. (1981): Arch. Gen. Psychiat. 38:363.
74. Selye, H. (1973): Amer. Scientist 61:692-699.
75. Shulman, R. (1980): Lancet ii:1085.
76. Spark, R. F., White, R. A. and Connolly, P. B. (1980): J. Amer. Med. Assoc. 243:750-755.
77. Spiker, D. G., Coble, P., Cofsky, J., Foster, F. G. and Kupfer, D. J. (1978): Biol. Psychiat. 13:485-488.
78. Spitzer, R. L., Endicott, J. and Robins, E. (1978): Arch. Gen. Psychiat. 35:773-782.
79. Van Moffaert, M. (1976): Acta Psychiat. Scand. 53:29-34.
80. Vogel, W., Klaiber, E. L. and Broverman, D. M. (1978): Prog. Neuropsychopharmacology 2:487-503.
81. Wagner, D. R. and Weitzman, E. D. (1980): Psychiat. Clin. North Am. 3:223-250.
82. Winokur, G., Behar, D., Van Valkenburg, C. and Lowry, M. (1978): J. Nerv. Ment. Dis. 166:764-768.

Neuroendocrinology and Psychiatric Disorder,
edited by G. M. Brown, et al.
Raven Press, New York 1984.

Pharmacoendocrine Studies of G.H., PRL, and Melatonin in Patients with Affective Illness

Stuart Checkley and Josephine Arendt

This review will cover the reported studies of growth hormone (G.H.), prolactin (PRL) and melatonin secretion in patients with affective illness. Within this field a particularly important issue is the use of neuroendocrine tests to assess the status of receptors involved in central neurotransmission. In this context the pharmacoendocrine studies of G.H. release are of particular promise and so these will be discussed in some detail.

Firstly, it is necessary to assess the role of the various neurotransmitters which are involved in the central regulation of G.H. release in man. Then it is necessary to consider how best to control for those biological influences (such as age and sex) which influence G.H. release. In the light of these issues the clinical studies will be assessed to see whether or not they indicate altered receptor status in patients with affective illness.

These issues will be discussed in some detail for G.H. and then more briefly in the case of PRL and melatonin.

THE ROLE OF NEUROTRANSMITTERS AND THEIR RECEPTORS IN REGULATING THE RELEASE OF G.H. IN MAN

The following section will primarily be devoted to human studies. Species differences will be mentioned when these cannot be explained by the use of anaesthetics and different doses of drug. Where extrapolation from human to animal studies is possible the animal studies will be quoted when they suggest possible mechanisms for the neuroendocrine responses which can be measured in man.

Noradrenaline and G.H.

Desipramine is a selective inhibitor of the re-uptake of noradrenaline and in man desimpramine stimulates the release of G.H. in a dose dependant manner (119). This effect must involve noradrenergic mechanisms as it is inhibited by the α-noradrenergic antagonists phentolamine (119) and yohimbine (120). Other drugs such as amphetamine, methylamphetamine, nomifensine and mianserine which increase intrasynaptic concentrations of noradrenaline also stimulate the release of G.H. in man (14, 121, 122) although these drugs also influence neurotransmitters other than noradrenaline. When these studies are considered together they suggest that noradrenaline exerts an excitatory influence over the release of G.H. in man.

Noradrenaline stimulates two types of post-synaptic receptor termed α- and β-adrenoceptors. In the sympathetic nervous system the stimulation of α- and β- adrenoceptors frequently has mutually antagonistic effects upon the function of target organs (3). It will be seen that a similar reciprocity between the effects of stimulating α- and β-adrenoceptors exists for control of G.H. release in man.

Effects of α-adrenoceptor agonists upon the release of G.H.

In man the release of G.H. is stimulated by the α-agonists clonidine (124), methoxamine (95), phenylephrine (95) and guanfacine (129). The G.H. response to methoxamine is inhibited by the α-antagonist phentolamine (95) and, in rhesus monkeys, the G.H. response to clonidine is inhibited by piperoxane (79). Thus the G.H. responses to these drugs depend upon their action at α-adrenoceptors (98).

Effects of α antagonists upon the release of G.H.

Just as drugs which stimulate α-adrenoceptors stimulate the release of G.H., so drugs which block α-adrenoceptors inhibit the release of G.H. Antagonists block the G.H. response to hypoglycemia (20, 95), to arginine (95), to vasopressin (92) to exercise (90) and to ECT (224). The G.H. responses to methylamphetamine (183) and to sleep (141) are apparently exceptions to this general rule: they are not inhibited by α antagonists.

Effects of β-adrenoceptor antagonists upon the release of G.H.

In this contect it is unfortunate that propranolol has been used as the sole β antagonist as propranolol also has important membrane stabilizing and 5-HT receptor blocking actions (49). When approximately 10 mg propranolol is given intravenously Caucasian subjects do not release G.H. (2, 20, 22, 150) although Japanese subjects do (95). When similar doses of propranolol are given to either Caucasian or Japanese subjects it enhances the G.H. responses to hypoglycemia (20, 99), to arginine (98), to glucagon (160), to exercise (90) and L-DOPA (150).

Effects of β-adrenoceptors agonists upon the release of G.H.

The direct effects of β agonists upon the release of G.H. are hard to distinguish from the inhibition of G.H. release which would be expected from the known effects of β agonists upon plasma concentrations of glucose and free fatty acids (150, 168).

Thus while it is clear that β-adrenoceptors mediate an excitatory influence over the release of G.H. the case for β-adrenoceptors exerting an inhibitory influence rests solely upon the effects of the non-selective β antagonist propranolol.

G.H. response to clonidine

Of the directly acting agonists and antagonists which have been mentioned so far clonidine is a particularly potent stimulant to the release of G.H. For this reason G.H. responses to clonidine have been and are being investigated in patients with affective illness: as will be seen later impaired responses have been found in many depressed patients.

Fortunately clonidine provokes a similar release of G.H. in rats, dogs, rhesus monkeys, baboons and presumably in other species too. The mechanisms involved in the G.H. response to clonidine have been studied in these animals and the extrapolation of results to man would seem reasonable.

Firstly, it is likely that the G.H. response to clonidine is mediated through the stimulation of brain (and possibly forebrain) structures rather than being mediated through the stimulation of peripheral or pituitary α-adrenoceptors. A pituitary site of action would appear unlikely as noradrenaline does not release G.H. from isolated pituitaries (18, 145). A peripheral action upon cardiovascular α-adrenoceptors is also unlikely as division of the cervical cord (and hence interruption of the sympathetic outflow) has no effect upon the G.H. response to clonidine even though the hypotensive effect of clonidine is abolished (74). More direct evidence for a central site of action comes from studies using anaesthetized dogs. Under these conditions the G.H. response to an intravenous injection of clonidine is inhibited by the injection of phenoxybenzamine into the third ventricle (140). Furthermore when the territories of the carotid and vertebral arteries are separated by occlusion of the basilar artery, then a small dose of clonidine only stimulates G.H. when given into the carotid artery: intravenous or intravertebral clonidine does not release G.H. (188). Thus, the G.H. response to clonidine is mediated through the stimulation of receptors within the forebrain.

The pharmacological properties of these receptors have been investigated in conscious non-human primates. In rhesus monkeys the G.H. response to clonidine is inhibited by the α_2 antagonist piperoxane (79). In baboons the G.H. response to clonidine is inhibited by the α_2 antagonists piperoxane, yohimbine and phenoxybenzamine: whereas the α_1 antagonist prazosin, had no effect (146). Thus receptors involved in the G.H. response to clonidine have the properties of peripheral (and possibly α_2) adrenoceptors. Clonidine is also a histamine agonist and studies are needed to investigate the possible involvement of histamine receptors in G.H. response to clonidine.

Finally α_2 adrenoceptors exist pre-and post-synaptically. To distinguish between the efects of clonidine upon pre-and post-synaptic α adrenoceptors, rats were pre-treated with reserpine to deplete presynaptic noradrenaline stores. Under these circumstances the G.H. response to clonidine was enhanced (64). These findings suggest that the G.H. response to clonidine can be mediated through the stimulation of post-synaptic α adrenoceptors.

Further studies are needed to justify the extrapolation of these findings in man but at the moment the suggestion is that G.H. responses to clonidine which may be measured in patients is mediated through the stimulation of post-synaptic α_2 adrenoceptors in the forebrain.

DOPAMINE AND G.H.

In man the release of G.H. is stimulated by a wide variety of dopamine agonists including apomorphine (123), bromocriptine (30, 54), piribedil (215), lergotrile (216) and lisuride (60).

Less selective dopamine agonists also release G.H. (14, 23, 25, 96, 183). The G.H. response to apomorphine must depend upon the stimulation of dopamine receptors as it is inhibited by the dopamine blocking drugs chlorpromazine (123), pimozide (125), clozapine (109) and haloperidol (185) but not by drugs with other actions such as benztropine (124), methysergide (125) and cyproheptidine (185). Similarly the G.H. response to bromocriptine and to lergotrile are both inhibited by dopamine blocking drugs (5, 216).

Although there is clear evidence for an excitatory dopaminergic control of G.H. release in man, such a system is not found in some experimental animals. It is particularly surprising that apomorphine does not stimulate the release of G.H. in conscious rhesus monkeys (42) and baboons (146). For this reason it is not possible to investigate the pharmacology of the dopamine receptors which regulate G.H. release. It has been suggested that at least some of the receptors that stimulate the release of G.H. must be outside the blood brain barrier (28, 133, 135): however these findings are disputed (31, 222).

5--HYDROXYTRYPTAMINE (5-HT) AND G.H.

Although the role of central noradrenaline and dopamine in the control of G.H. release can be defined in man the role of 5-HT is less certain. Much of this uncertaintly is due to the lack of specificity of the clinically available 5-HT agonists and antagonists. Thus virtually all of the 5-HT antagonists are histamine antagonists: cyproheptidine also has atropinic properties and both cyproheptidine and metergoline block dopamine receptors (63, 77, 204). Furthermore, there is uncertainty as to whether the 5-HT antagonists cross the blood brain barrier (102) and alter the firing of 5-HT neurones (55).

A role for 5-HT in the central regulation of G.H. release was suggested by reports that the G.H. response to hypoglycemia was inhibited by the 5-HT antagonists cyproheptidine and methysergide (19, 155, 201). However these findings are disputed (115). Cyproheptidine has been reported to inhibit G.H. responses to 5-HTP (171), to L-DOPA (57, 202), to exercise (201) and to argine (171) and sleep (47). These last two findings conflict with the reports that the G.H. responses to arginine and sleep are enhanced by the 5-HT antagonists metergoline (179) and methysergide (156).

Unfortunately the clinically available 5-HT agonists are equally lacking in potency and specificity. Thus 5-hydroxytryptophan (5-HTP) the immediate precursor of 5-HT, is known to displace endogenous stores of noradrenaline and dopamine as well as 5-HT. These may be important in the G.H. response to 5-HTP as this is blocked by the α-adrenergic antagonist phentolamine (170) as well as by cyproheptidine (171). In fact only high doses of 5-HPT stimulate the release of G.H. (13, 89, 97, 233) and high doses of 5-HPT have euphoric side effects which themselves could be the stimulus to the release of G.H.

L-tryptophan is a more selective though less potent stimulus to the release of 5-HT from nerve terminals. L-tryptophan stimulates a small but variable release of G.H. (94, 167, 237) which suggests a weak 5-HT excitatory influence over the release of G.H.

A third strategy for investigating the role of 5-HT in regulating G.H. release is to give drugs which block the re-uptake of 5-HT. It has been seen that drugs which block the uptake of noradrenaline are potent and reliable stimuli to the release of G.H. In contrast drugs such as chlorimipramine and zimeldine which selectively block the uptake of 5-HT have little effect upon the release of G.H. (121, 122, 208). If chlorimipramine and zimeldine block 5-HT uptake as potently as desmethylimipramine and nomifensine block catecholamine uptake, then these findings demonstrate that the release of G.H. is more influenced by catecholamines than by 5-HT.

GABA AND G.H.

In man the release of G.H. is stimulated by a number of GABA mimetic drugs including gamma hydroxybutyric acid (209), gamma amino beta hydroxybutyric acid (71) and diazepam (207). The findings that the G.H. response to diazepam is inhibited by the GABA agonist sodium valproate (118) may suggest that GABA is involved in the G.H. response to diazepam. However other transmitters must be involved as the G.H. response to diazepam is also inhibited by the neuroleptic pimozide (118).

OPIATE RECEPTORS AND G.H.

Morphine and β-endorphin do not stimulate the release of G.H. in man (37, 75). However the synthesic enkephalin analogue DAMME does release G.H. although DAMME also causes stressful side effects, and whether or not naloxone prevents the G.H. response to DAMME remains controversial (206, 226).

Naloxone (10 mg i.v.) has been reported to inhibit the G.H. response to arginine (164). Smaller doses of naloxone did not influence the G.H. responses to hypoglycemia (203, 227) and apomorphine (127). The G.H. response to exercise was inhibited by naloxone in two studies (153-203).

These findings contrast with the animal literature where virtually all opiate agonist and antagonist drugs respectively stimulate and inhibit the release of G.H. (163). It would appear that in man opiate receptors exert a rather weak excitatory influence over the release of G.H. This influence may only be investigated in patients by giving large doses of agonist drugs.

HISTAMINE AND G.H.

Although no histamine agonist can be given to human subjects a variety of antagonists are available and appear to have little if any influence upon the release of G.H. The G.H. responses to arginine and hypoglycemia are influenced by neither meclastine nor dexchlorphenir-amine (179) while the G.H. response to L-DOPA was unaffected by diphenhydramine and cimetidine even though it was inhibited by betazole (33).

PROSTAGLANDINS

It remains uncertain whether or not prostaglandins influence G.H. release as the administration of different prostaglandin synthesis inhibitors has different effects upon G.H. release, even in the same patients. Thus acetylsalicylic acid inhibited the G.H. response to hypoglycemia while indomethacin did not (38). In another study indomethacin had no effect upon the G.H. response to arginine (223). In a third study the infusion of prostaglandin PGE2 stimulated the release of G.H. possibly because the infusion resulted in stressful side effects (100).

ACETYLCHOLINE AND G.H.

It is uncertain whether or not acetylcholine influences the release of G.H. in man. The peripherally acting antagonist methscopolamine has been reputed to inhibit the G.H.response to sleep and to hypogly-cemia (156). However in another study the centrally acting antagonist atropine had no effect upon the G.H. response to hypoglycemia (21).

The agonist physostigmine does not release G.H. except at doses which cause stressful side effects (193).

Conclusion

The release of G.H. is controlled by excitatory α-adrenergic dopaminergic, GABA-ergic and opiate influences and probably by an inhibitory β-adrenergic influence. The functioning of each of these systems can be investigated using pharmacoendocrine tests of the functioning of each type of receptor. However the results of such studies will only be meaningful when all of the other influences upon G.H. release are held constant. A review of these other influences will now be made.

BIOLOGICAL VARIABLES INFLUENCING G.H. RELEASE

The major episodes of G.H. release are linked to the onset of slow wave sleep but episodic release also occurs spontaneously and in response to stressful and other stimuli. The spontaneous release of G.H. imposes a major constraint upon studies of G.H. release because G.H. is known to inhibit its own release (1, 195). For this reason patients with 'raised' baseline G.H. concentrations are excluded from studies of G.H. release, and in this way one third of any study population is lost. Further studies are needed to define the most conservative criteria for a 'normal' baseline which will not interfere with the size or measurement of subsequent G.H. response. Conventional practice is to exclude patients with plasma G.H. concentrations of greater than 3 or 5 ng/ml at the time of giving the test drug but this practice is arbitrary.

Effects of age

The spontaneous secretion of G.H. as studied by 24 hour smapling is maximal during adolescence and then declines throughout life so that some elderly subjects secrete little G.H. at all (70).

Studies of G.H. responses to drugs such as L-DOPA, apomorphine, desipramine and clonidine in depressed patients include data suggestive of impaired G.H. responses to test drugs with increasing age (72, 85, 119, 121, 152, 192). Although G.H. responses to some stimuli are not influenced by age (35) it would seem wise to control for age in any clinical study of G.H. release.

Effects of peripheral hormones upon G.H. responses

G.H. release is enhanced by oestrogen and so varies markedly throughout the menstrual cycle before declining in the menopause. To control for this variation pre-menopausal women are usually excluded from studies of G.H. release. Post menopausal women whether normal or depressed have small G.H. responses and are therefore inconvenient for study.

Cortisol inhibits the release of G.H. at least in patients with Cushing's Syndrome (213) (Thompson et al. 1972) although it remains to be seen whether or not the smaller increase in cortisol secretion which is found in depression alters G.H. release.

Other influences upon G.H. release

Many of the other physiological and pathological influences upon G.H. release can be excluded from neuroendocrine investigations. Thus patients with obesity, starvation, pregnancy, the puerperium, or with debilitating medical illnesses should all be excluded (44). Patients with alcoholism should also be excluded (41) and Matussek has shown that a daily intake of 2 litres of beer is sufficient to impair G.H. responses (152). Psychotropic drugs interfere with G.H. release and a three week washout period is assumed to be sufficient to exclude such effects: no formal study of this issue has been reported. Benzodiazepines are given as night sedation even though they are known to stimulate the release of G.H. (207) and to have half lives sufficiently long to be still active the next day. For these reasons studies are needed to investigate the neuroendocrine effects of the previous night's sedation. Finally, G.H. is one of the pituitary hormones which are secreted in response to acute "stress" (51). However little is known of the neuroendocrine effects of the chronic and non-specific stresses which are associated with psychiatric illness and for this reason the G.H. responses of patients with affective illness should be compared with those of patients with other psychiatric illnesses.

Conclusion

In pharmacoendocrine studies of G.H. release it is necessary to control for effects of age, ovarian function and chronic stress as well as to exclude the influence of drugs, baseline G.H. release, starvation, obesity, pregnancy and medical illness. The following review of studies of G.H. release in depressed patients will examine the adequacy of the control groups that were employed.

G.H. RELEASE IN DEPRESSION

G.H. response to hypoglycemia

Of the available provocative stimuli hypoglycemia has been used most extensively in depressed patients. Unfortunately depressed patients are relatively resistant to the hypoglycemic action of insulin. Consequently although depressed patients tend to have smaller G.H. responses than do recovered patients (52, 62, 81, 165, 190) in each study the depressed patients had less hypoglycemia. Similarly although patients with endogenous depression may have smaller G.H. responses than patients with reactive depression (52, 165) they also become less hypoglycemic. Only one study has matched depressed patients individually with controls for age, for sex and for degree of hypoglycemia (82): in this study 10 depressed patients had smaller G.H. responses than did 10 normal subjects.

G.H. responses to L-DOPA

No differences were found in the G.H. responses to L-DOPA when 22 male depressives were matched for age with normal male subjects and when 18 post menopausal female depressives were matched for age with normal post menopausal subjects (192). A second report of normal G.H. responses to L-DOPA in depressed patients (80) also included 7 patients with bipolar depressive illness had G.H. responses which were greater than those of manic patients of unipolar depressives and of normal subjects: however data on the age and sex of these groups was not given.

G.H. responses to amphetamine

Nine endogenous depressives had smaller G.H. responses to d-amphetamine (0.1 mg/kgm weight) than did 21 normal subjects and 7 reactive depressives (13). However these groups were not matched for age and the raw data presented by the authors suggest that the G.H. response to d-amphetamine is attenuated with age and that 7 patients with endogenous depression had similar G.H. responses to 7 normal subjects with whom they could be individually matched for age and sex. Halbreich found no significant difference between the G.H. responses to amphetamine of depressed and normal subjects who were matched for age and sex (88).

In another study no difference was found between the G.H.responses to methylamphetamine of 20 patients with endogenous depression and those of 10 recovered depressives, 6 reactive depressives, 8 psychotic patients and 10 neurotic patients (43).

G.H. responses to clonidine

G.H. responses to clonidine were significantly less in 10 patients with endogenous depression than in 22 normal subjects, in 12 patients with reactive depression and in 10 patients with schizophrenia; however the patients with endogenous depression were older than the controls (152). In another study the responses of 10 patients with endogenous depression were compared with the responses to 10 normal subjects individually matched with the patients for age and sex. In 9 of the comparisons the depressed patients had a smaller G.H. response than did the control who was matched for age and sex (45). Similarly impaired G.H. responses to clonidine have been found in other depressed patients who were included in other studies (46, 199). To date 25 drug free depressed patients have had smaller G.H. responses to clonidine than have 21 age matched controls.

G.H. responses to desipramine

G.H. responses to desipramine (75 mg i.m.) have been measured in normal subjects, in patients with reactive depression and in patients with endogenous depression (119, 121). Desiprmaine did not release G.H. from post menopause depressives and from post menopausal normal women, but desipramine was a ptoent and reliable stimulus for the secretion of G.H. in all other subjects. Patients with endogenous depression had significantly smaller responses than either the normal subjects of the patients with reactive depression. Among the published raw data can be found 8 pairs of endogenous depressives and normal subjects who are individually matched for age and sex. In 7 cases the response of the depressed patient is less than that of the control subject.

G.H. responses to 5-HTP

A small group of 6 depressed patients had a smaller G.H. response to 5-HTP (200 mg orally) than did 7 normal subjects and 4 manic patients (210). In a second study (175) subjects were pretreated with benserazide before treatment with 5-HTP (2 mg/kgm i.v. over 1 hour) 7 depressed patients tended to have delayed G.H. responses to this treatment when their responses were compared to those of 8 normal subjects. In both of these studies the patients were older than the controls.

G.H. response to apomorphine

G.H. responses to apomorphine (0.75 mg s.c.) have been reported to be normal in two studies of depressed patients (36, 72) in neither of which were depressed patients closely matched with controls for age and sex.

G.H. responses to sleep

Only 1 out of 6 drug free depressed patients secreted a pulse of G.H. during slow wave sleep (196). Rubin (186) has also found abnormal G.H. release in sleeping depressed patients but has pointed out that these findings may be a direct effect of the broken sleep that accompanies depression.

G.H. responses to thermal stimulation

Eight out of 12 depressed patients had inadequate G.H. responses to being placed in a hot bath (at 37° for 15 mins and then at 43° for 15 mins) as compared to only 3 of 10 normal volunteers (196). It is not clear how closely matched were the depressed and normal subjects.

Paradoxical G.H. responses to TRH

TRH does not release G.H. in normal subjects but may do so in patients with acromegaly, liver disease and anorexia nervosa. An anomalous G.H. release has also been reported in studies of depressed patients (24, 148, 211). However placebo controls have not yet been employed to exclude the possibility that the rather variable G.H. variable responses which were seen in these depressed patients were spontaneous events.

G.H. responses in patients with hypomania

Although impaired G.H. responses to hypoglycemia have been found in some hypomanic patients (36, 76) the patients and controls were not matched for degree of hypoglycemia. Carroll (34) has reviewed some very preliminary studies of G.H. responses to L-DOPA, apomorphine and 5-HTP in hypomanic patients. The numbers of patients studied were so small that meaningful conclusions could not be drawn. Multi-centre studies may be needed to obtain sufficient numbers of drug free hypomanic patients.

OVERVIEW OF STUDIES OF G.H. RELEASE IN DEPRESSION

Age and ovarian status strongly influence the size of G.H. responses to test stimuli. These influences are best controlled for when patients and controls are individually matched for age and ovarian status.

G.H. responses to many stimuli are impaired in patients with endogenous depression although the influence of depression may be less than the combined influences of age and sex. If this is so then G.H. responses cannot be used for diagnosing endogenous depression unless normal values are available for a wide range of age groups and for differing states of ovarian activity. For similar reasons studies of G.H. release are unlikely to be useful in biological studies of the classification of depression. Further constraints upon studies of G.H. release come from the need to employ stringent drug free criteria and to exclude patients with raised baseline G.H. concentrations. In these ways G.H. is of less interest to psychiatry than is the more robust hypothalamic-pituitary adrenal axis.

However from a pharmacoendocrine viewpoint the position is reversed and G.H. is the pituitary hormone of greatest interest to psychiatry. Neuroendocrine tests of G.H. release are available for assessing the status of α-adrenoceptors, of dopamine receptors, of opiate receptors and of the bendiazepine-GABA receptor complex. Furthermore, many of these neuroendocrine models can be studied both in experimental animals and in patients and in this way they can be used to study pharmacological questions such as the mechanism of action of electroconvulsive therapy (199) and tricyclic antidepressants (46).

To date the main application of G.H. studies has been to look at central α-adrenoceptor and dopamine receptor status. Some patients with endogenous depression have impaired G.H. responses to drugs which stimulate α-adrenoceptors: some have apparently normal G.H. responses to the dopamine agonist apomorphine. Further studies are needed using other control groups and different stimuli. At the moment the main results reviewed in this section are consistent with a defect at α-adrenoceptors in brain regions regulating the release of G.H. in patients with endogenous depression.

II PROLACTIN

A similar but briefer review will now be made of the biological factors which influence prolactin release and of the role of neurotransmitters in controlling prolactin secretion. The reported studies of prolactin release will then be assessed in the light of these general sections.

FACTORS INFLUENCING THE SECRETION OF PROLACTIN

The release of prolactin is influenced by many of the factors whose influence upon the release of G.H. has been discussed in detail. Thus estrogen facilitates the release of prolactin which is increased in females from puberty until after the menopause (83, 214). A mid cycle rise may also occur and a striking increase is seen in pregnancy (214) and for the duration of lactation. The sex difference is not evident in old age when low plasma prolactin concentrations are found in male and female subjects (214). The release of prolactin is closely entrained to non-REM sleep and plasma concentrations build up through the hours of sleep and then decline over the next day (187). Like G.H. PRL is secreted episodically and in response to psychological "stress" (51). The release of both hormones is impaired in the obese, in alcoholics and in the medically ill (43). It follows from these observations that each of the above factors should be controlled for in any study of prolactin release in depression.

THE ROLE OF NEUROTRANSMITTERS AND THEIR RECEPTORS IN REGULATING THE RELEASE OF PROLACTIN IN MAN

Dopamine and Prolactin (PRL)

It is well established that the release of PRL is tonically inhibited by a central mechanism in which dopamine is involved. Thus in man as in experimental animals the secretion of PRL is stimulated by dopamine antagonists (12, 48, 132, 189) and is inhibited by dopamine and by dopamine antagonists (15, 123, 216). Indeed a competitive inhibition between the effects of dopamine infusions and the effects of neuroleptic drugs can be demonstrated in man (133).

Identical effects of dopamine agonists and antagonists can be detected *in vitro* when these drugs are added to isolated pituitary glands (146, 200). Pituitary lactotropes are endowed with dopamine receptors (29) and it would appear that the PRL response to a dopamine agonist or antagonist provides a measure of the status of the dopamine receptor on pituitary lactotropes. Dopamine receptors within the median eminence (174) and other brain regions (107) are also involved in the regulation of PRL release but are unlikely to exert a major influence upon the prolactin response to drugs which act directly at dopamine receptors upon the lactotrope.

NORADRENALINE AND PROLACTIN

In general noradrenaline would appear to have little if any influence upon the release of PRL in man. The α-adrenoceptor agonist guanfacine has been reported to inhibit the PRL response to hypoglycemia (130) although neither guanfacine nor clonidine alters the spontaneous secretion of PRL (124, 130). Desipramine is a potent and selective inhibitor of the re-uptake of noradrenaline and stimulates the release of G.H.: it has no effect upon basal PRL levels (122).

5-HYDROXYTRYPTAMINE (5-HT) AND PROLACTIN

A number of human studies have shown that the release of PRL can be stimulated by 5-HT agonists and inhibited by 5-HT antagonists. However the effects are often slight and are not always replicated and so it would appear that any excitatory 5-HT control is weaker than the inhibitory dopamine control.

Thus l-tryptophan stimulated the release of prolactin in some studies (144, 237) although not in others (67, 73, 78, 94, 202, 231). Similarly 5-hydroxytryptophan (5-HTP) stimulated the release of PRL when given in large doses (233); smaller doses had no effect (89).

Fluoxetine and zimeldine are indirectly acting 5-HT agonist drugs which selectively block the re-uptake of 5-HT. Neither drug releases PRL (149, 208) although fluoxetine has been reported to enhance the PRL response to hypoglycemia (149). These findings are also consistent with the presence of a weak facilitatory influence of 5-HT upon PRL release. In experimental animals 5-HT agonists release PRL more consistently although larger doses are used and these may cause stressful side effects which themselves would stimulate the release of PRL. Such side effects did not occur in the human studies which have been reviewed.

The 5-HT antagonist cyproheptidine has been reported to inhibit the PRL responses to l-tryptophan (144), to sleep (155), to nursing (50) but not to hypoglycemia (115). The PRL response to nursing is also inhibited by the 5-HT antagonists methysergide and metergoline (50). Methysergide and metergoline also reduced prolactin levels in normal subjects before and after treatment with pimozide (69).

In conclusion there would appear to be a weak facilitatory serotonergic influence upon the release of PRL in man. At present there is no selective 5-HT agonist which can be used as the stimulus for a neuroendocrine test of 5-HT receptor function in patients.

ACETYLCHOLINE AND PROLACTIN

Anticholinergic drugs do not influence the spontaneous secretion of PRL (Sachar et al. 1978; Lal and Nair, 1979) although they do antagonize the PRL response to neuroleptic drugs (Lal and Nair, 1979; Halbreich et al. 1980).

Physostigmine only stimulates the release of PRL when it also causes stressful side effects (194). Thus although there may be a cholinergic dopaminergic interaction in the tuberoinfundibular as in other dopamine systems, acetylcholine would not appear to exert a direct effect upon the release of PRL.

GABA AND PROLACTIN

In man the secretion of PRL is stimulated by the GABA mimetic drugs gamma hydroxybutyric acid (209), gamma amino beta hydroxybutyric acid (71) and muscimol (212). Thus in man GABA would appear to exert a facilitatory influence over the release of PRL as well as of G.H. Unfortunately the underlying mechanisms are not amenable to study in experimental animals where GABA drugs inhibit PRL release (128, 181).

Opiate Receptors and Prolactin

In man the secretion of PRL is stimulated by morphine (217), by methadone (66), by the enkephalin analogue DAMME (206, 226) and by β-endorphin (37). However, the opiate antagonist naloxone reduced neither the basal nor the provoked release of prolactin in man (104, 127, 153, 164, 203, 227) which is surprising as in experimental animals naloxone inhibits and opiate agonists stimulate the release of PRL (154). In view of this species difference it may be wise not to extrapolate to man the results of animals studies investigating the interaction between opiate and dopamine receptors in the regulation of PRL release (154).

HISTAMINE AND PROLACTIN

Plasma concentrations of PRL rise promptly after the intravenous injection of the H_2 histamine antagonist cimetidine (27, 32, 53, 59). This effect is not obtained when cimetidine is added to rat pituitary cells *in vitro* (59) suggesting that the effect of cimetidine upon PRL is mediated through the blockade of central histamine H_2 receptors.

PROLACTIN RELEASE IN DEPRESSED PATIENTS

At present most reported studies show little or no change in the plasma concentrations of PRL in fasting depressed patients studied between 0900 and 1000 hours (75, 80, 81, 84, 158). However two of these groups found lower PRL levels in bipolar depressives. There are also two reports of raised PRL concentrations (148, 191) and two reports in which prolactin levels rose during treatment with antidepressants (10 172).

Two 24 hour catheter studies have found defective sleep-related PRL release in depressed patients (158, 186) although one study found an essentially normal release of PRL during sleep (84). However even if some depressed patients fail to release PRL normally at night this could be a direct effect of their disturbed sleep and need not have any other biological significance (187). Halbreich's patients had unexpectedly raised evening prolactin concentrations (84) which would be consistent with a phase advance of the circadian rhythm of PRL release: however the studies by Mendlewicz (158) and by Rubin (186) did not replicate this finding.

Prolactin responses to TRH

There are two reports of impaired PRL responses to TRH in depression

(61, 158) of which one (158) provided control for menopausal status. One other study which did not apparently control for menopausal status found normal responses (148). Two studies found similar PRL responses to TRH in depressed and recovered patients (81, 148). This literature contrasts with the clearer evidence of impaired TSH responses to TRH in depression.

Prolactin responses to other stimuli

In response to physostigmine (0.22 mg/kgm i.v.) 7 depressed patients had larger PRL responses than did 15 patients with other psychiatric diagnoses (105). However the depressed patients had different psychological responses to the physostigmine (and more nausea) and they were not necessarily matched for age, sex and manapausal status.

In response to morphine (5 mg i.v.) 10 depressed patients had smaller prolactin responses than 6 control subjects (65). However many of the depressed patients had received psychotropic drugs one week before the study.

The peripherally acting decarboxylase inhibitor carbidopa stimulates the release of PRL presumably by inhibiting the synthesis of dopamine in the median eminence. In a study of male and female, unipolar and bipolar depressives and normal subjects, impaired PRL responses to carbidopa were found in a group of 6 female bipolar depressives (75). L-DOPA has been reported to suppress plasma PRL levels normally in depressed patients (191). Similar findings were reported in a second study (80): this contained a subgroup of 8 bipolar depressives who showed an exaggerated suppression, although appropriate controls for the subgroup were not employed. Further evidence of normal pituitary dopamine receptor function in depression comes from Coppen's findings of normal PRL responses to bromocriptine (44).

OVERVIEW OF STUDIES OF PROLACTIN RELEASE IN DEPRESSION

Few studies control for the effects of age, ovarian status and drugs upon the release of PRL. Those which do suggest that the spontaneous secretion of PRL is essentially normal during the day but abnormal during the night. However, it remains to be seen whether or not the defective nocturnal release of PRL in depression is a direct effect of impaired sleep.

The pharmacological control of PRL release is dominated by an inhibitory dopaminergic influence which acts predominantly at the pituitary. This mechanism would appear to function normally in depressed patients in whom PRL release is normally suppressed by L-DOPA.

Apart from the strong inhibitory dopaminergic control of PRL release there are excitatory GABA-ergic and opiate influences and adequately controlled studies of these systems are needed in depressed patients.

III MELATONIN

Within a pharmacoendocrine review of affective disorders, studies of melatonin release are included more for their future promise than for their past achievements. The subject has been held back by the impractical and insufficiently sensitive nature of the early bioassays with a consequent lack of knowledge of the clinical endocrinology of melatonin and a lack of dynamic tests of pineal function. Progress in all of these areas is now rapid. There is reasonable agreement between the results of most radioimmunoassays for melatonin (5) and comparison is possible with the absolute determination of melatonin using gas chromatography - mass spectometer (GCMS) techniques (137). As will be seen in the next section it has recently become apparent that the secretion of melatonin varies greatly among normal individuals and furthermore time of the year, menstrual cycle, body weight, intense light and age may all influence its secretion. Finally although no pineal function test has been found the nocturnal release of melatonin is to some extent a natural test of pineal function.

BIOLOGICAL FACTORS INFLUENCING THE SECRETION OF MELATONIN

Light is the main influence upon the release of melatonin in experimental animals and probably in man as well. In animals the secretion of melatonin follows a 24 hour rhythm whereby melatonin is regularly secreted during the hours of darkness but not during the light (16, 180). This rhythm is endogenous and persists in total darkness (182). Normally it is entrained to the light - dark cycle as light inhibits the synthesis and release of melatonin (112, 238). In man too light inhibits the release of melatonin although intense light is needed (139). whether or not some melatonin is secreted during the day time in less intense light remains disputed (8, 136).

In animals which breed seasonally plasma concentrations of melatonin show marked seasonal variations (4, 7). A smaller seasonal variation in human melatonin levels has been reported (Arendt et al. 1977; Birau et al. 1981). Even though further studies are needed to define the details of the seasonal rhythm of human melatonin secretion, it is clear that seasonal variation requires control in any human study of melatonin secretion. The seasonal variation in the reproductive activity of man is slight but significant (Reinberg, 1974) and puberty represents the main change in sexual activity. It is therefore interesting that marked changes in melatonin secretion have been reported at this time (Silman et al. 1979) although it is perhaps surprising that these changes have been restricted to male subjects. However reports at variance with these findings have appeared (Sizonenko et al. 1980) and clearly further study is required. Plasma melatonin concentrations in the early morning have been reported to vary throughout the menstrual cycle (230) suggesting either a phase-shift or a change in total secretion. Total secretion is assessed by 6-hydroxymelatonin estimation reportedly does not change during the menstrual cycle (68). Clearly the possible influence of the menstrual cycle should be considered when designing human studies. There is general agreement in the literature that melatonin secretion varies greatly between individuals (8, 142) while remaining relatively constant within individuals implying that large populations are required for statistical analyses, or that individuals should be used as their own controls in experimental situations.

Finally in a study of normal subjects a positive correlation was found between body weight and plasma melatonin concentrations (6).

In summary human studies of melatonin should control for effects of body weight, menstrual cycle, puberty and both circannual and circadian variation. As melatonin release is entrained to the light dark cycle but not to sleep (106) it is necessary to control for time of day but not for the effects of broken sleep.

THE ROLE OF NEUROTRANSMITTERS IN REGULATION OF THE RELEASE OF MELATONIN NORADRENALINE

In experimental animals the pineal gland is usually considered to be innervated by post-ganglionic fibres which originate in the superior cervical ganglion (109, 110) although there is evidence for some central innervation in ferrets and rats. The preganglionic fibres are part of the sympathetic outflow from the spinal cord and the central connections of the preganglionic fibres include the suprachiasmatic nucleus and the retinohypothalamic tract. The normal synthesis of melatonin is dependent upon the integrity of these structures (161, 162). The postganglionic fibres terminate around β-adrenoceptors upon pinealocytes. Pineal glands can be cultured in vitro when the β-agonists isoprenaline and noradrenaline can be shown to stimulate the activity of adenylate cyclase (228), the formation of cyclic AMP (56, 205), the production of N-acetyltransferase (111) and the synthesis and release of melatonin (11). Drugs which indirectly stimulate β-adrenoceptors have been shown to increase the secretion of melatonin in vivo (236).

In man the secretion of melatonin is dependent upon the integrity of the autonomic nervous system (221) and the cervical cord (116). The nocturnal release of melatonin is dependent upon normal β-adrenoceptor function as it is inhibited by propranolol (91, 220). For these reasons it would appear that the secretion of melatonin is dependent upon β-adrenoceptor function in man just as it is in animals.

It is therefore disappointing that in general β agonists fail to release melatonin in man. The direct agonist isoprenaline has been tested (136) as have the indirectly acting drugs L-DOPA (221), tyramine, dopamine (136), imipramine, tranylcypromine and methylamphetamine (6). Chronic treatment with desipramine may stimulate the release of melatonin as in patients who had been treated with desipramine, a positive correlation could be found between plasma concentrations of desipramine and melatonin (81): however other explanations for this correlation are available. In general drugs which release melatonin in animals fail to do so in man possibly because larger doses are used in the animal studies than is safe in clinical studies. When clinically relevant doses of antidepressant drugs are given to rats then they fail to stimulate acutely the release of melatonin (60).

In animals presynaptic α-adrenoceptors have been demonstrated in noradrenergic nerve endings within the pineal (173, 176). Whether or not clonidine (which stimulates presynaptic α-adrenoceptors) inhibits the release of melatonin remains to be seen and the apparent enhancement of noradrenergic pineal stimulation in vitro by phentolamine (114) has not be explored in vivo.

OTHER NEUROTRANSMITTERS AND MELATONIN

As well as noradrenaline, octopamine (103), histamine (143), GABA (151), dopamine (177) and serotonin (103) are all to be found in the pineal although only noradrenaline and octopamine are thought to be within nerve endings. At present only noradrenaline is implicated in the neural control of melatonin release.

MELATONIN RELEASE IN PATIENTS WITH AFFECTIVE ILLNESS

A definitive study of melatonin secretion in affective illness would require that patients and controls be matched for each of the variables whose influence of melatonin secretion has been discussed already. Such studies are in progress. The reported studies do not control for all of the necessary variables.

One early study compared 5 untreated depressed patients with 5 normal subjects of the same age and measured the urinary secretion of melatonin (using a bioassay) from urinary samples taken during daytine and night-time (106). The patients and controls excreted similar quantities of melatonin, both excreted more melatonin at night and sleep deprivation had no influence upon the secretion of melatonin. No control was made for any effects of time of the menstrual cycle, time of year, sex, body weight, or any non-specific effect of mental illness upon melatonin.

There then followed a series of reports in which plasma melatonin concentrations were measured using radioimmunoassays. Wirz-Justice and Arendt (234) studied 6 patients with unipolar depression and 7 with bipolar depression. Samples were taken at 8.00 a.m. when the unipolar depressives had significantly lower plasma melatonin concentrations than the controls. The bipolar depressives and the controls all had similar plasma melatonin concentrations at 8.00 a.m. This study controlled for time of year, but not for body weight, age or stage of menstrual cycle.

Three of these depressed patients were treated with maprotiline. None responded, and all had similar (low) plasma melatonin concentrations (235).

In another study four depressed patients were studied by 24 hour sampling firstly when depressed and secondly while taking antidepressant medication when they had recovered. Similar mean values for plasma melatonin concentrations were obtained on the two occasions. Five normal subjects tended to have higher plasma melatonin concentrations during the dark phase, although no demographic or other details about these controls are given (157).

One single patient was studied in winter firstly when well and secondly when depressed. Plasma melatonin concentrations were estimated on four occasions during the night and on each occasion a lower value was obtained from the patient when she was depressed (232). In a further study of depressed patients this group have found an inverse correlation between the nocturnal secretion of melatonin and escape from dexamethasone depression (233).

To date only one group have measured plasma melatonin concentrations over a 24 hour period in patients with affective illness and using a GCMS assay for melatonin. Three patients were studied under these conditions and had higher mean melatonin levels when manic than when depressed (138). A fourth manic patient was also studied and the four had significantly higher melatonin levels than four normal subjects. The longitudinal comparison controlled for age and sex but neither comparison controlled for effects of drugs, body weight, time of the menstrual cycle ot time of the year. Elsewhere Lewy (136) has noted a phase advance of the 24 hour melatonin rhythm in mania as compared to in depression and in depression as compared to in normal subjects. He has also noted that the nocturnal release of melatonin was more readily depressed by light than was the case in normal subjects. Full details of these studies have not been published and so it is not yet possible to assess the controls that were employed.

SUMMARY OF REVIEW

The central issue running through this review is the use of pharmacoendocrine tests in which neuroreceptor function is measured as the pituitary hormone response to the stimulation of specific neuroreceptor agonist. Such a strategy is considered valid under the following conditions:

i) several drugs which stimulate a specific neuroreceptor should release the hormone in question:

ii) this response should be inhibited by drugs which block the specific neuroreceptor:

iii) evidence from animal and/or human studies should confirm that the neuroreceptors are within the brain.

Neuroendocrine tests of G.H. release which meet the first two criteria are available for α-adrenoceptors, for dopamine receptors and for opiate receptors. Tests of PRL release which meet the criteria are available for dopamine and opiate receptors. No pharmacoendocrine test of melatonin release is available.

Most of the pharmacoendocrine tests to localize the receptors have been studied in experimental animals. The dopamine receptors regulating PRL release are of course predominantly in the pituitary while the α-adrenoceptors regulating G.H. release are undoubtedly in the brain (74, 140). The opiate receptors regulating G.H. and PRL release are also located within the brain (154).

Such pharmacoendocrine tests are considered to provide a valid measure of neuroreceptor status when all other influences regulating hormone release are held constant. The practical difficulties involved in finding suitable patients and controls are well known and account for the relatively slow accumulation of reliable data in this field.

Patients with endogenous depression have impaired G.H. responses to α-agonists, while the G.H. responses to dopamine agonists may be normal. Studies are needed of the G.H. and PRL responses to opiate and GABA agonists in patients with endogenous depression. The presently available data suggests that patients with endogenous depression may have impaired α-adrenoceptor status at least in neuroendocrine systems.

As well as providing baseline measures of receptor status these pharmacoendocrine tests can also monitor receptor status during drug treatment (46) or ECT (199). In this way they can be used to test pharmacological hypotheses both in patients and in experimental animals.

None of the pharmacoendocrine tests of G.H. release are recommended for diagnostic purposes as only drug-free patients with normal baseline G.H. levels can be used and as controls must be provided for the effects of age and ovarian function.

REFERENCES

1. Abrams, R. L. (1971): J. Clin. Invest. 50:3940-3950.
2. Abramson, E. A., Arky, R. A. and Woeber, K. A. (1966): Lancet ii:1386-1388.
3. Ahlqvist, R. P. (1948): Am. J. Physiol. 153:586-600.
4. Arendt, J. (1979): Prog. Brain Res. 52:249-259.

5. Arendt, J. (1981): In: Melatonin: current status and perspectives, edited by N. Birau and W. Schloot, pp.3-8. Pergamon Press, Oxford.
6. Arendt, J. unpublished observations.
7. Arendt, J., Wirz-Justice, A. and Bradtke, J. (1977): Neurosci. Letters 7:327-330.
8. Arendt, J., Wirz-Justice, A., Bradtke, J. and Koruemark, M. (1980): Ann. Clin. Biochem. 16:307-312.
9. Arendt, J., Symons, A. M. and Land, C. A. (1981): Experientia (in press).
10. Asnis, G. M., Nathan, R. S., Halbreich, N., Halpern, F. S. and Sachar, E. J. (1980): Am. J. Psychiatry 137:1117-1118.
11. Axelrod, J., Shein, H. M. and Wurtman, R. S. (1969): Proc. Natl. Acad. Sci. USA 62:554-559.
12. Barraclough, C. A. and Sawyer, C. H. (1959): Endocrinology 65: 563-571.
13. Benkert, O., Laakmann, G., Souvatzoglou, A. and Von Werder, K. (1973): J. Neural Transm. 34:291-299.
14. Besser, G. M., Butler, P.W.P., Landon, J. and Rees, L. (1969): Br. Med. J. iv:528-530.
15. Besser, G. M., Parke, L., Edwards, C.R.W., Forsyth, I. A. and McNeilly, A. S. (1972): Br. Med. J. iii:669-672.
16. Binkley, S., MacBridge, S. E., Klein, D. C. and Ralph, C. L. (1975): Endocrinology 96:848-853.
17. Birau, N., Birau, M. and Schloot, W. (1981): In: Melatonin: current status and perspectives, edited by N. Birau and W. Schloot, pp.287-296. Pergamon Press, Oxford.
18. Birge, C. A., Jacobs, L. S., Hammer, C. T. and Daughaday, W. H. (1970): Endocrinology 86:120-130.
19. Bivens, C. H., Lebovits, H. E. and Feldman, J. M. (1973): N. Eng. J. Med. 289;236-239.
20. Blackard, W. G. and Heidingsfelder, S. A. (1968): J. Clin. Invest. 47:1407-1414.
21. Blackard, W. G. and Waddell, C. C. (1969): Proc. Soc. Exp. Biol. Med. 131:192-196.
22. Blackard, W. G. and Hubbell, G. J. (1970): Metabolism 19:547-552.
23. Boyd, A. E., Lebovitz, H. E. and Pfeiffer, J. B. (1970): N. Eng. J. Med. 283:1425-1429.
24. Brambilla, F., Smeraldi, E., Sacchetti, E., Negri, F., Cocchi, D. and Muller, E. E. (1978): Arch. Gen. Psychiatry 35:1231-1238.
25. Brown, W. A., Corriveau, D. P. and Ebert, M. H. (1978): Psychopharmacology 58:189-195.
26. Buckler, J.H.M., Hold, A. M., Taberner, M. and London, D. R. (1969): Br. Med. J. iii:153-154.
27. Burland, W. C., Gleadle, R. I., Lee, R. M. and Rowley-Jones, D. (1978): Br. Med. J. 1:717.
28. Burrow, G. N., May, P. B., Spaulding, S. W. and Donabedian, R. K. (1977): J. Clin. Endocrinol. Metab. 45:65-72.
29. Calabro, M. A. and Macleod, R. M. (1978): Neuroendocrinology 25: 32-46.
30. Camanni, F., Massara, F., Belforte, L. and Molinatti, G. M. (1975): J. Clin. Endocrinol. metab. 40:363-366.
31. Camanni, F., Massara, F., Belforte, L., Rosatello, A. and Molinatti, G. M. (1977): J. Clin. Endocrinol. Metab. 44:465-473.
32. Carlson, H. E. and Ippoliti, A. F. (1977): J. Clin. Endocrinol. Metab. 45:367-370.

33. Carlson, H. E. and Chang, R. J. (1980): Clin. Endocrinol (Oxf). 12:461-466.
34. Carroll, B. J. (1979): In: Manic illness, edited by B. shopsin, pp.163-176. Raven Press, New York.
35. Cartlidge, N.E.F., Black, M. U., Hall, M.R.P. and Hall, R. (1970): Geront. Clin. 12:65-70.
36. Caspar, R. C., Davis, J. M., Pandey, G. N., Garver, D. L. and Dekirmenjian, H. (1977): Psychoneuroendocrinology 2:105-114.
37. Catlin, D. H., Poland, R. E., Gorelick, D. A., Gerner, R. H., Hui, K. K., Rubin, R. T. and Li, C. H. (1980): J. Clin. Endocrinol. Metab. 50:1021-1025.
38. Cavagnini, F., Di Landro, A., Invitti, C., Raggi, V., Alessandrini, P., Pinto, M., Girotti, G. and Vigo, P. (1977a): Metabolism 26: 193-200.
39. Cavagnini, F., Invitti, C., di Landro, A., Tenconi, L., Maraschini, C. and Girotti, G. (1977b): J. Clin. Endocrinol. Metab. 45: 579-584.
40. Cavagnini, F., Benetti, G., Invitti, C., Namella, G., Pinto, M., Lazza, M., Dubini, A., Marelli, A. and Muller, E. E. (1980): J. Clin. Endocrinol. Metab. 51:789-792.
41. Chalmers, R. J., Bennie, E. H., Johnson, R. H. and Kinnell, H. G. (1977): Psychol. Med. 6:607-611.
42. Chambers, J. W. and Brown, G. M. (1976): Endocrinology 98:420-428.
43. Checkley, S. A. (1979): Psychol. Med. 9:107-116.
44. Checkley, S. A. (1980): Psychol. Med. 10:35-53.
45. Checkley, S. A., Slade, A. P. and Shur, E. (1981): Br. J. Psychiatry 138:51-55.
46. Checkley, S.A., Slade, A. P., Shur, E. and Dawling, S. (1981): Br. J. Psychiatry 138:248-251.
47. Chihara, K., Kato, Y., Maeda, K., Matsukura, S. and Imura, H. (1976): J. Clin. Invest. 57:1393-1403.
48. Coppola, J. A., Leonard, R. G., Lippman, W., Perrini, J. and Ringler, L. (1965): Endocrinology 77:485-490.
49. Costain, D. W. and Green, A. R. (1978): Br. J. Pharmacology 64: 193-200.
50. Crosignani, G., Lombroso, G. C., Mattei, A., Caccamo, A. and Trojsi, L. (1979): J. Clin. Endocrinol. Metab. 48:335-337.
51. Curtis, G. C. (1979): In: Mind and Coucer Prognosis, edited by B. A. Stoll, pp.61-73. John Wiley and Sons Ltd.,
52. Czernik, A., Kleesiek, K. and Steinmeyer, E. M. (1980): Der Nervenarzt 51:662-667.
53. Daubresse, J. C., Meunier, J. C. and Ligny, G. (1978): Lancet i: 99.
54. Dammacco, F., Regillo, N. and Tafaro, E. (1976): Horm. Metab. Res. 8:247-248.
55. Deakin, J.F.W. and Green, A. R. (1978): Br. J. Pharmacol. 64: 201-209.
56. Deguchi, T. (1973): Mol. Pharm. 9:184-190.
57. Delitala, G., Masala, A., Alagna, S. and Devilla, L. (1975): Biomedical Express 23:406-409.
58. Delitala, G., Stubbs, W. A., Yeo, T., Jones, A. and Besser, G. M. (1979): Br. J. Clin. Pharmacol. 7:117-119.
59. Delitala, G., STubbs, W. A., Wass, J.A.H., Yeo, T., Jones, A., Williams, S., Besser, G. M., La Brooy, S. A. and Misiewicz, J. J. (1978): Lancet ii:1054-1055.

60. Delitala, G., Wass, J.A.H., STubbs, W. A., Jones, A., Williams, S. and Besser, G. M. (1979): Clin. Endocrinol. ii:1-9.
61. Ehrensing, R. H., Kastin, A. J., Schalch, D. S., Friesen, H. G., Vargas, J. R. and Schally, A. V. (1974): Am. J. Psychiatry 131: 714-718.
62. Endo, M., Endo, J., Nishikubo, M., Yamaguchi, T. and Hatotani, N. (1974): In: Psychoneuroendocrinology, edited by N. Hototani, pp.22-31. S. Karger, Basel.
63. Enjalbert, A., Hamon, M., Bourgoin, S. and Brockaert, J. (1978): Mol. Pharmacol. 14:11-23.
64. Eriksson, E., Dellborg, M., Eden, S. and Modigh, K. (1980): In: Abstracts of the 12th CINP Congress, Goteborg, Sweden, June 1980. Pergamon Press, Oxford.
65. Extein, I., Pottash, A.L.C., Gold, M.S., Sweeney, D. R., Martin, D. M. and Goodwin, F. K. (1980): Am. J. Psychiatry 137:845-846.
66. Exstein, I., Pickar, D., Gold, M. S., Gold, P. W., Pottash, A.L.C., Sweeney, D. R., Ross, R. J., Rebard, R., Martin, D. and Goodwin, F. K. (1981): Psychopharmacol. Bull. 17:29-32.
67. Faber, J., Hagen, C., Keirkegaard, C., Lauridsen, U. B. and Moller, S. E. (1977): Psychoneuroendocrinology 2:413-415.
68. Fellenberg, A. J., Pillipou, G. and Seamark, R. F. (1980): Biomed. Mass Spectrom. 7:84-87.
69. Ferrari, C., Caldara, R., Romussi, M., Rampini, P., Telloli, P., Saatar, S. and Curtarelli, G. (1978): Neuroendocrinology 25: 319-328.
70. Finkelstein, J. W., Roffwarg, H. P., Boyar, R. M., Kream, J. and Hellman, L. (1972): J. Clin. Endocrinol. Metab. 35:665-670.
71. Fioretti, P., Melis, G. B., Paoletti, a. N., Parodo, G., Caminiti, F., Corsini, G. U.and Martini, L. (1978): J. Clin. Endocrinol. Metab. 47:1336-1340.
72. Frazer, A. (1975): In: Biological Psychiatry, edited by J. Mendels, pp.7-26. Wiley, New York.
73. Frazer, W. M., Tucker, H. S., Grubb, S. R., Wigand, J. P. and Blackard, W. G. (1979): Horm. Metas. Res. 11:149-155.
74. Ganong, W. F., Wise, B. L., Reid, I. A., Holland, J., Kaplan, s., Shackleford, R. and Borezka, A. T. (1978): Neuroendocrinology 25:105-110.
75. Garfinkel, P. E., Brown, G. M., Warsh, J. J. and Stancer, H. C. (1979): Psychoneuroendocrinology 4:13-20.
76. Garver, D. L., Pandey, G. N., Dekirmenjian, H. and Deleon-Jones, F. (1975): Am. J. Psychiatry 132:1149-1159.
77. Gilbert, J. C. and Goldberg, L. I. (1975): J. Pharmacol. Exp. Ther. 193:435-442.
78. Glass, A. R., Smallridge, R. C., Schaaf, M. and Dimond, R. C. (1980): Psychoneuroendocrinology 5:261-265.
79. Gold, M. S., Danabedian, R. K. and Redmond, J. R. (1978): Psychoneuroendocrinology 3:187-194.
80. Gold, P. W., Goodwin, F. K., Wehr, T., Rebar, R. and Sack, R. (1976): Lancet ii:1308-1309.
81. Gregoire, F., Brauman, H., de Buck, R. and Corvilain, J. (1977): Psychoneuroendocrinology 2:303-312.
82. Gruen, P. H., Sachar, E. J., Altman, N. and Sassin, J. (1975): Arch. Gen. Psychiatry 32:31-33.
83. Guyda, H. J. and Friesen, H. G. (1923): Pediatr. Res. 7:534-540.

84. Halbreich, U., Grunhans, L. and Ben-David, M. (1979): Arch. Gen. Psychiatry 36:1183-1186.
85. Halbreich, U., Asnis, G., Halpern, F., Tabrizi, M. A. and Sachar, E. J. (1980): Psychoneuroendocrinology 5:339-344.
86. Halbreich, U., Sachar, E. J., Nathan, R. S., Asnis, G. M. and Halpern, F. S. (1980): Psychopharmacology 72:61-65.
87. Halbreich, U., Weinberg, U., Stewart, J., Klein, D. F., Weitzman, E. D. and Quitkin, F. M. (1981): Psychiatry Research 4:109-113.
88. Halbreich, U. (personal communication).
89. Handwerger, S., Plonk, J. W., Lebovitz, H. E., Bivens, C. H. and Feldman, J. M. (1975): Horm. Metabol. Res. 7:214-216.
90. Hansen, A. P. (1971): J. Clin. Endocrinol. Metab. 33:807-812.
91. Hansen, T., Heyden, T. and Sundberg, L. (1977): Lancet ii:309-310.
92. Heidingsfelder, G. V. and Blackard, W. F. (1968): Metabolism 17: 1019-1024.
93. Henninger, G. R., Mueller, P. S., and Davis, L. S. (1975): J. Nerv. Ment. Dis. 161:421-431.
94. Hyyppa, M. T., Jolma, T., Liira, J., Langvik, V-A. and Kytomaki, O. (1979): Psychoneuroendocrinology 4:29-35.
95. Imura, H., Kato, Y., Ikeda, M., Morimoto, M. and Yawata, M. (1971): J. Clin. Invest. 50:1069-1079.
96. Imura, H., Nakai, Y., Matsuyama, S. and Matsuyama, H. (1973): Horm. Metabol. Res. 5:41-45.
97. Imura, H., Nakai, Y., and Yoshimi, T. (1973): J. Clin. Endocrinol. Metab. 36:204-206.
98. Imura, H., Nakai, Y., Kati, Y., Yoshimoto, Y. and Moridera, K. (1973): In: Endocrinology, edited by R. O. Scow, pp.156-162. Excerpta Medica, Amsterdam.
99. Imura, H., Nakai, Y., Kato, Y., Yoshimoto, Y. and Moridera, K. (1974): Horm. Metabol. Res. 6:343-346.
100. Ito, H., Momose, G., Katayama, T., Tagashi, H., Ito, L., Nakajima, H. and Jakai, Y. (1971): J. Clin. Endocrinol. Metab. 32:857-859.
101. Jacobs, L. S., Snyder, P. J., Wilber, J. F., Utiger, R. D. and Daughaday, W. H. (1971): J. Clin. Endocrinol. Metab. 33:996-998.
102. Jacoby, J. H., Poulakos, J. J. and Bryce, G. F. (1978): Psychopharmacology 17:299-306.
103. Jaim-Etcherverry, G. and Zieher, L. M. (1975): J. Neurochem. 25: 915-918.
104. Janowsky, D., Judd, L., Huey, L., Toitman, N. and Parker, D. (1979): Psychopharamcology 65:95-97.
105. Janowsky, D.S., Risch, C., Parker, D., Huey, L. and Judd, L. (1980): Psychopharmacol. Bull. 16:29-30.
106. Jimerson, D. C., Lynch, J. H., Post, R. M., Wartman, R. J. and Bunney, W. E. (1977): Life Sci. 20:1501-1508.
107. Kamberi, I. A., Mical, R. S. and Porter, J. C. (1970): Experientia 26:1150-1151.
108. Kansal, P. C., Buse, J., Talbert, O. R. and Buse, M. G. (1972): J. Clin. Endocrinol. Metab. 34:99-105.
109. Kappers, J. A. (1960): Z. Zellforsch 52:163-215.
110. Kappers, J. A. (1965): In: The Structure and Function of the Epiphysis Cerebri, Progress in Brain Research Vol. 10, edited by J. Ariens Kappers and J. P. Schade, Elsevier, Amsterdam.
111. Klein, D. C., Berg, G. R. and Weller, J. (1970): Science 168: 979-980.

112. Klein, D. C. and Weller, J. L. (1972): Science 177:532-533.
113. Klein, D. C. and Weller, J. L. (1972): In: International Congress Series No.256, p.52. Excerpta Medica, Amsterdam.
114. Klein, D. C and Weller, J. L. (1973): J. Pharmacol. Exp. Ther. 186:516-527.
115. Kletzsky, O. A., Marrs, R. P. and Nicoloff, J. T. (1980): Clin. Endocrinol. (Oxf) 13:231-234.
116. Kneisley, L. W., Maskowitz, M. A. and Lynch, H. J. (1978): J. Neural. Transm. 13:311-323.
117. Koulu, M., Jammintausta, R. and Dahlstrom, S. (1979): J. Clin. Endocrinol. Metab. 48:1038-1040.
118. Koulu, M., Lammintaustra, R., Kangas, L. and Dahlstrom, S. (1979): J. Clin. Endocrinol. Metab. 48:119-122.
119. Laakmann, G. (1980): Der Nervenarzt 51:725-732.
120. Laakmann, G. (1980): Abstracts of the 12th CINP Congress, Goteborg, Sweden, June, 1980. Pergamon Press, Oxford.
121. Laakmann, G. (Personal communication).
122. Laakmann, G. and Benkert, O. (1978): In: Depressive Disorders, edited by S. Garattini amd F. K. Schattauer. Verlag, Stuttgart.
123. Lal, S., De la Vega, C. E., Sourkes, T. L. and Friesen, H. G. (1973): J. Clin. Endocrinol. Metab. 37:719-724.
124. Lal, S., Tolis, G., Martin, J. B., Brown, G. M. and Guyda, H. (1975): J. Clin. Endocrinol. Metab. 41:827-832.
125. Lal, S., Guyda, H. and Bikadoroff, S. (1977): J. Clin. Endocrinol. Metab. 44:766-770.
126. Lal, S. and Nair, N.P.V. (1979): In: Neuroendocrine Correlates in Neurology and Psychiatry, edited by E. E. Muller and A. Agnoli, pp. 179-185. Elsevier/North Holland Biomedical Press, Amsterdam.
127. Lal, S., Nair, N.P.V., Cervantes, P., Pulman, J. and Guyda, H. 1979): Acta Psychiatr. Scanc. 59:173-179.
128. Lamberts, S.W.J. and Macleod, R. M. (1979): Proc. Soc. Exp. Biol. Med. 158:10-13.
129. Lancranjan, I. and Marbach, P. (1977): Metabolism 26:1225-1230.
130. Lancranjan, I., del Pozo, E. and Ohnhaus, E. (1978): J. Clin. Endocrinol. Metab. 47:671-674.
131. Langer, G., Heinze, C., Reim, B. and Matussek, N. (1976): Arch. Gen. Psychiatry 33:1471-1475.
132. Langer, G., Sachar, E. J., Halpern, F. S., Gruen, P. H. and Solomon, M. (1977): J. Clin. Endocrinol. Metab. 45:996-1002.
133. Langer, G., Sachar, E. J. and Halpern, F. S. (1978): Psychoneuroendocrinology 3:165-169.
134. Leblanc, H., Lachelin, G.C.L., Abu-fadil, S. and Yen, S.S.C. (1976): J. Clin. Endocrinol. Metab. 43:668-674.
135. Leebaw, W.F., Lee, L. A. and Woolf, P.D. (1978): J. Clin. Endocrinol. Metab. 47:480-487.
136. Lewy, A. J. (1981): In: Melatonin: Current Status and Perspectives, edited by N. Birau and W. Schloot, pp.397-400. Pergamon Press, Oxford.
137. Lewy, A. J. and Markey, S. P. (1978): Science 201:741-743.
138. Lewy, A. J., Wehr, T. A., Gold, P. W. and Goodwin, F. K. (1979): In: Biological Psychiatry Today, edited by J. OBiols, C. Ballus, E. Gonzalez-Monchus and J. Pujol, pp.563-565. Elsevier, Amsterdam.
139. Lewy, A. J., Wehr, J. A., Goodwin, F. K., Newsom, D. A. and

Markey, S. P. (1980): Science 210:1267-1269.
140. Lovinger, R., Holland, J., Kaplan, S., Grumbach, M. M., Boryczka, A. T., Shackelford, R., Salmon, J., Reid, I. A. and Ganong, W. F. (1976): Neuroscience 1:443-450.
141. Lucke, C., and Glick, S. M. (1971): J. Clin. Endocrinol. Metab. 32:729-736.
142. Lynch, H. J., Wurtman, R. J., Moskowitz, M. A., Archer, M. C. and Ho, M. H. (1975): Science 187:169-171.
143. Machado, A.B.M., Faleiro, L. C. and Dasilva, D. A. (1965): Z. Zellforsch. Mikrosk. Anat. 65:521-525.
144. MacIndoe, J. H. and Turkington, R. W. (1973): J. Clin. Invest. 52:1972-1978.
145. MacLeod, R. M. (1969): Endocrinology 85:916-923.
146. McWilliams, J., Meldrum B. S. and Checkley, S. A. (unpublished data).
147. Macleod, R. M. and Lehemeyer, J. E. (1974): Endocrinology 94: 1077-1085.
148. Maeda, K., Kato, Y., Ongo, S. and Chihara, K., Yoshimoto, Y., Yamaguchi, N., Kuromaru, S. and Imura, H. (1975): J. Clin. Endocrinol. Metab. 40:501-503.
149. Masala, A., Delitala, G., Devilla, L., Alagna, S. and Rouasio, P. P. (1979): J. Clin. Endocrinol. Metab. 49:350-352.
150. Massara, F. and Camanni, F. (1972): J. Endocrinol. 54:195-206.
151. Mata, M. M., Schrier, B. K., Klein, D. C., Weller, J. L. and Chiou, C. Y. (1976): Brain Res. 118:383-394.
152. Matussek, N., Ackenheil, M., Hippius, H., Muller, F., Schroder, H-Th., Schultes, H. and Wasilewski, B. (1980): Psychiatry Research 2:25-36.
153. Mayer, G., Wessel, J. and Kobberling, J. (1980): Clin. Endocrinol. 13:413-416.
154. Meites, J., Bruni, J. F., Van Vugt, D. A. and Smith, A. F. (1979): Life Sc. 24:1325-1336.
155. Mendelson, W. B., Jacobs, L. S., Reichman, J. D., Othmer, E., Cryer, P. E., Trivedi, B. and Daughaday, W. H. (1975): J. Clin. Invest. 56:690-697.
156. Mendelson, W. B., Sitaram, N., Wyatt, R. J., Gillin, J. C. and Jacobs, L. S. (1978): J. Clin. Invest. 61:1683-1690.
157. Mendlewicz, J., Linkowski, P., Branchey, Ltd., Weinberg, U., Weitzman, E. D. and Branchey, M. (1979): Lancet ii:1362.
158. Mendlewicz, J., Van Cauter, E., Linkowski, P., L'Hermite, M. and Robyn, C. (1980): Life Sci. 27:2015-2024.
159. Merimee, T. J. and Fineberg, S. E. (1971): J. Clin. Endocrinol. Metab. 33:896-902.
160. Mitchell, M. L., Suvunrungsi, P. and Sawin, C. T. (1971): J. Clin. Endocrinol. Metab. 32:470-475.
161. Moore, R. and Rapport, R. L. (1970): Neuroendocrinology 7: 361-374.
162. Moore, R. Y. and Klein, D. C. (1974): Brain Res. 71:17-33.
163. Morley, J. E. (1981): Metabolism 30:195-209.
164. Morley, J. E., Baranetsky, N. G., Wingert, T. D., Carlson, H. E., Hershman, J. M., Melmed, S., Levin, S. R., Jamison, K. R., Weitzman, R., Chang, R. J. and Varner, A. A. (1980): J. Clin. Endocrinol. Metab. 50:251-257.
165. Mueller, P. S., Henninger, G. R. and McDonald, R. K. (1969): Arch. Gen. Psychiatry 21:587-594.

166. Mullen, P. E., Linsell, C. R., Leone, R. M., Silman, R. E., Smith, L., Hooper, R.J.L., Finnie, M. and Parrot, J. (1981): In: Melatonin: Current Status and Perspectiveness, edited by N. Birau and W. Schloot, pp.337-342. Pergamon Press, Oxford.
167. Müller, E. e., Brambilla, F., Cavagnini, F., Peracchi, M. and Panerai, A. (1974): J. Clin. Endocrinol. Metab. 29:1-5.
168. Muller-Hess, R., Geser, C. A., Jequier, E., Felber, J. P. and Vannotti, A. (1974): Acta Endocrinol. 75:260-273.
169. Nair, N.P.V., Lal, S., Cervantes, P., Yasa, R. and Guyda, H. (1979): Neuropsychobiology 5:136-142.
170. Nakai, Y., and Imura, H. (1974): endocrinol. Jpn. 21:493-497.
171. Nakai, Y., Imura, H., Sakurai, H., Kurahachi, H. and Yoshimi, T. (1974): J. Clin. Endocrinol. Metab. 38:446-449.
172. Nielsen, J. L. (1980): Neuropsychobiology 6:52-55.
173. O'Dea, R. F. and Zats, M. (1976): Proc. natl. Acad. Sci. USA 73:3398-3402.
174. Ojeda, S. R., Harms, P. G. and McCann, S. M. (1974): Endocrinology 94:1650-1657.
175. Oshima, N., Kumashiro, H., Takahashi, Y., Kaneko, M., Numata, Y., Watanabe, A., Tago, H., Itagaki, S. and Takaya, Y. (1980): Abstracts of the 12th CINP Congress, Goteborg, Sweden, June, 1980. Pergamon Press, Oxford.
176. Pelayo, F., Dubocovich, M. L. and Langer, S. Z. (1978): Nature 274:76-78.
177. Pelligrino de Iraldi, A. and Zieher, L. M. (1966): Life Sci. 5: 149-154.
178. Pontiroli, A. E., Viberti, G. S., Tognetti, A. and Pozza, G. (1976): Horm. Metabol. Res. 8:106-108.
179. Pontiroli, A. E., Viberti, G., Vicari, A. and Pozza, G. (1976): J. Clin. Endocrinol. Metab. 43:582-586.
180. Quay, W. B. (1964): Proc. Soc. Exp. Biol. 115:710-713.
181. Racagni, G., Apud, J. A., Locatelli, V., Cocchi, D., Nistico, G., diGiorgio, R. M. and Muller, E. C. (1979): Nature 281:710-713.
182. Ralph, C. L., Mull, D., Lynch, H. J. and Hedlund, L. (1971): Endocrinology 89:1361-1366.
183. Rees, L., Butler, P.W.P., Gosling, C. and Besser, G. M. (1970): Nature 228:565-566.
184. Reinberg, A. (1974): In: Circannual Clocks: Annual Biological Rhythms, edited by E. T. Pengelly, pp.423-507. Academic Press, New York.
185. Rotrosen, J., Angrist, B., Gershon, S., Paquin, J., Branchey, L., Oleshansky, M., Halpern, F. and Sachar, E. J. (1979): Br. J. Psychiatry 135:444-456.
186. Rubin, R. T. (Personal communication).
187. Rubin, R. T. and Poland, R. E. (1981): In: Neuroendocrine Perspectives Vol. 1, edited by R. M. Macleod and E. E. Muller. Elsevier, Amsterdam (in press).
188. Rudolph, C., Kaplan, S. L. and Ganong, W. F. (1980): Neuroendocrinology 31:121-128.
189. Sachar, E. J. (1978): In: Psychopharmacology: A Generation of Progress, edited by M. A. Lipton, A. De Mascio and K. R. Killam, pp.499-507. Raven Press, New York.
190. Sachar, E. J., Finkelstein, J. and Hellman, L. (1971): Arch. Gen. Psychiatry 25:263-269.

191. Sachar, E. J., Frantz, A. B., Altman, N. and Sassin, J. (1973): Am. J. Psychiatry 130:1362-1367.
192. Sachar, E. J., Altman, N., Gruen, P. H., Glassman, A., Halpern, F. S. and Sassin, J. (1975): Arch. Gen. Psychiatry 32:502-503.
193. Sachar, E. J., Gruen, P. H., Altman, N., Halpern, F. S. and Frantz, A. G. (1976): In: Hormones Behaviour and Psychopathology edited by E. J. Sachar, pp.161-176. Raven Press, New York.
194. Sachar, E. J., Gruen, P. H., Altman, N., Langer, G. and Halpern, F. S. (1978): In: The Nature of Schizophrenia, edited by L. C. Wynne, pp.95-104. John Wiley, New York.
195. Sakuma, M. and Knobil, E. (1970): Endocrinology 86:890-894.
196. Schilkrut, R., Chandra, O., Osswald, M., Ruther, E., Baartusser, B. and Matussek, N. (1975): Neuropsychobiology 1:70-79.
197. Silman, R. E., Leone, R. M., Hooper, R.J.L. and Preece, M. A. (1979): Nature 282:301-303.
198. Sizonenko, P. C., lenko, H. L., Lang, V., Anbert, M. and Paunier, L. (1981): Abstract. International Symposium on Bremen, 1980.
199. Slade, A. P. and Checkley, S. A. (1980): Br. J. Psychiatry 137: 217-221.
200. Smalstig, E. G., Sawyer, B. D. and Clemens, J. A. (1974): Endocrinology 95:123-129.
201. Smythe, G. A. and Lazarus, L. (1974): J. Clin. Invest. 54: 116-121.
202. Smythe, G. A., Compton, P. J. and Lazzrus, L. (1976): In: Growth Hormone and Related Peptides, edited by A. Pecile and E. E. Muller, pp.222-225. Excerpta Medica, Amsterdam.
203. Spiler, I. J. and Molitch, M. E. (1980): J. Clin. Endocrinol. Metab. 50:516-520.
204. Stone, C. L., Wenger, H. C., Ludden, C. T., Stravorski, J. M. and Ross, C. A. (1961): J. Pharm. Exp. Therm. 131:73-84.
205. Strada, S., Klein, D. C., Weller, J. and Weiss, B. (1972): Endocrinology 90:1470-1576.
206. Stubbs, W. A., Delitala, G., Jones, A., Jeffcoate, W. J., Edwards, C.R.W. and Ratter, S. J. (1978): Lancet ii:1225-1227.
207. Syvalahti, E.K.G. and Kanto, J. H. (1975): Int. J. Clin. Pharmacol. 12:74-82.
208. Syvalahti, E., Nagy, A. and van Praag, H. M. (1979): Psychopharmacology 64:251-253.
209. Takahara, J., Yunoki, S., Yakushiji, W., Yamauchi, J., Yamane, Y. and Ofuji, T. (1977): J. Clin. Endocrinol. Metab. 44:1014-1017.
210. Takahashi, S., Kondo, H., Yoshimura, M. and Ochi, Y. (1974): In: Psychoneuroendocrinology, edited by N. Hatotani, pp.32-38. S. Karger, Basel.
211. Takahashi, S., Kondo, H. and Yoshimura, M. (1975): Folia Psychiatr. Neurol. Jpn. 29:215-220.
212. Tamminga, C. A., Neophytides, A., Chase, T. N. and Frohman, L. A. (1978): J. Clin. Endocrinol. Metab. 47:1348-1351.
213. Thompson, R. G., Rodriquez, A., Kowarski, A. and Blizzard, R. M. (1972): J. Clin. Invest. 51:3193-3199.
214. Thorner, M. O. (1977): In: Clinical Neuroendocrinology edited by L. Martin and G. M. Besser, pp.320-363. Academic Press, New York.
215. Thorner, M. O., Wass, J.A.H., Jones, A., Bloom, S. R. and MacLeod, R. M. (1976): Abstract 5th International Congress of

Endocrinology, Abstract No.860.
216. Thorner, M. O., Ryan, S. M., Wass, J.A.H., Jones, A., Bouloux, J. P., Williams, S. and Besser, G. M. (1978): J. Clin. Endocrinol. Metab. 41:372-378.
217. Tolis, G., Hickey, J. and Guyda, H. (1975): J. Clin. Endocrinol. Metab. 41:797-800.
218. Tolis, G., Dent, R. and Guyda, H. (1978): J. Clin. Endocrinol. Metab. 47:200-204.
219. Torella, R., Giugliano, D., Siniscalchio. N., Sgambato, S. and D'Onofrio, F. (1979): Metabolism 28:887.
220. Vaughan, G. M., Pelham, R. W., Pang, S. F., Loughlin, L. L., Wilson, K. M., Sandock, K. L., Vaughan, M. K., Koslow, S. H. and Reiter, R. J. (1976): J. Clin. Endocrinol. Metab. 42:752-764.
221. Vaughan, G. M., McDonald, S. D., Jordan, R. M., Allen, J. P., Bell, R. and Stevens, E. A. (1979): Psychoneuroendocrinology 4: 351-362.
222. Verde, G., Oppizzi, G., Colussi, G., Cremascoli, G., Botalla, L., Muller, E. E., Silvestrini, R., Chiodini, P. G. and Liuzzi, A. (1976): Clin. Endocrinol. 5:419-423.
223. Vierhapper, H., Bratusch-Marrain, P. and Waldhausl, W. (1980): J. Clin. Endocrinol. Metab. 50:1131-1134.
224. Vigas, M., Wiedermann, V., Nemeth, S., Jurcovicova, J. and Zigo, L. (1976): Neuroendocrinology 21:42-48.
225. Vivien-Roels, B., Arendt, J. and Bradtke, J. (1979): Gen. Comp. Endocrinol. 37:197-210.
226. von Graffenfried, B., del Pozo, E., Rowbicek, J., Krebs, E., Poldinger, W., Burmeister, P. and Kerp, L. (1978): Nature 272: 729-730.
227. Wakabayashi, I., Demura, R., Miki, N., Ohmura, E., Miyoshi, H. and Shiznme, K. (1980): J. Clin. Endocrinol. Metab. 50:597-599.
228. Weiss, B. and Costa, E. (1968): J. Pharmacol. Exp. Ther. 161: 310-319.
229. Wetterberg, L. (1979): Prog. Brain Res. 52:539-547.
230. Wetterberg, L., Arendt, J., Paunier, L., Sizenenko, P. C., Van Doselaar, W. and Heyden, T. (1976): J. Clin. Endocrinol. Metab. 42:752-764.
231. Wiebe, R. H., Handwerger, S. and Hammond, C. B. (1977): J. Clin. Endocrinol. Metab. 45:1310-1312.
232. Wetterberg, L., Beck-Friis, J., Aperia, B. and Petterson, N. (1979): Lancet ii:1361.
233. Wetterberg, L. and Eriksson, O. (1981): In: Melatonin: Current STatus and Perspectives, edited by N. Birau and W. Schloot, pp.15-20. Pergamon Press, Oxford.
234. Wirz-Justice, A., Puhringer, W., Lacoste, V., Graw, P. and Gastpar, M. (1976): Pharmakopsychiatr. Neuropsychopharmakol. 9: 277-288.
235. Wirz-Justice, A. and Arendt, J. (1979): In: Biological Psychiatry Today, edited by J. Obiols, C. Ballus, E. Gondalez-Mondus and J. Pujol, pp.294-300. Elsevier, Amsterdam.
236. Wirz-Justice, A. and Arendt, J. (1980): Lancet i:425.
237. Wirz-Justice, A., Arendt, J. and Marston, A. (1980): Experientia 36:442-444.
238. Woolf, P. D. and Lee, L. (1977): J. Clin. Endocrinol. Metab. 45: 123-133.
239. Wurtman, R. J., Axelrod, J. and Phillips, L. S. (1963): Science 142:1071-1073.

Neuroendocrinology and Psychiatric Disorder,
edited by G. M. Brown, et al.
Raven Press, New York 1984.

Findings in Affective Disorders Relevant to the Thyroid Axis, Melanotropin, Oxytocin, and Vasopressin

Arthur J. Prange, Jr. and Peter T. Loosen

Psychoendocrinology has relevance therapeutically as well as diagnostically, but this brief review will concentrate only on the diagnostic capability of psychoendocrinology pertaining to affective disorders. Other clinical entities will be referenced where findings are relevant for contrasts to affective disorders. The hormones to be considered are those of the thyroid axis, thyrotropin releasing hormone (TRH), thyrotropin (thyroid stimulating hormone,(TSH), thyroxine (T_4), L-triiodothyronine (T_3); the intermediate lobe of the pituitary gland, melanocyte stimulating hormone (MSH, melanotropin); and the posterior pituitary gland, oxytocin (OXY) and vasopressin (VP). References to these hormones studied in animals will be cited to amplify clinical findings or to suggest new avenues for clinical research.

Clinical researchers have alluded to the utility of diagnostic psychoendocrinology, though no endocrine finding has yet been established as necessary to the diagnosis of any psychiatric entity. Some have been advanced as more or less reliable state markers of an illness, and another has been proposed as an occasional trait marker, but all psychiatric diagnoses presently depend upon the display of characteristic behavioural abnormalities. Indeed, this caveat can be entered for all somatic findings in psychiatry and not only for those which are endocrinological.

I. HORMONES OF THE THYROID AXIS

A. TRH

This tripeptide, the first hypothalamic hypophysiotropic hormone identified, appears, after intravenous administration, to exert antidepressant effects, though this conclusion is contraversial (58). TRH evokes the release by the anterior pituitary gland of TSH and prolactin (5) and, in some circumstances, growth hormone (7). One report suggests that in depressed patients TRH in spinal fluid may be elevated (31). This finding, if verified, could resonate with the finding of a diminished TSH response to injected TRH described (see section on TSH, which follows). That is, excessive stimulation by TRH could lead to down-regulation of pituitary thyrotrophs and a sluggish response to subsequent stimulation.

B. TSH

This polypeptide, like other anterior pituitary gland hormones, has varied amino acid composition from species to species (76). TSH has been employed as a stimulus (independent variable) and studied as a response (dependent variable).

In an early study we showed that if 10 International Units of bovine

TSH were given intramuscularly to women with unipolar depression, their antidepressant response to dubsequent imipramine (IMI) treatment was enhanced (53), the release of thyroid hormones (see below) being a sufficient explanation for the event. More apposite to the present context of diagnostic psychoendocrinology, it was found that the thyroidal responses of these women were normal; 24 hours after 10 I.U. of TSH total serum T_4 doubled over baseline values. No abnormality in thyroid reserve was demonstrated.

As a dependent variable TSH has been studied in two ways, naturalistically and experimentally. In depressed patients unpertubed by treatment, Weeke and Weeke (70, 71) and Golstein et al. (20) have assessed the diurnal variations of the hormone and compared the results to findings in normal subjects. Both groups of investigators found an absent nocturnal rise of TSH in depressed patients. The former group reported that the severity of this disturbance was directly related to the severity of depression, severely depressed patients showing virtually no nocturnal TSH increase. Golstein et al. (20), studying unipolar and bipolar depressed patients, found that the absence of a nocturnal rise of TSH is a characteristic of unipolar patients.

More attention has been devoted to the response of TSH to TRH administration, and we have reviewed these data in detail (40, 52, 56). In the so-called TRH test, the tripeptide is given orally or intravenously, the latter being generally perferred as it avoids the potential problem of differential absorption. At baseline before TRH injection and at regular intervals thereafter one measures the serum levels of TSH, and prolactin and growth hormone, if desired. Only TSH responses will be considered here.

In 1972 we first reported our experience in giving TRH (0.6 mg I.V.) to 10 women with unipolar depression. Two women showed a virtually null response while another was bnormally low. Hyperthyroidism, the usual explanation for such findings, was excluded in these patients by usual means (54). There are now 41 studies involving in toto 917 patients that show that about 25% of patients with primary depression show a blunted TSH response to TRH stimulation. Four studies pertaining to 20 patients have not confirmed this finding (40). The generalization of a 25% incidence of the fault in depressed patients is based on a conservative criterion, intended to exclude false positives from the group to be designated as non-responders. We have required that patients show a maximum rise over respective baseline (max ΔTSH) of less than 5 μU/ml, a rise less than that seen in a large series of age- and sex-matched controls.

The TSH abnormality in depression seems not to be a function of increasing age (6, 41, 65), previous drug intake (9, 30, 41) or severity of illness (23, 24, 45). In a similar way, elevation of thyroid hormones, which would cause increased negative feedback on the pituitary, does not provide an explanation; depressed patients who show the TSH fault are almost always euthyroid. Some may, paradoxically, have a blunted TSH response and low thyroid hormone levels (22, 65), suggesting a disturbance in feedback dynamics. Circulating thyroid hormones normally inhibit the TSH response; when they are low, an exaggerated response is expected. The concept of a disturbed feedback relationship is further supported by our preliminary finding (44) that pretreatment with a single oral dose of thyroid hormones attenuates the TRH-induced TSH response in normal subjects but not in those depressed patients who do not show spontaneous blunting.

There are at least four questions as to the possible utility of the blunted TSH response in depression.

First, is it informative as to best treatment choice, to treatment outcome, or to prognosis? To date, no data are available on the usefulness of the TRH-test as regards treatment choice. The TRH test has, however, been used to predict both outcome to standard antidepressant treatment (tricyclics, ECT) and prognosis for early relapse after remission induced by such treatment. In these studies TRH was administered in depression and during recovery, the change in maximumΔTSH between first and second testing serving as the endocrine variable. It was found that an increased maximum Δ TSH on second testing correlated well with a favourable clinical response (6, 35). Furthermore, a persistently low maximum Δ TSH allowed prediction of early relapse, usually within six months (26). The latter finding, however, has not been confirmed (35).

Second, is a blunted TSH response valuable either as a trait marker or as a state marker? In several studies the TRH test was performed during the state of depression and again after clinical remission. In six studies (6, 21, 22, 26, 47, 67) the TSH response, being reduced in depression, normalized upon recovery. Two studies (29, 45) reported the persistence of some blunted responses into remission while five additional studies (2, 11, 41, 47, 50) found the persistence of nearly all blunted response. These data suggest that in depression, a blunted TSH response is sometimes a trait marker and sometimes a state marker. The fact that, as a state marker, the abnormal response can occur in depression without persisting into remission suggests that the endocrine changes that underlie it may play a role in the pathophysiology of depression.

As a trait marker the sensitivity of TSH blunting must be less than 25%, for this is its approximate frequency in depressive attacks and only to some lesser depree does it persist. Specificity, of course, is also imperfect, as with other putative trait markers in psychiatry, but the exceptions to specificity are interesting. Apart from depression (and certain states of physical illness), TSH blunting occurs in anorexia nervosa, mania and alcoholism (40), all of which bear some relationship to depression. The absence of blunting in schizophrenia confers a degree of specificity to the finding within mental disorders (40). An efficient means of assessing TSH blunting as a trait marker is to study its distribution in the relatives of an affected (i.e. depressed) proband. Brambilla and her colleagues (6) have made a start in this direction. They found two of six phenotypically normal, healthy relatives of an affected proband to show blunting. While this suggests that TSH blunting is sometimes heritable, it remains to be shown that "blunted" relatives show a higher frequency of depression than "non-blunted" relatives.

Third, does a blunted TSH response to TRH aid in the distinction of diagnostic subtypes of depression? Findings have been contradictory. Comparison of the TSH responses in primary vs. secondary depression has been reported to indicate (2, 6, 16, 30, 50) or not to indicate (15, 33, 65) that the fault occurs only in primary depression. A similar lack of concensus obtains if one compares the TSH response in unipolar vs. bipolar patients. However, in the majority of reports (1, 4, 11, 30, 41, 45, 47) no significant difference emerged. Taken together, these data indicate that the TRH test presently does not aid in the distinction between primary and secondary depression or between unipolar and bipolar subgroups.

Fourth, does a blunted response provide clues to the pathogenesis of depression in the patients in whom it is identified? The mechanism of the blunted TSH response is not well understood. At present, two interpretations of the fault seem most plausible. A thorough discussion of supporting data, as well as the shortcomings of these interpretations are beyond the scope of this paper and has been given in a recent review (40). Here it may suffice to say that the first hypothesis describes the fault as being the result of chronic TRH hypersecretion. In this case, the receptor sites on the thyrotroph cell are thought to be downregulated with resulting lowered sensitivity to TRH administration. The second hypothesis suggests that the fault is caused by excessive inhibition of the thyrotroph by substances from the brain such as somatostatin, neurotensin and dopamine.

A third interpretation - TSH blunting construed as the result of high serum cortisol levels - has already been examined and can be rejected. It is well known that elevation of serum cortisol reduces the TSH response both in patients with endocrine disorders and in normal subjects (49, 59). Because activation of the pituitary-adrenocortical axis, presumably from limbic stimulation, is a hallmark of primary depression (10), it was important to investigate possible relationships between serum cortisol elevation and TSH blunting. In a preliminary study we reported that cortisol elevations were, in fact, correlated with TSH blunting in a small sample of unipolar depressed women (42, 43). However, other investigators who subsequently addressed this point in depressed patients found no such relationship (16, 27, 35, 50, 63). Thus, it appears doubtful that adrenal activation accounts for more than a small fraction of TSH blunting during episodes of depression.

C. T_3 and T_4

These hormones will be considered together because it is convenient to do so, because we are ignorant of important distinctions between them in patients with affective disorders, and because T_3 is mainly derived from $T_4$4, by monodeiodination.

The thyroid state of depressed patients has been reported to be elevated, normal or diminished, the vast majority of patients being euthyroid by presently accepted criteria. Dewhurst (12), Whybrow et al. (75), Loosen and Prange (39), and Kirkegaard and Faber (28) reported thyroid indices to be somewhat elevated but within the normal range in depressed patients. Whybrow et al. (75) noted that degree of thyroidal activation was positively correlated with excellence of subsequent antidepressant response to IMI treatment.

Rybakowski and Sowinski (62) found diminished T_4 values in nine depressed patients. Rinieris et al. (61) studied 25 depressed patients, five of whom showed a subnormal FT_4 Index and total T_4.

The following authors have found the thyroid values of depressed patients to be in the normal range: Leichter et al. (37); Kirkegaard (30); Karlberg et al. (24); Hatotani et al.(22); and Gregoire et al. (21).

These data considered together suggest to us not that the thyroid axis plays no role in depression but rather the possibility that thyroid findings in a given patient may reflect the phase of illness, and that the thyroid axis is interacting with a medley of other biological factors pertinent to that patient. Another source of variance, characteristic of depressed patients, has received inadequate attention and that is nutritional status. Starvation reduces the conversion of T_4 to T_3

and may affect thyroid hormone binding (64). That the thyroid axis may play a dynamic role in the depression process is further supported by three observations: T_3 added to IMI accelerates the antidepressant response, at least in women (55); recovery from a depressive episode has been reported to be followed by hyperthyroidism (32, 38); patients with frank hypothyroidism are often clinically depressed (74).

In systematic studies of groups of manic patients thyroid indices have been reported to be low or normal but not, to our knowledge, high. Rybakowski and Sowinski (62) studied six manic patients and found the FT_4 Index and Total T_4 values to be lower than in controls. Kirkegaard et al.(30) found reduced serum T_3 levels in 14 manic patients. Rinieris and colleagues (61) found the thyroid indices of 15 manic patients to be normal. It should be noted that the usual affective changes in hyperthyroid patients is not the simple converse of usual affective changes in depressed patients. Although hypothyroid patients are often depressed, hyperthyroid patients typically do not show mania but instead a tense dysphoria (74). Whybrow and Prange (73) have offered a detailed view of the role of the thyroid axis in affective disorders.

II. MSH, A HORMONE OF THE INTERMEDIATE LOBE OF THE PITUITARY GLAND IN ANIMALS

This hormone stimulates melanophore expansion in primitive vertebrates producing skin darkening. In man, MSH appears to be absent except during fetal life (60). The hormone is found in animals with a discrete intermediate lobe, e.g. the rat, but even in such species its function is obscure (3). αMSH is more important than β MSH and is perhaps the only active form of the hormone. Activities attributed to β MSH are probably the properties of β-lipotropin (66), the former being embedded in the sequence of β- lipotropin. MSH consists of 13 amino acids. It is identical with the first 13 amino acids of adrenocorticotropin (ACTH). Peptides designated, for example, ACTH 4-10 are identical with MSH 4-10. Thus many peptide sequences can properly be referred to as fragments of ACTH or as fragments of MSH. This has caused confusion. There is evidence to suggest that in the frog the release of MSH is inhibited by pro-leu-gly-NH, (MSH-release inhibiting factor, MIF-I), though this substance has no such effect in mammals (66).

Fragments of αMSH, usually designated as fragments of ACTH 1-13, have been given to normal humans and to psychiatric patients with different diagnoses, often with the result of improved attention (58). To our knowledge such trials have not been done in depressed or manic patients.

MIF-I has been given to patients with Parkinson's disease, and most results have been positive (58). The tripeptide has also been given to depressed patients with positive results (13, 14). Thus, though man appears to lack MSH, and MIF-I could hardly be its physiological inhibitor, MIF-I may nevertheless exert non-endocrinological effects. Such effects are well-described in animals (57).

III. THE POSTERIOR PITUITARY GLAND HORMONES

The two hormones of the posterior pituitary gland, OXY and VP, are synthesized in nerve cell bodies in brain nuclei and transported within long axons to the gland, from which they are secreted into the general vascular circulation in response to specific stimuli. Accumulating evidence suggests that terminals of axons bearing these hormones can be found in areas of brain other than the posterior pituitary gland (8).

A. Oxytocin

This nanopeptide consists of a six member ring and a three amino acid side chain. The side chain is pro-leu-gly-NH_2, the structure of MIF-I, which exerts behavioural effects in animals and probably in Parkinson's disease and depression. Because much of what in brain has been identified as MIF-I may in fact by OXY (46), behavioural studies of OXY in man would seem in order. It should also be noted that OXY increases dramatically during parturition, following which mental morbidity is common.

OXY causes uterine contraction and milk ejection. In the virgin, female rat, Pedersen and Prange (51) have recently shown that intracerebroventricularly administered OXY produces a full spectrum of maternal behaviour that is dose-related and estrogen dependent.

B. VP

This peptide differs from OXY only by the substitution of one amino acid in the ring structure and another in the side chain (68). The role of VP in the regulation of animal behaviour has been extensively studied (69). A leading finding is this: rats with hereditary absence of VP only poorly maintain learned avoidance responses, and this deficit is readily reversed by administration of VP or many analogs of VP (69).

In preliminary studies analogs of VP appear effective in treating the memory loss of elderly men (36) and of patients suffering post-traumatic memory deterioration (48). Weingartner et al. (72) recently suggested that the VP analog, 1-desamino-8-D-arginine-vasopressin (DDAVP) causes beneficial effects in cognitively impaired as well as cognitively unimpaired adults. DDAVP also appeared to partially reverse ECT-induced retrograde amnesia. Furthermore, VP is elevated in human pain states without changes in plasma osmolality (25). For these and related reasons, Gold et al. (17) have postulated that VP may be functionally deficient in depressed states and funtionally overactive in mania. However, VP appears to possess ACTH releasing properties (34), and since ACTH is presumably elevated in some depressed patients (10), one might plausibly suggest that VP would be elevated in these same patients. Gold and his colleagues (19) studied these relationships by examining VP in CSF. Here it is important to recall, however, that CSF VP may not reflect neurohypophysial VP and may therefore be irrelevant to ACTH (and cortisol) changes. In any case, they reported that in CSF arginine VP (AVP) levels are lower in drug free unipolar and bipolar depressed patients than in controls. Furthermore, they observed that, in patients with bipolar depression, both the CSF levels of AVP and the plasma AVP response to hypertonic saline injection are lower in the depressed phase than in the manic phase. When DDAVP was administered to depressed patients, cognitive performance and depressive symptomatology were found to be improved (19).

SUMMARY

This brief review has been addressed to a variety of hormones. Among them the four hormones of the thyroid axis bear especially close functional relations. It is in this system, of the ones considered, that findings relevant to the affective disorders are most numerous. Studies of T_3 and T_4 suggest the dynamic involvement of the thyroid axis in affective disorders, but by themselves do little to characterize it. Studies of TRH as a dependent variable are meager, but its use as a means of evoking the response of TSH has proven useful. In depressed patients the TSH reponse is often blunted. At present it appears that when the TSH reponse to TRH increases on subsequent testing, this augurs well for a favourable clinical response to be the treatment in effect. Conversely, a blunted response that persists into remission may be associated with early depressive relapse. Further study of the TSH response may lead to both theoretical and practical clinical progress.

ACKNOWLEDGEMENTS

This research was supported in part by Public Health Service Career Scientist Award MH-22536 (AJP).

REFERENCES

1. Amsterdam, J. D., Winokur, A., Mendels, J. and Snyder, P. (1979): Lancet ii:904-905.
2. Asnis, G. N., Nathan, R. S., Halbreich, U., Halpern, F. S., Sachar, E. J. (1980): Lancet i:424-425.
3. Bennett, H. P. and McMartin, C. (1979): Pharmacol. Rev. 30:247-292.
4. Bjorum, N. and Kirkegaard, C. (1979): Lancet ii:694.
5. Bowers, C. Y., Friesen, H. G., Hwang, P., Guyda, H. Y. and Folkers, K. (1971): Biochem. Biophys. Res. Commun. 45:1033-1041.
6. Brambilla, F., Smeraldi, E., Bellodi, L., Sachetti, E. and Mueller, E. (1980): In: Progress in Psychoneuroendocrinology, edited by F. Brambilla, G. Racagni and D. deWied, pp.235-245. Elsevier/North Holland Biomedical Press, New York.
7. Brown, G. M., Seggie, J. A., Chambers, J. W. and Ettigi, P. G. (1978): Psychoneuroendocrinology 3:131-153.
8. Buijs, R. M., Velis, D. N. and Swaab, D. F.(1980): In: Adaptive Capabilities of the Nervous system, Vol. 53, edited by P. McConnell, G. J. Boer, H. C. Romyn, N. E. van de Poll and M. A. Corner, pp. 159-167. Elsevier/North Holland Biomedical Press, Amsterdam.
9. Burger, H. G. and Patel, Y. C. (1977): In: Clinical Neuroendocrinology, edited by L. Martini and G. M. Besser. Academic Press, New York.
10. Carroll, B. J., Mendels, J. (1976): In: Hormones, Behavior and Psychopathology, edited by E. J. Sachar. Raven Press, New York.
11. Coppen, A., Montgomery, S., Peet, M. and Bailey, J. (1974): Lancet ii:433-434.
12. Dewhurst, K. E., Eklabir, D. J., Exley, D., Harris, G. W. and Mendelbrote, B. M. (1968): Lancet ii:1160-1162.
13. Ehrensing, R. H. and Kastin, A. J. (1974): Arch. Gen. Psychiatry 30:63-65.
14. Ehrensing, R. H. and Kastin, A. J. (1978): Amer. J. Psychiatry 135:562-566.
15. Ettigi, P. G., Brown, G., Seggie, J. A. (1979): Psychosom. Med. 41:203-208.
16. Gold, M. S., Pottash, A.L.C., Ryan, N., Sweeney, D. R., Davies, R. K. and Martin, D. M. (1980): Psychoneuroendocrinology 5:147-155.
17. Gold, P. W., Goodwin, F. K. and Reus, V. I. (1978): Vasopressin in affective disorders. Lancet ii:1233.
18. Gold, P. W., Goodwin, F. K., Wehr, T. and Rebar, R. (1977): Amer.

J. Psychiatry 134:1028-1031.
19. Gold, P. W., Goodwin, F. K., Ballenger, J. C., Post, R. M., Weingartner, H. and Robertson, G. L. (1981): Intern. J. Mental Health 9:91-107.
20. Golstein, J., Van Cauter, E., Linkowski, P., Vanbaelst, L. and Mendlewicz, J. (1980): Life Sci. 27:1695-1703.
21. Gregoire, F., Brauman, H., de Buck, R. and Corrilain, J. (1977): Psychoneuroendocrinology 2:303-312.
22. Hatotani, N., Nomura, J., Yamaguchi, T. and Kitayama, J. (1977): Psychoneuroendocrinology 2:115-130.
23. Hollister, L. E., Davis, K. L. and Berger, P. A. (1976): Arch. Gen. Psychiatry 33:1393-1396.
24. Karlberg, B. E., Kjellman, B. F. and Kagedol, B. (1978): Acta psychiatr. scand. 58:389-400.
25. Kendler, K. S., Weitzman, R. E. and Fisher, D. A. (1978): Clin. Endocrinol. 8:89-94.
26. Kirkegaard, C. and Bjorum, N. (1980): Lancet i:152.
27. Kirkegaard, C. and Carroll, B. J. (1980): Psychiatry Research 3: 253-264.
28. Kirkegaard, C., Faber, J. (1981): Acta endocrinologica 96:199-207.
29. Kirkegaard, C., Norlem, N., Lauridsen, U. B., Bjorum, N. and Christiansen, C. (1975): Arch. Gen. Psychiatry 32:1115-1118.
30. Kirkegaard, C., Bjorum, N., Cohn, D. and Lauridsen, U. B. (1978): Arch. Gen. Psychiatry 35:1017-1023.
31. Kirkegaard, C., Faber, J., Hummer, L. and Rozowski, P. (1979): Psychoneuroendocrinology 4:227-235.
32. Kleinschmidt, H. J. and Waxenberg, S. E. (1956): J. Mt. Sinai Hosp. N.Y. 23:131-153.
33. Keonig, G., Langer, G., Schoenbeck, G., Schuessler, M. and Reiter, H. (1980): Proc. XI internatl. Congr. Soc. Psychoendocrinology, Florence, Italy, p.74.
34. Krieger, D. and Zimmerman, E. (1977): In: Clinical Neuroendocrinology, edited by L. Martini and G. M. Besser, pp.364-388. Academic Press, New York.
35. Langer, G., Schoenbeck, G., Koenig, G., Reiter, H., Schussler, M., Aschauer, H. and Lesch, O. (1980): In: Progress in Psychoneuroendocrinology, edited by F. Brambilla, G. Racagni and D. deWied, pp.197-208. Elsevier/North Holland Biomedical Press, New York.
36. Legros, J., Gilot, P., Seron, X., Claessers, J., Adam, A., Moeglen, J. M., Audibert, A. and Berchier, P. (1978): Lancet i:41.
37. Leichter, S. B., Kirstein, L. and Martin, N. D. (1977): Amer. J. Psychiatry 134:1270-1272.
38. Lidz, T. (1949): Psychom. Med. 2:2-8.
39. Loosen, P. T. and Prange, A. J., Jr. (1980): Psychoneuroendocrinology 5:63-80.
40. Loosen, P. T. and Prange, A. J., Jr. (1982): Amer. J. Psychiatry 139:405-416.
41. Loosen, P. T., Prange, A. J., Jr., Wilson, I. C., Lara, P. P. and Pettus, C. (1977): Psychoneuroendocrinology 2:137-148.
42. Loosen, P. T., Prange, A. J., Jr. and Wilson, I. C. (1978): Amer. J. Psychiatry 135:244-246.
43. Loosen, P. T., Prange, A. J., Jr., and Wilson, I. C. (1978): Prog. Neuro-Psychopharm. 2:479-486.
44. Loosen, P. T., Wilson, I. C., Prange, A. J., Jr. (1980): J. Affective Disorders 2:267-278.
45. Maeda, K., Kato, Y., Ohgo, S., Chihara, K., Yoshimoto, Y.,

Yamaguchi, N., Korumaru, S. and Imura, H. (1975): J. Clin. Endocrinol. Metab. 40:501-505.
46. Manberg, P. G., Youngblood, W. W. and Kizer, J. S. (1981): Brain Research (submitted).
47. Mendlewicz, J., Linkowski, P. and Brauman, H. (1979): Lancet ii: 1079-1080.
48. Oliveros, J. C., Jandoli, M. K., Timsit-Berthler, M., Reny, R., Benghezala, A., Audibert, A., and Moeglen, J. M. (1978): Lancet i:42.
49. Otsuki, M., Dakoda, M. and Baba, S. (1973): J. Clin. Endocrinol. Metab. 36:95-102.
50. Papakostas, V., Fink, M., Lee, J., Irwin, P. and Johnson, L. (1981): Psychiatry Res. 4:55-64.
51. Pedersen, C. A. and Prange, A. J., Jr. (1979): Proc. Nat'l. Acad. Sci. USA 76:6661-6665.
52. Prange, A. J., Jr. (1977): In: Phenomenology and Treatment of Depression, edited by W. E. Fann, I. Karacan, A. D. Pokorny and R. L. Williams, pp.1-15. Spectrum Publishing Co., New York.
53. Prange, A. J., Jr., Wilson, I. C., Knox, A., McClane, T. K. and Lipton, M. A. (1970): Amer. J. Psychiatry 127:191-199.
54. Prange, A. J., Jr., Wilson, I. C., Lara, P. P., Alltop, L. B. and Breese, G. R. (1972): Lancet ii:999-1002.
55. Prange, A. J., Jr., Wilson, I. C., Breese, G. R. and Lipton, M. A. (1976): In: Hormones, Behavior and Psychopathology, edited by E. J. Sachar, pp.41-67. Raven Press, New York.
56. Prange, A. J., Jr., Lipton, M. A., Nemeroff, C. B. and Wilson, I.C. (1977): Life Sci. 20:1305-1318.
57. Prange, A. J., Jr., Nemeroff, C. B., Lipton, M. A., Breese, G. R., and Wilson, I. C. (1978): In: Handbook of Psychopharmacology, Vol. 13, edited by L. L. Iversen, S. D. Iversen and S. H. Snyder, pp.1-107. Plenum Publishing Corporation, New York.
58. Prange, A. J., Jr., Loosen, P. T. and Nemeroff, C. B. (1979): In: New Frontiers of Psychotropic Drug Research, edited by S. Fielding, pp.117-189. Futura Publishing Co., Inc., Mt. Kisko, New York.
59. Re, R. N., Kourides, I. A., Ridgway, E. C., Weintraub, B. D. and Maloof, R. (1976): J. Clin. Endocrinol. Metab. 43:338-345.
60. Rees, L. H. (1977): In: Clinical Neuroendocrinology, edited by L. Martini and G. M. Besser, pp.401-441. Academic Press, New York.
61. Rinieris, P. M., Christodoulou, G. N., Sourateoglou, A., Koutras, D. A. and Stefanis, C. N. (1978); Comp. Psychiatry 19:561-564.
62. Rybakowski, J. and Sowinski, J. (1973): Lancet i:889.
63. Sachar, E. J., Halbreich, U., Asnis, G., Nathan, S. and Halpern, F. S. (1980): In: Progress in Psychoneuroendocrinology, edited by F. Brambilla, G. Racagni and D deWied, pp.265-272. Elsevier/North Holland Biomedical Press, New York.
64. Schimmel, M., Utiger, R. D. (1977): Ann. Int. Med. 87:760-768.
65. Takahashi, S., Kondo, H., Yoshimura, M. and Ochi, Y. (1974): Folia Psychiat. Neurol. Jap. 28:355-365.
66. Thody, A. J., Lever de Vries, C. H. and Tilders, J. H. (1980): Acta Endocrinologica 93:300-305.
67. Tsutsui, S., Yamazaki, Y., Namba, T. and Tsushima, M. (1979): J. Int. Med. Res. 7:138-146.
68. Valiquette, G. (1980): In: The Endocrine Function of the Brain, edited by Motta, M., pp.385-417. Raven Press, New York.

69. van Wimersma Greidanus, Tj. B., and deWied, D. (1977): In: Biochemical Correlates of Brain Structure and Function, edited by A. N. Davison, pp. 215-248. Academic Press, London.
70. Weeke, A. and Weeke, J. (1978): Acta psychiatr. scand. 57:281-289.
71. Weeke, A. and Weeke, J. (1980): Acta psychiatr. scand. 62:69-74.
72. Weinberger, H., Gold, P., Ballenger, J. C., Smallberg, S. A., Summers, R., Rubinow, D. R., Post, R. M. and Goodwin, F. K. (1981): Science 211:601-603.
73. Whybrow, P. C. and Prange, A. J., Jr. (1981): Arch. Gen. Psychiatry 38:106-113.
74. Whybrow, P. C., Prange, A. J., Jr. and Treadway, C. R. (1969): Arch. Gen. Psychiatry 20:48-63.
75. Whybrow, P. C., Coppen, A., Prange, A. J., Jr., Noguera, R. and Bailey, J. E. (1972): Arch. Gen. Psychiatry 26:242-245.
76. Wilbur, J. G. (1979): In: Endocrinology, vol. 1, edited by L. J. DeGroot, G. F. Cahill, Jr., W. E. O'Dell, L. Martini, J. T. Potts, Jr., D. H. Nelson, E. Steinberger and A. i. Winegrad. Grune and Stratton, New York.

Neuroendocrinology and Psychiatric Disorder,
edited by G. M. Brown, et al.
Raven Press, New York 1984.

Pituitary-Adrenocortical Dysfunction in Severe Depressive Illness

John W. Kendall

One long-range goal in psychiatry has been to develop biological tests of specific disorders. Such tests would hopefully permit more accurate diagnosis, predict outcome, and lead to an eventual understanding of the pathogenesis of the disorders. The discovery of increased pituitary-adrenocortical activity in some patients with severe depressive illness (melancholia, endogenous depression) and the subsequent further refinement of testing of this endocrine abnormality has provided what is probably the most specific laboratory test now available in clinical psychiatry. The earlier recognition in depressive illness of increased plasma cortisol metabolites by Board and co-workers (2) and increased cortisol secretion by Gibbons (8) was followed by the discovery of resistance of the pituitary-adrenocortical axis to feedback inhibition (4, 5), a finding which has subsequently been studied extensively and refined as a test. Of the various cortisol-associated abnormalities in depression the resistance to dexamethasone suppression has received the greatest attention.

In the past five years, groups led by Carroll (7), Brown (3), Holsboer (10) and others, have applied the dexamethasone suppression test to more than 1,000 patients and have standardized it, so that it is now a highly specific and reasonably sensitive indicator of endogenous depression (7). While it is not yet clear that the test can distinguish subtypes of the disorder, it does appear to have predictive value (7). Other cortisol-associated abnormalities, such as the altered circadian rhythmicity of plasma cortisol concentration (22), have received considerable attention but have not been as reliable diagnostic indicators of severe depressive illness (3).

In this discussion, I will comment on some features of pituitary-adrenocortical dysfunction and its testing from an endocrinologist's perspective. I will call particular attention to the strikingly similar problem the disciplines of endocrinology and psychiatry face in trying to understand the etiologies of pituitary-dependent Cushing's syndrome (Cushing's Disease) and severe depressive illness, respectively. Also, I will call attention to certain points about the application of the dexamethasone suppression test, which I believe, after reviewing the recent literature, seem to need emphasis.

Comparison of Cushing's Disease and Severe Depressive Illness

It has long been recognized that there is a similarity between the pituitary-adrenocortical hyperactivity of Cushing's Disease and severe depressive illness. Table 1 lists some of the pituitary-adrenocortical abnormalities in pituitary-dependent Cushing's syndrome and in severe depressive illness. It is apparent that the hypercortisolemic derangements are *qualitatively* extraordinarily similar and differ primarily in degree. This is not surprising since they share portions of the final common pathway of the hypothalamic-pituitary-adrenal axis. The point of

TABLE 1. Pituitary-Adrenocortical Dysfunction in Pituitary-Dependent Cushing's Syndrome and in Severe Depressive Illness

	Pituitary-Dependent Cushing's	Severe Depression Illness
Elevated plasma cortisol	+	+
Increased cortisol secretion	+	+
Abnormal cortisol rhythm	++	+
Resistance to Dexamethasone Suppression	+ to ++++	0 to ++
Diminished Cortisol Response to Hypoglycemia	+	+
Improvement of Dexamethasone Suppression test	uncommon	common
Physical and Other Signs of Cortisol Excess	+ to ++++	0

overlap in the chain of events beginning in the brain and ending in adrenal cortisol secretion appears to be located in the corticotroph since all of the abnormalities listed in the table can be explained by shared defects in the pituitary corticotroph and/or its controlling systems.

The quantitative differences in pituitary-adrenalcortical activity are such that, for whatever reason, the derangement in pituitary-adrenocortical drive is more intense in Cushing's Disease than in depressive illness. For example, as contrasted with Cushing's Disease, in severe depressive illness the mean plasma cortisol concentration is usually only slightly elevated (21). The circadian rhythm is only subtly altered, and a larger proportion of depressed patients display dexamethasone suppressibility of the plasma cortisol concentration to less than 5 ug/dl at 8 a.m. (7).

The cortisol-associated problems of severe depressive illness and Cushing's Disease do appear to differ qualitatively in two respects. The peripheral clinical features of cortisol excess are not reported to be present in severe depressive illness as they are in classical Cushing's Disease. Thus, signs of protein wasting (ecchymoses, striae, osteoporosis), carbohydrate intolerance, and fat redistribution, which are characteristic of Cushing's Disease are notably lacking in classical descriptions of depression. From an endocrinological perspective this is puzzling since even very mild persistent hypercortisolemia in Cushing's Disease produces at least a few typical features of the disorder. The described absence of these signs in depressive illness perhaps is attributable to the very mild degree of the adrenal overactivity, or alternatively, to a shorter overall duration of exposure to elevated cortisol concentrations than is the case in Cushing's Disease. Yet this explanation is discomfiting because some patients with classical physical stigmata of Cushing's Disease present with histories of very recent onset of symptoms and only minimally elevated plasma cortisol values. Another alternative possibility is that patients with severe depressive illness have not been systematically examined for quantifiable correlates of cortisol excess. For example, corticosteroid administration produces mild carbohydrate intolerance in normal individuals (13) and therefore the hypercortisolemia of depressive illness would be expected to produce at lease a mild degree of carbohydrate intolerance. To my knowledge subtle changes in glucose tolerance have not been sought in active depressive illness.

The other apparent qualitative difference in the pituitary-adrenal axis between Cushing's Disease and severe depressive illness is the greater frequency of normalization of the cortisol disorder with remission of the latter disease. Spontaneous remiisions of pituitary suppressibility do occur in Cushing's Disease, but are uncommon (17, 19). Switches from depression to mania are characteristic of bipolar depressive disease and are often accompanied by normalization of the cortisol-associated abnormalities (6). Furthermore, therapeutic remissions of severe depressive illness are also frequently accompanied by normalization of the pituitary-adrenocortical axis (9). These cited differences between severe depressive illness and Cushing's Disease may well reflect instrinsic differences in the etiologies of the two disorders.

Can the pituitary-adrenocortical derangements of these two disorders help to establish their underlying etiologies? While not yet providing the ultimate causal explanations, knowledge of the cortisol abnormalities in severe depressive illness has contributed to a broadening of the spectrum of possible causes of Cushing's Disease, just as studies of the pathogenesis of the latter are aiding in clarifying some aspects of depressive illness. Our knowledge of the endocrinology of depressive illness has provided an argument for one of the main hypotheses for the cause of Cushing's Disease. There appear to be three main theories for the excess ACTH secretion of Cushing's Disease: 1) Cushing's Disease may be an intrinsic pituitary problem with the defect residing in the pituitary corticotroph. This possibility is supported by the knowledge that approximately 80% of patients with this disorder have a pituitary tumor and that remission can follow selective excision of a pituitary tumor; 2) Cushing's Disease may be due to a primary hypothalamic abnormality, such as over-secretion of corticotropin releasing factor into the hypophseal portal system with resultant hyperstimulation of normal pituitary corticotrophs. This possibility is attractive because it would account for those cases of Cushing's Disease without demonstrable pituitary tumors and could even account for pituitary tumors if they were secondary to the hyperstimulatory effect of the releasing factor; 3) Cushing's Disease might be a result of brain neurotransmitter excess or deficiency (e.g. norepinephrine and/or serotonin) acting on the pituitary directly or more likely through stimulation or disinhibition of corticotropin releasing factor secretion. This explanation gains support from the reported favourable responses to serotonin antagonists in some cases of Cushing's Disease (16) and from the oft-cited hypothesis that some abnormality of neurotransmitter function underlies the pituitary-adrenocortical hyperactivity in depressive illness. However, it is exactly at this point that our knowledge of Cushing's Disease stops. We can hypothesize that Cushing's Disease and depressive illness share some abnormalities of neuroendocrine control (at least in one or more of their individual variants) but we lack evidence to draw definitive conclusions. Nonetheless, through continued comparison of advances made in understanding each disorder, knowledge derived from one will continue to add to our understanding of the other.

Comments on the Dexamethasone Suppression Test

The dexamethasone suppression test as presently employed in the laboratory evaluation of endogenous depression has a high degree of specificity and is fairly sensitive. According to Carroll and associates (7), if one combines the appropriate dexamethasone dosage (1 mg at midnight), chooses the most favourable sampling times for obtaining plasma cortisol levels (4 p.m. and 11 p.m.), and selects a plasma cortisol value of 5 ug/dl as the diagnostic criterion, one achieves a 96% specificity and 67% sensitivity in the diagnosis of severe depressive illness (7). That is, abnormal tests will be found in only 4% of non-depressives and normal tests in only 33% of severe depressives.

The test as presently recommended by Carroll's group takes advantage of the difference in the pattern of suppression of plasma cortisol by dexamethasone between normals and depressives particularly during the phase of recovery from suppression. The pattern of recovery in depressives has been operationally termed "early escape" (3, 6). After examining many patterns of responses in the dexamethasone suppression test both in the literature and in our own experience, published in the rat (12, 14, 15) and unpublished in man, it is my interpretation that the "escape" phenomenon is an expression of quantitatively greater resistance to suppression which is more easily distinguished from normal suppression during the recovery period (at 4 p.m. and 11 p.m.) than it is at the nadir (8 a.m.) of the plasma cortisol concentration. This point is emphasized by Carroll (6) and is illustrated in Figure 1, which shows selected patterns of cortisol responses to dexamethasone administration at typical sampling times over a 24-hour period. (The illustration while selected from a larger series of patients with "rule out" Cushing is supported by other data including the example shown in Fig. 2 Chapter 11). Some patients show virtually complete resistance to suppression throughout the 24-hour sampling period. The response in normal individuals is complete suppression lasting about 24 hours. Others with abnormal suppressibility display a spectrum of suppression. The greatest spread of values and the largest absolute differences from normal occur at 4 p.m. and 11 p.m. Note however, that there is also a gradient of resistance to suppression at 8 a.m. Thus "escape" might be properly regarded as an operational description of a quantitative difference rather than as a phenomenon unique to depression. Early escape is also seen in Cushing's Disease in those individuals who show partial suppression at 8 a.m. While authors who have used the term "escape" have not ascribed pathological specificity to it, this reviewer senses that such an overinterpretation could become linked to its application in depressive illness through tradition.

Carroll and associates (7) have called attention to some important caveats in the use and interpretation of the dexamethasone test. I believe some of them deserve special emphasis. First, it is important to bear in mind the exclusion cirteria. The list is rather lengthy and includes pregnancy, high dose estrogens, severe weight loss, hepatic enzyme inducing states (drugs in particular), uncontrolled diabetes mellitus, major physical illness (i.e. any severe stress), and, of course, other states of cortisol excess (Cushing's syndrome). Chronic renal failure (17, 24) and excess alcohol intake (20, 23) must be added to those recently listed by Carroll and co-workers (7). Second, the test

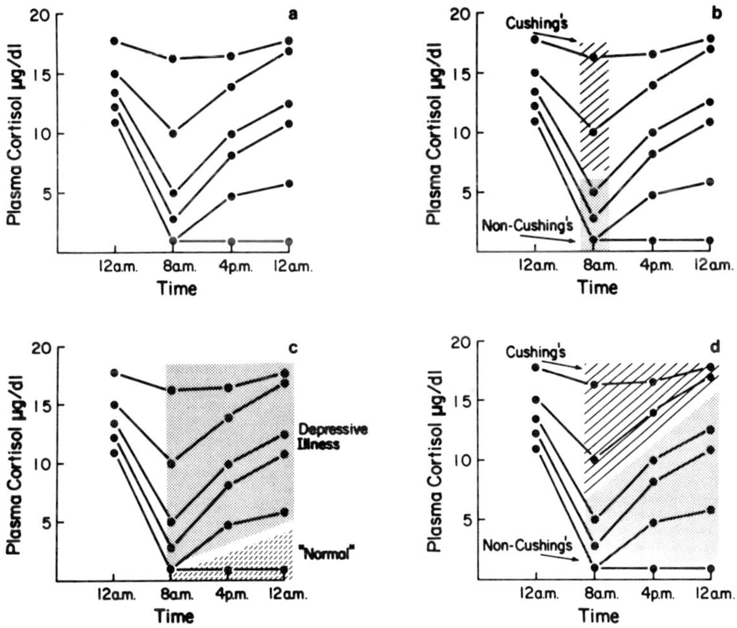

FIG. 1. Patterns of suppression of plasma cortisol concentration following a single dose of dexamethasone administered at midnight from a series of patients studied to "rule out" Cushing's syndrome. Note the graded resistance to suppression illustrated in 1a. In the diagnostic evaluation of possible Cushing's syndrome the finding of failure of suppression to less than 6 ug/dl at 8 a.m. is taken as presumptive evidence of the diagnosis (Fig. 1b). This test is merely an abbreviation of the now standardized test for depression (Fig. 1c). Note that the limits for a positive test in depressive illness (Fig. 1c) differ from those in Cushing's syndrome (Fig. 1d), but that the difference is quantitative rather than qualitative.

must be employed in a rigidly standardized fashion. To be optimally sensitive and specific for severe depressive illness Carroll's group has recommended the use of a 1 mg dose of dexamethasone. It must be recognized that one cannot casually substitute 0.5 mg or 2 mg because these doses will alter the specificity and sensitivity of the test. This is due to the fact that these doses are close to the steep portion of the dose-response curve for effecting cortisol suppression and any change in dose will alter response. In addition to the dose of dexamethasone, the time points for blood sampling and for drug administration must also be rigidly controlled. A final point is that while Carroll's group has provided data indicating there is no difference in results obtained between in-patient and out-patient use of the test (7), experience with other tests which have been shown to be interfered with by the stress of hospitalization, such as the serum prolactin determination (11), suggests that continued evaluation of the interchangability of the in- and out-patient data is warranted.

In addition to the negative feedback effect of glucocorticoids, at any moment the plasma cortisol concentration is the net product of a multitude of variable influences. These include factors producing the circadian and pulsatile secretion of ACTH, the interposition of stressful events, and the distribution, binding and metabolism of cortisol. Thus, in addition to the controlled variable in the suppression test, that is, the comparatively weak feedback effect produced by the low dose of dexamethasone, these uncontrolled variables can be expected to markedly influence the final cortisol concentration. To all of this must be added the variance of the laboratory cortisol determination (commonly there is 5-10% interassay variation). For these reasons, endocrinologists who work up patients suspected of having Cushing's syndrome regard the overnight dexamethasone suppression test as a screening test. If an abnormal test is obtained it is usually repeated. Or, if the index of diagnostic suspicion is high, other tests are ordered such as those using urinary cortisol or its metabolites as an end-point, since these provide an integrated value. Thus, there is an important increase in diagnostic confidence gained by replication of the test or by other tests of hyperfunction of the pituitary corticotroph. Serial testing is also very advantageous as has been demonstrated recently by a number of groups who have studied the use of the dexamethasone suppression test in the diagnosis of severe depressive illness.

REFERENCES

1. Bigos, S. T., Robert, F., Pelletier, G. and Hardy, J. (1977): J. Clin. Endocrinol. Metab. 45:1251-1260.
2. Board, F. A., Persky, H. and Hamburg, D. A. (1956): Psychosom. Med. 18:324-333.
3. Brown, W. A., Johnston, R. and Mayfield, D. (1979): Am. J. Psychiat. 136;543-547.
4. Butler, P.W.P. and Besser, G. M. (1968): Lancet i:1234-1236.
5. Carroll, B. J., Martin, F.I.R. and Davies, B. (1968): Brit. Med. J. iii:285-287.
6. Carroll, B. J., Curtis, G. C. and Mendels, J. (1976): Arch. Gen. Psychiat. 33:1039-1044.
7. Carroll, B. J., Feinberg, M. F., Greden, J. F., Tarika, J., Albala, A. A., Haskett, R. F., James, N. McI., Kronfol, Z., Lohr, N., Steiner, M., de Vigne, J. P. and Young, E. (1981): Arch. Gen. Psychiat. 38:15-22.
8. Gibbons, J. L. (1964): Arch. Gen. Psychiat. 10:572-575.
9. Greden, J. F., Albala, A. A., Haskett, R. F., James, N. McI., Goodman, L., Steiner, M. and Carroll, B. J. (1980): Biol. Psychiat. 15:449-458.
10. Holsboer, F., Klein, H., Bender, W. et al. (1980): In: Progress in Neuropharmacology, edited by A. Carlsson, J. Engel and C. G. Gottfries, pp.180. Pergamon Press, New York.
11. Kellett, J. and Friesen, h. G. (1980): In: Pituitary Microadenomas, edited by G. Faglia, M. A. Giovanelli and R. M. MacLeod, pp.265-275. Academic Press, New York.
12. Kendall, J. W. (1961): Proc. Soc. Exp. Biol. Med. 107:926-928.
13. Kendall, J. W., Liddle, G. W., Federspiel, C. F. and Cornfield, J. (1962): J. Clin. Invest. 42:396-403.
14. Kendall, J. W. (1971): In: Frontiers in Neuroendocrinology, edited by L. Martini and W. Ganong, pp.177-207. Oxford University Press, New York.

15. Kendall, J. W., Egans, M. L., Stott, A. K., Kramer, R. M. and Jacobs, J. J. (1972): Endocrinology 90:525-530.
16. Krieger, D. T., Amorosa, L. and Linick, F. (1975): N. Engl. J. Med. 292:893-896.
17. Liddle, G. W., Giansiracusa, J. E. and Bennett, L. L. (1953): Metabolism 2:411-420.
18. McDonald, W. J., Golper, T. A., Mass, R. D., Kendall, J. W., Porter, G. A., Girard, D. E. and Fischer, M. D. (1979): J. Clin. Endocrinol. Metab. 48:92-95.
19. Pasqalini, R. Q. and Gurevich, N. (1956): J. Clin. Endocrinol. Metab. 16:406-410.
20. Rees, L. H., Besser, G. M., Jeffcoate, W. J., Goldie, D. J. and Marks, V. (1977): Lancet i:726-728.
21. Rubin, R. T. and Poland, R. E. (1981): In: this volume.
22. Sachar, E. J., Hellman, J., Roffwarg, H. P., Halpern, F. S., Fukushima, D. K. and Gallagher, T. F. (1973): Arch. Gen. Psychiat. 28:19-24.
23. Smals, A. G., Kloppenborg, P. W., Njo, K. T., Knoben, J. M and Ruland, C. M. (1976): Brit. Med. J. ii:1298.
24. Wallace, E. Z., Rosman, P., Toshav, N., Sacerdore, A. and Balthazar, A. (1980): J. Clin. Endocrinol. Metab. 50:46-51.

Neuroendocrinology and Psychiatric Disorder,
edited by G. M. Brown, et al.
Raven Press, New York 1984.

Critical Evaluation of the Clinical Neuroendocrine Findings in Affective Disorders

G. Tolis

A. R. T. Rubin and R. E. Poland (Chapter 11)

a. Pituitary adrenocortical axis

The data reviewed by these investigators can be divided into two parts:

i. 24 hour (circadian) pattern of plasma cortisol levels.
ii. suppressibility of plasma cortisol to dexamethasone.

I. The nychthermeral plasma cortisol values, determined at 30 minute intervals, in unipolar depressives show:

a^1: normal circadian amplitude (see Fig. 1 in Chapter 11)

a^2: increased area under the curve when compared to matched for age healthy females (see Fig. 1 in Chapter 11)

a^3: a shift to the left (phase advance) in cortisol secretion during night so that the increase in hormone levels begins several hours earlier than in control subjects (see Fig. 1 in Chapter 11).

II. The suppressibility of the pituitary-adrenal axis was tested in one patient prior to and during drug treatment of her depression by determining plasma cortisol in blood drawn at 8 a.m., 4 p.m. and 11 p.m. after the patient had ingested 1 mg dexamethasone the night before. In that patient, the authors clearly demonstrate that the non-suppressible axis at the acute phase of the disease changed its autonomy and gradually became fully suppressed at a time correlating with drug induced clinical remission (Fig. 2 in Chapter 11).

The approaches used by the above investigators, namely multiple blood sampling and data collection in a standard manner at various phases of a disease represent today the ideal clinical investigational method for assessment of the hypothalamic-pituitary-adrenal axis with minimal risk and maximum efficiency. This dual approach may provide clues with respect to the chronobiology of depressive disorder i.e. whether there is a temporal dissociation between nycthemeral rhythm and adrenocortical suppressibility. Although the data tend to indicate that the dexamethasone test alone might provide most of the information needed, i.e. be used as an ancillary diagnostic test for endogenous depression and possibly help predict remission or relapse potentially, it may be that the demonstration of phase advance in nocturnal cortisol secretion can also be used as a marker of sleep-wake cycle disturbances. Whether this finding, when positive, can be used to diagnose depressive disorders at an early stage among patients with early awakening needs to be evaluated.

Finally, it should be mentioned that in patients with non-suppressibility to dexamethasone it is necessary to exclude diagnosis of

Cushing's Syndrome. This can be done by measuring 24 hour urine for free cortisol, morning cortisol and AcTH levels and determination of serum potassium and bicarbonate. In the hirsute and/or obese and/or hypertensive female, the determination of blood DHEA, DHEA-S and/or 17 ketosteroid levels in urine is required to exclude an androgen glucocorticoid producing adrenal tumor (adenoma or carcinoma).

b: Pituitary-Gonadal Function

As stated by the authors the available data (including their own) are limited. Among the problems in interpreting the few reported findings are 1) the lack of information concerning the clinical status of these patients i.e. if male are they impotent, do they have normal libido? If they are females, do they have regular or irregular menses? Amenorrhea? Hirsutism? 2) The incompleteness in the evaluation of the hypothalamic-pituitary-gonadal axis i.e. measurements of testosterone without LH or vice versa.

I. For the male patient

In addition to obtaining a proper history of fertility and sexual function prior to the onset of the disease, the patient should be given a detailed sexual questionnaire aimed in documenting changes in libido and/or erectile potency. In patients complaining of decreased potency (complete impotence or inability to maintain an erection) determination of penile pressure will exclude or document the presence of vascular insufficiency (as this may occur either in association with diabetes, renal failure, Leriche's syndrome or following the intake of drugs that interfere with peripheral neurotransmitter function such as antihypertensive medications). Once such vasculotoxic conditions have been ruled out, one should proceed to the recording of nocturnal erections with the use of a penile tumescence plethysomographic device. Documenting the presence of nocturnal erections in a patient claiming impotence points to the existence of a major psychogenic component in its etiopathogenesis.

The minimal endocrine work-up will consist of the blood determination of serum FSH, LH, PRL* and testosterone either in a single blood sample or in an integrated manner i.e. measurements of FSH, LH and testosterone in blood drawn at frequent time intervals (Chapter 11) or after the administration of an LH/FSH secretagogue such as LHRH.

Measurements of plasma testosterone in serial blood samples suggest that the mean levels are lower in depressed than controls although not always statistically different (Chapter 11); studies based on single blood samples have reported no differences in the levels of patients as contrasted to controls or to the patients after treatment (p. 15 in Chapter 11). The combination of the finding of low LH and testosterone in Dr. Rubins' study suggests a central defect accounting for the low testosterone level. Although another study also reported low plasma testosterone (Chapter 11 - Vogel's) the finding by this investigator of elevated plasma estradiol is puzzling; since the production of testicular estrogens is also under LH control one would expect normal or low levels. Whether the reported patients had abused ethanol or had other liver or renal disorders was not reported in that study.

Measurements of serum gonadotropins in man are often of little value if done on a single blood sample (note that healthy adults may have

*(see Chapter 3)

levels indistinguishable from those of hypopituitary patients). serial blood samples at 20 minute intervals for 6 hours may provide information about the existence of pulsatility and allow a quantitative estimate. Determination of 24 hour or overnight urine gonadotropins provides a means for indirectly assessing production. Repetition of the above strategies during the remission of the depressive disorder should enable the investigator to better characterize the quantitative and qualitative differences in gonadotropin secretion in depression. These may include FSH-LH imbalance. Measurements of FSH and LH responses to a 100 μg bolus of LHRH would not be expected to provide much insight since this dose (used by both Dr. Rubin and Dr. Ettigi) is too large to detect subtle pituitary abnormalities. It has been repeatedly shown that even patients with hypogonadism due to pituitary tumors may show a normal FSH/LH release to 100 μg LHRH. An alternate strategy would be to use two doses 25 μg and 100 μg with the aim to document the sensitivity threshold with the lower dose and probably to evaluate the releasable and reserve pool of gonadotropins with the higher dose. An additional level of sophistication in one use of the LHRH test is to study responses to a 6 hr infusion. Some patients with pituitary prolactinomas will show a normal FSH/LH response to 100 μg LHRH bolus injection but an abnormal response to a 6 hr infusion thus suggesting a decrease in the LH reserve pool. Thus, better determination may result from use of graded LHRH doses and prolonged infusion.

<u>II</u>. For the female patient

One has to direct investigations differently when evaluating a premenopausal and post-menopausal females. If the patient is premenopausal and bleeds at monthly intervals, the only investigation justified is that of evaluating whether the women ovulates and has a normal luteal function. This is accomplished by measuring plasma progesterone on days 21 and 23 of the cycle. If the patient complains of spaniomenorrhea (she bleeds every 2-4 months) then investigations are required to exclude the co-existence of polycystic ovarian syndrome (PCO). These include determination in blood of E1, E2, D4-androstenedione and testosterone and measurements of LH, FSH either in serial blood samples for a 3 hour minimum period and/or after the administration of 100 μg LHRH. The finding of elevated estrogens and androgens and enhanced LH response to LHRH should raise very strong suspicion of the existence of PCO and will require further work-up with ovarian ultrasonography and laparoscopy.

If a patient in the reproductive age has secondary amenorrhea that has persisted for 6 months or more, one has to exclude the presence of a pituitary adenoma (prolactin secreting or non-secretory) or a hypothalamic-stalk infiltrate (usually accomplished with the help of highly refined computed tomography of the sellar area) or anorexia nervosa as common pathologic conditions leading to amenorrhea in the non-medicated patient. If these situations are excluded and the patient does not have a primary ovarian disorder such as radiation or chemotherapy of Hodgkin's disease or autoimmune oophoritis - (conditions associated with high serum gonadotropins) the investigation should include serial measurements of serum FSH and LH and assessment of FSH and LH responses to a 6 hour infusion of LHRH rather than a standard 100 g bolus (the latter is more often used for convenience). Determination of basal estradiol, estrone and testosterone levels performed on single blood samples are expected to be low in amenorrheic women with depression since the presumed defect is a decrease in LHRH release mechanism. One finding of elevated E2 and testosterone is not compatible with low LH profile and should point to an altered gonadotropin output as seen in polycystic ovary syndrome. In this respect, the data of Dr. Vogel (p. 16) should not be considered typical until a full evaluation of the adrenal-ovarian status of these patients, excluding other pathological conditions, is provided. In the event that one demonstrates a low episodic secretion of LH and a satisfactory pituitary LH output - as tested with LHRH, one could study the effect of intravenously administered naloxone on the LH profile; a restoration or enhancement of LH secretion by naloxone can then be taken as evidence of an increased opiergic tone which most likely leads to suprahypophyseal amenorrhea by depressing monaminergic input to the LHRH secreting neurons.

In the post-menopausal woman, administration of LHRH and measurements of LH/FSH responses is not the method of choice. Rather, determination of serum FSH/LH in serial blood samples (see ref. by Dr. Altman) during the acute phase and during remission would be expected to provide the most useful information about hypothalamic-gonadotropic regulation. The ability of exogenous opiates to lower LH secretion in healthy menopausal women suggests that the naloxone testing previously described may be a relevant method in assessing the role of endogenous opiates in suppressing LH release in depressed menopausal women.

B. S. Checkley and J. Arendt (Chapter 12)

1. Assessment of GH release

To date the evaluation of GH secretion in depressed patients has been done primarily using drugs acting at the C.N.S.; few studies have employed "physiological" stimuli such as sleep and thermal environment. In general - as discussed in great detail by Dr. Checkley - the available data do not allow the researcher-clinician to use GH-testing as an adjuvant mean to diagnose depressive disorders or predict relapse or entering into remission. One of the factors seems to be related to failure to match patients with controls with respect to age and sex. Yet, it is of interest that most of the depressed patients tend to show a decreased GH output at least when drugs or procedures are used which operate via central noradrenergic receptors. The question may now be asked: if a patient has decreased GH response to desmethyl imipramine while depressed and no improvement when the disease is in remission, does this imply trait disorder? Such data are not as yet available. When they become available the psychiatrist-researcher has to realize that for reasons not entirely clear, normal individuals may show different response patterns to different secretagogues. We believe that in terms of accuracy and small false negative result-yield, insulin induced hypoglycemia, apomorphine and des-methylimipramine are the best tests of GH-reserve. The availability for clinical studies of synthetic GH releasing factor (as announced by the group of Dr. Guillemin's of the Salk Institute during the June 1982 Annual Meeting of the Endocrine Society and reported in Science 218:585, 1982) will provide a direct means to assess the status of pituitary somatotropes. Finally, as far as the reported "paradoxical" GH responses to TRH we need to exclude placebo effect and spontaneous variations in level. When this is done,

one should attempt to find out whether the TRH responders are more responsive to particular neuropharmacotherapeutic agents.

2. Assessment of PRL release

Studies have been performed using physiological and pharmacological means with the objective of stimulating or inhibiting PRL secretion. The use of TRH is an unfortunate choice because it acts directly upon the lactotropes and gives no clues to the hypothalamic control of PRL which should be the main focus. Insulin induced hypoglycemia will accomplish that but to date extensive studies have not been published. For the drugs inhibiting PRL secretion the use of levodopa again informs one of the status of the lactotrope dopamine receptors; a better method for assessment of central dopaminergic input would be to measure PRL levels after levodopa-carbidopa combination (250-25 mg). Bromocriptine is a very potent direct pituitary-lactotrope supressant and it is unlikely therefore that its use will be of discriminating value. Finally as far as physiological stimuli is concerned, sleep remains the most reliable one but it necessitates EEG recording to document its "normalcy"; if the sleep architecture is disturbed i.e. narcolepsy, epilepsy, anorexia nervosa then the hormonal correlates are difficult to interpret. Finally, in order to explore the possible involvement of opiergic circuits in maintaining elevated PRL levels during the late afternoon hours (discussion on Halbreich's data) an infusion of a low dose naloxone (0.8 mg/hr) should be done prior to the expected rise rather than at 8 a.m. (as it has been done by the Fair Oaks group). To summarize, the available data base on different strategies than suggested above do not indicate that monitoring of PRL is a worthwhile marker in depressive disorders. Whether PRL levels and dynamics determined during treatment with antidepressants or ECT can be of predictive value to therapy remains to be determined.

C. A. J. Prange, Jr. and P. T. Loosen (Chapter 13)

In approximately 50% of depressed patients, a blunted response of the pituitary thyrotropes to TRH can be demonstrated, although basal thyroid hormone (T4 and T3) and TSH values are within normal range (3, 9, 12).

The TRH test is not used frequently although it could lead to the identification of a treatable disorder, i.e. biochemical subclinical hypothyroidism. It requires the administration of synthetic TRH and the determination of TSH blood at given intervals (usually every 15 minutes for one hour). This test evaluates the ability of the pituitary thyrotropes to release TSH which presumably reflects among other variables the status of the endogenous TRH receptors. The findings of subnormal TSH rise after TRH is thought to characterize patients with endogenomorphic depression (-DSM III) and it has been suggested that the normalization of the response may parallel clinical remission (12, 2).

The reasons why there is such an abnormality in the thyrotropes of depressed patients are not clear. We can offer the following hypotheses based on the physiological knowledge concerning the regulation of TSH secretion. The main neuroactive substance that activates the thyrotropes to synthesize and release TSH is the naturally occurring hypothalamic peptide TRH. The neurotransmitters governing its secretion have not been clearly identified. The thyroid hormones, when in excess, and the glucocorticoids are capable of suppressing its release from the hypothalamic nuclei. AT the level of the thyrotropes four substances are known to inhibit their ability to respond to TRH or to inhibit spontaneous release of TSH. These are a) thyroid hormones, b) glucocorticoids, c) somatostatin, and d) dopamine. Given that spontaneous TSH release occurs at night time, it was postulated that this may in part be associated with the falling glucocorticoid levels. If this were so, an absence of circadian TSH rhythm should be expected in patients with Cushing's syndrome, in patients ingesting glucocorticoids, and in some patients with unipolar depression. The observation that the administration of various dopamine-receptor blocking agents such as haloperidol, metoclopramide, clebopride stimulates TSH release more intensely at night than during the day (Table 1) suggests to us that the circadian control of TSH secretion is affected not only by glucocorticoids but also by endogenous dopamine*. The evaluation of TSH release by TRH and antidopaminergic agents in a circadian manner and the correlation of the findings to the endogenous cortisol values and to the dexamethasone suppression test may help elucidate the hormone-neurotransmitter interaction in the control of thyrotrope function in affective disorders which are characterized by considerable heterogeneity insofar as thyroid-pituitary relations is concerned (9, 3).

In order to assess the functional status of the hypothalmic-pituitary-thyroid axis in depressed patients other investigations have determined the serum concentrations of T4 and TRH - induced TSH changes in forty-five patients with psychotic and neurotic depression (9, 13). Blood levels of T4 were lower in psychotic (n:25) than neurotic (n:20) patients who were sex and age matched (1). In addition, psychotic patients had lower levels of Free Thyroxine Index (FTI) as compared with 240 euthyroid controls, none suffering mental illness (1). A reverse relationship could also be demonstrated between FTI and the score for depression as estimated by the Hamilton Depression Rating Scale (HDRS). The mean (SD) values for FTI and HDRS were: Neurotic, FTI 2.6 0.8, HDRS 26.7 1.7 and Psychotic, FTI 1.9 0.5, HDRS 36.6 4.1. In these groups of patients, one could not demonstrate a difference between the TSH or PRL blood levels prior to and 30 minutes after the administration of 200 ng TRH i.v. either at 14.00 or 24.00 hours. Among the patients with psychotic depression, it was found that those with involutional depression responded more than those with unipolar type of depression (3). This finding indicates that there is a heterogeneity of the psychotic depressives from a neuroendocrine standpoint and may help explain some of the discrepant data in "pooled" depressives.

To sum up the available data, it appears that a group of patients with unipolar depression exhibits a blunted response to TRH. But what is a blunted response? Drs. Wetterberg's, Prange's and Extein's groups consider a blunted response if TSH rises to less than 3, 5 and 7 uU/ml respectively after the administration of 400-600 ug TRH. On the other hand the group of Drs. A. Winokur and J. Amsterdam reported at the meeting of the International Society of Psychoneuroendocrinology in Montreal (May 1981) age-adjusted minimum and maximum

*For a recent review of the role of dopamine in TSH regulation see Scanlon, M. F., Lewis, M., Weightman, D. R., Chan, Y. and Hall, R. The Neuroregulation of Human Thyrotropin Regulation. Frontiers in Neuroendocrinology, Vol. 6, edited by L. Martini and W. F. Ganong. Raven Press, New York, 1980, pp.333-380.

TABLE I. Circadiem Responses of Thyrotropes and/or Lactotropes to Various Secretagogues in Healthy Subjects

Hormone Response	Time of Day			Substance Administered	Reference (no)
	02.00	10.00	18.00	TRH	
TSH	++	+	+		
Prl	+	+	+		
	14.00	24.00		TRH	6
TSH	+	+			
Prl	++	+			
	Sleep S.W.S.		REM	TRH	8
TSH	++		+		
Prl	+		+		
	09.00	18.00		Insulin induced Hypoglycemia	4
Prl	+	++			
	09.00	18.00		Haloperidol	5
Prl	+	+			
	09.00	24.00		Clebopride	7
TSH	+	++			
Prl	+	+			
	11.00	23.00		Metochlopramide	10
TSH	+	++			
Prl	+	+			

responses to TRH and pointed out the need for the collected of age and sex adjusted normal data. Concerning the question whether a blunted response is indicative of state or trait disorder, one way to evaluate this is to study the TRH responses in familial pure depressives and their relative; to assess genetic factors i.e. HLA and A B O grouping and to demonstrate persistence of the blunted response despite normalization of other parameters such as D.S.T. which are thought to represent a state disorder marker. Hypothalamic pituitary disorders, Cushing's disease-central or related to an adrenal adenoma and last but not least subclinical hyperthyroidism - as seen in the presence of a toxic thyroid nodule - should be excluded. In the presence of a non-blunted response to TRH even when there is an escape from dexamethasone (D.S.T. non suppressor) it will be of great value to follow-up the TRH test in order to establish whether the TRH will evoke a larger TSH rise. If this were the case then we would have to conclude that the so called non-blunted TSH rise was certainly subnormal for that given patient. From previous experiments we know that administation of T_4 or T_3 in normal volunteers will decrease the TSH response to TRH even if it was normal before and will still be normal i.e. TSH prior to treatment: 11 uU/ml; TSH after 2 weeks treatment with L-thyroxine: 6 uU/ml. The investigator must be familiar with the concept of individuality and the need to periodically assess the endocrine gland responses to a given challenge so that a misinterpretation of test-data is avoided. As to whether the TRH test can be used as predictor of outcome and guide for drug selection (see discussion also by Dr. Prange), the available information does not allow any conclusion.

REFERENCES

1. Belmaker, R. H., Kon, M., Ebstein, R. P. and Dasberg, H. (1980): Biolog. Psychiat. 15:3-8.
2. Kirkegaard, C., Norlem, N., Lanridsen, U. B., Bjorum, N. and Christiansen, C. (1975): Arch. Gen. Psychiat. 32:1115-1118.
3. Martinos, A., Papachristou, D., Rinieris, P., Souvatzoglou, A., Koutras, D. and Stefanis, C. (1980): Paper presented at the International Symposium on Depression in Athens (in press).
4. Nathan, R. S., Sachar, E. J., Langer, G., Tabrizi, M. A. and Halpern, F. S. (1979): J. Clin. Endocrinol. Metab. 49:231-235.
5. Nathan, R. S., Pezel, J., McCarthy, T. and Jarrett, D. (1982): In: Proceedings of the 3rd International Congress on Human Prolactin, edited by G. Tolis et al. Raven Press (in press).
6. Perez-Lopez, F. R., Gomez, A. G. and Abos, M. D. (1981): Acta Endocrinol. 97:7-11.
7. Perez-Lopez, F. R., Couzalez-Moreno, C., Abos, M., Andonegui, J. and Corvo, R. (1982): Acta Endocrinol. (in press).
8. Peters, J. A., Santa-Cruz, F., Tower, B. B. and Rubin, R. T. (1981): J. Clin. Endocrinol. 52:975-981.
9. Rinieris, P., Christodoulou, G., Souvatzoglou, A., Koutras, D. and Stefanis, C. (1978): Acta Psychiat. Scand. 58:56-60.
10. Scanlon, M. F., Weetman, A. P., Lewis, M., Pourmand, M., Rodriguez-Arnao, M. D., Weightman, D. R. and Hall, R. (1980): J. Clin. Endocrinol. 51:1251-1256.
11. Stefanis, C., Lykouras, E., Garelis, E. and Varsou, E. (1979): In: Biological Psychiatry Today, edited by J. Obiols, C. Ballus, E. Gonzalz Monclus and J. Pujol, pp.149-154. Elsevier North Holland.
12. Tolis, G. (1982): In: Proceedings of International Symposium on Depression, edited by C. Stefanis. Plenum Press.

Neuroendocrinology and Psychiatric Disorder,
edited by G. M. Brown, et al.
Raven Press, New York 1984.

Summary Overview: Affective Disorders—Endocrine Features

Eugenio E. Müller

Depressive illness includes a heterogeneous group of disorders having dissimilar etiology, symptomatology and response to treatment, though, likely, sharing in common a central neurotransmitter disturbance. It is therefore understandable that in this syndrome there exist several abnormalities in the secretion pattern of the anterior pituitary hormones and/or in the feedback action of peripheral target endocrine gland hormones, activities for which a normal functioning of central nervous system (CNS) transmitters is mandatory (see ref. 2 for review). The neuroendocrine component in depressive illness represents an important biologic correlate in the disease which can be exploited for understanding the etiologies, providing new information in the differential diagnosis of several types of depression and, possibly, predicting the treatment response.

The first speaker of the Session, Dr. R. Rubin (Chapter 11) discussed data on endocrine changes in the hypothalamo-pituitary adrenal-cortical and gonadal axis in the endogenous subtype of major depression (melancholia), a type of depression characterized by a specific cluster of symptoms, a prolonged course, often a family history of similar illness and, generally, a responsiveness only to somatic therapies.

Among other anterior pituitary hormones, adrenocorticotropin (ACTH) presents with a prominent circadian variation, as does its target hormone cortisol; the lowest blood levels of both hormones occur in the early hours of sleep and then rapidly increase in the latter few hours of sleep to a maximum at the time of awakening. Adrenal cortical activity is increased in both the apathetic as well as in anxious depressives throughout the entire 24 hrs and especially during the sleep period, (the difference compared to normals being particularly evident between 2400 and 0300h), with ensuing circadian blunting of ACTH and cortisol rhythmicity. Increased corticosteroid secretion far from being a mere reflection of anxiety and dysphoria would be secondary to an underlying disturbance of brain function and would usually return to normal following successful treatment.

Dr. Rubin then focused in his presentation on a laboratory test of neuroendocrine function that is highly specific for melancholia, and is a marker of the hyperactivity of the ACTH-cortisol axis i.e., the dexamethasone (DEX) suppression test (DST). Both inpatients and outpatients with endogenous depression have an abnormal early escape of plasma cortisol concentrations during a 24-hr overnight DST, i.e., they often show an early increase in serum cortisol 16 and 24 hrs post-administration of DEX (0.5-2.0 mg p.o.). The DST is now being used widely for the diagnosis of endogenous depression (1). Since differing procedures have been adopted for the DST in various centers, the test needs standardization for general use. Dr. Rubin delineated various aspects of the test procedure i.e., the dose of DEX (1.0 mg), number and timing of blood samples (800, 1600 and 2300 of the second day), the criterion value of plasma cortisol for judging a test result as abnormal ($>$5 μg/dL). In many clinical settings the DST has a high degree of specificity i.e., it recognizes 90-95% of true depressives but lower sensitivity, about 60-70% i.e., 30-40% of true depressives have a normal DST, therefore the overall diagnostic confidence i.e. the proportion of abnormal test results that are true-positive for endogenous depression is high. Moreover, the DST does possess predictive validity, i.e. conversion of abnormal DST response to normal is associated with a good prognosis after treatment, while failure of the DST to convert to normal is associated with early relapse. Construct validity of the test stems from several observations i.e. abnormal DST responses return to normal on complete recovery or following a switch from depression to mania and are related significantly to a positive history of depression. In the final part of his presentation Dr. Rubin dealt with the secretion patterns of the pituitary gonadotropins and their peripheral target gonadal hormones, a problem which may have a particular relevance in the illness, since decreased sexual drive is part of the symptom cluster of endogenous depression. In all, data presented suggest a dysfunction of the hypothalamo-pituitary gonadal function with reduced plasma titers of LH, testosterone, and increased levels of estradiol in depressed men, and reduced LH, but increased estradiol and testosterone, in depressed women. However, these findings invite further studies evaluating both gonadotropins and gonadal steroids in the same blood samples (in only few studies this was performed) and a better understanding of the psychohormonal importance of reduced LH and testosterone in depressed men.

Particularly relevant to Dr. Rubin's presentation is that of Dr. Kendall (Chapter 14) who addressed himself to comment from an endocrinological viewpoint on some features of pituitary-adrenocortical dysfunction in severe depressive illness viewed in comparison with pituitary-adrenocortical hyperactivity of pituitary-dependent Cushing's syndrome (Cushing's Disease). As pointed out by Dr. Kendall there are no major qualitative differences in the hypercortisolemia of the two disease states, the differences being especially in degree, i.e. the derangement being more intense in Cushing's disease. The milder degree of the adrenal overactivity or alternatively the shorter duration of exposure to hypercortisolemia may explain the otherwise perplexing finding that peripheral clinical features of cortisol excess are present in Cushing's Disease are lacking in severe depressive illness. However, in the latter condition searching for subtle biochemical correlates (e.g. carbohydrate intolerance) may be worthwhile. Another qualitative difference between the two pathologic states is the frequently encountered normalization of the cortisol disorder with remission or with the switch to mania which is present in severe depressive illness in contrast with the more enduring cortisol associated abnormalities of Cushing's Disease. Since tricyclic antidepressants or electroconvulsive therapy (ECT) may improve or even normalize abnormal DST responses in depressives (vide supra), it may well be that Dex in depressives exerts its feedback inhibition at a site which is susceptible to CNS-directed therapeutic remedies. In Cushing's Disease, a primary defect in the pituitary corticotroph with DEX exerting its feedback action mainly on a pituitary locus may explain why spontaneous remissions of pituitary suppressiblity are uncommon. It is obvious that these differences may throw light on the different etiologies of the two disorders; therefore, comparison of advances made in understanding each disorder will continue to add knowledge to our understanding of the other. In the final part of his presentation Dr. Kendall placed special emphasis in commenting on some of the important caveats in the use and interpretation of the DST as recently suggested by Carroll and colleagues (1981) (vide supra Dr. Rubin's presentation).

A logical corollary to the notion that individual anterior pituitary hormones are under control by brain neurotransmitters is the use of neuroendocrine tests to assess the status of receptors involved in central neurotransmission. To be valid this pharmacoendocrine strategy should meet at least two criteria: 1) drugs which stimulate, even though through different mechanisms, a specific neuroreceptor should release the hormone in question; 2) this response should be inhibited by drugs which block the specific neuroreceptor. This central issue was running through Dr. Checkley's presentation which focused especially on the pharmacoendocrine studies of growth hormone (GH) release (Chapter 12). He described first the role of neurotransmitters and their receptors in the regulation of the release of GH in man; briefly, GH is controlled by excitatory α-adrenergic, dopaminergic, GABAergic and opiate influences and, likely, by inhibitory β adrenergic influences. The functioning of each of these systems can be investigated using pharmacoendocrine tests of the functioning of each type of receptor. However, as Dr. Checkley cautioned; results of such studies will be meaningful when all of the other biological (spontaneous GH release, sex, age, etc.) and physiopathological (stress, obesity, starvation, drug intake, medical illness) influences on GH release are held constant. Such variables were not adequately considered in the past studies in depressive patients.

In view of the many factors which influence the size of GH responses to test stimuli, GH responses cannot be used for diagnosing endogenous depression or classifying depression subtypes but can provide an invaluable aid for: 1) assessing the status of α-adrenoceptors, dopamine (DA) and opiate receptors, etc. and 2) their possible modifications during the course of ECT or antidepressant therapy. In this way GH responses can provide useful information on the mechanism of action of ECT and antidepressants.

Along this line recent findings obtained with clonidine, a potent stimulant of α_2-adrenoceptors are of particular interest. GH response to clonidine are significantly impaired in patients with endogenous depression when compared to age-and sex-matched controls. This suggests a defect at α_2-(postsynaptic?) adrenoceptors in brain regions regulating the release of GH. However, after 3 weeks of institution of antidepressant therapy, the GH response to clonidine in depressed patients is significantly enhanced, while the drug's sedative and hypotensive effects are significantly inhibited. The potential importance of these studies for understanding the type of brain deficit underlying the disorder and therapy-induced changes does not escape attention.

Hormones of the thyroid axis may play an important role in modulating catecholamine neurotransmission in the CNS and thus may serve as a mechanism of physiological adjustment or defense during times of adaptive demand (3). Because of the possibility that depressive illness may often involve a diminished availability of norepinephrine

(NE) at central adrenergic receptor sites, adequate mobilization of thyroid hormones during the course of the disease may be crucial to increase NE receptor sensitivity (providing the person with an adaptive advantage) and thus maintain the system compensated (3). In his presentation Dr. Prange dealt mainly with the diagnostic aspect of thyroid hormones in affective illness (Chapter 13). Investigation of the hypothalamo-pituitary-thyroid (HPT) axis in persons with depression has shown that about one third have increased levels of circulating thyroid hormones that decrease with recovery from the illness. Indices of elevated thyroid function correlate with a rapid recovery from depression, when the individual is treated with tricyclic drugs that increase the availability of catecholamines. In this vein has also to be viewed the finding that thyrotropin (TSH) given to depressed women enhances their antidepressant response to subsequent imipramine treatment. Dr. Prange than addressed himself to considering TSH as a dependent variable and, namely, its response to the hypothalamic tripeptide TSH-releasing hormone (TRH). Early reports that administration of TRH produced a brief antidepressant effect led to an extensive series of studies of the effects of TRH in depressive patients. While the alleged antidepressant effect of TRH remains controversial the original finding that the TSH response to TRH (600 μg i.v.) is blunted in 25% of patients with primary depression (maximum ΔTSH $<$ 5 μU/ml) has been confirmed in 38 studies involving 781 patients. As with the DST response, the TRH test may be useful for the clinician in identifying the active and remitted state of the illness, while no firm data are available on the usefulness of the TRH test in guiding choice of treatment and distinguishing between primary and secondary depression or unipolar and bipolar subgroups. Regarding the pathophysiologic significance of a blunted TSH response, this important issue is still unresolved, though there are several possible explanations for this finding. They include: 1) a state of hyperthyroidism-however, no correlation has been found between increased levels of thyroid hormones and the TSH response to TRH in depressives, 2) chronic TRH hypersecretion with ensuing down regulation of the receptor sites on the thyrotroph cell; 3) a "disordered" function of the thyrotroph cell secondary to causes such as somatostatin or neurotensin hypersecretion, or a hyperdopaminergic state (so-called "sick" thyrotroph cell syndrome) and, finally 4) a negative feedback influence exerted by elevated levels of cortisol. No one of these mechanisms can account satisfactorily for the altered neuroendocrine response.

Interestingly, apart from depression and certain states of physical illness i.e., acute starvation, TSH blunting also occurs in cognate mental disorders e.g. anorexia nervosa, mania and alcoholism but not in schizophrenia, thus providing a certain degree of specificity to this finding.

Dr. Prange then turned out to consider briefly the state of peripheral thyroid hormones in affective illness. Although the mean value of any thyroid index for a group of depressed patients is apt to fall within normal limits, inspection of data from individual subjects frequently discloses elevated thyroid indices (see <u>also supra</u>). By contrast, biochemical evidence of hypothyroidism has been occasionally revealed by other studies. In all these findings suggest that the state of thyroid function in a given subject is apt to reflect the particular stage of illness he or she is facing and that adequate mobilization of thyroid function is associated with clinical recovery from depression, whereas poor mobilization is associated with prolonged illness (see also ref. 3).

REFERENCES

1. Carroll, B. J., Feinberg, M., Greden, J. F., Tarika, J., Albala, A.A., Haskett, R. F., James, N. M., Kronfol, Z., Lohr, N., Steiner, M., Pauld de Vigne, J., and Young, E. (1981): Arch. Gen. Psychiatry 38: 15-22.
2. Müller, E. E., Nistico, G., and Scapagnini, U. (1978): In: Neurotransmitters and Anterior Pituitary Function. Academic Press, New York.
3. Whybrow, P. C., and Prange, jr. A. J. (1981): Arch. Gen. Psychiatry 38: 106-113.

Neuroendocrinology and Psychiatric Disorder,
edited by G. M. Brown, et al.
Raven Press, New York 1984.

Discussion: Affective Disorders—Endocrine Features

Seymour Reichlin

I would like to suggest that we may be failing to obtain useful information about possible psychiatric or neurologic abnormalities in "normal" patients who are non-responders. From 15 to 20%, or sometimes up to 40% of "normal" individuals tested as volunteers fail to respond to one or other provocative stimulus to GH release. The endocrinologist in charge usually discards these patients as unsuitable for study without considering neural differences in these individuals.

Laurence S. Jacobs; I think that the TRH test is more consistent than many other provocative tests talked about, such as L-dopa and hypoglycemia induced GH release. For growth hormone responses especially, normal individuals may fail to respond to 15-20% of this, and the response varies 15-20% from day to day in the same individual. This variation is presumably neurally based, while the more consistent TSH responses to TRH are the result of direct stimulation of the pituitary.

Dr. J. Davis

I'd like to comment on the significance of "abnormal" values in normal controls. This is a difficult problem and I don't think it is appropriate to eliminate from the normal control group individuals with abnormal values. It is a statistical problem. We simulated random selection processes by taking a thousand samples of a situation where we would draw with random numbers 20 in the experimental group and 20 in the control group - and we did this a thousand times. We then dropped the three highest values from the normal control group. These were then compared with our experimental group. Normally one would expect to have significant differences 5 or less times out of 100 times, but if you purge the control group of the three highest values, you can get a statistically significant difference between two similar groups 50% of the time.

In studies of physiological responses in psychiatric patients differences will appear if we deliberately purge the control group of a couple of values; this creates a systematic error.

Dr. Reichlin: I think it is of importance to emphasize that none of the provocative tests we do follow a normal distribution. Not a single one of the responses reported this morning is normally distributed, and this heterogeneity is especially noted in all the growth hormone reserve tests. I don't think we have dealt adequately with statistical evaluation of this kind of data.

Dr. Puig-Antich

I would like to comment again on the normal group. It was apparent this morning, as well as from data reported in the literature, that for growth hormone and TSH responses, if not for cortisol, the question of trait vs state is unsettled. In order to answer this, it is essential for future studies to have two groups of normals. All the normals should be assessed as completely as the patients are and should have family histories taken, with assignment to two groups - one with a family history for depression or alcoholism and other antisocial personality, and the other without such positive family history. Only under these circumstances will we be able to provide accurate controls for the presence of a trait.

Stuart A. Checkley

May I reply on the question of the normal subject with an absent growth hormone response? One problem relates to dose. I am sure that if we push up the dose of clonidine, for instance, more of the normal subjects would respond - and this would be true for apomorphine too. But if we push up the dose, we will encounter other problems. We will encounter various side effects, including retching and vomiting, and the hypertensive patients might become comatose. As a result, the whole test procedure would become much less specific, as well, of course, as being ethically unacceptable. So I think I prefer it as it is now. For this reason, I think one has to be at the bottom end of the dose-response curve, which is also a good position on the dose-response curve to pick up abnormalities - so I personally am not bothered by the problem of the non-responder.

John W. Kendall

One of the possible causes of non-response is the presence of occult pituitary disease. For example, Gerry Burrows and his colleagues at Toronto have evaluated pituitary glands at autopsy for the prevalence of tumors. They have found that about 25% of adult patients harbor a pituitary tumor at least 0.2 mm or greater in size. A study done at the Mayo Clinic in the 1930's, involving 1000 pituitaries, found small pituitary tumors in more than 20% of individuals. One patient actually had 11 pituitary tumors. We should not necessarily assume that we are always dealing with a normal gland in a seemingly normal person.

Barry Sherman

The accepted criteria for a normal cortisol response to a 1.0 mg dose of dexamethasone given at 11:00 p.m. are given as anywhere from 5-10 µg/dl. These values were derived from visual examination of results that in general employed older methods for measurement of serum cortisol rather than currently accepted methods such as competitive protein binding or radioimmunoassay. It is somewhat surprising that results from large numbers of healthy subjects or patients have never been submitted to statistical analysis.

We recently analyzed a large data set derived from an experiment in which 1 mg of dexamethasone was given at 11:00 p.m. and serum cortisol was measured at 8:00 a.m. the following morning. The postdexamethasone serum cortisol concentrations were not normally distributed but followed a gamma distribution in healthy subjects. Most values fell near the level of detectability. The 95% confidence limits indicated an upper value for serum cortisol of 1.8 µg/dl after dexamethasone. We found this to be true of obese as well as normal weight subjects, as well as a large population of manic patients.

If an 8:00 a.m. postdexamethasone serum cortisol value of 2 µg/dl is considered normal, then patients with values between 2.1 and 5 should be regarded as suspicious for nonsuppression. Such individuals might demonstrate early "escape" from the effects of dexamethasone when subsequent samples are obtained at 4:00 p.m. or later.

There is evidence that values obtained using radioimmunoassay methods for serum cortisol may give higher values than the competitive protein-binding method used in our laboratory. For this reason, criteria for normal responses should be determined in individual laboratories.

Bernard Carroll

I would like to make a couple of comments about the dexamethasone work that has been discussed. One is to emphasize at this point that our data and those of Barry Sherman and Martin Shaffer strictly refer to medically 'clean' patients. There are a wide variety of medical conditions and drugs, as Dr. Kendall has emphasized, that will technically interfere with the test. Among our in-patients, this amounted to 20% of available subjects, so it is important to keep this in mind. Dr. Kendall referred to the possibility that we may be able to improve the sensitivity of the test by repeating it. He pointed out the variability of dexamethasone testing in Cushing's disease, and we now have data on test re-test/reliability that confirms that it does vary in the direction that Dr. Kendall predicted. The test for reliability is around 95% for the non-melancholic, non-endogenous cases. It is more in the order of 71% for the melancholy group, so that by doing two tests it is possible to pick up more like 80% of the melancholy patients at the same level of diagnostic confidence. Re-test reliability between episodes of depression is again in the 90% range - so that is useful.

Dr. Rubin and Dr. Sherman have raised questions, about using the psychiatric diagnosis as the basis of classification of responders and non-responders. Should we hold the clinical diagnostic category as the independent variable and look at endocrine markers, or should we reverse the dependencies and try to define the homogeneous group by biological indices? All I want to say about this is that we are presently in the dialectic phase of redefining melancholia and endogenous depression and will eventually emerge with a small group of biologic markers that can be added to clinical criteria to provide a more comprehensive definition of the illness. This is exactly what happened with other conditions in medicine such as thyrotoxicosis, hypothyroidism and myocardial infarction. Exactly what the laboratory markers will be has yet to be worked out. One final comment about the site of action of the disturbance in pituitary-adrenal feedback in depression should be made. I think we can agree with what Dr. Kendall and others have said, namely that the locus of dexamethasone suppression is in the pituitary, but that is not to say that the pathology is at the pituitary level. The best model for this is the demonstration that you can dexamethasone-suppress a normal person, then give him an insulin tolerance test, and then he will have an absolutely normal cortisol and ACTH response. And you can do the same thing with drugs that act strictly at the CNS level, such as physostigmine, as I mentioned earlier. So it is our belief that this disturbance is not of pituitary origin but a limbic system disinhibition of the axis.

Eugenio E. Müller

Among the battery of tests that can be useful as diagnostic aids in primary affective disorders, no one has mentioned the deranged growth hormone response to TRH and LHRH that we and Brambilla observed in at least 60 to 70% of patients. This response is present only in primary affective disorders and not in secondary depression. Dr. Brambilla is now following up the relatives of these patients and there is apparently some deranged response in these as well. As has been pointed out by Dr. Tolis, TRH administration but only in large doses of 1 mg or more blunts the L-dopa induced growth hormone response and there is a hypothalamic site of action of TRH. We think that the TRH-induced growth hormone increase is a fairly good indicator of 'deranged' neurotransmission in the CNS but that this effect is exerted directly at the level of the anterior pituitary. The TRH response can be an indicator of disturbances in the central nervous system the understanding of which will give us better insight on the pathogenesis of this disease. I doubt that dexamethasone works at the level of the pituitary. I say this because the abnormal response is normalized by administration of antidepressant drugs and there is no evidence that antidepressant drugs modulate pituitary function directly. There are corticosterone receptors within the limbic system which are modulated by monoamines. Nevertheless, I find it difficult to understand how the administration of a drug that acts on the CNS is capable of restoring the pituitary site of response to dexamethasone.

Robert M. Rose

One of the things that is perplexing about the dexamethasone test is that there is no continuum of response. The more seriously ill patients do not show more profound impairment of dexamethasone suppression and there is no correlation with the Hamilton scores, for example. Why is it that among those who do escape suppression, there is no relationship between the magnitude of illness and magnitude of cortisol abnormality?

Robert T. Rubin

I believe that the range of Hamilton scores we have tried to correlate with cortisol hypersecretion is really too restricted, and we are in the middle range of a bi-variant normal distribution. But we could expand the scale if we included things such as indices of suicidality, dimensions of psychotic depression and that sort of thing. I speculate that it is the extremes of the clinical circumstance that really yield the positive correlations between psychological and endocrine abnormality. I would like to respond to Dr. Müller's comments. In contrast to his statements, we believe that there is no specific growth hormone response to TRH in depressed patients. We sampled blood for a long period of time before and after TRH and have found a random distribution of values (slide shown) in 19 of 22 patients.

Next I would like to respond to Dr. Carroll. I certainly agree that we are in a dialectic phase and that we need both clinical and biochemical independent variables from time to time, and that we must ultimately combine the two. If we use only biochemical markers, we run the risk of widening the range of the diagnosis by virtue of the non-specificity of each of the tests. When a test is used more and more frequently, the small amount of its non-specificity increases the prevalence of the illness in the population. We will ultimately combine both the clinical the the biochemical criteria to better define our diagnostic groups.

Peter E. Stokes

With regard to the dexamethasone escape phenomenon, I would add one further bit of evidence for this being due to an influence above the level of the pituitary. But there may also be an influence acting on the pituitary gland. Some years ago, we described the effect of ECT on the hypothalamic-pituitary adrenocortical axis. When pre- and post-ECT cortisol levels were compared as a percentage of initial value we noted that individuals whose initial cortisol levels were low had high values following ECT, and those whose initial cortisol levels were high went only a bit higher or went down. I think that this argues more for a central than a pituitary effect. Similar data have been reported for hypoglycemia induced cortisol release.

Phil Gold

My comments relate to our recent work on vasopressin and neurohypophysial hormones in depression. Vasopressin and other posterior pituitary hormones are synthesized in the CNS and are widely distributed throughout the brain, via CSF and axonal transport. They also are released into the peripheral blood where they can be measured in minute quantities. Within the brain, they are considered as neuromodulators - they affect electrical activity and may influence biological rhythms and neuroendocrine functions. In our current work, we have devised a paradigm to evaluate vasopressin function; we measure levels in the CSF and in plasma using osmotic stimulation and have been able to show that the intensity of the response to the osmotic stimulus is reproducible and inheritable in monozygotic twins. Vasopressin levels in CSF are reduced, and vasopressin response to hypertonic saline decreased in depression as compared with mania. This observation is of interest because vasopressin is a peptide with behavioural effects - influencing cognition in normal and depressed subjects, and possibly in demented patients. With respect to the question about why vasopressin might be low in depression (in which ACTH secretion is inappropriately high) if it is an ACTH releasing factor, we are presenting a poster this afternoon that shows that in anorexia nervosa there is a dissociation between vasopressin secretion into the CSF and into the plasma. There is also a suggestion that there are different populations of neurons that secrete into the CSF and into the plasma, and that these may be modulated by some of the same physiological stimuli, but there are a number of differences in regulation of the two neuronal systems. Secretion into CSF is mediated by the paraventricular and perhaps by the suprachiasmatic nuclei whereas secretion into the plasma is mediated by the supraopticohypophysial tract and the neuronal connections from the supraopticohypophysial tract to the median eminence. If you give hypertonic stimuli, you do not raise ACTH or cortisol, indicating that the osmoreceptor does not seem to regulate the neurohypophysial AVP with corticotropin releasing factor properties. To explain the fact that CSF levels of vasopressin are lower and that hypertonic stimuli release lesser amounts of vasopressin into the plasma in depression there seems to be an alteration in one or more of the neuromodulators that influences osmoregulation in depressed patients. What we are doing now is investigating the neuromodulation of osmoregulation, and we have looked at opiate agonists and antagonists, lithium, carbamazepine and some of the tricylic antidepressants.

Alfred J. Lewy

I think we would all agree that a state marker should have high sensitivity, high specificity, and , as Dr. Rose has just pointed out, it would be nice if it was correlated with the severity of illness. For trait markers, on the other hand, you would not expect high specificity, even though a segment of the normal population would carry that trait.

I think we have to distinguish between state markers and trait markers, when we evaluate specificity.

Seymour Reichlin: Can I take my prerogative as Chairman to ask a question? Is depression a stress? All the discussions of today have blurred the definition. In the abnormalities described, which are rather striking, are we seeing specific 'stress-induced' changes in the brain-pituitary axis, or are we seeing a disturbance more characteristic of depression? I wonder if the experts could comment on that?

Bernard J. Carroll

I think we put this question to rest about six years ago, with respect to the dexamethasone work. The best evidence that cortisol hypersecretion in depression is not simply stress-related comes from prospective studies in which we identify neuroendocrine disturbances appearing several days prior to new episodes of depression, in rapid cycling of polymanic depressives and up to three weeks before depression in people with predictable seasonal episodes. So it is almost as though we have in these people a signal of limbic system disturbance, preceding overt behavioural manifestations. In patients, there is associated stress and distress along with the underlying neuroendocrine disturbance, and the same is true for patients with medical disorders. This is where specificity of the dexamethasone test really helps, because both depressed and non-depressed psychiatric patients have non-specific stress-related elevations of baseline cortisol. This is why baseline cortisol values lack diagnostic utility.

Neuroendocrinology and Psychiatric Disorder,
edited by G. M. Brown, et al.
Raven Press, New York 1984.

Pituitary Adrenal Regulation in Relation to Affective Disorders

Donald S. Gann, Catherine F. Allen-Rowlands, David A. Bereiter, and Paul M. Plotsky

Altered adrenal cortical activity is a frequent concomitant of depression (see chapter 11 - Rubin). Reports have noted both alterations in the normal circadian rhythms of ACTH and cortisol possibly related to a similar alteration of the sleep-wake cycles (31), and an early escape from suppression of pituitary ACTH secretion by dexamethasone (8). However, thirty to forty percent of depressed patients do not exhibit this escape phenomenon. Brown and associates (5, 6) have suggested that the pituitary escape from dexamethasone suppression may be related to deficiencies of specific neurotransmitters active within the pathways controlling release of ACTH, and have proposed that the choice of antidepressive medication should be related to the presence or absence of the escape phenomenon. The underlying assumption is that one form of depression is associated with deficiency of norepinephrine that normally inhibits release of ACTH, and that this is associated with escape from dexamethasone. Other depressed patients who do not demonstrate escape from dexamethasone are presumed to have deficiency of serotonin that normally stimulates release of ACTH. The present paper will consider this hypothesis in light of a current understanding of brainstem pathways involved in the control of release of ACTH.

NEURAL CONTROL OF ACTH

Brainstem regions mediating release of ACTH in the cat have been defined through extensive neuroanatomic studies (11, 14, 22, 35, 36, 37), using low level electrical stimulation. Specific areas in the medulla, pons, midbrain and hypothalamus were associated with facilitation or inhibition of ACTH release, measured within 1-6 minutes of stimulation. These regions have been related to the distribution of neurons that have been shown to be responsive to hemodynamic (11) and, to pain stimulation (24). The pathways are illustrated diagramatically in Figure 1. Primary neural afferents from baroreceptors located in the arteries and atria appear to terminate in the lateral solitary complex. Bereiter and associates (3) have recently found a pain afferent response to tooth-pulp stimulation that terminates on some of these same neurons in the cat. Some secondary projections extend medially to anterolateral and posterior-medial nucleus intercalatus in the solitary complex. From this area cells project rostrally to principal locus ceruleus and locus subceruleus. The finding of Lefcourt and associates (19) that discrete lesions of this portion of the dorsal pons can prevent the ACTH response to hemorrhage suggests that a considerable portion of the hemodynamic input must pass through this small region. At the pontine level there is a projection which traverses medially from the locus ceruleus to the dorsal raphe nucleus and to a portion of dorsal tegmental nucleus (26). The principal locus ceruleus is facilitatory for ACTH, whereas the locus subceruleus and raphe complex appear to be inhibitory for ACTH (37). From these pontine regions, the facilitatory pathways probably project through the midbrain and into the hypothalamus through the dorsal longitudinal fasciculus or through the medial forebrain bundle. Neurons in the dorsal pathway appear to terminate in periventricular and parvicellular nuclei of the hypothalamus. Neurons in the ventral pathway appear to terminate in suprachiasmatic, ventromedial, dorso-medial, paraventricular and arcuate nuclei. The inhibitory pathways travel through the midbrain via the ventral tegmental tract and mammillary peduncle and appear to terminate in the posterior hypothalamic area and in the dorsal hypothalamic area. Thus, at each level of the brainstem there are multiple parallel pathways, some facilitatory and some inhibitory (11). The evidence suggests that the total pathway, however, is oligosynaptic; so that it should be possible to consider the modes of chemical neurotransmission involved in the ascending projection.

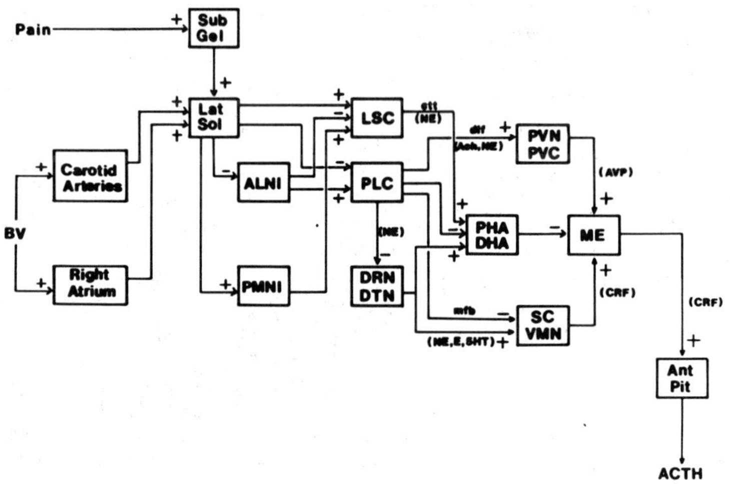

FIG. 1. Principal areas in the medulla, pons, midbrain and hypothalamus which may inhibit (-) or facilitate (+) the release of ACTH following pain and/or a blood volume stimulus: ME=median eminence; ANT PIT = anterior pituitary; LAT SOL = lateral solitary nucleus; ALNI = anterolateral nucleus intercalatus; PMNI = posteromedial nucleus intercalatus; LSC = locus subceruleus; PLC = principal locus ceruleus; DRN = dorsal raphe nucleus; DTN = dorsal tegmental nucleus; DLF dorsal longitudinal fasciculus; MP = mammillary penduncle; CTT = central tegmenal tract; MFB = medial forebrain bundle; PVN = paraventricular nucleus; PVC = parvicellular nucleus; SC = suprachiasmatic nucleus; VMN = ventromedial nucleus (dorsomedial, arcuate, periventricular, and premammillary nuclei may be included in the block with SC and VMN); PHA = posterior hypothalamic area; DHA = dorsal hypothalamic area. Associated neurotransmitters and peptides implicated the neural control of ACTH secretion: NE = norepinephrine; E = epinephrine; Ach = acetylcholine; AVP = arginine vasopressin; 5HT = serotonin; CRF = corticotrophin releasing factor.

Areas of the forebrain limbic system including the amygdala have been implicated both in affective disorders and in the modulation of both tonic and stress induced pituitary-adrenal function. Disruption of important hypothalamic afferents from the limbic system have produced alterations in pituitary-adrenal activity. Allen and Allen (1) reported that bilateral lesions destroying the medially directed amygdalo-hypothalamic fibers abolished amygdaloid facilitation of neurogenic stress-induced signals (leg break), but not signals from systemic stresses (ether). However, destruction of the fornices and stria terminalis did not block the adrenocortical stress response.

Bilateral destruction of the medial forebrain bundle, which contains important limbic-hypothalamic projections abolished adrenocortical rhythmicity (23). Bilateral transection of the fornices (38), bilateral hippocampectomy (38), or septal ablation (39) does not permanently impair the plasma corticosterone rhythm in the rat. On the other hand, the amgdaloid complex appears to exert an inhibitory influence on adrenalcorticoid activity (32). Furthermore, Allen-Rowlands and Allen (unpublished observations) have shown that bilateral knife cuts which disrupted the direct medial projecting amgdalo-hypothalamic fibres without significant injury to the medial forebrain bundle abolished diurnal rhythmicity of plasma corticosterone in the rat. Basal steroid levels remained intermediate between the normal AM-PM levels up to 3 weeks following disruption of the medially directed amygdalo-hypothalamic fibres (Fig. 2). Unilateral knife cuts were ineffective. Neural structures in the limbic system that project to the lateral hypothalamus have been shown to participate in the steroid feedback control of pituitary ACTH secretion. The hippocampus and septum appear to have a greater affinity for steroids than do other sites in the brain (25). Bilateral radio frequency lesions of a direct medial projecting portion of the ventral amygdalo-hypothalamic pathway blocked compensatory hypersecretion of ACTH following adrenalectomy (2). However, unilateral lesions, septal ablation or bilateral destruction of the stria terminalis were ineffective. The evidence suggests that the limbic system, in particular the amygdalar complexes, are involved in the extrahypothalamic modulation of pituitary ACTH secretion.

NEUROTRANSMITTERS INVOLVED IN THE CONTROL OF ACTH

The various ascending pathways to the hypothalamus in the brainstem summarized above appear to arise from areas where there are cell bodies containing epinephrine, norepinephrine, acetylcholine and serotonin (11). The posterior medial nucleus intercalatus is roughly congruent with area A2 of Dahlström and Fuxe (9) which is described as sending adrenergic fibres through the medial forebrain bundle into the ventral basal hypothalamus without synapsing. The anterolateral nucleus of locus ceruleus and locus subceruleus contains noradrenergic neurons, as do the tegmental nuclei. Noradrenergic neurons and cholinergic neurons are found in the locus ceruleus, and serotoninergic neurons are found in the nucleus of the dorsal raphe. The latter projects directly through the medial forebrain bundle into the suprachiasmatic nucleus (4). The anterolateral locus ceruleus and locus subceruleus project through the central tegmental tract and mamillary peduncle into the hypothalamus and the projection may be coincident with the intermediate noradrenergic bundle of Maeda and Shimizu (21). There is some evidence that locus ceruleus projects through a dorsal pathway described as cholinergic by Lewis and Shute (30) or as noradrenergic by others (28). The medial forebrain bundle itself contains ACTH facilitatory and ACTH inhibitory components (7). The studies of Ganong (12) and of Van Loon (33) suggest that norepinephrine inhibits the release of ACTH in response to trauma. The work of Vernikos-Danellis (34) suggests that serotonin exerts an inhibitory influence in control of ACTH.

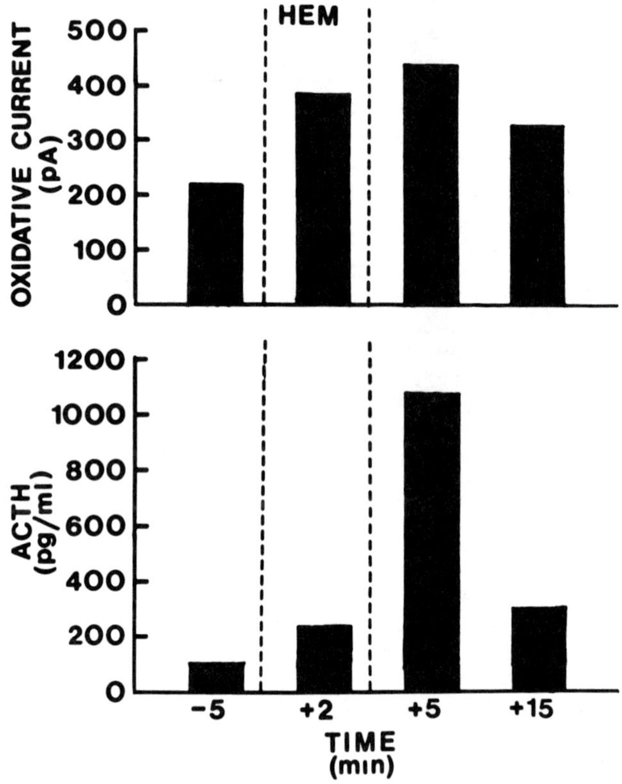

FIG. 2. Effect of bilateral or unilateral destruction of direct medial-projecting amygdalo-hypothalamic fibres on plasma corticosterone concentration in the AM(0800) or PM(1600) compared to intact controls. The height of the bar represents the mean and the vertical line above the bar the standard error. The number in each group is indicated by N. Bilateral lesions abolished the AM-PM difference of resting plasma corticosterone.

Jones and colleagues (17) have studied the release of corticotropin releasing factor by isolated explants of hypothalamus. In this preparation, acetylcholine and serotonin appear to stimulate release of CRF whereas norepinephrine and GABA appear to inhibit release of CRF. Kaneko and Hiroshige (18) have suggested that serotonergic pathways mediate extrahypothalamic control of slow or level sensitive feedback whereas noradrenergic pathways mediate extrahypothalamic control of fast or rate sensitive feedback. On the other hand, Sato and his co-workers (29) have advanced evidence that rate sensitive feedback may be localized in the median eminence itself. Hsu et al. (16) found a paradoxical response to L-Dopa, a precursor of norepinephrine, such that administration of L-Dopa potentiated ACTH release in response to metapyrone.

The above results allow one to formulate a set of conjectures concerning the interrelationship or specific facilitatory or inhibitory pathways controlling ACTH and neurotransmitters that might be associated with these pathways. The conflicting evidence indicates that both norepinephrine and serotonin may be associated with either facilitation or inhibition of ACTH release. However, epinephrine appears likely to be associated only with inhibition of ACTH, and acetylcholine has been associated only with facilitation of ACTH release. The exact nature of the physiologic interrelationships of the neurotransmitters in the control of pituitary ACTH secretion remain to be elucidated. Up to the present time no studies have been reported of in vivo measurements of changes in neurotransmitter to any specific portion of the brain correlated with changes of ACTH in response to a physiologic stimulus. Such studies have been initiated recently by Plotsky and Bereiter in our laboratory. They have been studying the release of ACTH in response to a small hemorrhage in cats with voltametric carbon microelectrodes placed in the region of the locus ceruleus. As shown in Figure 3, hemorrhage (10 ml/kg) produces an increase in ACTH that is paralleled by an increase in oxidative current in the locus ceruleus which is related to the release of catecholamines. Since locus ceruleus contains no epinephrine or dopamine, it is inferred that there is an increase in norepinephrine parallel to that of ACTH. Although preliminary, these studies point to the need for direct localized in vivo measurements of n neurotransmitter flux associated with changes in ACTH release, before inferences can be made concerning the roles of specific neurotransmitters in the modulation of release of ACTH.

Prange and Loosen (27) have pointed out (chapter 13) the hypothesis of Gold et al. (13) that vasopressin may be deficient in depression. Vasopressin has been implicated in the release of CRF (15) or in potentiation of ACTH release of the pituitary (40) or as a CRF itself (41). Recent evidence suggests that vasopressin released by the paraventricular nucleus acts at the level of the median eminence (10) via a direct projection from the paraventricular nucleus to the median eminence described by Zimmerman (41). The common theme of all investigations of the effects of vasopressin on ACTH release is that the peptide plays a facilitatory role. Thus, vasopressin deficiency in the median eminence cannot account for escape from dexamethasone suppression or for the phase advance in the circadian rhythm. It is also important to point out that some vasopressinergic neurons are distributed to many parts of the neurais other than median eminence.

SUMMARY

The findings discussed herein are consistent with the general finding that specific neurotransmitters are involved in the control of ACTH release in response to a variety of physiologic stimuli, of feedback inhibition of ACTH release by steroids, and of circadian release of ACTH. However, these findings suggest also that it would be premature to infer the in vivo action of a specific neurotransmitter from a change in the pattern of release of ACTH. Such inferences by Brown et al. (5, 6) that have led to the use of different antidepressant medications on the basis of the pituitary-adrenocortical response to the dexamethasone suppression test, may be somewhat tenuous. Their hypothesis, however, may be important for further elucidation of the physiological control of ACTH, in that they may point to relationships among specific neurotransmitters that are associated with steroid suppression and with circadian rhythm of pituitary activity. However, the underlying neural substrates remain to be determined. Finally, one cannot exclude the possibility that affective disorders may modulate the activity of hypothalamic loci involved in the control of the release of ACTH, perhaps through projections from the limbic areas described above. Descending projections from these limbic areas to areas such as the locus ceruleus and the dorsal raphe may also modify sleepwake patterns. Since these latter areas have been implicated in the control of ACTH release, the projections to them may also render the system less susceptible to steroid suppression and may alter the circadian activity. Thus, it is possible that the effects of various affective disorders upon the pituitary-adrenal system are not only the result of actions upon those neural structures that are directly involved in the control of the system, but are also the result of effects upon the limbic areas or higher centers whose descending activity can modulate these structures.

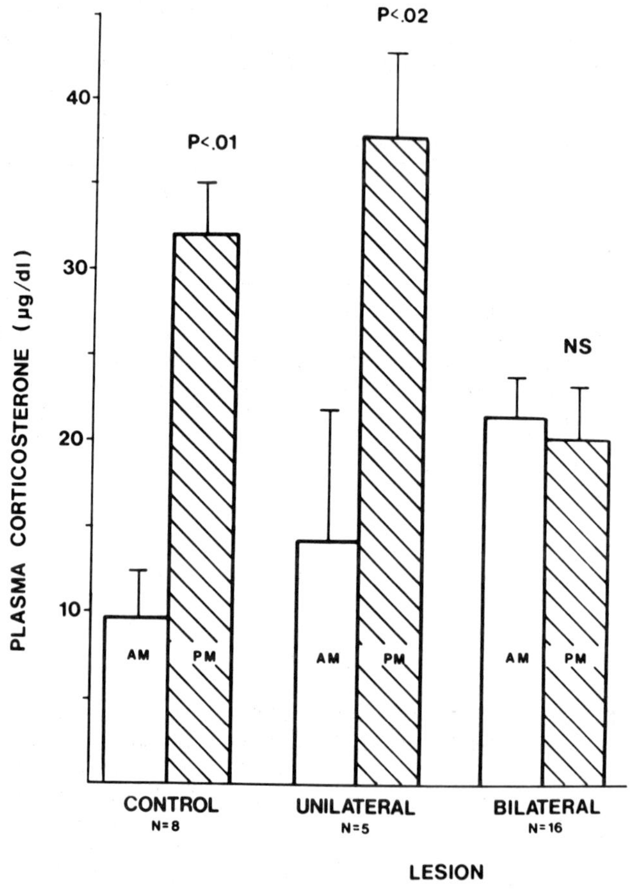

FIG. 3. Oxidative current recorded from a voltametric microelectrode stereotaxically placed into the locus ceruleus of the cat. The current corresponds to the oxidation wave occurring at +0.15 V (vs. AG/AgCl) which represents oxidation of catecholamines at the electrode surface. The current signal and peripheral ACTH levels rise following a 3 min duration 10 ml/kg hemorrhage.

REFERENCES

1. Allen, J. P. and Allen, C. F. (1974): Neuroendocrinology 15:220-230.

2. Allen, J. P. and Allen, F. C. (1975): Neuroendocrinology 19:115-125.
3. Bereiter, D. A., Plotsky, P. M. and Gann, D. S. (198): Neurosci. Abstr. 7:333.
4. Bloom, F. E., Hopper, B. J., Siggins, G. R., Barker, J. L. and Nicol, R. A. (1972): Fed. Proc., Am. Soc. Expt. Biol. 31:97-106.
5. Brown, W. A., Haier, R. J. and Qualls, C. B. (1980): Lancet i: 928-929.
6. Brown, W. A., Haier, R. J. and Qualls, C. B. (1981): Psychopharm. Bull. 17(1):88-90.
7. Carlson, D. E., Dornhorst, A. and Gann, D. S. (1981): Endocrinology 107:961-969.
8. Carrol, B. J., Feinberg, M., Gredin, J. F., Tarika, J., Albala, A. A., Haskett, R. F., James, N., Kronfol, Z., Hohr, N., Steiner, M., deVigne, J. P. and Young, E. (1981): Arch. Gen. Psychiat. 38: 15-22.
9. Carlson, D. E., Dornhorst, A., Seif, S. M., Robinson, A. G. and Gann, D. S. (1982): Endocrinology 110: 680-682.
10. Dahlstrom, A. and Fuxe, K. (1964): Acta Physiol. Scand. 62:1-55.
11. Gann, D. S., Ward, D. G. and Carlson, D. E. (1978): Rec. Prog. in Horm. Res. 34:357-400.
12. Ganong, W. F. (1972): In: Brain-Endocrine Interaction, Median Eminence: Structure and Function, edited by J. M. Knigge, D. E. Scott and A. Weindl, pp.254-266. Karger, Basal.
13. Gold, P. W., Goodwin, F. K. and Reus, V. I. (1978): Lancet ii: 1233-1236.
14. Grizzle, W. E., Dallman, M. F., Schramm, L. P. and Gann, D. S. (1974): Endocrinology 95:1450-1461.
15. Hedge, G. A. Yates, M. B., Marcus, R., Yates, F. E. (1966): Endocrinology 79:328-340.
16. Hsu, T. H., Hsu, C. K. and Gann, D. S. (1976): Endocrinology 99: 1115-1118.
17. Jones, M. T. and Hillhouse, E. W. (1977): Ann. N.Y. Acad. Sci. 297:536-560.
18. Kaneko, M. and Hiroshige, T. (1978): Am. J. Physiol. 234:R46-R51.
19. Lefcourt, A. M., Ward, D. G., Santana, H., Rudrow, V.S. and Gann, D. S. (1979): Neurosci. Abst. 5:451.
20. Lengvari, I. and Halasz, B. (1973): Neuroendocrinology 11:191-196.
21. Maeda, T. and Shimizu, N. (1972): Brain Res. 36:19-35.
22. Maran, J. W., Carlson, D. E., Grizzle, W. E., Ward, D. G. and Gann, D. S. (1978): Endocrinology 103:957-970.
23. Moore, R. Y., and Qavi, H. B. (1971): Experientia 27:249-250.
24. Morita, N., Tamai, Y. and Tsjimoto, T. (1977): Brain Res. 134: 158-160.
25. McEwen, B. S., Weiss, J. M. and Schwartz, L. S. (1969): Brain Res. 16:227-241.
26. Palkovits, M. and Jacobowitz, D. M. (1974): J. Comp. Neurol. 157: 29-42.
27. Prange, Jr., A. J. and Larsen, P. T. (1981): In: present volume.
28. Roizen, M. F. and Jacobowitz, D. M. (1976): Brain Res. 101:561-568.
29. Sato, T., Sato, M., Shinsako, J. and Dallman, M. F. (1975): Endocrinology 97:265-274.
30. Lewis, P. R. and Shute, C. C. (1967): Brain 90:521-540.
31. Spiker, D. G., Coble, P., Dofsky, J., Foster, F. G. and Kupfer, D. J. (1978); Biol. Psychiat. 13:485-488.
32. Taylor, A. N. and Branch, B. J. (1971): Exp. Neurol. 31:391-401.

33. Van Loon, G. R. (1974): Adv. Neurol. 5:479-486.
34. Vernikos-Danellis, J. and Berger, P. A. (1973): In: Serotonin and Behavior, edited by J. Barchas and E. Usdin, pp.173-177. Academic Press, New York.
35. Ward, D. G. and Gann, D. S. (1976): Endocrinology 99:1213-1219.
36. Ward, D. G., Bolton, M. G. and Gann, D. S. (1978): Endocrinology 102:1147-1154.
37. Ward, D. G., Grizzle, W. E. and Gann, D. S. (1976): Endocrinology 99:1220-1228.
38. Wilson, M. and Critchlow, V. (1974): Neuroendocrinology 13:29-40.
39. Wilson, M. and Critchlow, V. (1974): Neuroendocrinology 14:333-344.40. Yates, F., S. M., Dhariwal, A.P.S. (1971): Endocrinology 88:3-15.
41. Zimmerman, E. A., Stillman, M. A., Recht, L. D., Antunes, J. L., Carmel, P. W. (1977): Ann. N.Y. Acad. Sci. 297:405-419.

19

Neuroendocrinology and Psychiatric Disorder,
edited by G. M. Brown, et al.
Raven Press, New York 1984.

Catecholamine Regulation of Growth Hormone and Thyrotropin in Mood Disorders

L. Cass Terry

A major thrust of psychiatric research in mood disorders has been to define biological characteristics that are useful diagnostically and therepeutically and that point to the pathophysiology of this disorder. The most prominent of the hypotheses implicates altered function of one or more monoamines acting as synaptic neurotransmitters in the central nervous system (CNS).

Support for the amine hypothesis derives from pharmacological, biochemical, behavioural, and neuroendocrine studies (6, 21). The most often mentioned amines are norepinephrine (NE) (128) and the indolamine, serotonin (96). Altered functions of dopamine (DA) (131) and acetylcholine (55) have also been considered. High concentrations of these amines in the hypothalamus and surrounding regions has been documented (49, 53, 93, 94) and there is convincing clinical evidence to implicate NE and DA in the regulation of pituitary growth hormone (GH) and thyrotropin (TSH) (40, 60, 61, 70, 79-83, 95, 123, 138, 142, 149).

The purpose of this chapter is to assess neuroendocrine strategies that have been used to test the catecholamine hypothesis in disorders of mood with reference to clinical investigations of regulation GH and TSH secretion. Emphasis is placed on the pathophysiologic features of mood disorders without necessarily supporting any preconceived theories.

EVALUATION OF CLINICAL NEUROENDOCRINE STUDIES

Although the neuroendocrine approach to mood disorders has considerable heuristic value, cognizance of its pitfalls is mandatory. A given hormonal response is usually regulated by an ensemble of neurotransmitters and hypothalamic hormones, rather than a single neural pathway. The hypothalamic-pituitary axis is the "final common pathway" where the effector is the pituitary and the measured response is the plasma level of one or more hormones. In clinical studies, it is difficult to ascertain whether a specific neurotransmitter or hypothalamic peptide is the mediator of that response. Measurement of biogenic amines or hypothalamic peptides in the peripheral circulation does not necessarily reflect events that occur across the blood-brain barrier.

Hormonal responses to different stimuli are mediated by different neurotransmitters, e.g. the GH response to insulin-induced hypoglycemia is inhibited by α-adrenergic blockade, but sleep-induced GH is not. It cannot be assumed that only one neurotransmitter mediates the hormonal response to a specific stimulus. Factors such as stress, age, gender, obesity, fasting, ethanol, sleep-deprivation, metabolic state, medical illnesses, and drugs also influence pituitary hormone secretion (79-83, 108, 123) and must be considered. This is particularly relevant when defining a matching control group.

Target gland hormones have feedback effects on the pituitary and hypothalamus, e.g., corticosteroids on adrenocorticotropin, T_3 and T_4 on TSH, and gonadal steroids on gonadotropins. Therefore, it is important to measure the target hormone concomitantly with its respective pituitary hormone.

Lack of familiarity with the specificity of a particular pharmacologic agent can lead to misinterpretation of its effects. It is naive to assume that a drug is responsible for the overall effects produced by a single action. Its other actions on the CNS may be as important as the particular action being tested.

Despite these caveats, neuroendocrine strategies appear to be of value as avenues to the study of hypothalamic and neurotransmitter function in mood disorders and as an approach to the assessment of brain effects of psychotropic drugs. They may also have some value as trait markers. What makes the observation of altered neuroendocrine function in mood disorders relevant to current neurobiologic research is that the same neurotransmitters that are implicated in the biochemical pathology of mood disorders - NE and DA - also play a role in the regulation of GH and TSH secretion.

SITES OF ACTION OF NEUROTRANSMITTERS

The concentrations of catecholamines and serotonin in the hypothalamus are higher than in most other regions of the brain (49, 54, 93, 94), and they are thought to be the primary central monoaminergic neurotransmitters that regulate neuroendocrine function (40, 60, 61, 70, 79-83, 95, 123, 138, 142, 149). The monoamines are concentrated in the hypophysiotropic area of the hypothalamus where the cell bodies of many of the peptidergic neurons that produce hypothalamic peptides are located (49). In addition, axons from monoaminergic neurons extend into the external lamina of the median eminence where they are in close contact with the peptidergic axons and the hypothalamic-pituitary portal system, which transports releasing factors and neurotransmitters to the pituitary.

There are several potential loci at which anterior pituitary hormone secretion could be influenced by neurotransmitters (95). One possibility is direct axoaxonic synapses between monoaminergic nerve terminals, which liberate a given neurotransmitter, and peptidergic terminals, which contain releasing or inhibiting factors. Secondly, direct axodendritic or axosomatic contacts between neuronal elements, or multisynaptic connections through monoaminergic neurons distant to the peptidergic neuron, are also possible. Thirdly, neurotransmitter release into the portal circulation could stimulate or inhibit directly pituitary hormone release or alter pituitary sensitivity to releasing/inhibiting factors. This appears to be the case with DA regulation of prolaction secretion. Alternatively, monoamines in the peripheral circulation might effect anterior pituitary function through a direct effect on the pituitary, or indirectly by affecting peripheral nerve pathways communicating with the CNS. Finally, neurons may contain both monoamines and peptides, the former affecting secretion of the latter.

With the exception of prolactin, there has been general agreement that the effects of neurotransmitters on anterior pituitary secretion are mediated by releasing and/or inhibiting hormones from the hypothalamus. However, more recent data suggests that neurotransmitters may have a direct pituitary action. Acetylcholine receptor sites have been reported to be present on rat and sheep anterior pituitaries (13, 125, 137, 143).

Also α_2-adrenergic receptors in cultures of bovine anterior pituitary cells showed close correlation with secretion of adrenocorticotropin (7). Furthermore, γ-aminobutyric acid was reported to directly inhibit prolactin release from isolated rat pituitaries in doses as low as 0.1 μg/ml (127), suggesting that this substance, in addition to DA, may have a prolactin-inhibiting factor capability (35, 44). Under certain conditions, DA also appears to inhibit TSH release through a direct effect on the pituitary (see section on TSH). Whether these effects are meaningful physiologically still remains to be determined.

GROWTH HORMONE

Plasma levels of GH, measured at frequent intervals throughout the day and night, show striking variations in man (12, 119, 151). Individual surges of GH secretion may reach levels of 20-60 ng/ml, the largest bursts occur during the first two hours of sleep (12, 119, 151). The number and magnitude of spontaneous GH bursts are age dependent, increasing during the growth spurt of adolesence and declining thereafter (38). Sleep-associated GH release is commonly absent in persons over 50 years of age (62, 87, 151).

The basis of these physiological variations in GH has been the subject of extensive investigations (70, 79-83). Factors such as sleep, exercise and stress, both physical and psychological, account for some of these fluctuations, but many GH surges are spontaneous. Abrupt changes in plasma GH levels are not caused by variations in glucose, amino acids nor free fatty acids (79, 81, 82, 145-147).

The profile of the secretory bursts of GH and their nonsuppressibility by potential metabolic regulators of growth hormone secretion suggest that the surges are the result of primary activation of GH secretion induced by neural mechanisms. Numerous studies in experimental animals support the concept that the physiologic GH secretory pattern is regulated by an intrinsic CNS rhythm that is dependent on neural structures located in the medial basal hypothalamus (70, 79-83). Furthermore, reflex GH secretion, associated with stress or related to sleep, probably requires neural input from higher centres such as the limbic system (70, 79-83).

A variety of other physiological and experimental stimuli affect GH (24, 25, 70, 79-83). These include gender, fasting, obesity, changes in plasma glucose, altered protein intake, prolonged bed rest (76), exercise, unpremedicated electroconvulsion (145, 146), amino acids (59), glucagon, vasopressin, adrenocorticotropin, gonadal steroids, corticosteroids, melatonin, alcohol (108), and hypoglycemia. Exogenously administered GH decreases the GH response to insulin-induced hypoglycemia (1), suggesting an autoregulatory mechanism for GH secretion. Intracerebroventricular GH administration to rats also inhibits pituitary GH release (136).

Neurotransmitters and GH Regulation (Figure 1)

Growth hormone is believed to be regulated by the release of both inhibitory (somatostatin) and excitatory (growth hormone-releasing factor) hormones (70, 79-83). In general, the effects of neurotransmitters on GH secretion are believed to be mediated at brain sites because direct application of biogenic amines to pituitary cells *in vitro* is without effect (82). The finding that several pharmacologic stimuli, particularly NE, DA and serotonin, affect GH secretion has led to extensive investigation of the role of neurotransmitters in normal and abnormal GH secretory states (40, 61, 80, 95, 123, 128, 149).

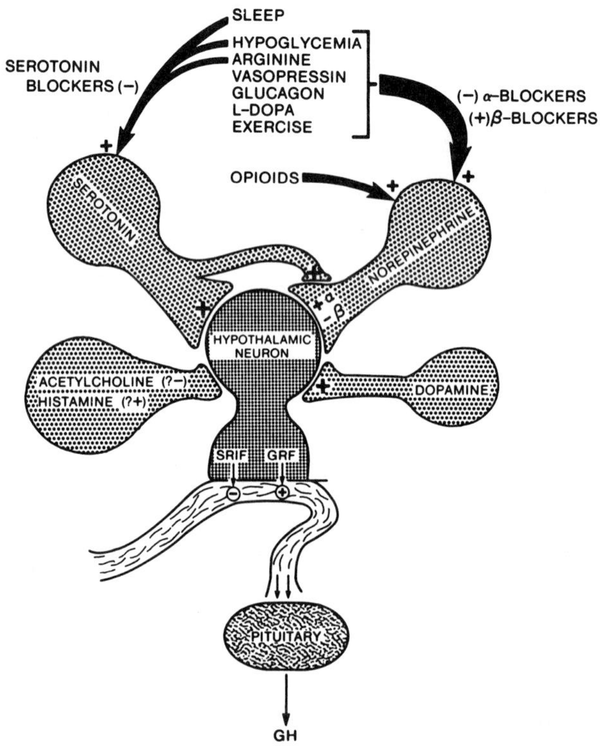

FIG. 1. Schematic representation of growth hormone (GH) regulation by biogenic aminergic and peptidergic neuronal systems. Somatostatin (SRIF): growth hormone-releasing factor (GRF).

Norepinephrine and Basal GH Secretion

Oral administration of L-dopa, the precursor of DA, NE and epinephrine (EPI), causes release of GH (13). Evidence that the L-dopa effect is mediated through its conversion to NE, or possibly EPI, is derived from experiments demonstrating that L-dopa-induced GH release is blocked by the α-adrenergic receptor blocker, phentolamine (58, 84). Other drugs such as amphetamines, methylphenidate, nomifensine and mianserine, which increase intrasynatpic levels of NE by increasing its turnover (2) and release, also stimulate GH secretion (14, 62, 63, 111). Inhibition of NE re-uptake by desmethylimipramine stimulates GH release, an effect that is inhibited by α-adrenergic blockade. Although several of these pharmacologic agents lack specificity, taken together, these results suggest that the central noradrenergic system stimulates GH secretion.

Administration of the α-adrenergic receptor agonists, clonidine, methoxamine, phenylephrine, and guanfacien stimulate GH in man (36, 52, 67, 72) and the effect of methoxamine is inhibited by phentolamine, an α-receptor blocker (52). Clonidine appears to act by activation of central α-adrenergic receptors (115). Thus, it seems clear that activation of α-adrenergic receptors in the CNS causes release of GH.

The role of β-adrenergic receptors in regulation of basal GH secretion is not defined well. Administration of NE or EPI, which activates α- and β- adrenergic receptors concomitantly, does not elevate plasma GH (10, 11, 84, 126). Furthermore, administration of propranolol alone has no effect on basal GH secretion (10, 11) but in combination with EPI increases GH (11) and this combined effect is blocked by phentolamine (84). L-dopa-stimulated GH release is also enhanced by propranolol (19, 52). In contrast, Japanese subjects were reported to release GH after administration of propranolol (51), an effect blocked by the β-receptor agonist, isoprenaline (52). Thus, in Caucasians, β-adrenergic receptors do not appear to have an important influence on basal GH secretion.

DA and Basal GH Secretion

L-dopa-stimulated GH is blocked by prior administration of chlorpromazine (90), suggesting a stimulatory effect of DA on GH. The DA agonists apomorphine, bromocriptine, CV 154, piribedil, lergotrile and lisuride also stimulate GH release (20, 29, 32, 64-66, 68, 97, 140, 141). Moreover, the enhancing effects of apomorphine and CB 154 on GH release are blocked by chlorpromazine, pimozide, clozapine and haloperidol (29, 65, 68, 97). Interestingly, benztropine (a DA uptake inhibitor with significant anticholinergic activity), methysergide (a 5HT blocker), and cyproheptadine (a 5HT receptor blocker with antihistaminic and anticholinergic activity) do not inhibit apomorphine-stimulated GH release (66, 68, 113), indicating that this is a specific effect due to activation of DA receptors.

Conversely, pimozide administration has no effect on basal GH secretion (27, 68) but enhances spontaneous GH fluctuations in diabetics (129). Less specific blockade of DA receptors with chlorpromazine decreases basal GH release (130), but this effect may be due to NE receptor blockade.

There is evidence that DA mechanisms act on both sides of the blood-brain barrier. L-dopa enhances GH release when administered with a peripheral inhibitor of dopa decarboxylase (78), and infusion of DA, which does not cross the blood brain barrier, either enhances (73, 74) or has no effect on basal GH (20). However, it is possible that DA exerts its effect by NE-receptor stimulation (42).

EPI and Basal GH Secretion

Several pharmacologic agents that activate NE neurotransmission may also have an effect on EPI. For example, L-dopa is a precursor of EPI, amphetamines stimulate EPI release, and clonidine and other α-receptor agonists may activate adrenergic receptors normally occupied by EPI. Until recently, it has been difficult to study the role of EPI in GH secretion because specific EPI agonists and antagonists were not available. Administration of adrenaline to humans has no effect on basal GH secretion (10, 11, 126). However, infusion of EPI produces multiple peripheral effects and the amount that crosses the blood brain barrier may be negligible.

Recent studies, designed to define the role of epinephrine in episodic growth hormone secretion show that the spontaneous surges of growth hormone in the rat are abolished by pretreatment with SK & F 64139 (25 and 50 mg/kg intraperitoneally), an agent that blocks synthesis of epinephrine in brain by inhibiting the enzyme, phenylethanolamine-N-methyl transferase (139). Inhibition of peripheral (adrenal) EPI synthesis with another agent (Sk & F 29661), which does not cross the blood brain barrier, has not effect on basal GH release. Growth hormone secretion can be restored in SK & F 64139-treated rats by administration of clonidine or antiserum to somatostatin. These findings suggest that epinephrine is involved in the generation of growth hormone pulses in the rat. Also, it is possible that the stimulatory effect of clonidine on growth hormone secretion is due to activation of α-adrenergic receptors that are occupied by epinephrine, rather than by norepinephrine. The regulatory role of the central EPI in human GH secretion remains to be determined.

Catecholaminergic Regulation of GH Secretion Induced by Various Stimuli

In general, most of the stimuli that cuase release of GH in man appear to be mediated by central α-adrenergic receptors. Growth hormone release induced by insulin-hypoglycemia, arginine, vasopressin, exercise, surgical stress, and electroconvulsion are antagonized by α-adrenergic blockade (10, 16, 46, 52, 146, 147). In contrast, β-adrenergic receptor blockade with propranolol enhances GH release induced by glucagon, vasopressin, insulin-hypoglycemia and exercise (2, 19, 47, 91). The role of β-adrenergic receptors in arginine-stimulated GH secretion is not clear (135). Thus, β-adrenergic receptor activation appears to have an inhibitory effect on certain types of stimuli that release GH.

Blockade of DA receptors with pimozide antagonizes the stimulatory effect of exercise and arginine on GH (129), suggesting that these responses may be mediated, in part, by DA. In addition, hypoglycemia-induced GH release is inhibited by chlorpromazine (130). In contrast, the infusion of DA causes a marked reduction in L-dopa- and insulin-induced GH secretion (74, 153). Thus, depending on experimental conditions, DA has both simulatory and inhibitory effects on GH release. The inhibitory action may be due to a pituitary effect.

Sleep-associated GH secretion is mediated by other mechanisms. Neither α- nor β-adrenergic receptor blockade has an effect on this phenomenon (77, 82). Administration of L-dopa also has no effect on GH release during sleep (26). The cholinergic system appears to play some role in sleep-releated growth hormone secretion. Methscopolamine, an anticholinergic agent with antimuscarinic properties, decreases sleep-induced growth hormone release (88), whereas piperidine, a cholinergic nicotonic receptor stimulator, enhances it (89). These effects suggest stimulatory roles for both muscarinic and nicotinic mechanisms in sleep-associated growth hormone release. Further studies are required to resolve this issue.

Overview of the Catecholaminergic Regulation of GH

Taken together these findings indicate that central α-adrenergic and dopaminergic stimulatory pathways, and an inhibitory β-adrenergic pathway, play a major role in the regulation of GH secretion. Furthermore, GH responses to certain pharmacological and physiological stimuli are mediated by different catechalamines and provide the opportunity to investigate involvement of selected neurotransmitter systems in various pathological states.

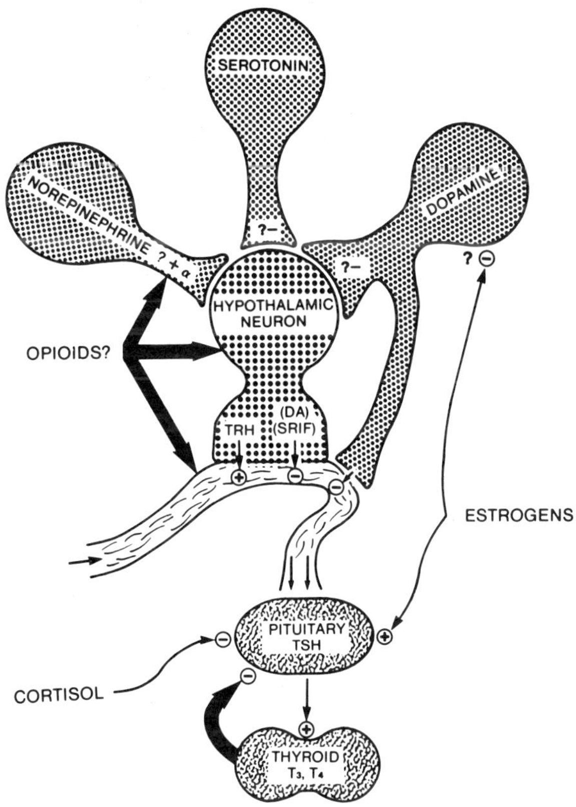

FIG. 2. Schematic representation of thyrotropin (TSH) regulation by amines, neuropeptides, and peripheral hormones. Thyrotropin-releasing hormone (TRH); somatostatin (SRIF); dopamine (DA); Tri- and tetraiodothyronine (T_3/T_4).

THYROID STIMULATING HORMONE (FIGURE 2)

A nyctochemeral rhythm in plasma TSH has been described (104, 123). Within this general pattern there appears to be more short-term fluctuations in TSH (3, 104) which represents an ultradian rhythm of TSH secretion and are possibly due to episodic bursts of TSH secretory activity. An important observation of the TSH circadian rhythm is that the elevation in basal TSH levels at night is not sleep-related, since it is detectable during the evening before the onset of sleep (23, 148). The mechanisms underlying the TSH secretory pattern are unknown, and both central and peripheral factors have been suggested (123).

The hypothalamus exerts a dominant stimulatory action over TSH secretion and this effect is believed to be mediated by the release of thyrotropin releasing hormone (TRH) into the hypothalamic-pituitary portal system. Although a specific thyrotropin release-inhibiting hormone has not been isolated, there is evidence to suggest that hypothalamic somatostatin and/or DA have such a role (123). Thus, the hypothalamic control over TSH has both stimulatory and inhibitory components.

While the dominant hypothalamic control over TSH is stimulatory via TRH, thyroid hormones exert a powerful, negative feedback control over TSH release (132). A decrease in T_3 and T_4 levels causes an elevation in basal and TRH-stimulated TSH levels and conversely, small increments in T_3 and T_4 reduce basal and TRH-stimulated TSH levels (50, 56, 116).

In addition, gonadal and adrenal steroids infludence TSH secretion. Females have a greater TSH response to TRH than males (4, 101, 103) and also show a greater response during the preovulatory than the luteal phase of the menstrual cycle (118). Administration of large doses of corticosteroids abolishes the nocturnal elevation (98, 127) and reduces both basal and TRH-stimulated TSH levels (110, 133). Although suppression of plasma cortisol with dexamethasone will lower overall basal TSH levels, it has no effect on the circadian pattern of TSH secretion (23). The roles of estrogen and glucocorticoids in the regulation of TSH secretion require further study and these factors must be kept in mind when interpreting neuroendocrine studies that involve TSH.

NE and TSH Secretion

There is little convincing evidence for direct central α- or β-adrenergic regulation of TSH release (9, 152). Isoproterenol, NE, phentolamine, propranolol (152) or clonidine (67) have no effect on basal TSH nor TRH-stimulated TSH secretion (152). The data are conflicting with respect to the effects of phentolamine on TSH. Under certain conditions, α-blockade with phentolamine suppresses the TSH response to TRH (99). Also phenoxybenzamine or propranolol have no effect on TSH secretion in cold-exposed young adults (39). Inhibition of NE and EPI synthesis with fusaric acid suppresses elevated TSH levels in hypothyroid patients but has no effect in normals (155). The possibility that α-adrenergic stimulation of TSH is increased in hypothyroid patients should be considered. Moreover, chronic β-receptor blockade causes a slight elevation in basal TSH levels, but this effect may be secondary to the known peripheral action of β-receptor blockers in reducing the conversion of T_3 and T_4 (150). Additional direct evidence is required to postulate a role for NE in central regulation of TSH secretion.

DA and TSH

The role of DA in the regulation of TSH secretion is not clear. L-dopa has no effect on TSH secretion in either normal (109) or in short-term hypothyroid individuals (112) but lowers TSH in long-standing hypothyroid patients (112) and when administered chronically inhibits TRH-induced TSH secretion (71, 134).

The effects of DA-receptor stimulation on TSH are variable. Apomorphine and bromocriptine have no effect on TRH-induced TSH levels (25, 48, 100) but it has also been reported that elevated basal TSH levels in hypothyroid patients were suppressed by bromocriptine as was acute suppression of the TSH response to TRH (41, 92, 154). Dopamine infusion acutely suppresses TSH response to TRH in normals (8, 17). Furthermore, DA infusion lowers basal TSH levels in both euthyroid and hypothyroid subjects (86), an effect that is inhibited by metoclopramide, a potent and specific DA-receptor blocker (30). Although these pharmacological studies suggest an inhibitory role for DA, they do not indicate the physiological significance of DA pathways in TSH regulation.

The effects of DA-receptor blockade on TSH are equally confusing. Chlorpromazine, sulpiride and metoclopramide do not affect basal TSH release in some studies (31, 57, 75, 102), whereas pimozide and chlorpromazine suppress TSH levels in euthyroid subjects (27, 34). In other studies, metoclopramide and sulpiride cause TSH release in hypothyroid (85, 120, 121) and euthyroid subjects (121, 122). TSH elevations are small in euthyroid compared to hypothyroid groups and females show greater TSH release than males after DA-receptor blockade (122). Also DA inhibition of TSH release is greater the lower the basal TSH level (122).

Since DA does not cross the blood brain barrier, DA-induced suppression of both basal (86) and TRH-stimulated TSH levels (8) is probably due to a direct action of DA on the pituitary or median eminence. The observation that domperidone, a specific DA-receptor antagonist that does not cross the blood brain barrier, releases TSH (123, 124) provides further evidence to support this concept.

Overview

There appears to be little evidence for a physiological role of NE in TSH regulation in man. Dopamine appears to have an inhibitory effect on TSH secretion that is most evident when the negative feedback effects of thyroid hormones are reduced. Also, DA may be a determinant of the rate and degree of TSH decline and is thus implicated in the circadian rhythm of TSH secretion. Finally, the inhibitory effect of DA on TSH is probably due to a direct effect on the pituitary and/or median eminence.

Furthermore, the major controlling factor in the regulation of TSH secretion is negative feedback exerted at the pituitary level by alterations in T_3 and T_4. Consequently, alterations in TSH secretion attributable to TRH and/or neurotransmitters should be derived from experiments in which circulating levels of thyroid hormones are unaltered.

INTERPRETATION OF GH STUDIES IN DEPRESSION

Studies of GH release in depression are reviewed in detail in another chapter (Checkley and Arendt, ref. 25) and other monographs (6, 21). Results of these studies are summarized in Figure 3.

Suppression of GH responses to insulin-induced hypoglycemia, desipramine and clonidine provide compelling evidence to support the hypothesis of decreased α-adrenergic neurotransmission. At present, it is difficult to provide a more concise localization of this putative central α-adrenergic defect.

Inhibition or alteration of postsynaptic α-receptors could explain suppression of GH responses to clonidine, desipramine, and insulin hypoglycemia. However, normal GH responses to L-dopa and methylamphetamine do not support this hypothesis unless their stimulatory effects on GH in depression are due to DA-receptor activation. This is possible since the GH response to apomorphine in depression is normal and methylamphetamine-induced GH release in normal subjects is not inhibited by α-antagonists (111). Moreover, L-dopa-induced GH in normals is blocked by chlorpromazine (90) in addition to α-antagonists (58, 84) suggesting that L-dopa can stimulate GH release by DA-receptor activation.

Data from experiments with non-human primates suggests that clonidine-induced GH release is mediated by activation of postsynaptic α_2-adrenergic receptors (25). With the increasing availability of selective

α_1 and α_2-receptor antagonists and agonists, it may be possible to characterize this phenomenon in humans. At present, there are no studies on involvement of β-adrenergic receptors in depression.

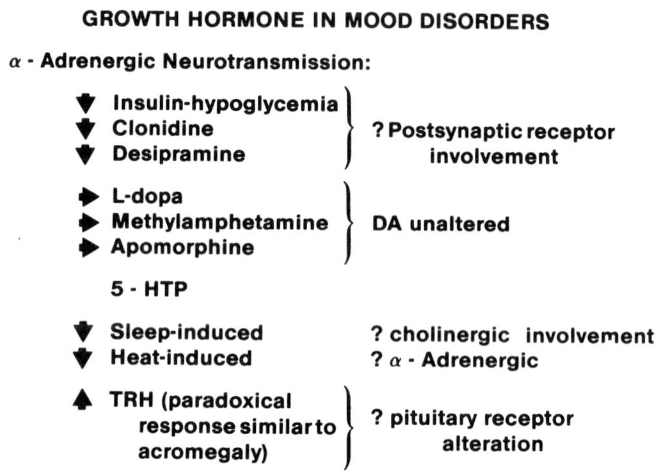

FIG. 3. Summary of the effects of mood disorders on growth hormone secretion (25). Arrows indicate the response compared to normal or control groups.

Alternate explanations for GH abnormalities in mood disorders are 1) impaired NE synthesis and release or 2) a change in pituitary receptor sensitivity. Decreased GH responses to insulin hypoglycemia and desipramine are compatible with the former hypothesis and the paradoxical GH response to thyrotropin-releasing hormone (TRH) supports the latter.

Basal GH levels are normal in depressed patients (22). This finding suggests that abnormalities in GH induced by various stimuli are not epiphenomena secondary to peripheral metabolic alterations. Also, since the GH response is blunted only after specific stimuli, it is probably not due to suppression by elevated levels of corticosteroids.

INTERPRETATION OF TSH STUDIES IN DEPRESSION

Studies of TSH secretion in depression are reviewed in another chapter (Prange and Loosen, ref. 107) and other monographs (21, 22). The results are summarized in Figure 4.

From a pathophysiologic standpoint, observations on TSH secretion in depression are less striking than those on GH. Except for TRH stimulation tests, very few pharmacoendocrine studies are described (21, 22).

The pathophysiologic significance of a decreased nocturnal TSH rise and blunted TSH response to TRH (21, 107) is not evident. It is not due to hypothalamic or pituitary hypothyroidism or negative feedback by thyroid hormones because the vast majority of patients are euthyroid (107). Also, it is doubtful that suppression of TRH-induced TSH release reflects a central neurotransmitter defect because TRH acts at the pituitary level. High doses of chlorpromazine enhance the TSH response to TRH (21) and this is consistent with the inhibitory effect of DA on TSH release. In contrast, apomorphine does not suppress this response (21). The significance of these results is not clear.

THYROTROPIN RELEASE IN DEPRESSION

↓ Nocturnal release

↓ TRH (25% in 1° depression)
(Also ↓ mania, anorexia nervosa, and acoholism)

→ Thyroid hormone and TRH levels

Suggests:
1. **Altered pituitary receptors (Tsh response to TRH is ↓ acromegaly)**
2. **↑ DA release**
3. **? ↑ SRIF**

FIG. 4. Summary of the effects of mood disorders on thyrotropin secretion (107). Arrows indicate the response compared to normal or control groups.

An alternate explanation for the blunted TSH response to TRH is the increased cortisol secretion that is often present in depression (114). High doses of adrenal steroids abolish the nocturnal TSH elevation and reduce both basal and TRH-stimulated TSH levels in normal subjects (98, 105, 110, 133). However, there is no clear relationship between plasma cortisol and TSH blunting in depressed patients (107).

There are several theories offered to explain the TSH response in depression (107). The most attractive one is similar to that proposed for the paradoxical GH response to TRH, that is altered pituitary receptor sensitivity. A similar phenomenon is seen in acromegaly where approximately 50% of patients have impaired or absent TSH responses to TRH despite clinical and biochemical evidence of euthyroid status (45, 53, 106). An alternate explanation is hypersecretion of DA, but there is no data available to support this concept.

SUMMARY

1. Catecholamines have a major role in the CNS regulation of GH secretion. Alpha-adrenergic and dopaminergic systems enhance and Beta adrenergic systems inhibit GH release under various experimental conditions.
2. Dopamine inhibits basal and TRH-induced TSH release most likely by a direct pituitary effect. There is no convincing evidence for central NE involvement in TSH secretion.
3. Neuroendocrine studies of GH secretion in mood disorders point to

a disturbance in central α-adrenergic neurotransmission.

4. Basal and TRH-induced TSH release are suppressed in depression, suggesting altered pituitary receptor sensitivity to TRH.

5. The lack of specificity of many of the drugs used and the extent of interaction and interdependence between many neuronal pathways frequently lead to difficulties in interpretation of results. All conclusions drawn from neuropharmacological studies should therefore be treated with caution.

ACKNOWLEDGEMENTS

I thank Linda McCreight, Dorothy Davis and Kristin Terry for excellent secretarial assistance. This work was supported by grants from the Veterans Administration and National Institutes of Health. The author is the recipient of a Clinical Investigator Award supported by the Veterans Administration.

REFERENCES

1. Abrams, R. L., Grumbach, M. M. and Kaplan, S. L. (1971): J. Clin. Invest. 50:940-950.
2. Abramson, E. A., Arky, R. A. and Woeber, K. A. (1966): Lancet 2: 1386-1388.
3. Alford, F. P., Baker, H.W.G., Burger, H. G., de Kretzer, D. M., Hudson, B., Johns, M.W., Masterton, J. P., Patel, Y. C. and Rennie, G. C. (1973): J. Clin. Endocrinol. Metab. 37:841-847.
4. Azizi, F., Vagenakis, A. G., Ingbar, S. H. and Braverman, L. E. (1975): Metabolism 24:691-694.
5. Azizi, F., Vagenakis, A. G., Portnay, G. I., Ingbar, S. H. and Braverman, L. E. (1975): J. Clin. Endocrinol. Metab. 40:157-159.
6. Baldessarini, R. J. (1981): A Summary of Biomedical Aspects of Mood Disorders. McClean Hospital, Boston, Ma.
7. Beulac-Baillargeon, L., DiPaolo, T., Raymond, V., Ginguere, V. and Labrie, F. (1980): Soc. Neurosci. Abstr. 6:29.
8. Besses, G. S., Burrow, G. N., Spaulding, S. W. and Donabedian, R. K. (1975): J. Clin. Endocrinol. Metab. 41:985-987.
9. Birk Launidsen, U., Faber, J., Friis, Th., Kirkegaard, C. and Nerup, J. (1976): Horm. Metab. Res. 8:406-407.
10. Blackard, W. G. and Heidingsfelder, S. A. (1968): J. Clin. Invest. 47:1407-1414.
11. Blackard, W. G. and Hubbell, G. J. (1970): Metabolism 19:547-552.
12. Boyar, R. (1978): In: The Hypothalamus, edited by S. Reichlin, R. J. Baldessarini and J. B. Martin, pp.373-386. Raven Press, New York.
13. Boyd, A. E., Lebovitz, H. E. and Pfeiffer, J. B. (1970): N. Engl. J. Med. 283:1425-1429.
14. Brown, W. A. and Williams, B. W. (1976): J. Clin. Endocrinol. Metab. 43:937-939.
15. Brown, G. M., Seggie, J. A., Chambers, J. W. and Ettigi, P. G. (1978): Psychoneuroendocrinology 3:131-153.
16. Buckler, J.M.H., Bold, A.M., Taberner, M. and London, D.R. (1969): Br. Med. J. 3:153-154.
17. Burrow, G. N., May, P. B., Spaulding, W. S. and Donabedian, R. K. (1977): J. Clin. Endocrinol. Metab. 45:65-72.
18. Burt, D. R. and Taylor, R. L. (1980): Neuroendocrinology 30:344-349.

19. Camanni, F., Massara, F. and Molinatti, G. M. (1974): Biomedicine 21:241-243.
20. Camanni, F., Massara, F., Belforte, L., Rosatello, A. and Molinatti, G. M. (1977): J. Clin. Endocrinol. Metab. 44:465-473.
21. Carroll, B. J. (1978): In: Psychopharmacology: A Generation of Progress, edited by M. A. Lipton, A. Dimascio and K. F. Killam, pp.487-497. Raven Press, New York.
22. Carroll, B. J., Curtis, G. C. and Mendels, J. (1976): Arch. Gen. Psychiatry 33:1039-1058.
23. Chan, V., Jones, A., Liendo-Ch., P., McNeilly, A., Landon, J. and Besser, G. M. (1978): Clin. Endocrinol. 9:337-349.
24. Checkley, S. A. (1980): Acta Psychiatric. Scand. 61:211-217.
25. Checkley, S. and Arendt, J. (1982): In: this volume.
26. Chihara, K., Kato, Y., Maeda, K., Ohgo, S. and Imura, H. (1976): Acta Endocrinol. 81:19-27.
27. Collu, R., Jequier, J.-C., Leboeuf, G., Letarte, J. and Ducharme, J. R. (1975): J. Clin. Endocrinol. Metab. 41:981-984.
28. Cooper, D. A. and Jacobs, L. S. (1977): J. Clin. Endocrinol. Metab. 44:404-407.
29. Dammacco, F., Rigillo, N., Tafaro, E., Gagliardo, F., Chetri, G. and Dammacco, A. (1976): Hormone Metab. Res. 8:247-248.
30. Delitala, G. (1977): Lancet 2:760-761.
31. Delitala, G., Masala, A., Alagna, S. and Devilla, L. (1975): IRCS Med. Sci. 3:274.
32. Delitalia, G., Wass, J. A., STubbs, W. A., Jones, A., Williams, S. and Besser, G. M. (1979): Clin. Endocrinol. (Oxf.) 11:1-9.
33. Delitala, G., Devilla, L. and Lotti, G. (1980): J. Clin. Endocrinol. Metab. 50:1127-1130.
34. DeWied, D. (1967): Pharmacol. Rev. 19:251-288.
35. Enjalbert, A., Ruberg, M., Arancibia, S., Fiore, L., Priam, M. and Kordon, C. (1979): Endocrinology 105:823-826.
36. Falkner, B., Onesti, G., Moshang, T. and Lowenthal, D. T. (1981): J. Clin. Pharmacol. 21:31-36.
37. Ferrari, C., Coldara, R., Barbieri, C., Testori, G., Benco, R., Trezzi, R., Crossignani, R. M. and Rompini, P. (1981): Neuroendocrinology 32:213-216.
38. Finkelstein, J. W., Roffwarg, H. P., Boyar, R. M., Kream, J. and Hellman, L. (1972): J. Clin. Endocrinol. Metab. 35:665-670.
39. Fisher, D. A. and Odell, W. D. (1969): J. Clin. Invest. 48:1670-1677.
40. Frohman, L. A. (1979): In: Endocrinology, Vol. 1, edited by L. J. DeGroot, G. F. Cahill, L. Martini, D. H. Nelson, W. D. Odell, J. G. Potts, E. Sternberger and A. I. Winegrad. Grune and Stratten, New York.
41. Fuxe, K. and Hokfelt, T. (1969): In: Frontiers in Neuroendocrinology edited by W. Ganong and L. Martini, pp.47-96. Oxford University Press, New York.
42. Goldberg, L. I., Volkman, P. H., Kohli, J. D. and Kotake, A. N. (1977): Adv. Biochem. Psychopharmacol. 16:251-256.
43. Goldstein, M., Lew, J. Y., Matsumoto, Y., Hokfelt, T. and Fuxe, K. (1978): In: Psychopharmacology: A Generation of Progress, edited by M. A. Lipton, A. DiMascio and K. F. Killam, pp.261-269. Raven Press, New York.
44. Grandison, L. and Guidotti, A. (1979): Endocrinology 105:754-759.
45. Hall, R. J., Ormston, B. J., Besser, G. M., Cryer, R. J. and

McKendrick, M. (1972): Lancet 1:759-763.
46. Hansen, A. P. (1971): J. Clin. Endocrinol. Metab. 33:807-812.
47. Heidingsfelder, S. A. and Blackard, W. G. (1968): Metabolism 17:1019-1024.
48. Hirvonen, E., Tanta, T. and Seppala, A. (1976): J. Clin. Endocrinol. Metab. 42:1024-1030.
49. Hokfelt, T., Elde, R., Fuxe, K., Johansson, O., Ljungdahl, H., Goldstein, M., Luft, R., Efendic, S., Nilsson, G., Terenuis, L., Ganten, D., Jeffcoate, S. L., Rehfeld, J., Said, S., Perez de la Mora, M., Possani, L., Tapia, R., Teran, L. and Palacios, R. (1978): In: The Hypothalamus, Vol. 56, edited by S. Reichlin, R. J. Baldessarini and J. B. Martin, pp.69-135. Raven Press, New York.
50. Ikeda, H. and Nagataki, S. (1976): Endocrinol. Jpn. 23:431-433.
51. Imura, H., Kato, Y., Ikeda, M., Morimoto, M., Yawata, M. and Fukase, M. (1968): J. Clin. Endocrinol. Metab. 28:1079-1081.
52. Imura, H., Kato, Y., Ikeda, M., Morimoto, M. and Yawata, M. (1971): J. Clin. Invest. 50:1069-1071.
53. Irie, M. and Tsushima, T. J. (1972): J. Clin. Endocrinol. Metab. 35:97-100.
54. Iversen, L. I., Iversen, S. D. and Snyder, S. H., editors (1978): In: Chemical Pathways in the Brain: Handbook of Psychopharmacology, Vol. 9. Plenum Press, New York.
55. Janowski, D. S., El-Yousef, M. K. and Davis, M. M. (1974): Psychosom. Med. 36:248-257.
56. Jubiz, W., Carlile, S. and Lagerquist, L. D. (1977): J. Clin. Endocrinol. Metab. 44:379-382.
57. Judd, S. J., Lazarus, L. and Smythe, G. (1976): J. Clin. Endocrinol. Metab. 43:313-317.
58. Kansal, P. C., Buse, J., Talbert, O. R. and Buse, M. G. (1972): J. Clin. Endocrinol. Metab. 34:99-105.
59. Knopf, R. F., Conn, J. W., Fagans, S. S., Floyd, J. C., Cuntsche, E. M. and Rull, J. A. (1965): J. Clin. Endocrinol. Metab. 25: 1140-1144.
60. Krieger, D. T. and Hughes, J. C. (1980): In: Neuroendocrinology. Sinauer, Sunderland, Ma.
61. Krulich, L. (1979): Ann. Rev. Physiol. 41:603-615.
62. Laakman, G. (1980): In: Psychoneuroendocrinology and Abnormal Behaviour, edited by J. Mendelewicz and H. M. Van Praag, pp.67-84. Karger, Basel.
63. Laakman, G., Schumaeker, G., Benkart, O. (1977): J. Clin. Endocrinol. Metab. 44:1010-1013.
64. Lal, S., de la Vega, C. E., Sourkes, T. L. and Friesen, H. G. (1972): Lancet 2:661.
65. Lal, S., de la Vega, C. E., Sourkes, T. L. and Friesen, H. G. (1973): J. Clin. Endocrinol. Metab. 37:719-724.
66. Lal, S., Martin, J. B., de la Vega, C. E. and Friesen, H. G. (1975): Clin. Endocrinol. 4:277-285.
67. Lal, S., Tolis, G., Martin, J. B., Brown, G. M. and Guyda, H. (1975): J. Clin. Endocrinol. Metab. 41:827-832.
68. Lal, S., Guyda, H. and Bikadoroff, S. (1977): J. Clin. Endocrinol. Metab. 44:766-770.
69. Lal, S. and Nair, N.P.V. (1979): In: Neuroendocrine Correlates in Neurology and Psychiatry, edited by E. E. Muller and A. Agnoli, pp.179-194. Elsevier-North Holland, Amsterdam.
70. Lal, S. and Martin, J. B. (1980): In: Handbood of Biological

Psychiatry: Part III Brain Mechanisms and Abnormal Behavior, edited by H. M. Van Praag, M. H. Lader, O. J. Rafaelsen and E. J. Sachar, pp.101-167.
71. Lamberg, B-A., Linnoila, M., Fogelholm, R., Olkinuora, M., Kotilaninen, P. and Saarinen, P. (1977): Neuroendocrinology 24: 90-97.
72. Lancranjan, I. and Marbach, P. (1977): Metabolism 26:1225-1230.
73. Leblanc, H., Lachelin, G.C.L., Abu-Fadil, S. and Yen, S.S.C. (1976): J. Clin. Endocrinol. Metab. 43:668-674.
74. Leeblaw, W.F., Lee, L. A. and Woolf, P. D. (1978): J. Clin. Endocrinol. Metab. 47:480-487.
75. L'Hermite, M., Denayer, P., Golstein, J., Vira-Soro, E., Vanhaelst, L., Copinschi, G. and Robyn, E. (1978): Clin. Endocrinol. 9: 195-204.
76. Lipman, R. L., Ulvedal, F., schure, J. J., Bradley, E. M. and Lecocq, F. R. (1970): Metabolism 19;980-987.
77. Lucke, C. and Glick, S. M. (1971): J. Clin. Endocrinol. Metab. 32:729-736.
78. Mars, H. and Genuth, S. M. (1973): Clin. Pharmacol. Therap. 14: 390-395.
79. Martin, J. B. (1977): In: Frontiers in Neuroendocrinology, edited by L. Martini and W. F. Ganong, Vol. 4, pp.129-168. Raven Press, New York.
80. Martin, J. B. (1980): Fed. Proc. 39:2902-2906.
81. Martin, J. B., Reichlin, S. and Brown, G. M. editors (1977): Clinical Endocrinology. Davis, Philadelphia, Pa.
82. Martin, J. B., Brazeau, P., Tannenbaum, G. S., Willoughby, J. O. Epelbaum, J., Terry, L. C. and Durand, D. (1978): In: The Hypothalamus, edited by S. Reichlin, R. J. Baldessarini and J. B. Martin, pp.329-372.
83. Martini, L. and Besser, G. M. (1977): In: Clinical Endocrinology. Academic Press, New Nork.
84. Massara, F. and Camanni, F. (1972): J. Endocrinol. 54:195-206.
85. Massara, F., Camanni, F., Felforte, L., Vergano, V. and Molinatti, M. (1978): Clin. Endocrinol. 9:419-428.
86. Massara, F., Camanni, F., Vergano, V., Belforte, L. and Molinatti, G. M. (1978): J. Endocrinol. Invest. 1:25-30.
87. Matussek, N., Ackenheil, M., Hippins, H., Muller, F., Schroder, H. T., Schultes, H. and Wasilewski, B. L. (1980): Psychiatry Res. 2: 25-26.
88. Mendelson, W. B., Jacobs, L. S., Sitarom, N., Wyatt, R. J. and Gillin, J. C. (1978): J. Clin. Invest. 61:1683-1690.
89. Mendelson, W. B., Lantigua, R. A., Wyatt, R. J., Gillin, J. C. and Jacobs, L. S. (1981): J. Clin. Endocrinol. Metab. 52:409-415.
90. Mims, R, B., Scott, C. L., Modebe, O. and Bethune, J. E. (1975): J. Clin. Endocrinol. Metab. 40:256-259.
91. Mitchell, M. L. and Suvunrungsi, P. and Sawin, C. T. (1971): J. Clin. Endocrinol. Metab. 32:470-475.
92. Moore, R. Y. and Bloom, F. E. (1978): Ann. Rev. Neurosci. 1:129-169.
94. Moore, R. Y. and Bloom, F. E. (1979): Ann. Rev. Neurosci. 2:113-168.
95. Müller, E. E., Nistico, G. and Scapagnini, Y., editors (1977): In: Neurotransmitters and Anterior Pituitary Function. Academic Press, New York.
96. Murphy, D. L., Campbell, I., Costa, J. L. (1978): In: Psychopharmacology: A Generation of Progress, edited by M. A. Lipton, A. DiMascio

and K. F. Killam, pp.1235-1247. Raven Press, New York.
97. Nair, N. P., Lal, S., Cervantes, P., Yassa, R. and Guyda, H. (1979): Neuropsychobiology 5:136-142.
98. Nicoloff, J. T., Fisher, D. A. and Appleman, M. D. (1970): J. Clin. Invest. 49:1922-1929.
99. Nilsson, K. O., Thorell, J. I. and Mikflet, B. (1974): Acta Endocrinol. 76:24-28.
100. Nilsson, K. O., Wide, L. and Hokfelt, B. (1975): Acta Endocrinol. 80:220-229.
101. Noel, G. L., Dimond, R. C., Wartofsky, L., Earll, J. M. and Frantz, A. G. (1974): J. Clin. Endocrinol. Metab. 39:6-17.
102. Onishi, T., Kiyai, K., Izumi, K., Nakanishi, H. and Kimahara, Y. (1975): J. Clin. Endocrinol. Metab. 40:30-32.
103. Ormston, B. J., Garry, R., Cryer, R. J., Besser, G. M. and Hall, R. (1971): Lancet 2:10-14.
104. Parker, D. C., Pekary, A. E. and Hershman, J. M. (1976): J. Clin. Endocrinol. Metab. 43:318-329.
105. Patel, Y. C., Alford, F. P. and Burger, H. G. (1972): Clin. Sci. 43:71-77.
106. Patel, Y. C. and Burger, H. G. (1973): J. Clin. Endocrinol. Metab. 37:190-196.
107. Prange, A. J. and Loosen, P. T. Raven Press, New York (in press).
108. Prinz, P. N., Roehrs, T. A., Vitaliano, P. P., Linnoila, M. and Weitzman, E. D. (1980): J. Clin. Endocrinol. Metab. 51:759-764.
109. Rapoport, B., Refetoff, S., Fang, V. S. and Friesen, H. G. (1973): J. Clin. Endocrinol. Metab. 36:256-262.
110. Re, R. N., Kourides, I. A., Ridgway, E. C., Weintraub, B. D. and Maloof, F. (1976): J. Clin. Endocrinol. Metab. 43:338-346.
111. Rees, L., Butler, P.W.P., Gosling, C. and Besser, G. M. (1970): Nature 228:565-566.
112. Refetoff, S., Fang, V. S., Rapoport, B. and Friesen, H. G. (1974): J. Clin. Endocrinol. Metab. 38:450-457.
113. Rotrosen, J., Angrist, B., Gershorn, S., Paquin, J., Branchey, L., Oleshansky, M., Halpern, F. and Sachar, E. J. (1979): Br. J. Psychiatry 135:444-446.
114. Rubin, R. T. and Poland, R. E. Raven Press, New York (in press).
115. Rudolph, C. D., Kaplan, S. L. and Ganong, W. F. (1980): Neuroendocrinology 2:121-128.
116. Saberi, M. and Utiger, R. D. (1974): J. Clin. Endocrinol. Metab. 39:923-927.
117. Sachar, E. J., Nathan, R. S., Asnis, G., Halbreich, Y., Tobnizi, M. A., Halpern, F. (1980): Acta Psychiatr. Scand. 61:201-210.
118. Sanchez-Franco, F., Garcia, M. D., Cacicedo, L., Martin-Zurro, A. and Escobar Del Ray, F. (1973): J. Clin. Endocrinol. 37:736-740.
119. Sassin, J. F., Parker, D. C., Mace, J. W., Gotlin, R. W., Johnson, L. C. and Rossman, L. G. (1969): Science 165-513-515.
120. Scanlon, M. F., Mora, B., Shale, D. J., Weightman, D. R., Heath, M., Snow, M. H. and Hall, R. (1977): Lancet 2:421-423.
121. Scanlon, M. F., Heath, M., Mora, B., Shale, D., Snow, M., Weightman, D. R. and Hall, R. (1978): J. Endocrinol. 77:31.
122. Scanlon, M. F., Rodriguez-Arnao, M. D., Pourmand, M., Weightman, D. R. and Hall, R. (1979): J. Endocrinol. Invest. (in press).
123. Scanlon, M. F., Lewis, M., Weightman, D. R., Chan, V. and Hall, R. (1980): In: Frontiers in Neuroendocrinology, Vol. 6, edited by L. Martini and W. F. Ganong, pp.333-380.

124. Scanlon, M. F., Weetman, A. P., Lewis, M., Pourmand, M., Rodriguez-Arnao, M. D., Weightman, D. R. and Hall, R. (1980): J. Clin. Endocrinol. Metab. 51:1251-1256.
125. Schaeffer, J. M. and Hsuch, A.J.W. (1980): Endocrinology 106: 1377-1381.
126. Schalch, D. S. (1967): J. Lab. Clin. Med. 69:256-269.
127. Schally, A. V., Redding, T. W., Arimura, A., Dupont, A. and Linthicum, G. L. (1977): Endocrinology 100:681-691.
128. Schidkraut, J. J. (1978): In: Psychopharmacology: A Generation of Progress, edited by M. A. Lipton, A. DiMascio and K. F. Killam, pp.1223-1234. Raven Press, New York.
129. Schwin, G., Schwarck, H., McIntosh, C., Milstrey, H.-R., Willms, B. and Koberling, J. (1976): J. Clin. Endocrinol. Metab. 43:1183-1185.
130. Sherman, L., Kim, S., Benjamin, F. and Kolodny, H. D. (1971): N. Engl. J. Med. 284:72-74.
131. Sjostrum, R. and Roos, B.-E. (1972): Eur. J. Clin. Pharmacology 4:170-176.
132. Snyder, P. J. and Utiger, R. D. (1972): J. Clin. Invest. 51: 2077-2084.
133. Sowers, R. J., Carlson, H. E., Brautbar, N. and Hershman, J. M. (1977): J. Clin. Endocrinol. Metab. 44:237-241.
134. Spaulding, S. W., Burrow, G. N., Donabedian, R. and Van Woert, M. (1972); J. Clin. Endocrinol. Metab. 35:182-185.
135. Strauch, G., Modigliani, E. and Bricaire, H. (1968): J. Clin. Endocrinol. Metab. 29:606-608.
136. Tannenbaum, G. S. (1980): Endocrinology 6:2117-2120.
137. Taylor, R. L. and Burt, D. R. (1979): Soc. Neurosci. Abstr. 5:406.
138. Terry, L. C. In: Functioning Pituitary Tumors: Diagnosis and Treatment, edited by J. Givens. Yearbook Medical Publishers, Chicago, Ill. (in press).
139. Terry, L. C., Crowley, W. R., and Johnson, M. D. (1982): J. Clin. Invest. 69:104-112.
140. Thorner, M. O. Wass, J. A., Rees, L. H. et al. (1976): Lancet 1: 588.
141. Thorner, M. O., Ryan, S. M., Wass, J.A.H., Jones, A., Bouloux, P., Williams, S. and Besser, G. M. (1978): J. Clin. Endocrinol. Metab. 47:372-378.
142. Tolis, G., Labrie, F., Martin, J. B. and Naftolin, F. (1979): In: Clinical Neuroendocrinology: A Pathophysiological Approach. Raven Press, New York.
143. Tolliver, J. M., Taylor, R. L. and Burt, D. R. (1981): Neuroendocrinology 32:33-37.
144. Van Praag, H. M. (1978): In: Handbook of Psychopharmacology, Vol. 13, edited by L. L. Iversen, S. O. Iversen and S. H. Snyder, pp.187-297. Plenum Press, New York.
145. Vigas, M., Stowasserova, N., Nemeth, S. and Jurcovicova, J. (1975): Hormone Res. 6:65-70.
146. Vigas, M., Wiedermann, V., Nemeth, S., Jurcovicova, J. and Zigo, L. (1976): Neuroendocrinology 21:42-48.
147. Vigas, M., Malatinsky, J., Nemeth, S. and Jurcovicova, J. (1977): Metabolism 26:399-402.
148. Weeke, J. (1973): Scand. J. Clin. Lab. Invest. 31:337-340.
149. Weiner, R. I. and Ganong, W. F. (1978): Physiol. Rev. 58:905-976.
150. Wiersinga, W. M. and Touber, J. L. (1977): J. Clin. Endocrinol. Metab. 45:293-298.

151. Weitzman, E. D. (1980): In: Neuroendocrinology, edited by D. T. Krieger and J. C. Hughes, pp.85-92. Sinauer, Sunderland, Ma.
152. Woolf, P. D., Lee, L. A. and Schalch, D. S. (1972): J. Clin. Endocrinol. Metab. 35:616-618.
153. Woolf, P., Lantigua, R., Lee, L. A. (1979): J. Clin. Endocrinol. Metab. 49:326-330.
154. Yap, P. L., Davison, N. McD., Lidgard, G. P. and Fyffe, J. A. (1978): Clin. Endocrinol. 9:179-183.
155. Yoshimura, M., Hachiya, T., Ochi, Y., Nagasaka, A., Takeda, A., Hidaka, H., Refetoff, S. and Fang, V. S. (1977): J. Clin. Endocrinol. Metab. 45:95-98.

Neuroendocrinology and Psychiatric Disorder,
edited by G. M. Brown, et al.
Raven Press, New York 1984.

Hypothalamic Releasing Hormones: Mechanisms Underlying Neuroendocrine Dysfunction in Affective Disorders

Ivor M.D. Jackson

The modern era of clinical neuroendocrinology can be said to date from the isolation of thyrotropin-releasing hormone (TRH) from the mammalian hypothalamus and the establishment of its structure by Guillemin, Schally and their respective co-workers (7, 9). Subsequently, these two groups characterized two other releasing hormones in the hypothalamus: luteinizing hormone releasing hormone or gonadotropin-releasing hormone (LH-RH or GnRH)(57) and growth hormone-release inhibiting hormone (somatostatin) (8) which like TRH proved to be simple peptides. LH-RH appears to regulate both LH and follicule-stimulating hormone (FSH) secretion. However, although TRH induces the release of both TSH and PRL, the evidence suggests that PRL secretion is regulated primarily by inhibitory control through a PRL-inhibitory factor (PIF), which appears to be the monoamine dopamine (DA) (34), and that another physiological PRL-releasing factor (PRF) may also exist. Somatostatin inhibits the secretion of both growth hormone (GH) and TSH and appears to be of physiological importance in the secretion of both, though the major regulatory factors appear to be a putative growth-hormone-releasing factor (GH-RF) and TRH, respectively. Adrenocorticotropin (ACTH) is regulated by a corticotropin-releasing factor (CRH) (54), the structure of which has been recently reported by Vale and his co-workers (68). The hypophysiotropic factors, or hormones, are synthesized by neurons in the hypothalamus, transported to nerve endings in the stalk-median eminence (SME), released into the interstitial space in contiguity with the primary portal capillary plexus, and distributed to the anterior pituitary by means of the portal circulation (Fig. 1). The hypothalamic peptidergic neurons are in turn regulated by neurotransmitters largely of the monoaminergic variety, dopamine (DA) norepinephrine (NE), and serotonin (5-HT), and much evidence suggests that the peptidergic neuron acts as a "neuroendocrine transducer" converting neural information from the brain into chemical information (69).

Since alteration in the metabolism of biogenic amines underlies the pathophysiology of affective disorders (58, 59), the hypothalamic-pituitary axis has been extensively investigated in patients with such psychiatric disturbances as a potential "window" through which brain function might be studied (16). Additionally, the recognition that the hypothalamic releasing hormones are part of a family of neural peptides with a widespread distribution throughout the central nervous system (CNS) (24) has led to the hypothesis that disturbances in neural peptide function, perhaps as a cause or consequence of disturbed CNS amine metabolism, might result in psychiatric or neuronal disorders (66). Although it was at first believed that the development of specific radioimmunoassay (RIA) for the releasing hormones would allow a direct evaluation of hypothalamic or brain function, it became clear that these substances are present in the systemic circulation in low concentrations and are

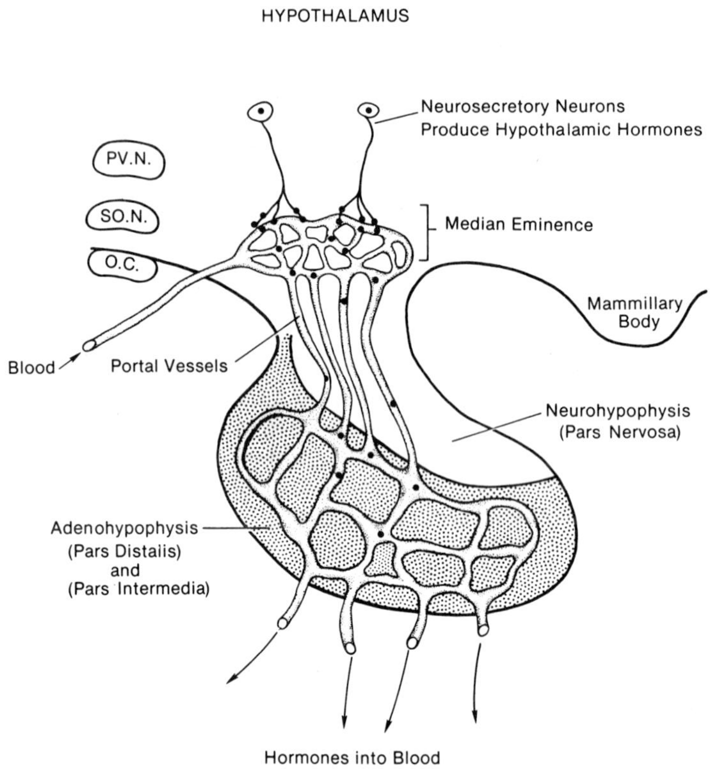

FIG. 1. Schematic representation of the hypothalamic-pituitary system.
P.V.N. = paraventricular nucleus
S.O.N. = supraoptic nucleus
O.C. = optic chiasm

rapidly degraded, thus making their measurement extremely difficult. Furthermore, since these peptides are found outside the nervous system altogether (24), it seems unlikely that measurement of these peptides in peripheral blood can be used to impute dysfunction in the hypothalamus or even CNS. The only exception to this view would be direct assay of pituitary-portal-vessel blood for these substances, and this circulation is inaccessible in intact man.

In recent years, a number of "biochemical markers" of endogenous depression have been identified (16) as a consequence of the widespread use of the dexamethasone suppression and TRH stimulation tests in depressed patients. These studies have revealed (a) impaired dexamethasone suppressibility of cortisol and (b) "blunted" TSH but "paradoxic" GH responses following TRH injection (Table 1). Other changes in pituitary function have included alterations in PRL and gonadotropin secretion especially in post-menopausal women. In this review, I will examine the role of the hypothalamic releasing hormones in these neuroendocrine responses.

TABLE 1. Abnormal Pituitary Hormone Responses to TRH Reported in Depression

	UNIPOLAR	BIPOLAR
TSH	BLUNTED	NORMAL[a]
PRL	BLUNTED[b]	BLUNTED[b]
GH	RISE	RISE

[a]Some studies fail to find TSH differences between depressive subtypes.

[b]Described in post-menopausal women. Other studies reveal no or variable PRL changes in depression.

CNS EFFECTS OF TRH: NEUROTRANSMITTER REGULATION OF CRF: DEXAMETHASONE SUPPRESSIBILITY

Extrahypothalamic Brain TRH

The widespread anatomic distribution of authentic TRH (25) throughout the CNS supports the view that this substance has a role in neuronal transmission (27) in addition to regulation of pituitary function. In the hypophysectomized mouse pretreated with pargyline, a monoamine oxidase (MAO) inhibitor, and then given L-dopa - an animal model for testing antidepressant drugs - TRH causes enhanced motor activity (49), however, a beneficial effect of TRH in human depression is controversial (50). Of note, CSF immunoreactive IR-TRH-like material (LM) has been reported increased in this disorder (30), a finding that suggests altered endogenous TRH metabolism. If the TRH LM measured represents the authentic tripeptide, the increased levels in the CSF may be interpreted as 'leakage' from functionally impaired neurons within the CNS.

In a number of neurophysiologic and neuropharmacologic paradigms TRH interfaces with the monoamine neurotransmitters in the CNS. TRH influences the excitatory or depressant effects of NE and acetylcholine (ACh) on single neurons, enhances cerebral NE turnover, magnifies the behavioural changes consequent on increased 5HT accumulation in rats and produces alteration of rotational activity in the rat (believed to be a DA mediated action) (see 70 for review). Thus, TRH may directly or indirectly influence the action of the established neurotransmitters, NE, DA, 5HT and ACh within the CNS. Such findings raise the possibility that TRH dysfunction could be implicated in the deranged monoamine metabolism of affective disorders (50, 70). Although lack of a consistent therapeutic response from TRH administration to depressed patients might be viewed as evidence against such an hypothesis, it should be noted that TRH (as well as other neural peptides) may have specific effects on neurotransmitter turnover only in selected brain regions (39). Thus, the beneficial effect of exogenous TRH in spinocerebellar ataxia in man has been postulated to result from an improvement in abnormal NE metabolism in the cerebellum and brain stem (67).

CRF Activity and Dexamethasone Suppressibility

There is much evidence that hypothalamic CRF activity is inhibited by

NE and stimulated by both ACh and 5HT - the latter through activation of cholinergic interneurons (28). Thus, the idea that CRF turnover might be enhanced in depression is consistent with the catecholamine hypothesis of depression - in which a deficiency of NE at functionally important brain receptor sites is postulated (58, 59). Further, increased serotonin turnover in unipolar depression has also been reported (60), which also could lead to increased CRF secretion.

Could endogenous brain TRH dysfunction play an etiologic role in the impaired dexamethasone suppressibility of depression? Much evidence has been marshalled to suggest that TRH within the brain may form an endogenous 'ergotropic' system (40) somewhat analagous to the opioid peptide system. TRH may influence the metabolism of each of the monoamines involved in CRF secretion from the hypothalamus and if this TRH 'ergotropic' system is a primary locus of dysfunction in human depression, secondary effects on CRF regulation could ensue. Further studies are required to test this hypothesis.

THE TSH AND PRL RESPONSE TO TRH IN AFFECTIVE DISORDERS

TSH Response

The pituitary release of TSH is primarily regulated by means of the negative feedback of thyroid hormone at the level of the thyrotrope (52). TRH is also involved in the physiologic regulation of TSH secretion and appears to act by determining the "set-point" at which thyroid hormone and TSH interact (52). Following the administration of TRH intravenously (iv) in a dose of 200 to 500 µg, a significant TSH release is obtained in normal subjects - the peak normally occurring 15 to 30 minutes following injection (22, 55). In states of thyroid overactivity, the TSH response is "flat" while in primary hypothyroidism a hyper-response is usually obtained (22, 55), so that the TRH test has proven to be useful in the appropriate clinical setting. However, the TSH response has also been found by a number of workers to be blunted in unipolar, though not bipolar, depression (19, 20), a finding reported to correlate with a beneficial response to electroconvulsive (ECT) therapy (17). (It should be noted, however, that other studies have not confirmed a role for the TRH test in delineating diagnostic subtypes of depression [see Prange and Loosen, Chapter 13]). The cause of the impaired TSH rise in depression has not been determined but it must be emphasized that an impaired TSH rise to TRH is not specific, for many conditions are associated with such a response (Table 2).

In most subjects with depression, thyroid hormone levels are within the normal range and no differences in the thyroid status of unipolar versus bipolar depressives are evident (19). However, reports of elevated thyroxine (T4) and free thyroxine index (FTI) with normal triiodothyronine (T3) levels have been reported in some depressed patients (12, 31). Could these patients be hyperthyroid? Morley et al. (41) recently described hyperthyroxinemia, accompanied by normal T3 and slightly raised TSH levels, induced by amphetamine and have drawn attention to the chemical similarity of amphetamine to phenylethylamine, an endogenous brain amine, which has been implicated in chronic paranoid schizophrenia. It is possible that a combination of central activation of the pituitary thyroid axis, along with enhanced conversion of T4 to T3 within the pituitary, in such subjects may expose the pituitary thyrotrope to "hyperthyroid" levels of T3 and result in a suppressed TSH response to TRH. Indeed, the pituitary thyrotrope is exquisitely sensitive to the suppressive effects of very slight increases in thyroid hormone levels induced by exogenous thyroid adminstration, despite concentrations remaining within the normal range (55). Patients with autonomous thyroid nodules, even if not thyrotoxic, frequently have a suppressed TSH response presumably because their ambient thyroid hormone levels are slightly raised though insufficient to cause thyrotoxicosis. Accordingly, thyroid gland size and consistency needs to be carefully assessed in the evaluation of TRH responsivity in depression. Hypopituitarism and pituitary tumors are frequently associated with a blunted TSH response, usually, though not always, in the context of secondary hypothyroidism (26, 63). Although not often viewed as a major diagnostic consideration in depressed subjects - primary organic disorders of the hypothalamus, pituitary and thyroid glands must be excluded in interpreting the TRH test. Repeated injections, or a continuous infusion, of TRH impairs the thyrotrope response to subsequent injections of TRH (65). This effect is probably consequent on (a) the slight increase in T3 induced by the TSH elevation and subsequent inhibition of TSH responsivity due to the negative feedback effect of thyroid hormone; (b) TRH itself appears to "down regulate" its own receptors (23). The overall effect leaves the thyroid levels within the normal range but the thyrotrope unresponsive to TRH injection. Consequently, if enhanced turnover of hypothalamic or brain TRH (27) occurs in depression, this could lead to increased central "drive" of the pituitary thyrotrope and resistance to exogenous TRH stimulation.

Glucocorticoids, both exogenous and endogenous, suppress the TSH response to TRH (46), and the high plasma levels of cortisol found in depression have been postulated to account for the impaired TSH rise in some depressed subjects (33). In this context, it is of relevance that CSF levels of 5 hydroxyindole acetic acid (5-HIAA) a metabolite of 5-HT- which stimulates hypothalamic CRF - shows a significant negative correlation with TSH response to TRH (20). However, in subsequent study, Kirkegaard and Carroll (29) found no correlation between serum TSH and Δ max TSH on the one hand, and serum and CSF cortisol or urinary excretion of cortisol on the other hand. Nevertheless, it seem likely to this author that the elevated levels of circulating cortisol play some role in the genesis of the blunted TSH response reported in unipolar depression. However, the fact that cortisol levels may be raised in bipolar depression (29), wherein abnormal TSH tests are described less frequently (3, 19, 20), demonstrates that glucocorticoid abnormalities do not account fully for the phenomenon.

Patients with acromegaly frequently show blunting of the TSH response to TRH (11), an effect that could be related to the high frequency of autonomous thyroid nodules in this condition. Additionally, GH administration to dwarfed children results in hypothyroidism with a suppressed TSH response (53). GH does not appear to influence pituitary thyrotrope secretion directly, but there is now much evidence to indicate that GH either directly (61) or via somatomedin C (4) can increase somatostatin secretion via a "short feedback" loop and by this means inhibit pituitary TSH secretion (62). Patients with anorexia nervosa (6) frequently have raised GH levels, though the serum GH is usually normal in primary endogenous depression. However, there is evidence of abnormal GH regulation in depression with a blunted rise following the usually provocative stimuli (insulin hypoglycemia, L-dopa), but a "paradoxic" increase in response to TRH stimulation (36) (see later). Whether the GH secretion rate, as distinct from basal serum concentrations, is increased in endogenous depression requires study to exclude the possibility that hypothalamic somatostatin secretion is enhanced in endogenous depression via such a "short feedback" mechanism. However, hypothalamic or brain somatostatin secretion could be increased in depression as a result of altered neurotransmitter and/or neural peptide metabolism and not involving the GH feedback loop. In this context, it is of interest that neurotensin, a tridecapeptide present throughout the mammalian brain inhibits TRH induced TSH release in the rat following intraventricular injection, possibly by stimulating somatostatin release (35). Starvation has been shown to blunt the TSH response to TRH, but the responsivity of the thyrotrope is preserved since potassium iodide (KI) administration, which has the effect of lowering circulating thyroid hormone levels through an effect at the thyroid gland level, restores the TSH response to normal (18). Such findings suggest that fasting induces metabolic effects which cause the thyroid hormone TSH interaction, to be "shifted to the right" and so inhibit a "normal" TSH rise. This development in fasting may be a teleologic response of the body which leads to suppression of the pituitary-thyroid axis and prevents catabolic consequences of thyroid activation. Relative caloric deprivation due to anorexia may be operative in some depressed patients, but whether KI administration would restore the TRH responsivity to normal in depressed subjects has not been reported.

In addition to TRH and somatostatin, there is evidence that a third hypothalamic factor DA plays a physiologic role in inhibiting TSH secretion (56). Enhanced hypothalamic DA secretion could be operative in depression but this possibility would need to be tested through examining the effect of DA antagonists (metoclopramide or domperidone) on the TSH response to TRH.

Renal failure (13) and alcohol withdrawal (50), conditions in which altered neurotransmitter milieu of the hypothalamic-pituitary system may be operative, are also associated with blunted TSH responses to TRH. Inhibition of prostaglandin synthesis (aspirin, indomethacin) also blunts the TSH response (51), a finding that points to a physiologic role for the prostaglandins in TSH secretion. Whether prostaglandin metabolism in the hypothalamic-pituitary axis is disturbed in depression is worthy of study.

Finally, it should be noted that sex hormone status can affect the TRH test. Thus, estrogen priming has been reported to enhance the TSH response to TRH (55) so that estrogen deficiency conversely may cause an impaired release. Old age in men, though not women, has been reported in one study to depress the TSH response to TRH (64). Accordingly, it can be seen that multiple factors including peripheral hormone levels (thyroid, cortisol, sex steroids, GH), neurotransmitter milieu (DA or possibly related chemicals), hypothalamic dysfunction (altered TRH, somatostatin, neurotensin, DA, prostaglandin secretion) could all affect the TSH response to TRH. Although it has been suggested that the blunted TSH response to TRH represents an "intrinsic" defect in the thyrotrope and may be a genetic marker for depression (3, 50), the reversibility of the suppressed TSH response in most subjects on cure of the depression makes this appear unlikely. The author favours alteration in one or more of the multiple factors (Table 2) that impinge upon TRH-TSH interaction as the underlying cause of the reduced TSH rise.

PRL Response

Conflicting results on PRL levels and response to TRH in patients with depression have been reported, low, normal and raised basal PRL levels, as well as increased, normal and suppressed responses to TRH administration have been described (see 32 for references). In one large study in which 27 unipolar and 24 bipolar depressive females were

TABLE 2. Factors Associated with a Blunted TSH Response to TRH

THYROID HORMONE (22,55).

- -Hyperthyroidism
- -Autonomous thyroid nodule(s)
- -Thyroid hormone treatment

TRH INFUSION (65)

HYPOPITUITARISM (26, 63)

PITUITARY TUMOR (26, 63)

CUSHING'S SYNDROME (46)
- -Glucocorticoid administration

ACROMEGALY (11)

GH TREATMENT (53)

SOMATOSTATIN INFUSION (62)

STARVATION (18)

RENAL FAILURE (13)

DEPRESSION (19, 20)

DOPAMINE INFUSION (5, 56)

PROSTAGLANDIN SYNTHESIS INHIBITORS (51)

ALCOHOL WITHDRAWAL (50)

AGING IN MALES (64)

matched with 38 controls, the PRL response to TRH was significantly blunted in both unipolar and bipolar post menopausal subjects but remained normal in all the premenopausal (unipolar and bipolar) depressed women (32). Linkowski et al. (32) postulate that discrepancies in different reports on the PRL status in depression results from failure to take into account both unipolar-bipolar dichotomy and menopausal status. In contrast to the findings in depression, an increased PRL response to TRH has been reported in patients with mania (38).

The underlying cause of the disturbances in PRL regulation in affective disorders is not clear. Increased activity of the hypothalamic tuberoinfundibular dopaminergic neurons or deficiency of central 5-HT pathways could account for the suppressed TRH induced PRL response. Although DA is the principal physiologic regulator of PRL secretion, it is now clear that a number of neurotransmitters which include gamma aminobutyric acid (GABA), 5-HT and histamine and neural peptides (vasoactive intestinal peptide (VIP), histidyl proline diketopiperazine - a metabolite of TRH-, β -endorphin, neurotensin and substance P) affect PRL secretion either directly at the pituitary level or at the hypothala-

TABLE 3. "Paradoxic" GH Responses to TRH

ACROMEGALY (26)
RENAL FAILURE (13)
HEPATIC DISEASE (48)
ANOREXIA NERVOSA (37)
DEPRESSION (36)
PRIMARY HYPOTHYROIDISM (21)
DIABETES MELLITUS (14)

mus (see 34 for review). Since it is likely that depression is a heterogenous disorder, disturbances in various brain neurotransmitter or neural peptide activities could each produce alterations in PRL secretion.

"PARADOXIC" GH RESPONSES TO TRH

TRH does not stimulate GH release in normal subjects but does so in about 50 percent of patients with unipolar and bipolar depression (36) as well as a number of other disorders which include acromegaly (26), renal failure (13), liver disease (48) and anorexia nervosa (37) (see Table 3 for complete list). Although abnormal TRH receptors on the tumerous somatotrope might be invoked to explain the GH rise in acromegaly (26), such an explanation does not obviously account for the situation in depression wherein during recovery the GH response does not occur (36). A common link in all these disorders exhibiting a paradoxic GH rise to TRH appears to involve an altered neurotransmitter milieu or some functional neurovascular disturbance in the brain-hypothalamo-pituitary axis, since an altered GH response to CNS acting stimuli such as glucose administration (paradoxic rise or impaired suppression) is also found in these conditions. Evidence in favour of such a view has been provided from studies emanating from Muller's laboratory (43, 44) showing that TRH releases GH from a pituitary transplanted under the kidney capsule of hypophysectomized rats at doses ineffective on the pituitary _in situ_. Furthermore, _in vivo_ in rats with surgical separation of the anterior pituitary from the hypothalamus, and _in vitro_ from normal rat pituitaries, a direct GH-releasing effect of TRH can be obtained. The PRL releasing effect of TRH is also blunted in such animals and is reminiscent of the blunted PRL response to TRH reported in post-menopausal depressed subjects (see previous section).

The failure of TRH to stimulate GH release _in vivo_ from the intact pituitary may involve somatostatin since passive immunization with somatostatin antiserum allows a TRH-induced GH rise to occur in the rat (47). Paradoxically, TRH has a central inhibitory effect on GH secretion for it prevents the sleep induced GH rise in normal humans (10). Overall these findings suggest that with respect to GH, TRH has a predominant effect on the CNS, probably via somatostatin to inhibit GH release from the adenohypophysis; however, when the central aminergic and/or peptidergic pathways are interrupted as postulated to occur in depression, the normal weaker stimulatory effect on the adenohypophysis becomes manifest. Whether somatostatin deficiency is the proximal cause of the GH response to TRH in depression is not known. A primary defect in hypothalamic somatostatin release, however, cannot account for the blunted TSH response in unipolar depression so that some additional factor in this sub-group such as increased turnover of the tuberoinfundibular dopaminergic system would need to be postulated in addition.

GONADOTROPIN SECRETION IN DEPRESSION

In post-menopausal women with unipolar depression, serum LH levels have been reported to be significantly lower than age matched controls (1). Studies in experimental animals suggest that this lowered LH is a consequence of hypothalamic NE deficiency since this monoamine appears to regulate hypothalamic LH-RH secretion. In gonadectomized female rats, administration of a blocker to DA β-hydroxylase (the enzyme responsible for the conversion of DA to NE) lowers LH levels. However, if such rats are then given dihydroxyphenylserine (DOPS), a direct precursor of NE, the circulating LH levels increase (45), presumably due to increased hypothalamic secretion of LH-RH, so that the decapeptide may be viewed as being under dual catecholaminergic regulation - DA being inhibitory and NE stimulatory to LH-RH release. Thus, the altered monoamine metabolism of depression is sufficient to account for the reduced LH levels in post-menopausal depressed women - though a number of other brain substances including prolactin, opioid peptides, and prostaglandins, known to affect LH-RH regulation (71) may additionally be disturbed in depression.

There is little data on LH-RH stimulation tests in depression. Ettigi et al. (15) infused LH-RH along with TRH to a group of males with primary unipolar depression and a group of males with secondary depression (depression preceded by a specific psychiatric disorder of another type). The LH response appeared normal in patients with unipolar depression but was much greater in the secondary depressives. The testosterone levels were subsequently reported to be similar in both groups (15a). The significance of this study in relation to the neurotransmitter regulation of the hypothalamic-pituitary-gonadal axis in various subsets of depression remains uncertain. In general however, the experience of many workers from different laboratories indicates that the gonadotropin response to LH-RH reflects the recent sex hormone status of the subject and poorly discriminates between pituitary and hypothalamic disorders (42). It appears doubtful to the author that LH-RH testing will make a significant contribution to our understanding of neuroendocrine regulation in depression.

SUMMARY

Altered metabolism of TRH, a neural peptide, which may form an endogenous brain ergotropic system, could be responsible for the disturbed biogenic amine metabolism in depression. Impaired dexamethasone suppression in this condition likely reflects increased hypothalamic CRF drive as a consequence of NE deficiency and/or 5-HT and ACh excess. The blunted TSH rise following TRH administration is not specific, but in the appropriate clinical setting has become a "chemical marker" for depression particularly of the unipolar type. The possible causes for this TSH response include changes in peripheral hormone (T4, cortisol) levels, hypothalamic or brain neural peptide (TRH, somatostatin, neurotensin) turnover, or biogenic amine (DA) metabolism. PRL responsivity to TRH stimulation is less clearly defined in affective disorders but the blunted rise reported in post-menopausal depressed woment could result from increased hypothalamic DA secretion. Studies in experimental animals suggest that the "paradoxic" GH rise to TRH in depression results from a "funtional disconnection" of the adenohypophysis from the rest of the brain, possibly due to the altered biogenic amine milieu in the CNS. This relative independence of the somatotrope from hypothalamic regulation (? somatostatin deficiency) may uncover normal 'weak' receptors on the somatotrope for TRH and lead to a GH rise. The lowered LH levels found in post-menopausal depressed females may be a consequence of NE deficiency which leads to reduced secretion of LH-RH from the hypothalamus.

ACKNOWLEDGEMENTS

Supported in part by NIH Grant AM 21863.

REFERENCES

1. Altman, N., Sachar, E., Gruen, P. H., Halpern, F. S. and Eto, S. (1975): Psychosom. Med. 37:274-276.
2. Asberg, M., Thoren, P., Traskman, L., Bertilson, L. and Ringberger, V. (1976): Science 191:478-480.
3. Asnis, G. M., Nathan, R. S., Halbreich, U., Halpern, f.S.H. and Sachar, E. J. (1980): Lancet 1:424-425.
4. Berelowitz, M., Szabo, J., Frohman, L. A., Firestone, S. and Chu, L. (1981): Science 212:1279-1281.
5. Besses, G. S., Burrow, G. N. and Spaulding, S. W. (1975): J. Clin. Endocrinol. Metab. 41:985-989.
6. Beumont, P.J.V., George, G.C.W., Pimstone, B. L. and Vinik, A. I. (1976): J. Clin. Endocrinol. Metab. 43:487-496.
7. Boler, J., Enzmann, F., Folkers, K., Bowers, C. Y. and Schally, A.V. (1969): Biochem. Biophys. Res. Comm. 37:705-710.
8. Brazeau, P., Vale, W., Burgus, R., Ling, N., Butcher, M., Rivier, J. and Guillemin, R. (1973): Science 179:77-79.
9. Burgus, R., Dunn, T., Desiderio, D. and Guillemin, R. (1969): C.R. Acad. Sci. (Paris) 269:1870-1873.
10. Chichara, K., Kato, Y., Maeda, K., Abe, H., Furomoto, M. and Imura, H. (1977): J. Clin. Endocrinol. Metab. 44:1094-1100.
11. Cobb, W. E., Reichlin, S. and Jackson, I.M.D. (1981): J. Clin. Endocrinol. Metab. 52:324-329.
12. Cohen, K. L. and Swigar, M. E. (1979): J. Am. Med. Assoc. 242: 254-257.
13. Czernichow, P., Dauzet, m. C., Broyer, M. and Rappaport, R. (1976): J. Clin. Endocrinol. Metab. 43:630-637.
14. Dasmahapatra, A., Urdanivia, E. and Cohen, M. P. (1981): J. Clin. Endocrinol. Metab. 52:859-862.
15. Ettigi, P. G., Brown, G. M. and Seggie, J. A. (1979): Psychosom. Med. 41:203-208.
15a. Ettigi, P. G. and Brown, G. M. (1979): In: Neuroendocrine Correlates in Neurology and Psychiatry, edited by E. E. Muller and A. Agnoli, pp.225-238. Elsevier/North Holland Biomedical Press, Amsterdam.
16. de la Fuente, J. R. and Rosenbaum, A. H. (1979): Mayo Clinic Proc. 54:109-118.
17. Furlong, F. W., Brown, G. M. and Beeching, M. F. (1976): Am. J. Psychiatry 133:1187-1190.

18. Gardner, D. F., Kaplan, M. M., Stanley, C. A. and Utiger, R. D. (1979): New Engl. J. Med. 300:579-584.
19. Gold, M. S., Pottash, A.L.C., Davies, R.K., Ryan, N., Sweeney, D. R. and Martin, D. M. (1979): Lancet 2:411-412.
20. Gold, P. W., Goodwin, F. K., Weher, T. and Rebar, R. (1978): Am. J. Psychiatry 134:1028-1032.
21. Hamada, N., Uoi, K., Nishizawa, Y., Okamoto, T., Hasegawa, K., Morii, H. and Wada, M. (1976): Endocrinol. Japon 23:5-10.
22. Hershman, J. M. (1974): New Engl. J. Med. 290:886-890.
23. Hinkle, P. M., Perrone, M. H. and Schonbrunn, A. (1981): Endocrinology 108:199-205.
24. Jackson, I.M.D. (1979): In: Hormones and Evolution, edited by E.J. W. Barrington, pp.723-789. Academic Press, London.
25. Jackson, I.M.D. (1980): Brain Res. 201:245-248.
26. Jackson, I.M.D. (1980): In: The Pituitary Adenoma, edited by K. D. Post, I.M.D. Jackson and S. Reichlin, pp.219-238. Plenum Press, New York.
27. Jackson, I.M.D. and Reichlin, S. (1979): In: Central Nervous System Effects of Hypothalamic Hormones and Other Peptides, edited by R. Collu, A. Barbeau, J. R. Ducharme and J.-G. Rochefort, pp.3-54. Raven Press, New York.
28. Jones, M. T., Hillhouse, E. and Burden, J. (1976): In: Frontiers in Neuroendocrinology, edited by L. Martini and W. F. Ganong, pp. 195-226. Raven Press, New York.
29. Kirkegaard, C. and Carroll, B. J. (1980): Psychiatry Res. 3:253-264.
30. Kirkegaard, C., Faber, J., Hummer, L. and Rogowski, P. (1979): Psychoneuroendocrinology 4:227-235.
31. Kirkegaard, C., Norlem, N., Lauridsen, U. B., Bjorum, N. and Christiansen, C. 91975): Arch. Gen. Psychiat. 32:115-118.
32. Linkowski, P., Brauman, H. and Mendlewica, J. (1980): Psychiat. Res. 3:265-271.
33. Loosen, P. T., Prange, A. J., Jr. and Wilson, I. C. (1978): Am. J. Psychiat. 135:244-246.
34. MacLeod, R. M. and Scapagnini, U., editors (1980): In: Central and Peripheral Regulation of Prolactin Function. Raven Press, New York.
35. Maeda, K. and Frohman, L. A. (1978): Endocrinology 103:1903-1909.
36. Maeda, K., Kato, Y., Ohgo, S. Chihara, K., Yoshimoto, Y., Yamaguchi, N., Kuromaru, S. and Imura, H. (1975): J. Clin. Endocrinol. Metab. 40:501-505.
37. Maeda, K., Kato, Y., Yamaguchi, N., Chihara, K., Ohgo, S., Iwasaki, Y., Yoshimoto, Y., Moridera, K., Kuromaru, S. and Imura, H. (1976): Acta Endocrinol. (Kbb) 8:1-8.
38. Maeda, K., Tanimoto, K., Yamaguchi, N., Iwasaki, Y., Chihara, K. and Fujita, T. (1979): New Engl. J. Med. 301:1400.
39. Malthe-Sorenssen, D., Wood, P. L., Cheney, D. L. and Costa, E. (1978): J. Neurochem. 31:685-691.
40. Metcalf, G. and Dettmar, P. W. (1981): Lancet 1:586-589.
41. Morley, J. E., Shafer, R. B., Elson, M. K., Slag, M. F., Raleigh, M. J., Brammer, G. L., Yuwiler, A. and Hershman, J. M. (1980): Ann. Int. Med. 93:707-709.
42. Mortimer, C. H. (1977): Clinics in Endocrinol. Metab. 6:167-179.
43. Müller, E. E., Panerai, A. E., Cocchi, D., Gil-Ad, I., Rossi, G. L. and Olgiatti, V. R. (1977): Endocrinology 100:1663-1671.
44. Müller, E. E., Salerno, F., Cocchi, D., Locatelli, V. and Panerai, A. E. (1979): Clin. Endocrinol. 11:645-656.
45. Ojeda, S. R. and McCann, S. M. (1973): Neuroendocrinology 12: 295-315.

46. Otsuki, M., Dakoda, M. and Baba, S. (1973): J. Clin. Endocrinol. Metab. 36:95-102.
47. Panerai, A. E., Giannattasio, G., Zanini, A., Melolesi, J., Rossi, G. L. and Muller, E. E. (1977): Program 59th Meeting Endocrine Society, Abstract 144, Chicago, Ill.
48. Panerai, A. E., Salerno, F., Manneschi, M., Cocchi, D. and Muller, E. E. (1977): J. Clin. Endocrinol. Metab. 45:134-140.
49. Plotnikoff, N. P., Prange, A. J., Breese, G. R., Anderson, M. S. and Wilson, I. C. (1972): Science 178:417-418.
50. Prange, A. J., Jr., Nemeroff, C. B., Loosen, P. T., Bissette, G., Osbahr, A. J., III, Wilson, I. C. and Lipton, M. A. (1979): In: Central Nervous Systems Effects of Hypothalamic Hormones and Other Peptides, edited by R. Collu, A. Barbeau, J. R. Ducharme and J.-G. Rochefort, pp.75-96. Raven Press, New York.
51. Ramey, J. N., Burrow, G. N. and Spaulding, S. (1976): J. Clin. Endocrinol. Metab. 43:107-114.
52. Reichlin, S., Martin, J. B. and Jackson, I.M.D. (1978): In: The Endocrine Hypothalamus, edited by S. L. Jeffcoate and J.S.M. Hutchinson, pp.230-269. Academic Press, New York.
53. Root, A. W., Snyder, P. J., Rezvani, I., DiGeorge, A. M. and Utiger, R. D. (1973): J. Clin. Endocrinol. Metab. 36:103-107.
54. Saffran, M. and Schally, A. V. (1955): Can. J. Biochem. 33:408-415.
55. Sawin, C. T. (1976): Pharmac. Ther. C. 1:351-366.
56. Scanlon, M. F., Weightman, D. R., Shale, D. J., Mora, B., Heath, M., Snow, M. H., Lewis, M. and Hall, R. (1979): Clin. Endocrinol. 10: 7-15.
57. Schally, A. V. (1978): Science 202:18-28.
58. Schildkraut, J. (1969): New Engl. J. Med. 281:197-201, 248-252, 302-306.
59. Schildkraut, J. (1978): In: Psychopharmacology: A Generation of Progress, edited by M. A. Lipton, A. Dimascio and K. F. Killam, pp.1223. Raven Press, New York.
60. Schlesser, M. A., Winokur, G. and Sherman, B. M. (1979): Lancet 1:739-741.
61. Sheppard, M. C., Kronheim, S. and Pimstone, B. L. (1978): Clin. Endocrinol. 9:583-586.
62. Siler, T. M., Yen, S.S.C., Vale, W. and Guillemin, R. (1974): J. Clin. Endocrinol. Metab. 38:742-745.
63. Snyder, P. J., Jacobs, L. S., Rabello, M. M., Sterling, F. H., Shore, R. N., Utiger, R. D. and Daughaday, W. H. (1974): Ann. Int. Med. 81:751-757.
64. Snyder, P. J. and Utiger, R. D. (1972): J. Clin. Endocrinol. Metab. 34:380-385.
65. Snyder, P. J. and Utiger, R. D. (1973): J. Clin. Invest. 52: 2305-2312.
66. Snyder, S. H. (1980): Science 209:976-983.
67. Sobue, I., Yamamoto, H., Konagaya, M., Iida, M. and Takayanagi, T. (1980): Lancet 1:418-419.
68. Vale, W., Spiess, J., Rivier, C. and Rivier, J. (1981): Science 213:1394-1397.
69. Wurtman, R. J. (1971): Neurosci. Res. Progr. Bull. 9:172-297.
70. Yarbrough, G. G. (1979): Prog. in Neurobiol. 12:291-312.
71. Yen, S.S.C. (1979): Hosp. Practice 14:83-97.

Neuroendocrinology and Psychiatric Disorder, edited by G. M. Brown, et al. Raven Press, New York 1984.

Assessment and Significance of Rhythm Disruptions in Affective Illness

Benjamin Rusak

Affective illnesses are often characterized by altered patterns of physiological function, including endocrine activity (17, 22, 27, 29, 30, 40, 42, 46). There are several reasons for evaluating these changes from the perspective of biological rhythms research. The first reason is that endocrine systems are generally rhythmic (2; Fig. 1) and their temporal structure is likely to be physiologically significant. For example, an increase in prolactin (PRL) levels at some phases of the daily cycle promotes fat deposition and gonadal changes in a number of vertebrate species, but the same treatment at other phases is ineffective (25). Melatonin injections can cause gonadal regression in photoperiodic species only at some circadian phases (44a). In general, the behavioural and physiological impact of altered hormone levels may depend on the presence of other hormones, on levels of neurotransmitters, and on other physiological parameters that vary with a daily rhythm.

Even a hormone such as luteinizing hormone (LH), the level of which may not fluctuate with a pronounced daily cycle in adult humans (but see 2), is released episodically. It has been suggested that the episodic character of LH release maintains LH receptor sensitivity of the gonads, since constant physiological levels of LH reduce gonadal responsiveness (5). Assessments of endocrine function that include measurements of hormone levels but fail to consider temporal aspects of hormone availability may ignore physiologically important information.

A second reason for concern with temporal patterns of hormone secretion is that erroneous conclusions about changes in hormone levels may result from sampling endocrine activity in populations with similar mean levels but altered rhythms of hormone release. A pathological condition or drug treatment that alters phasing of a daily rhythm can readily confound a research design that involves sampling at only one daily phase. Advances or delays in a rhythm relative to clock time may lead to mistaken conclusions that hormone levels have either increased or decreased, depending on the time of sampling. Fig. 2 illustrates a hypothetical example in which a phase shift can result in opposite conclusions both of which are erroneous.

A number of discrepant reports on hormonal levels in depression have been published. PRL levels are reported to be elevated or reduced in depression (4, 24) and PRL responses to thyrotropin releasing hormone have been described in different studies as "[e]levated, normal and blunted" (24). Consideration of the daily phase of sampling and the use of rhythm profiles rather than single measurements are particularly important in studies of affective disorders, since there are many suggestions in the literature that sleep, cortisol and other physiological rhythms are phase shifted during depression (17, 22, 29, 30, 36).

The possibility that rhythms in depressed patients are phase-shifted

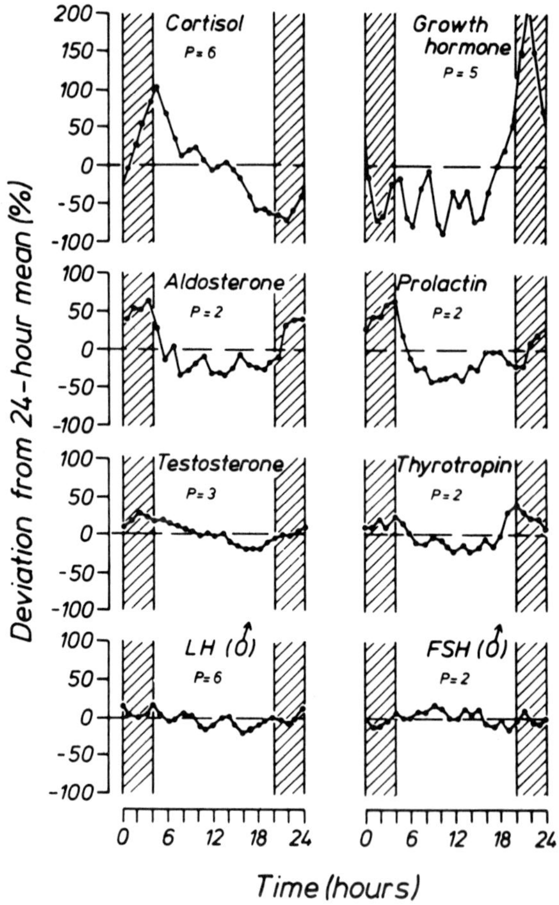

FIG. 1. A variety of daily endocrine rhythms in humans, compiled by Aschoff (2). Copyright, 1979, Raven Press. Reprinted by permission.

creates a problem for the analysis of endocrine responses to drug treatment even when daily profiles of endocrine activity are obtained. In the dexamethasone (DEX) suppression test, the drug is typically given near midnight and suppression of corticosteroid (CS) secretion measured at intervals thereafter; depression is associated with the escape of cortisol release from DEX suppression (36). There is evidence that the amplitude of stress-induced CS release under DEX suppression varies with the time of day of DEX administration in rats (9). Researchers should be alert to the possibility that drugs administered at a single clock time might have different effects in patients and controls because a phase shift in patients ensures that they are, in fact, treated at a different physiological time.

A third reason for studying endocrine rhythms is the possibility that they will reveal abnormalities in circadian regulatory mechanisms which play a role in the etiology of disorders such as bipolar affective illness. The inherent cyclicity of the illness (35, 48), the reported constraint on the daily phase at which mood switches occur (41), and the occasional appearance of 48hr cycles of mood change (6, 35), all hint at the involvement of physiological oscillatory processes. In addition, many treatments that are useful in alleviating the symptoms of affective disorders also have a significant impact on circadian mechanisms (see below).

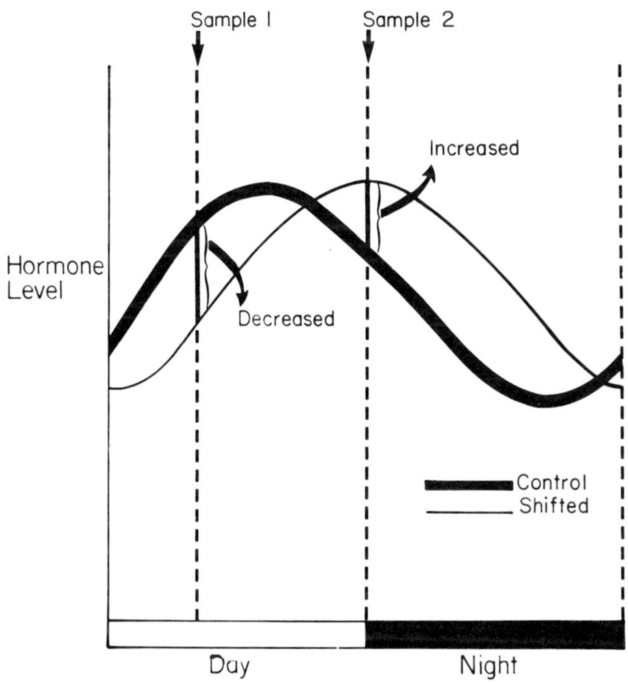

FIG. 2. A phase difference between two populations can give the erroneous impression of a change in hormone levels. In this hypothetical example an endocrine rhythm in a clinical population is phase shifted relative to control subjects. Although mean hormonal levels are similar in the two groups, single samples drawn at different times may lead to the conclusion that levels are decreased or increased in the clinical population.

In summary, assessment of endocrine rhythm disorders in depression is important for several reasons: (1) Since the rhythmicity of endocrine function is itself physiologically significant, the detection of abnormal rhythms of endocrine activity is as important a goal as the detection of abnormal levels. (2) A daily profile of hormone levels provides a more reliable index to the level of endocrine function than any single measure, particularly if an illness is associated with changes in rhythm phasing and wave form. (3) The intrinsic rhythmicity of bipolar affective illness and its characteristic rhythm abnormalities suggest that biological rhythms may be important in the etiology of the illness.

ASSESSING ENDOCRINE RHYTHMICITY

The analysis of endocrine rhythms depends on the use of appropriate research designs and statistical tests. But the choice of research designs and statistical tools depend in turn on the researcher's model of the system being studied. If one conceives of the endocrine system as being in a homeostatically regulated steady-state, a single, arbitrarily timed sample of its function may seem adequate. If one conceives of it as subject to episodic, ultradian, and circadian fluctuations in activity (2), samples obtained every 20 min over several days will seem barely adequate to characterize its behaviour. An analysis of the issues involved in assessing disrupted rhythms should, therefore, begin with a statement of our current conception of the mechanisms regulating normal circadian rhythms.

1. Circadian Control of Endocrine Activity

The presence of a hormonal rhythm can be demonstrated by samplig circulating levels throughout a 24 hr period. It is generally assumed, although not often established, that these regular daily rhythms are the product of an endogenous circadian mechanism. A rigorous demonstration of circadian involvement requires evidence that the rhythm persists (free-runs) under constant environmental conditions with a period near 24 hr. The function of temporal cues in the natural environment, predominantly lighting cycles, is to synchronize otherwise freerunning rhythms to an exact 24 hr period (entrainment). Adrenal corticosteroid (CS) secretion in rodents is a well-studied example of a true circadian rhythm (13) that can be used to illustrate the complexity of the intact system and the difficulties inherent in studying disrupted rhythms.

In mammals, both the generation and photic synchronization of circadian rhythms, including that of CS secretion, depend on the integrity of the hypothalamic suprachiasmatic nuclei (SCN). The results of a variety of studies involving ablations, electrical stimulation, and recording of neural and metabolic activity in the SCN are consistent with the conclusion that the SCN function as a dominant oscillator in the mammalian circadian system (28, 38, 39). However, this conclusion conceals a great deal of the complexity of the intact system that is relevant to understanding the characteristics of disrupted rhythms.

Despite the critical role of the SCN, there is evidence from studies in both rodents and primates that circadian oscillators exist outside the SCN as well (19, 28a, 37). In fact, the circadian system of mammals is best understood as a complex of mutually and hierarchically coupled oscillators (33). The function of the SCN appears to be to maintain the integrity of a population of partially autonomous oscillators in the nervous system (37, 38). The mechanisms that intervene between this oscillator complex and particular effector systems are virtually unexplored. In order to produce a daily CS rhythm, the activity of neurons containing corticotrophin-releasing factor (CRF) must ultimately be regulated by a light-entrained SCN rhythm, but it is not known whether this control is direct or mediated through other oscillator systems, nor whether CRF neurons also show a degree of intrinsic rhythmicity (18).

The pulsatile character of the release of many hormones, including CRF, (18) adds still another aspect to the mechanisms regulating CS rhythms. The circadian input to this system probably acts either by shortening the period or by increasing the amplitude of a high-frequency oscillation in CRF activity. In addition, the possibility exists that circadian rhythmicity is an intrinsic feature of other levels in the neuroendocrine axis connecting the hypothalamus to the adrenals. Circadian rhythms of CS secretion persist in hamster adrenal glands cultured in vitro under constant conditions (1).

Given the complexity of the mechanisms that generate normal endocrine rhythms, the observation of a disrupted rhythm in CS secretion in a clinical disorder is susceptible to a variety of interpretations. Causes of the abnormal rhythms may range from defects in central mechanisms responsible for rhythm generation and entrainment to changes in adrenal rhythms of sensitivity to trophic hormones or other inputs. As an indication of problems of interpretation encountered in the analysis of clinically observed rhythm disorders, it may be useful to examine a situation in which circadian rhythms are disrupted experimentally.

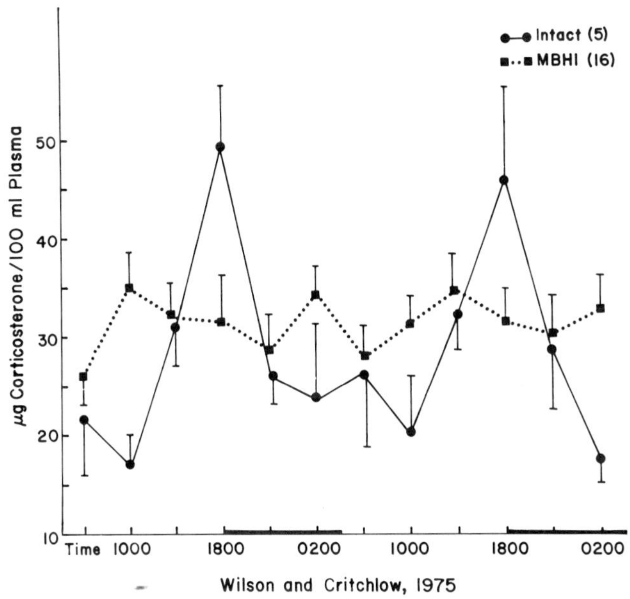

FIG. 3. Daily patterns of circulating corticosterone levels in intact rats and in rats with knife cuts that isolate the medial basal hypothalamus (MBHI). The 10 hr daily dark phase is indicated by the dark bars on the abscissa. Grouped data from MBHI rats does not show a rhythm in corticosterone levels. From Wilson and Critchlow (50); copyright, 1975, S. Karger AG. Reprinted by permission.

2. Suprachiasmatic Lesions and Rhythm Disruptions

Ablation of the SCN eliminates the capacity for the generation of intact circadian rhythms and severely disrupts photic entrainment (28, 39). Similar effects are produced by knife cuts that separate the SCN from the mediobasal hypothalamus (MBH) (28, 50). The daily pattern expressed as mean values of circulating CS levels measured in a group of rats with such knife cuts appears to be flat (Fig. 3). However, serial blood samples taken repeatedly from individual rats over 44 hr periods show excursions of CS levels which are as large as those of controls, but which are not phased appropriately or consistently with respect to the illumination cycle (50; Fig. 4).

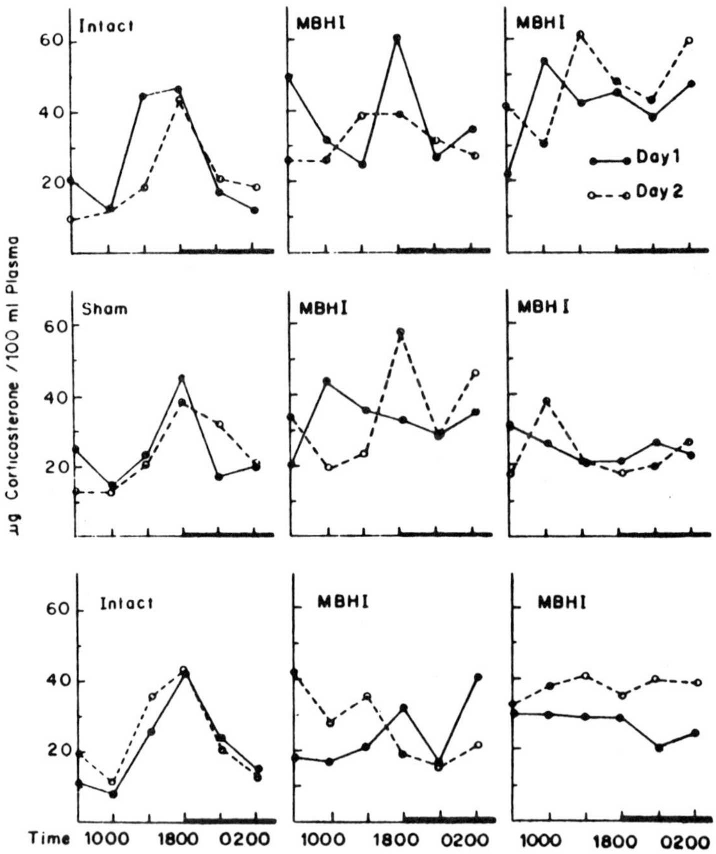

FIG. 4. Daily patterns of circulating corticosterone (CS) sampled repeatedly from individual rats. Intact and sham-operated rats have clear daily CS rhythms; rats with isolations of the medial basal hypothalamus (MBHI) generally have excursions of CS levels which are as large as those of intact animals but which are inappropriately and unstably phased relative to the LD cycle indicated on the abscissa. Compare to Figure 3. From Wilson and Critchlow (50); copyright, 1975, S. Karger AG. Reprinted by permission.

These observations eliminate the possibility that after MBH isolations CS is secreted at a uniform intermediate rate throughout the day, but they do not discriminate among a number of other possibilities. The lack of normal rhythmicity may reflect any of several mechanisms: failure of entrainment of circadian and ultradian oscillators; adrenal responses to an unentrained endogenous oscillator combined with the exogenous influence of photic or other rhythmic inputs; or dissociations among a number of oscillators, perhaps at different levels of physiological control. The 44 hr sampling time used in this study is too brief to permit tests of these hypotheses.

Sampling CS from rodents for a longer period of time may not be possible, but long-term, continuous recordings can be obtained for behavioural rhythms, such as that of activity. Although behavioural and endocrine rhythms are undoubtedly subject to different intervening control mechanisms, both are affected by SCN lesions, and the technical advantages of behavioural rhythms make them a useful source of ideas about the nature of the physiological consequences of SCN lesions. A few of the generalizations that have emerged from research on SCN lesions and behavioural rhythms may be relevant to understanding the nature of rhythm disruptions in general (see 28, 39 for reviews).

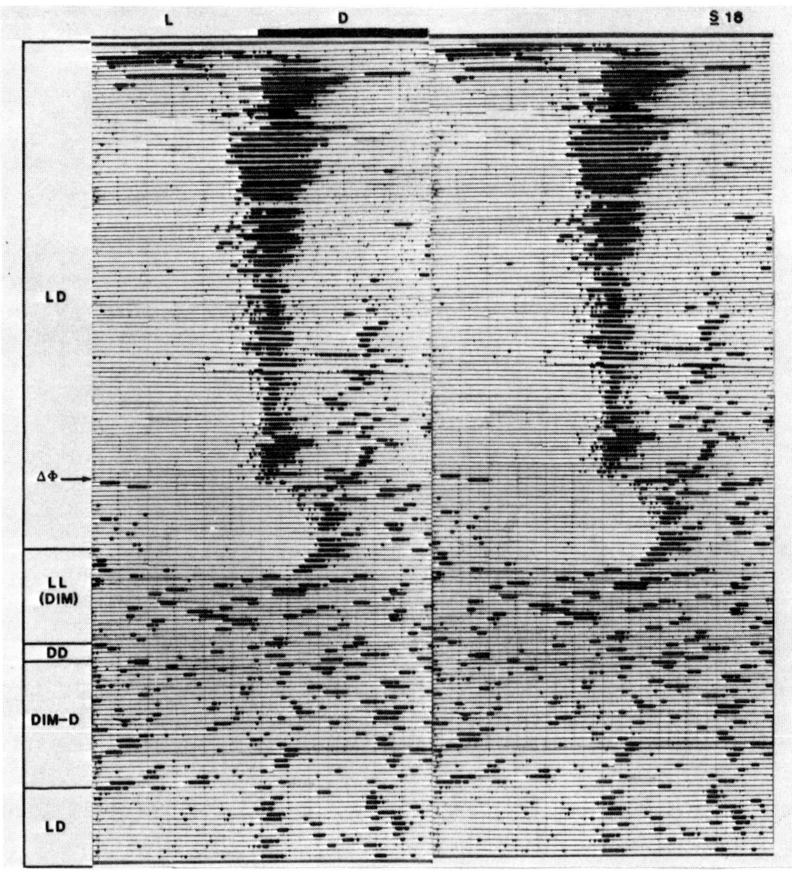

FIG. 5. Wheel-running activity record of a hamster with a lesion of the suprachiasmatic nuclei. The 24 hr record is double-plotted with the original light-dark (LD) cycle indicated above the record. The LD cycle is delayed by 4 hr ($\Delta\Phi$) and then changed to constant dim illumination (LL), constant darkness (DD) and to a low-contrast cycle (DIM-D) before the original LD cycle is restored. The hamster's activity synchronizes to the LD cycle but the rhythm breaks down in constant conditions. The breakdown results from a dissociation among oscillators with different periods that follows the imposition of constant lighting (LL). From Rusak (37); copyright, 1977, Springer Verlag. Reprinted by permission.

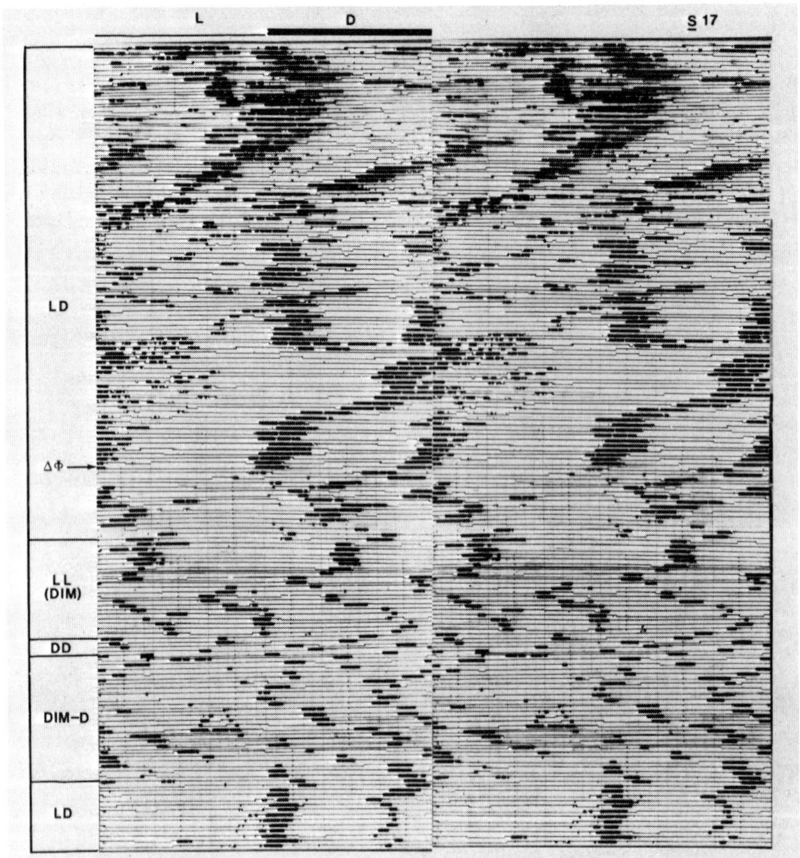

FIG. 6. Activity record of a hamster with a lesion of the suprachiasmatic nuclei. For details, see Figure 5. The hamster's activity is sometimes unstably synchronized to the lighting cycle but it is characterized by the appearance of multiple rhythmic components that are not integrated into a stable circadian pattern. From Rusak (37); copyright, 1977, Springer Verlag. Reprinted by permission.

First, the mammalian circadian system is comprised of multiple oscillators; rhythm disruptions appear to reflect a lack of normal integration among these oscillators (Fig. 5). Second, the dissociations and interactions that occur among other oscillators after SCN ablation are unstable and generate a variety of changing patterns over time (Fig. 6). Finally, external rhythmic events may resynchronize oscillators and restore some overt rhythms. For example, illumination cycles can synchronize activity in some SCN-ablated hamsters (37; Fig. 5) and food restriction cycles can synchronize CS secretion in SCN-ablated rats (19).

Depressed people and SCN-ablated rodents are obviously different, but the conclusions about disrupted rodent rhythms can provide some important lessons for the analysis of endocrine activity in depressed people. One clear lesson is that when rhythm disruptions are suspected it is essential to examine data from individuals before grouping data from a population that may be heterogeneous. If rhythm disruptions are characterized by idiosyncratically unstable coupling among oscillators and partial synchronization to environmental cycles, grouped data will obscure the individual patterns. The result will be a flat group curve that may not reflect the data from any individual in that group.

Ideally, data from individuals should be collected over a fairly long period of time. It is possible to monitor behavioural and some physiological rhythms in people continuously for many days. If data collection can only be continued for a few days, it is important to repeat the measurements at intervals to assess the stability of any observed pattern. Finally, an ideal study would permit assessment of rhythms in both the presence and absence of a variety of potential external synchronizers. This procedure can help discriminate rhythm abnormalities attributable to the rhythm generating mechanism from those attributable to the mechanisms of external synchronization.

3. Problems of Analysis

Meeting all of these criteria in clinical studies is difficult and expensive. Among the technical problems are those of obtaining a sufficiently detailed record of physiological activity over a long period and of collecting these data from appropriate control subjects and patients under similar conditions. Finding an appropriate control population is critical, especially when studying endocrine rhythms which are likely to be influenced by variables such as age, sex, reproductive status, daily routine and history of drug exposure. The use of a within-subjects design may be helpful in controlling for these factors, but baseline measures on appropriate control subjects are still necessary for interpretation of the results.

When continuous longitudinal monitoring of an individual is not feasible, the use of a single cross-sectional assessment of endocrine patterns in a potentially heterogeneous group should at least be abandoned in favour of repeated assessments in individuals over a number of weeks. Whatever necessary compromises are made, the strength of the conclusions drawn should reflect the degree to which the experimental design has approached the ideal.

Another issue in experimental design is the use of descriptive and inferential statistics to assess rhythmicity. There are a variety of methods available which may be more or less appropriate depending on the quantity and form of the data to be analyzed (11, 43). Some analytic methods are useful only for long time series, so there has been considerable interest in the development of techniques for assessing rhythmicity in short time series such as might be readily obtained in a clinical setting (7, 43). The danger in the uncritical application of these methods to the analysis of rhythm disorders is that disrupted rhythms are unlikely to be stationary in time. A rhythm whose amplitude measured over a single cycle meets the criteria for statistical significance might not be representative of any longer interval that might be sampled.

This problem can be illustrated in an experimentally induced disruption of normal cycles. If one were to choose for analysis a single day or even a few days from the activity record of an SCN-ablated hamster, one could find statistically significant 24 hr or 12 hr rhythms or a lack of significant rhythmicity (Fig. 6). None of these cross-sectional assessments provides a very useful description of the status of the animal's circadian system. The unstable patterns generated by the interactions of a population of oscillators that do not maintain normal phase relations to each other or to environmental cycles are only detectable in a detailed longitudinal profile.

Rhythm disruptions in affective illness probably reflect uncoupling or unusual coupling among oscillators and environmental synchronizers. The analysis of these rhythms should begin with long-term recordings that will permit a detailed description of rhythm abnormalities, their persistence and stability over time. These descriptive data can give insights into which research designs and statistical techniques would be most useful for determining where in the complex hierarchy of endocrine and circadian control mechanisms the critical defects occur.

ETIOLOGY OF AFFECTIVE DISORDERS

1. The Hypothesis of Circadian Involvement

Any physiological characteristic that distinguishes patients with affective illness from a control population is of interest because of its potential for use in diagnosis and treatment choice. But the most exciting possibility is that the distinguishing characteristic, for example, rhythm abnormalities, might be a primary manifestation of the mechanism that also generates the behavioural and affective symptoms. Since the possibility that changes in physiological oscillators may be involved in the etiology of affective disorders has been raised repeatedly (20, 32, 35, 48), it is worth considering some of the evidence that has led to this suggestion.

The idea that biological oscillators are involved in affective illness is undoubtedly derived from the cyclicity of symptoms displayed, particularly by patients with bipolar illness (35). The regularity of the attacks of depression and mania and their apparent independence from environmental factors suggest that the illness is endogenously triggered and that internal timing mechanisms are involved. The reported rhythm in timing of mood switches (41), the sleep abnormalities seen in depression (22, 32, 42), and the disruption of other daily rhythms (17, 26, 27, 29, 30, 46) also contribute to the hypothesis of circadian involvement.

These observations do not alone provide very strong support for the hypothesis. The timing of mood switches may reflect a non-specific influence of rhythms in endocrine and neural activity that modulate the probability of mood changes on a daily basis. The timing constraint need not imply that disrupted circadian oscillators are critical components of the mood-switching mechanism. The rhythm abnormalities of depressed patients may prove to be important but they have not been well documented. In many studies appropriate control procedures were not used, so it is uncertain which of the reported abnormalities are independent of prior or concurrent drug exposure, age, sex, activity level and other variables (17, 26, 27, 29, 46).

Other evidence relevant to the proposition that abnormal circadian rhythms are involved in affective illness is provided by consideration of the treatments that ameliorate the condition. One such treatment is the administration of lithium salts which reduces endogenous mood swings in some patients. The fact that lithium also slows circadian oscillations (21) led Kripke to suggest that abnormally fast circadian oscillations in some physiological functions may be the target of the lithium effects (20).

His hypothesis suggests that unusual phase relations among oscillators engendered by the fast freerun of some rhythms and the stable entrainment of others trigger mood changes in susceptible individuals. The observation that affective illness is more common in older people is consistent with the evidence that they are more susceptible to internal desynchronization among rhythms during temporal and social isolation (49). It is possible that a change in the frequency of circadian rhythms with age is involved since there is evidence for an age-related increase in frequency of rhythms in some mammals (34). In support of his hypothesis, Kripke presented preliminary evidence that some rhythms appear to freerun in manic-depressives under conditions that should be adequate to entrain normal circadian oscillators(20).

Another treatment that has been reported to improve symptoms of depression is total sleep deprivation or selective REM deprivation (8, 12, 16, 23, 31, 32, 44, 47). Although the results obtained in different studies have been inconsistent, a large number of severely depressed patients show at least transient mood improvement after sleep deprivation (8, 12, 16). It is surprising that a treatment which may produce mild dysphoria in healthy subjects should produce any improvement in severely depressed patients (12, 16).

Various mechanisms have been proposed to account for the therapeutic effects of sleep deprivation, including the resetting of abnormally phased circadian oscillators (31). The involvement of sleep-related oscillators is an attractive possibility because sleep abnormalities accompany depression and because chemical antidepressants also influence REM sleep (14). However, the transience of the observed improvement suggests either that the critical phase shifts are rapidly reversed or that temporary changes in another mechanism are responsible for mood improvement. One problem with the hypothesis is that there is little indication in the literature dealing with circadian rhythms that preventing overt expression of the sleep-wake cycle can feed back on and modify the phase of an underlying circadian oscillator, although one set of observations could be so interpreted (10).

Another therapeutic technique has been explored by Wehr et al. (48) based on their observation that sleep patterns change in patients cycling between depressed and manic states. They noted that the switch out of depression was accompanied by an advance of the beginning of activity, while depression was characterized by relatively delayed activity onsets. They mimicked the phase advance characteristic of mood improvement by forcing a shift of the sleep-wake cycle of a depressed patient and they observed marked, but transient, mood improvement.

An enforced change in sleep time in normal subjects does not improve mood, but has mild dysphoric effects, just as sleep deprivation does (12, 45). In each case, the effectiveness of the treatment does not depend on its general mood-elevating characteristics. The contrasting effects on depressed and normal people suggest rather that the treatments are influencing a specific mechanism that functions differently in the two groups. The possibility that these behavioural antidepressants operate through effects on circadian oscillators is strengthened by evidence that chemical antidepressants of different types, such as clorgyline and imipramine, also modify basic features of circadian organization in animals (52).

2. Testing the Hypothesis

These several lines of indirect evidence lead to the conclusion that the mechanisms that generate circadian rhythms and those that function abnormally in endogenous affective disorders are somehow closely linked. This conclusion is still far short of the assertion that circadian mechanisms are etiologically important in affective illness. The general hypothesis that some rhythms slip from normal entrainment and thereby periodically achieve abnormal phase relations to other internal rhythms will not be amenable to an adequate test until the relevant rhythms are identified. Both Kripke et al. (20) and Wehr et al. (48) found that changes in the phasing of body temperature rhythms tracked mood changes in their patients, but the significance of this observation has not been elucidated.

One attraction of the hypothesis that circadian abnormalities are etiologically important in affective illness is its emphasis on the functional importance of particular timing relations among endocrine and other physiological rhythms. The examples cited earlier of hormones having radically different effects at different daily phases (25, 44a) indicate the importance of temporal relations in the neuroendocrine system.

Another attractive feature of the hypothesis is its reliance on a plausible pathogenic mechanism: the breakdown of both environmental and mutual coupling of oscillators. There is evidence in both animals and people that coupling among oscillators in the mammalian circadian system can break down. The experimental examples of the loss of normal integration in the circadian system are attributable to unusual environmental conditions (15, 49) or to neural damage (37), but the likelihood that spontaneous dissociations occur under normal environmental conditions has hardly been explored.

Given the attractiveness of the hypothesis, it remains to be explained why treatments that presumably affect rhythms are not more successful. The transient and variable effectiveness of sleep deprivation and phase shifting probably reflect both the lack of specificity and the transient nature of the treatments. If some oscillators are phased abnormally because of their intrinsic periods, a treatment which shifts an observable rhythm such as sleep may incidentally bring the unidentified critical oscillators into appropriate phase relations, but with time they will re-establish their pathogenic phase relations because of their unchanged natural periods.

On the other hand, continuous lithium treatment may permanently lengthen the period of an oscillator with too short a natural period, but it will also lengthen the periods of other oscillators. In some patients, it may be impossible to find a dosage level that slows abnormal oscillators sufficiently without driving the periods of normal oscillators outside the limits that permit their stable entrainment. In other patients, the physician must identify the correct dosage without feedback from the unidentified rhythms whose phasing is presumably critical to achieving therapeutic results. It would obviously be useful to identify the systems that are functionally abnormal and to develop the necessary pharmaceutical, behavioural or dietary tools to affect those systems with some degree of specificity.

As a first step it will be necessary to monitor a large number of rhythms in patients and control subjects over long periods of time. These data will provide essential information about the functional clusters of rhythms as well as an indication of which rhythms fail to maintain stable phase relations to the environment and to each other. Coupled with an understanding of the basic neural and endocrine mechanisms that regulate these rhythms, this information should permit the development of treatments aimed as exclusively as possible at the regulators of the identified aberrant rhythms. It would be satisfying to find that those treatments that specifically correct the rhythm abnormalities are also effective antidepressants. However, even if the treatments were ineffective, their development and trial would be valuable in providing a more adequate test of the hypothesis of circadian involvement than has so far been possible.

CONCLUSIONS

The study of the neuroendocrine features of affective disorders in relation to biological rhythms is likely to confer a variety of benefits Among these are more reliable estimates of the levels of endocrine activity and more meaningful assessments of the functional integrity of the endocrine system.

It is also possible that research on rhythm disorders in patients and on the physiological mechanisms underlying normal rhythmicity will yield effective treatment paradigms based on the regulation of internal oscillators. Despite some indirect evidence for the importance of circadian abnormalities in the etiology of affective illness, this remains an exciting but uncertain possibility.

ACKNOWLEDGEMENT

Preparation of this chapter was aided by grant A-0305 from NSERC of Canada.

REFERENCES

1. Andrews, R. V. (1968): Comp. Biochem. Physiol. 26:179-193.
2. Aschoff, J. (1979): In: Endocrine Rhythms, edited by D. T. Krieger, pp.1-61. Raven Press, New York.
3. Boulos, Z., Rosenwasser, A. and Terman, M. (1980): Behav. Brain Res. 1:39-65.
4. Checkley, S. and Arendt, J. (1981): In: this volume.
5. Desjardins, C. (1981): Biol. Reprod. 24:1-21.
6. Dirlich, G., Kammerloher, A., Schulz, H., Lund, R., Doerr, P. and von Zerssen, D. (1981): Biol. Psychiat. 16:163-179.
7. Drescher, K., Timm, J., Rensing, L., Graf, G. and Cornelius, G. (1980): J. Interdiscipl. Cycle Res. 11:69-83.
8. Duncan, W. C., Jr., Gillin, J. C., Post, R. M., Gerner, R. H. and Wehr, T. A (1980): Biol. Psychiat. 15:879-889.
9. Dunn, J. D. and Carrillo, J. (1978): J. Endocr. 76:63-66.
10. Eastman, C. E. (1980): Circadian Rhythms of Temperature, Waking and Activity in the Rat: Dissociation, Desynchronizations and Disintegrations. Ph.D. Thesis, University of Chicago.
11. Enright, J. T. (1981): In: Handbook of Behavioural Neurobiology, Vol. 4, edited by J. Aschoff, pp.21-39. Plenum Press, New York.
12. Gerner, R. H., Post, R. M., Gillin, J. C. and Bunney, W. E., Jr. (1979): J. Psychiat. Res. 15:21-40.
13. Gibbs, F. P. (1976): Am. J. Physiol. 231:817-821.
14. Gillin, J. C., Wyatt, R. J., Fram, D. and Snyder, F. (1978): Psychopharmacology 59:267-272.
15. Hoffmann, K. (1971): In: Biochronometry, edited by M. Menaker, pp.134-146. Nat. Acad. Sci., washington.
16. King, D. (1977): Dis. Nerv. Syst. 38:873-879.
17. Kramer, B. A. and Katz, J. L. (1978): J. Clin. Psychiat. 39:439-444.
18. Krieger, D. T. (1979): In: Endocrine Rhythms, edited by D. T. Krieger, pp.123-142. Raven Press, New York.

19. Krieger, D. T., Hauser, H. and Krey, L. C. (1977): Science 197: 398-399.
20. Kripke, D. F., Mullaney, D. J., Atkinson, M. and Wolf, S. (1978): Biol. Psychiat. 13:335-351.
21. Kripke, D. F. and Wyborney, V. G. (1980): Life Sci. 26:1319-1321.
22. Kupfer, D. J. (1976): Biol. Psychiat. 11:159-174.
23. Kvist, J. and Kirkegaard, C. (1980): Acta Psychiat. Scand. 62: 494-502.
24. Linkowski, P., Brauman, H. and Mendlewicz, J. (1980): Psychiat. Res. 3:265-271.
25. Meier, A. H. (1975): In: Hormonal Correlates of Behaviour, Vol. 2, edited by B. Eleftheriou and R. L. Sprott, pp.469-549. Plenum Press, New York.
26. Mendlewicz, J., Van Cauter, E., Linkowski, P., L'Hermite, M. and Robyn, C. (1980): Life Sci. 27:2015-2024.
27. Moody, J. P. and Allsopp, M.N.E. (1969): Brit. J. Psychiat. 115: 923-928.
28. Moore, R. Y. (1979): In: Endocrine Rhythms, edited by D. T. Krieger, pp.63-87. Raven Press, New York.
28a. Moore-Ede, M. C., Lydic, R., Czeisler, C. A., Fuller, C. A. and Albers, H. E. (1980): Soc. Neurosci. Abst. 6:708.
29. Nikitopoulou, G. and Crammer, J. L. (1976): Brit. Med. J. 1: 1311-1314.
30. Niskanen, P., Nuttunen, M., Tamminen, T. and Jääskeläinen, J. (1976): Brit. J. Psychiat. 128:67-73.
31. Pflug, B. (1976): Acta Psychiat. Scand. 53:148-158.
32. Pflug, B. and Tölle, R. (1971): Int. Pharmacopsychiat. 6:187-196.
33. Pittendrigh, C. S. (1974): In: The Neurosciences: Third Study Program, edited by F. O. Schmitt and F. G. Worden, pp.437-458. MIT Press, Cambridge, Mass.
34. Pittendrigh, C. S. and Daan, S. (1974): Science 186:548-550.
35. Richter, C. P. (1965): Biological Clocks in Medicine and Psychiatry, Thomas, Springfield.
36. Rubin, R. T. and Poland, R. E. (1981): In: present volume.
37. Rusak, B. (1977): J. Comp. Physiol. 118:145-164.
38. Rusak, B. (1982): In: Vertebrate Circadian Systems; Structure and Physiology, edited by J. Aschoff, S. Daan, and G. Groos, pp.62-74. Springer, New York.
39. Rusak, B. and Zucker, I. (1979): Physiol. Rev. 59:449-526.
40. Sachar, E. J., Hellman, L., Roffwarg, H. P., Halpern, F. S., Fukushima, D. K. and Gallagher, T. F. (1973): Arch. Gen. Psychiat. 28:19-24.
41. Sitaram, N., Gillin, J. C. and Bunney, W. E., Jr. (1978): Acta Psychiat. Scand. 58:267-278.
42. Sitaram, N., Nurnberger, J. I., Jr., Gershon, E. S. and Gillin, J. C. (1980): Science 208:200-201.
43. Sollberger, A. (1970): J. Interdiscipl. Cycle Res. 1:49-88.
44. Svendson, K. (1976): Acta Psychiat. Scand. 54:184-192.
44a. Tamarkin, L., Westrom, W. K., Hamill, A. I. and Goldman, B. D. (1976): Endocrinology 99:1534-1541.
45. Taub, J. M. and Berger, R. J. (1974): Psychosomat. Med. 36:164-173.
46. Van Cauter, E. and Mendlewicz, J. (1978): Life Sci. 22:147-156.
47. Vogel, G. W., Vogel, F., McAbee, R. S. and Thurmond, A. J. (1980): Arch. Gen. Psychiat. 37:247-253.
48. Wehr, T. A., Wirz-Justice, A., Goodwin, F. K., Duncan, W. and Gillin, J. C. (1979): Science 206:710-713.

49. Wever, R. (1979): The Circadian System of Man. Springer, New York.
50. Wilson, M. M. and Critchlow, V. (1975): Neuroendocrinology 19: 185-192.
51. Wilson, M. M. and Greer, M. A. (1977): Proc. Soc. Exp. Biol. Med. 154:69-71.
52. Wirz-Justice, A., Wehr, T. A. and Groos, G. (1981): In: Vertebrate Circadian Systems: Structure and Physiology, edited by J. Aschoff, S. Daan, and G. Groos, pp.183-193. Springer, New York.

Neuroendocrinology and Psychiatric Disorder,
edited by G. M. Brown, et al.
Raven Press, New York 1984.

Discussion: Affective Disorders—Neural Mechanisms Underlying Endocrine Features

Seymour Reichlin

Bernard J. Carroll

Dr. Rusak suggested that phase shifting might be related to and was the basis of dexamethasone non-suppression in depressed individuals. Indeed, it is critical that you give the steroid at a specific period in the circadian cycle. This is not a new idea in the psychoendocrinology of depressed patients, as we tested that hypothesis back in 1968. The best estimate of phase advance is that it is about 3 hours - it could not possibly be greater than that. We administered dexamethasone at two times once at midnight and then once at 9.0 p.m. in the same group of patients, and found absolutely no difference in lack of suppressibility. So I think this really rules out phase shifting as an explanation of non-suppression.

I want to make one final comment on the dexamethasone test, related to Bob Rose's earlier question about the relationship between severity of illness and intensity of test abnormalities. In cross-sectional studies, we see no real relationship, although if you follow individual patients you will see some parallel improvement - both in severity and in the test results. It is important to underline that whatever this test is telling us, it is only indirect information about some disturbance in the limbic system. It is not directly linked to the etiology of the psychiatric disorder, and is only an indirect indicator. This explains the lack of relationship to severity - a little like having EEG recordings where the severity of the electrical disturbance does not really correlate with the severity of the behavioural disorder, such as in limbic epilepsy. This also means, I think, that ideas about two distinct sub-groups of patients that can be identified with this particular test should be held somewhat cautiously. It may be just the insensitivity of the tests that suggests that there are two distinct subgroups of patients.

John M. Davis

My comments relate to the quantitative nature of the dexamethasone suppression test. Dexamethasone suppression is abnormal in some depressed patients but not all. An important question is why the degrees of impairment does not correlate quantitatively with the degree of the depression? In the subtype which has dexamethasone abnormality, it seems to correspond quantitatively as they recover, as found by Dr. Carroll and ourselves, and it may well be that if you could separate trait from state, certain patients with the dexamethasone abnormality would correspond quantitatively, while others would have depression with a different disease who will not respond.

Seymour Levine

In the days when we thought we knew a lot, we thought that there was a very nice correlation between ACTH and corticosteroids and we built very nice models of feedback systems. But Mary Dallman has shown clear-cut corticoid rhythms in rats and what is barely an ACTH rhythm if any at all. In fact, there are circumstances in which there is no apparent ACTH rhythm and a very clear corticoid rhythm.

We observed in the rat extremely high corticosterone levels (with values of 500-600 micrograms/%), while ACTH responses are only one quarter of that. (The implication here is that one cannot be sure that measurement of adrenal secretion accurately reflects ACTH secretion under all circumstances. Ed.).

Herbert Meltzer

I want to mention some of our findings (to be presented in the poster session) that may provide a clue to the localization of the mechanism responsible for dexamethasone suppression test (DST) abnormalities in depression. A few months ago, we became aware that there is much information in the literature indicating that corticosteroids can suppress prolactin secretion in man and laboratory animals. As we had some pre and post-DST samples in depressed patients and normal controls, we looked at the relationship between failure to suppress cortisol and prolactin. To our supprise, we found there is a very close correlation between this failure to suppress cortisol and failure to suppress prolactin. Thirteen out of our 16 cortisol non-suppressors were also prolactin non-suppressors, and 36 of 45 of the suppressors, which included 9 normal controls and 26 of 36 patients, did show a decrease in prolactin - (in morning samples). If, the effect of corticosteroids is directed at the pituitary level as has been known in vitro studies, the effect of cortisol can possibly be localized to the pituitary.

The second point to come of of our study relates to ACTH data. We are quite confident about our assay, even though there are a great many problems associated with ACTH assays. Nevertheless, our findings are consistent with the work from Carroll and Kierkegard and others, that ACTH levels are normal in depressed patients. We studied 29 depressed patients, of whom there were 12 non-suppressors and 17 suppressors; there was no difference in ACTH levels prior to dexamethasone, either in the suppressors, the non-suppressors or the normal controls. All groups suppressed their ACTH levels at 8 hours after dexamethasone, but at 16 hours the real difference emerged for the non-suppressors. They showed escape, ACTH levels returning almost to pre-dexamethasone levels at this time whereas the other two groups did not. To the extent that high ACTH levels might have been expected in hypothalamic hyperfunction, we did not see it in this group.

Dr. D. Gann

I have two comments about the mechanisms of DST's. Although glucocorticoids can unmistakably act on isolated pituitary glands in vitro, in no way can you infer from this that the effect of steroid in the whole animal (or man) is at the pituitary. That is the problem Dr. Kendall and I have been squabbling about for 15 years. Glucocorticoids exert clear-cut effects on both the central nervous system and on the pituitary. To argue that one or another is dominant, you must be able to measure things other than at the last step in the process, i.e. glucocorticoid secretion. In the cast of ACTH release you have to be able to measure CRF. To the extent that this has been done CRF has been reported to accumulate in response to steroids, suggesting that they block CRF release and later CRF synthesis. These findings, which are compatible with there being an exclusive effect on the pituitary, do not answer the question of which is dominant.

The other thing I would like to point out is that there is some evidence from Dr. Dallman's laboratory (and some from our own laboratory published by Newland) indicating that adrenal sensitivity to ACTH can be regulated by mechanisms that are independent of ACTH. There is a rhythm to this sensitivity and this can be disrupted, just as you can disrupt the rhythm for ACTH release, so that some of what has just been said can be explained by that sort of mechanism.

Seymour Reichlin: Dr. Gann, on the basis of the neurophysiological work you presented earlier can you explain the blunted dexamethasone test in depression?

Dr. Gann: I think that there are several possibilities, but there is no direct evidence. Kaneko and Hiroshige*(1978) have made several suggestions about the extra hypothalamic inhibition of ACTH release and have suggested that norepinephrine is implicated in fast feedback and serotonin in slow feedback - in both cases they suggest that steroids increase the inhibitory drive on the CRF neuron. This is compatible with old work from Martini's laboratory in the mid-1960's suggesting that mid-brain implantation of steroid inhibits the steroid response to leg break stress and to ether.

We have recently found that cortisol is taken up by the magnacellular neurons of the mid-brain, at just about the site where Martini's group put the steroid. So it could be that a feedback is really, at least in part, driven from outside the hypothalamus and that it represents activation of the inhibitory pathway - but all I can say is that it is possible but not proven.

M. E. Ted Quigley

One thing that has become very apparent today is that little is known about gonadotropin release in patients with depression, and as indicated earlier by Dr. Rusak, assessment of biological rhythms in these patients might be very meaningful.

Pulsatile gonadotropin release in animals is mediated by a hypothalamic mechanism - the GNRH being released into the portal circulation in pulses. One way to evaluate hypothalamic function more specifically would be to measure pulsatile release of GNRH in post-menopausal women and in normal males. If indeed we see an 'apparent' decrease in gonadotropin levels - and I say apparent because we should be very skeptical of a single sample in a post-menopausal women where there are marked fluctuations in pulsatile activity, with a tendency to decrease with age - we should look for the many other factors that George Tolis has alluded to, namely the weight factor and the hot flushes, as further evidence of a hypothalamic dysfunction. Just looking at the frequency and the amplitude of LH pulses in this very common dysfunction is not adequate. What is natural menstrual function in women with dpression and off medications? What is the fertility of patients who are depressed when off the medication?

*Kaneko, M. and Hiroshige T. (1978): Site of fast, rate-sensitive feedback inhibition of adrenocorticotropin secretion during stress. Am. J. Physiol. 234:R46-R51.

Francesca Brambilla

I have evaluated gonadotropin secretion in post menopausal depressed women by taking samples for three hours, from 8:30 a.m. until 12, every 15 minutes at the beginning and then every 30 minutes. We did not see any spiking. The values were always very low, with absolutely no difference from one point to another. In answer to Dr. Quigley's question, menstrual irregularity in women of fertile age with depression is infrequent. Even when the depression is very severe, to the point of suicide, only occasionally does amenorrhea occur. And there is apparently no difference in ovulation in depressed women. They get pregnant like other women.

Dr. Van Loon

My comment deals with possible animal models of the DST in depression. Results identical with that seen in dperessed patients by Sachar can be produced in rats by administering methyltyrosine, which depletes norepinephrine. This drug leads to decreased dexamethasone suppressibility. It may be useful in analysing mechanisms of the abnormality in man by injecting it into specific brain areas.

Seymour Reichlin: Now, I wish to make a next-to-the-last-day summarizing statement. Studies of pituitary regulation in psychiatric disease have been used in many contexts, all of which were illustrated in this conference. As has been said repeatedly, the pituitary is seen by some as the window on the brain, and this has its greatest potential impact in the evaluation of schizophrenia. This is the case because a clear-cut hypothesis has been formulated that states that dopamine receptors are disturbed in schizophrenia and because virtually all neuroleptic agents raise prolactin levels through a dopamine antagonist effect. It is logical for us therefore to scrutinize prolactin and growth hormone regulation, as these are the principal hormones which have a clear-cut dopamine regulating component, in order to find out more about the nature of schizophrenia. Dr. Meltzer told us that for the most part schizophrenics have relatively normal regulation of prolactin and growth hormone, and that although it sounds like a 'negative finding', it is perhaps an exceedingly positive finding. Putting this another way, we can also look at what is good about a schizophrenic. Prolactin regulation for one thing, thus indicating that if dopamine function is abnormal it is not generalized. Also, we have learned from Dr. Moore's beautiful presentation that, all dopaminergic neurons are not alike. I think this is an important insight about the tubero-infundibular (T-1) dopaminergic system: although it secretes dopamine, it clearly operates according to different rules than the mesolimbic and the mesocortical system. The T-1 system responds to hormonal feedback while the others do not. The T-1 system also has different pre-synaptic receptors for dopamine. I think this is a general lesson for pharmacologic coding in the brain. The nature of the secretory products of a neuron does not define its total function. We see this for the classical neurotransmitters and certainly it is true for the neuropeptides. Somatostatin, for example, occurs in 3 or 4 different kinds of cells in the central nervous system, each one of which is probably regulated in a different way.

Dr. Moore made another point which, to me, was extremely important. Although the prolactin response has been taken as a good empirical test of the adequacy of neuroleptics, the neuropharmacologist may be overlooking major classes of drugs which act on the mesolimbic system, but not on the tuberoinfundibular systems. The tuberoinfundibular effects of neuroleptics which include lactation and amenorrhea are only an annoyance; what is really important in evaluation of potentially valuable new drugs is activation of receptors that will differentially modify the extrapyramidal system and the cortical system.

A last point about the pituitary as a window to the brain: the pituitary in fact is a window darkly seen, because there are multiple links in the neuroendocrine chain between brain and hormone response and multiple interactions at each of the links. This is a challenge for the neuroendocrinologist, as much as for the clinical psychoneuroendocrinologist, because it will take much more basic information to learn how to detect complexities of function.

The second level of abstration that has run through this conference is the utilization of studies of pituitary function as models of stress response. One of the most important concepts arising from the study of adrenal responses to stress is the concept of adaptation as proposed by Hans Selye.

There are many ways to study models of stress. The adrenal is not the only stress model, and the other models are not consonant with one another. Cardiovascular responses are different from adrenal activation, as is autonomic activation, as judged by the psychogalvanic reflex and by behavioural changes. Even endocrine responses show different patterns of reaction and adaptation. If one is going to use pituitary secretion as a model of human stress resource, it should be put in the context of other stress models. We look at the pituitary only as a marker of the stress response, with all its advantages and disadvantages. Perhaps we have been too much captivated by Hans Selye into thinking that the hormone was the message - that is, the hormone was the destructive agent, and therefore we should pay much more attention to it. We would do better if we just thought of the hormone as a symbolic inference of what was going on - perhaps no more important than any other stress response.

Now, I am going to go to another level of abstraction - namely pituitary responses as a marker of abnormality. It has been pointed out, particularly by Dr. Carroll, that one of the most important aspects of the dexamethasone suppression test, other than the fact it is a quite reliable indicator of depression, is that it is a test of some very indirect measure of a pathological process. Nevertheless, it is a marker of an 'organic' abnormality which has been confirmed in many laboratories. There are precious few of these "hard" markers in clinical psychiatry and leaving aside the question of its underlying mechanism it is a tremendously important thing to have something like this. It will probably be useful for establishing a diagnosis, and as the Winokur-Sherman group has shown, as an indication of the genetic background of certain types of depressed patients. Other markers that are important are the blunting of TSH response to TRH and also qualitatively abnormal tests such as abnormal cortisol rhythms and paradoxical responses to TRH and to L-dopa. Each will be useful as a marker and also as a wedge for the basic neuroendocrinologist because it is just as important to find out why and how one gets an atypical or qualitatively different response, as to provide a marker in psychiatric disease.

I would like to go a step further. Abnormal neuroendocrine responses observed in medical illness are in themselves extremely interesting in telling us how to understand disturbed function in psychiatric illness. For example, we do not know why patients with anorexia nervosa release growth hormone in response to TRH. We do not know why there are changes in renal insufficency, hepatic insufficiency, hypothyroidism, alcoholism and obesity. In the process of studying these, we may make it easier for the clinical psychoneuroendocrinologist to understand the nature of the problem in mental disorder.

We had the privilege today, with the help of Drs. Gann, Kendall and Jackson, to get into the 'black box'. The white box, the patient's behaviour and communication, is out where everybody can see it but the black box is what is really going on inside the head to cause the observed abnormalities in function. I am really overwhelmed with how little we know after all these years of research. There are so many questions and so few answers. Dr. Rusak I think gave an extremely important talk about rhythems - not just a cautionary talk, but actually a recognition that there are internal oscillators of extreme importance and that we are just beginning to understand what they mean. And even more important, their extension into clinical medicine is just beginning - not just to psychiatric disease which we have been talking about, but to other illness as well.

There is considerable evidence that the occurance of hypertension, peptic ulcer and even arthritis may be related to time of day and time of year, but how those seasonal rhythms are expressed is not clear. The biggest problem is in associating anatomical pathways with neuropharmalogical coding and with functional states. Dr. Checkly mentioned that he did not care particularly where the alpha receptor was, because he could still use certain endocrine functions as predictive tests which work largely to classify patients and to follow their course. He expressed this point very well - you can do quite well in following patients without knowing precisely what is going on pharmacologically. But just think how much better it would be if we know what was inside the black box, and how it actually interfaced with the white one.

I would also like to say a word about the use of non-adrenohypophysial hormonal markers. Some like the catecholamines are old but have only become useful because of recently developed technology. The pineal gland secretes melatonin under the influence of catecholamines, which are modified through the superior cervical ganglion, unequivocally defined by beta-receptor control. We do not know if that system is regulated in the same way as the other catecholaminergic systems in the body. But here is a hormone marker that escapes the constraints of the tuberoinfundibular system and that lies outside the brain.

Other potentially valuable markers include the neurohypophysial secretions. Neurohypophysial hormones have the advantage of being secreted only from neural structures, unlike catecholamines and gut-brain peptides. Additionally a whole array of cerebrospinal fluid amines, metabolites and peptides can be detected. Unfortunately, they can only be sampled through the spinal fluid and we do not as yet really know all the factors that govern their entry into the CSF or their exit. They are very difficult to follow clinically because of problams in getting volunteers and repeated sampling in patients. Informed consent is very difficult, and so certain important avenues of investigation are, of practical purposes, closed to us. We have to develop new ways of measuring brain peptide secretion directly.

Let us quickly consider other challenges, one of the most important of which to the clinical psychoneuroendocrinologist is the significance and definition of 'normal'. One of the points brought out in Dr. Brambilla's work is that in any class of patients the response to a given test depends on the HLA type of the individual. This is to my knowledge the first example of an attempt to associate a genetic marker with a characteristic neuropharmacological response. This is an area that really should be developed further. There are now literally hundreds of chromosomal markers, which can be identified by relatively non-invasive techniques in the human. Perhaps you can correct me, but to my knowledge none of these have been associated with abnormal endocrine responses to provocative stimuli. Conceivably, blunted TRH tests for example in normals are phenotypic expressions of a gene which we have not yet begun to look at.

Another point made was the difficulty and work involved, not only in making repeated and long-term longitudinal measurements, but also in the fact that for each of the drugs studied, there has to be well established clinical pharmacology. Dr. Davis mentioned the importance of determining dose-response curves and blood levels of relevant hormones over time and space. This involves a lot of work, and though tedious and costly it is exceptionally important. It is a wonder that the dexamethasone test was ever discovered, considering all these problems.

Now, lastly, and perhaps the most interesting part of all the topics we talked about, though inconclusively, is the mechanism of cognition and of effect, the brain/mind problem and the analysis of internal physiological events as they relate to what patients feel and to what the endocrinologist measures.

Neuroendocrinology and Psychiatric Disorder, edited by G. M. Brown, et al.
Raven Press, New York 1984.

Hypothalamic Hypogonadotropism in Weight-Loss-Associated Amenorrhea[1]

Robert A. Vigersky

Amenorrhea is a prominent, though not invariable, symptom of women with anorexia nervosa. In fact, a wide spectrum of menstrual disorders may be seen ranging from sparse and/or irregular menses to frank amenorrhea (31). The amenorrhea is usually secondary, i.e. occuring after menarche and the institution of cyclic menses. However, the apparent increase in the incidence of this disorder with its presentation at earlier ages has produced a greater frequency of primary amenorrhea. In both cases, it is often the symptom of amenorrhea that brings the anorectic to medical attention, perhaps through their ignorance of how intimately amenorrhea is related to their weight loss and/or eating behaviour. An issue of great debate and importance to the understanding of the etiology of the amenorrhea is the frequency with which this symptom occurs prior to the weight loss. Fries (16) reviewed this issue and found that 16% of women became amenorrheic preceding other symptoms while another 55% developed amenorrhea coincident with the beginning of the abnormal eating behaviour or with only minimal weight loss. This has been recently confirmed by Morimoto et al. (32) who have studied pre-morbid weight, weight at onset of amenorrhea, minimum weight, and weight at the return of menses in 6 patients with anorexia nervosa. They found that amenorrhea occurred in 50% of those with minimal, if any weight change. These observations together with those showing that menses may not return in some women after weight gain (25), suggest that the development of amenorrhea is multi-factorial and demonstrate the wide individual variation with respect to the importance that weight loss, per se, plays.

The failure to menstruate in anorexia nervosa is due to the low and non-cyclic levels of ovarian sex steroid secretion (vide infra). Serum estradiol levels are usually at or below the level of detection of the radioimmmnoassay (46). The hypoestrogenic state is the cause of the vaginal atrophy often seen in these women and the resultant dyspareunia in many of those who are sexually active. It is not clear how much of the decrease in sexual activity seen in anorexia nervosa can be attributed to the dyspareunia, as opposed to the disinterest in sex seen in the majority of these women. The hypoestrogenism of women with this disorder is not associated with hot flashes as is seen in menopausal or hypopituitarism gonadal failure. The difference may reflect the hypothalamic etiology of the hypogonadotropism in anorexia nervosa.

While there has been general agreement that the amenorrhea of AN is due to hypogonadotropic hypogonadism, the mechanism of the gonadotropin deficiency is still unclear. One possibility, of course, is that there

[1]The opinions or assertains contained herein are the private views of the author and are not to be construed as official or reflecting the views of the Department of the Army or the Department of Defense.

is some specificity to the hypogonadotropism of AN, i.e., the same process that affects eating behaviour also influences gonadotropin secretion - perhaps by way of a common neurotransmitter abnormality. Alternatively, the hypogonadotropism may be non-specific, i.e., related to the weight loss per se, as the two factors may interact. For this reason, it is useful to study the effects of more modest amounts of weight loss in patients without the "distorted and implacable attitude toward foods and body image" present in AN (12). Such a group of women are those with "simple weight loss", a term coined to describe individuals with none of the psychologic aberrations of anorexia nervosa, but who have lost small to moderate amounts of weight within the normal range (45). This weight loss is usually deemed appropriate by parents, peers, and physicians, but they come to medical attention for evaluation of secondary amenorrhea. The incidence of this disorder is unknown, but is likely to be even higher than that of AN which in England is estimated to be 1 in 100 girls, ages 16 to 18 (8). Though psychologically distinct, anorexia nervosa and simple weight loss seem to represent points on the spectrum that, according to Fries (16) includes dieting due to neurotic fixation on weight and/or food intake and anorectic behaviour. Two other factors, exercise and stress, frequently found in AN patients need to be considered as important variables in the pathogenesis of the hypogonadotropism. For this reason, data dealing with gonadotropin abnormalities in exercise and stress-induced amenorrhea will also be considered in this review.

Menses and Fatness

The relationship of weight to menstrual function is a complex one. Frisch (17) investigated the relationship of menarche to pubertal weight gain, and of weight gain after weight loss to the resumption of menses. She found that menarche is directly correlated with fatness (or weight for a particular height) (17). As an index of fatness she used the equation of Mellits and Cheek. After weight-loss induced amenorrhea, resumption of menses was found to be related to this function, though generally occuring at a slightly higher weight than did menarche. A useful nomogram to calculate these parameters of body fat is shown in Figure 1. This figure should only serve as a general guideline, however, particularly in light of recent data from Morimoto et al. (32) who have shown that while the weight at the time amenorrhea developed and at the time menses resumed were similar, if not identical, in 6 patients with anorexia nervosa, this weight was well below the 10th precentile in 2 women and above the 25th percentile in another 2. Thus, each individual may have her own critical body weight for menstruation. Since a) most studies do not provide weights at the time of amenorrhea and at the resumption of menses and b) these data are on Japanese women while Frisch's data are on American women, it remains to be seen how universal these observations may be. Figure 1 should thus be used with understanding that it may be fallacious to equate the achievement of the minimum weight for height with the obligation to resume menses. As Frisch (17) has noted, increasing weight and fatness is necessary but may not be sufficient for menses to return. Other factors, such as stress and exercise (vide infra) may play important roles in explaining the failure of 50% of anorexic women to resume menstruation after regaining weight (3, 38). Similarly, weight loss cannot explain the frequent onset of secondary amenorrhea (71%) before, or coinciding with, the onset of eating abnormalities (16).

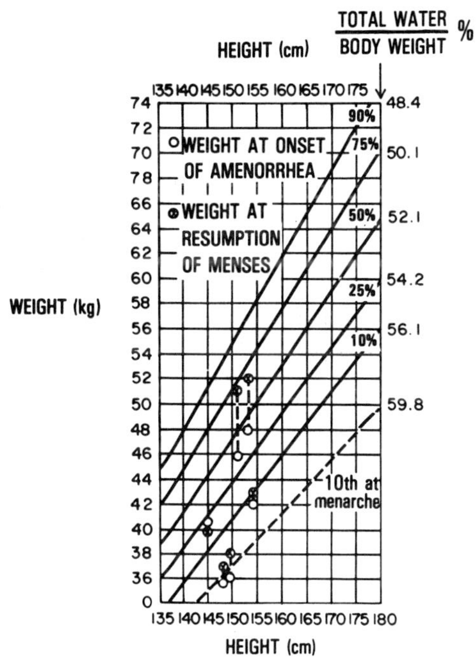

FIG. 1. Minimal weight necessary for a particular height for restoration of menstrual cycles is indicated on the weight scale by the 10th percentile diagonal line of TW/BWt%, 56.1%, as it crosses the vertical height line. The 10th percentile at menarche is shown by the dashed line. The symbols indicate the weight at the time of amenorrhea ○ and the weight at the time of the resumption of menses ⊗ of 6 patients of Morimoto et al. (32). Modified from Frisch (17).

Gonadotropins in Anorexia Nervosa

The proximate cause of the amenorrhea in weight loss is the decreased and noncyclic nature of ovarian secretion of sex-steroids. This hypogonadism has been shown by numerous investigators to be due to hypogonadotropism (1, 5, 14, 19, 24, 29, 31, 35, 41, 44, 48, 49). It is the etiology of the hypogonadotropism that has been under the intensive investigation. While serum LH and FSH are lower in AN, both gonadotropins respond to the hypothalamic releasing factor LRH (or GnRH). This response may be either blunted or in the normal range and has a pre-pubertal pattern, i.e., the FSH response is greater than that of LH (1, 14, 29, 31, 32, 41, 45, 49). These results implicate suprahypophyseal factors as being responsible for the low basal serum gonadotropin levels. Further proof of the integrity of the pituitary (and the ovary) lies in the demonstration that chronic LRH administration (via pulsatile i.v. or i.m. administration or via i.v. infusion) restores LH responsiveness to LRH to a normal pubertal or post-pubertal pattern and may induce ovulation (1, 29, 33, 52). Hypothalamic, rather than pituitary, dysfunction is also suggested by the delayed peak in LH and FSH after LRH (45), the abnormal response of LH to clomiphene citrate (1, 4, 24, 28), and failure to demonstrate a positive feedback after estrogen adminstration (47).

Finally, these abnormalities of gonadotropin regulation occur concomitantly with abnormalities of specific hypothalamic functions such as temperature regulation and water regulation (44). The 24 hour pattern of secretion of gonadotropins resembles that seen prepubertally or during puberty (25, 35).

Men with AN manifest hypogonadotropic hypogonadism similar to that in women has been found. Anorexia nervosa in males is rare, probably representing less that 5% of all patients with this disorder. Though over 75 cases of male anorexia nervosa have been reported, endocrine data particularly with regard to the hypothalamic-pituitary-gonadal axis, is scanty (7, 22). The reports of Hurd et al. (23), Garfinkle et al. (19), and my own observations indicate men with anorexia nervosa have low plasma testosterone levels and low plasma LH and FSH concentrations. Pirke et al. (35) demonstrated that there was a pubertal LH secretory pattern in one 18 year old man with anorexia nervosa. The LH and FSH response to LRH has not been previously reported in male anorexia nervosa. In a 19 year old man, serum LH rose from 2.3 to 10.3 mIU/ml and FSH from 4.3 to 12.4 mIU/ml after 100 ug of LRH. The time of the peaks LH and FSH levels was 45 and 120 minutes, respectively (Vigersky, R.A., unpublished data). This blunted and delayed response is similar to those of the women with this disorder. Therefore, it would seem, that men and women with anorexia nervosa have the same cause of their hypogonadism. However, these findings are quite different from the changes seen in men with protein-calorie malnutrition (43). The reason for these differences is unclear at the present, but may relate to dietary composition rather than total caloric content.

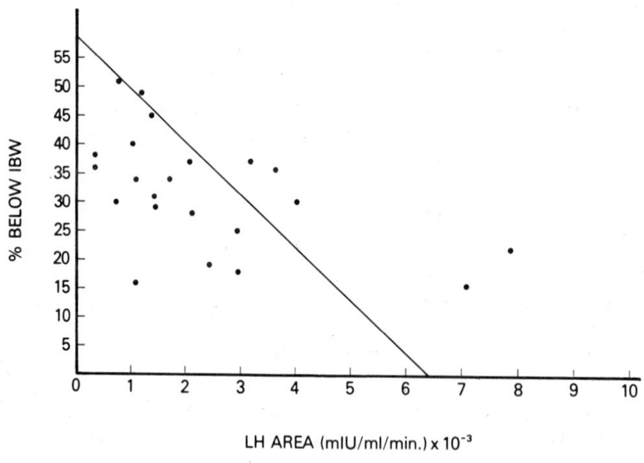

FIG. 2. Linear regression analysis of the area under the LH response curve after the injection of 10 ug LRH i.v. as a function of thinness (% below ideal body weight - IBW) in patients with anorexia nervosa = 0.56; $p < 0.05$.

In order to shed light on the relationships of fatness and weight to hypothalamic-pituitary-gonadal function, several investigators have studied: 1) the severity of the gonadotropin abnormalities with respect to the degree of weight loss in anorexia nervosa; 2) anorexia nervosa patients before and after "nutritional rehabilitation"; and 3) patients with simple weight loss. Basal levels of LH and FSH are correlated with the severity of weight loss or percent body fat in some studies (5, 24). Furthermore, the gonadotropin responses to LRH (24, 45) and clomiphene citrate (23) are correlated with the severity of weight loss (45) (Figure 2 and 3). Basal serum LH concentration, the circadian pattern of LH, and the LH response to LRH all improve in patients with anorexia nervosa who gain weight (5, 14, 32, 35, 41, 48). However, why some women who regain their body weight do not resume menses is not clear. Of interest in this regard is the study by Katz et al. (25) which shows persistence of pre-pubertal or pubertal pattern of LH secretion in anorexia nervosa patients who have regained weight but retain their abnormal eating behaviour. Thus, their amenorrhea, while being hypothalamically mediated, may be due to imput from higher centres. Finally, patients with simple weight loss have levels of basal LH and FSH which are intermediate between normal and AN (46). The kinetics of the response of gonadotropins to LRH i.e., the time of maximal peak serum level, is also related to weight loss and is of intermediate severity in the simple weight loss group (45) (Figure 4).

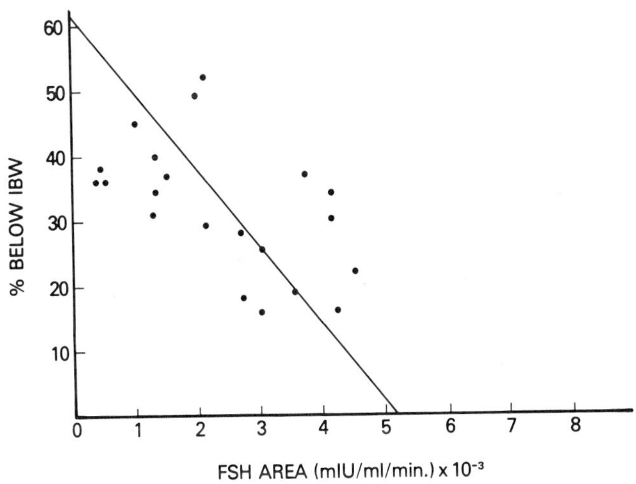

FIG. 3. Linear regression analysis of the area under the FSH response curve after the injection of 10 ug LRH i.v. as a function of thinness (% below ideal body weight - IBW) in patients with anorexia nervosa. r - 0.47; $p < 0.05$.

These observations about gonadotropins support the hypothesis that the endocrine and hypothalamic abnormalities in anorexia nervosa are related to weight loss. Further support comes from the demonstration that the severity of abnormalities of hypothalamic function in AN such as temperature regulation are correlated with the severity of weight loss (44). However, since amenorrhea persists in some women despite weight gain, other factors (as yet undefined) are obviously important for the resumption of menses, i.e. weight gain is necessary but not sufficient.

Mechanisms of Weight-Induced Changes in Gonadotropin Secretion

How weight changes induce these abnormalities in hypothalamic function is unclear. With respect to gonadotropin regulation, fat per se may be a factor, since *in vitro* it actively metabolizes androstenedione and

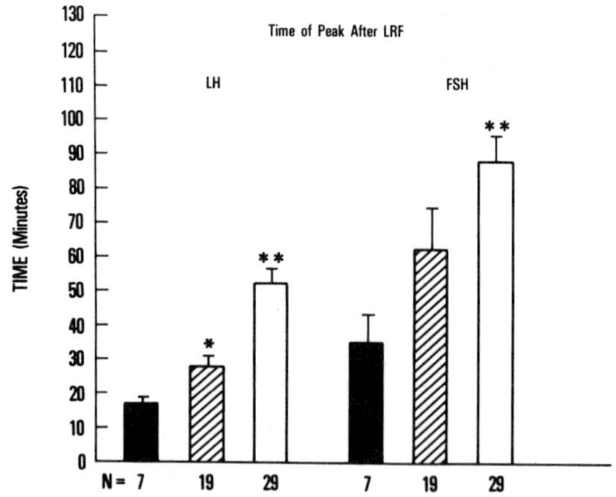

FIG. 4. The (mean ± SE) time of peak serum luteinizing hormone (LH) and follicle stimulating hormone (FSH) levels after 10 ug of LRH in normals (■) and patients with secondary amenorrhea associated with simple weight loss (▨) and anorexia nervosa (□). $^*p < 0.01$; $^{**}p < 0.01$.

testosterone to estrone and estradiol, respectively (34, 39). Obese women appear to have increased conversion of androgens to estrogens and decreased α-hydroxylation of estradiol, while women with anorexia nervosa have increased α-hydroxylation (13, 20, 42). Such changes in sex steroid metabolism may influence hypothalamic LRH synthesis and/or secretion. However, extrapolation from studies done in obese or normal women to patients with anorexia nervosa may not be valid. For instance, Boyar et al. (6) have shown an inverse relationship between body weight and gonadotropins in Turner's syndrome. Serum levels of sex steroids were unmeasurable and 24-hour urinary excretion of these steroids showed no correlation with serum gonadotropin levels or weight. Beitins et al. (2) have demonstrated no change in serum gonadotropin levels and an increase in urinary gonadotropins (due to increased serum clearance) in fasting obese post-menopausal women. Graham et al. (21) have recently found abnormally low serum LH in only 2 of 6 obese women after significant weight loss. Finally, Smith et al. (43) have shown that men with protein-calorie malnutrition respond to weight loss with an increase in gonadotropins which decreased to normal with weight gain. This is quite different from the observations in men with anorexia nervosa. These and other studies suggest that weight loss and gonadotropin regulation are related in complex and, as yet, poorly understood ways. Katz et al. (25) have proposed that weight loss (and decreased fat) and hypothalamic changes may both be a reflection of different aspects of the nutritional deprivation, the former being total caloric content and the latter biogenic amine content.

Exercise-Induced Amenorrhea

Strenuous exercise is one of the common means that patients with AN use to reduce and maintain their body weight. Therefore, it seems appropriate to consider the effects of exercise on menstrual function and gonadotropins. Numerous studies in the last 20 years have documented the high incidence of menstrual abnormalities in women engaged in strenuous exercise. The type of exercise seems to influence the frequency of these abnormalities. For instance, women engaged in activities in which a prolonged expenditure of energy is required have, in general, a higher incidence of amenorrhea then those engaged in activities requiring frequent, short bursts of energy (10). Long distance runners and professional ballet dancers, examples of the former group, have recently been studied by several investigators (9, 11, 18, 30, 40). Feicht et al. (11) found that women long distance runners have a 35% overall incidence of secondary amenorrhea and that there was correlation between the distance run per week and the incidence of amenorrhea. Dale et al. (9) found a 34% incidence of oligo- or amenorrhea among 90 women who ran more than 30 miles per week at 7.5 - 9.5 min/mile. The incidence in 24 "joggers" (5 - 30 miles per week at 10.5 - 11.5 min/mile) was 23%. Young professional ballet dancers have a 28% incidence of primary or secondary amenorrhea and a later age at menarche than normal women (18).

The mechanism of the amenorrhea in these women is complex. Schwartz et al. (40) found that prior menstrual disorders are more common in amenorrheic runners than in runners who menstruate normally. But, the amenorrheic women in this study were also lighter, leaner and faster than their menstruating counterparts. The loss of weight and body fat, as in anorexia nervosa, appear to be contributing factors. Dale et al. (9) found that runners had significantly lower body fat compared to controls (17.1% vs. 24.1%; p 0.05), with "joggers" being intermediate (21.3%). Evidence is mounting that suggests it is the physical exertion itself which produces the amenorrhea. Warren (50) proposed that, in addition to achieving a critical weight for height, girls must have a net positive "energy" balance. Thus, the "energy drain" imposed by vigorous ballet practice prevents menarche (accounting for the later age at menarche in ballet dancers) or induces secondary amenorrhea (50). When ballet dancers do not practice because of vacation or injury, menses resume despite no change in body weight. Finally, other factors, such as the composition of the diet and stress, may modulate the incidence of amenorrhea in exercising women. For example, Schwartz et al. (40) report a lower protein content despite higher total caloric intake in amenorrheic runners compared to runners with normal menses. The amenorrheic women also felt their routine was more "stressful".

Only scanty and conflicting endocrine data exists at present. McArthur et al. (30) found low basal serum estradiol, LH and FSH levels with either a normal or hyperresponse of the gonadotropins and estradiol to LRH in 3 normal weight, amenorrheic runners. Warren (50) also found low basal serum LH and FSH concentrations in amenorrheic ballet dancers. However, Schwartz et al. (40) found slightly higher levels of serum LH in their amenorrheic runners compared to normal runners, with basal serum FSH and estrogen levels indistinguishable between the groups.

Stress-Induced Amenorrhea

Stress-induced amenorrhea is a poorly defined, yet frequently used, diagnosis used to describe the numerous women whose menses have ceased in association with a disruptive situational event. Hypothalamic dysfunction was proposed as the mechanism for this disorder by Klinefelter et al. (26) and Reifenstein (37). Reifenstein (37) went on to suggest that the amenorrhea was the somatic representation of "overt or latent psychological disturbances". Therefore, the term "psychogenic" amenorrhea has been used synonymously with "stress-induced" and "hypothalamic" amenorrhea.

The frequency with which stressful events are related to the appearance of secondary amenorrhea is difficult to determine. No prospective study on this subject has been performed. However, the postal survey of 2000 women, conducted by Fries et al. (15), is instructive. They found a 3.1% overall incidence of secondary amenorrhea. Forty-one women were further questioned as to factors surrounding the onset of amenorrhea and they were compared to 61 controls. Stressful events such as bereavement, family conflicts or illness, etc., were significantly more common in the amenorrheic group than the controls (34.4% vs. 11.5% p 0.05). However, amenorrhea was multifactorial in these women (as it is in amenorrheic women discontinuing oral contraceptives) with weight loss, psychotropic drug use, and cessation of oral contraceptive use, being present in some of the same women.

The concomitant presence of several other possible factors in stress-induced amenorrhea has made the investigation of the etiology of the disorder difficult, if not impossible. In fact, no endocrine studies of a "pure" stress-induced amenorrhea group exists. Several studies do exist, however, which have shown low or non-cyclic serum LH levels, normal pituitary gonadotropin responses to exogenous LRH, and abnormal positive and negative feedback responses to estradiol in patients with "hypothalamic" amenorrhea (27, 36, 51). Undoubtedly, individuals with "pure" stress-induced amenorrhea are included in these series.

CONCLUSIONS

The data gathered by numerous investigators unequivocally demonstrate that the amenorrhea seen in anorexia nervosa results from hypogonadotropic hypogonadism, anorexia being at the end of a spectrum of progressive gonadotropin deficiency (and reversion to pre-pubertal status) related to weight loss per se. The etiology of the hypogonadotropism remains unclear, though it is most likely hypothalamically mediated. It has become apparent, however, that it is more than merely an effect of the weight loss alone. It has been recognized that psychologic stress and physical exertion which themselves produce amenorrhea (probably via hypothalamic mediation), are important factors in the life of an anorexic patient. Whether the effects of weight loss, exercise, and stress are synergistic or additive and whether they are mediated through a common (neurotransmitter) pathway remains to be determined.

ACKNOWLEDGMENTS

I am indebted to Dr. Lynn Loriaux and Mortimer B. Lipsett for their guidance and encouragement and to Mrs. Barbara Kuffler for her expert secretarial assistance.

REFERENCES

1. Aono, T., Kinugasa, T., Yamamoto, T., Miyake, A. and Kurachi, K. (1975): Acta Endocrinologica 80:630-641.
2. Beitins, I. Z., Shah, A., O'Loughlin, K., Johnson, L., Ostrea, T. R., Van Wart, J. and McArthur, J. W. (1980): J. Clin. Endocrin. Metab. 51:26-34.

3. Bell, E. T., Harkness, R. A., Loraine, J. A. and Russell, G.F.M. (1966): Acta Endocrinologica 51:140-148.
4. Beumont, P.J.V., Carr, P. J. and Gelder, M. G. (1976): Psychological Medicine 3:495-501.
5. Beumont, P.J.V., George, G.C.W., Pimstone, B.L. and Vinik, A. I. (1976): J. Clin. Endocrin. Metab. 43:487-496.
6. Boyar, R.M., Ramsey, J., Chipman, J., Fevre, M., Madden, J. and Marks, J. (1978): N. Engl. J. Med. 298:1328-1331.
7. Crisp, A. H. and Toms, D. A. (1972): Brit. Med. J. 1:334-338.
8. Crisp, A. H., Palmer, R. L. and Kalucy, R. S. (1976): Brit. J. Psychiat. 128:549-554.
9. Dale, E., Gerlach, D. H. and Wilhite, A. L. (1979): Obstet. and Gynecol. 54:47-53.
10. Erdelyi, G. J. (1976): The Physician and Sportsmedicine 4:79-81.
11. Feicht, C. B., Johnson, T. S., Martin, B. J., Sparkes, K. E. and Wagner, W. W. (1978): Lancet 2:1145-1147.
12. Feighner, J. P., Robins, E., Guze, S. B., Woodruff, R. A., Jr., Winokur, G. and Munoz, R. (1972): Archives of Gen. Psychiat. 26: 27-63.
13. Fishman, J., Boyar, R. M. and Hellman, L. (1975): J. Clin. Endocrin. Metab. 41:989-991.
14. Frankel, R. J. and Jenkins, J. S. (1975): Acta Endocrinologica 78:209-221.
15. Fries, H., Nillius, S. J. and Pettersson, F. (1974): Am. J. Obstet. and Gynec. 118:473-479.
16. Fries, H. (1977): In: Anorexia Nervosa, edited by R. A. Vigersky, pp.163-176. Raven Press, New York.
17. Frisch, R. E. (1977): In: Anorexia Nervosa, edited by R. A. Vigersky, pp.149-161. Raven Press, New York.
18. Frisch, R. E., Wyshak, G. and Vincent, L. (1980): N. Engl. J. Med. 303:17-19.
19. Garfinkel, P. E., Brown, G. M., Stancer, H. C. and Moldofsky, H. (1975): Arch. Gen. Psychiat. 32:739-744.
20. Glass, A. R., Burman, K. D., Dahms, W. T. and Boehm, T. M. (1981): Metabolism 30:89-104.
21. Graham, R. L., Grimes, D. L. and Gambrell, R. D. (1979): Southern Medical Journal 72:1259-1261.
22. Hay, G. G. and Leonard, J. C. (1970): Lancet 2:574-576.
23. Hurd, H. P., II, Palumbo, P. J. and Gharib, H. (1977): Mayo Clinic Proceedings 52:711-716.
24. Jeuniewic, N., Brown, G. M., Garfinkel, P. E. and Moldofsky, H. (1978): Psychosom. Med. 40:187-198.
25. Katz, J. L., Boyar, R., Roffwarg, H., Hellman, L. and Weiner, H. (1978): Psychosom. Med. 40:549-567.
26. Klinefelter, H. F., Jr., Albright, F. and Griswold, G. C. (1943): J. Clin. Endocrin. 3:529-544.
27. Lachelin, G.C.L. and Yen, S.S.C. (1978): Am. J. Obstet. Gynec. 130: 825-831.
28. Marshall, J. C. and Fraser, T. R. (1971): Brit. Med. J. 4:590-592.
29. Marshall, J. C. and Kelch, R. P. (1979): J. Clin. Endocrin. Metab. 49:712-718.
30. McArthur, J. W., Bullen, B. A., Beitins, I. Z., Pagano, M., Badger, T. M. and Klibanski, A. (1980): Endocrine Research Communications 7:13-25.
31. Mecklenburg, R. S., Loriaux, D. L., Thompson, R. H., Anderson, A. E. and Lipsett, M. B. (1974): Medicine 53:147-159.

32. Morimoto, Y., Oishi, T., Hanasaki, N., Miyatake, A., Sato, B., Norma, K., Kato, H., Yano, S. and Yamamura, Y. (1980): Endocrinologica Japonica 27:191-200.
33. Nillius, S. J., Fries, H. and Wide, L. (1975): Am. J. Obstet. Gynec. 122:921-928.
34. Nimrod, A. and Ryan, K. J. (1975): J. Clin. Endocrin. Metab. 40: 367-372.
35. Pirke, K. M., Fichter, M. M., Lund, R. and Doerr, P. (1979): Acta Endocrinologica 92:193-204.
36. Rakoff, J. S., Rigg, L. A. and Yen, S.S.C. (1978): Am. J. Obstet. Gynec. 130:807-812.
37. Reifenstein, E. C. (1946): Med. Clin. N. Am. 30:1103-1114.
38. Russell, G.F.M. (1972): Postgraduate Med. J. 48:10-13.
39. Schlindler, A. E., Ebert, A. and Friedrich, E. (1972): J. Clin. Endocrin. Metab. 35:627-630.
40. Schwartz, B., Rebar, R. W. and Yen, S.S.C. (1980): Fertility and Sterility 34:306 (Abstract).
41. Sherman, B. M., Halmi, K. A. and Zamudio, R. (1975): J. Clin. Endocrin. Metab. 41:135-142.
42. Siiteri, P. K. and MacDonald, P. C. (1973): In: Handbook of Physiology, Section 7, Vol. II, edited by R. O. Greep, pp.615-629. American Physiological Society, Washington, D.C.
43. Smith, S. R., Chhetri, M. K., Johanson, A. J., Radfar, N. and Migeon, C. J. (1975): J. Clin. Endocrin. Metab. 41:60-69.
44. Vigersky, R. A., Loriaux, D. L., Andersen, A. E. and Lipsett, M. B. (1976): Clin. Endocrin. Metab. 5:517-535.
45. Vigersky, R. A., Loriaux, D. L., Andersen, A. E., Mecklenburg, R. S. and Vaitukaitis, J. L. (1976): J. Clin. Endocrin. Metab. 43:893-900.
46. Vigersky, R. A., Andersen, A. E., Thompson, R. H. and Loriaux, D. L. (1977): N. Engl. J. Med. 297:1141-1145.
47. Wakeling, A., De Souza, V. and Beardwood, C. J. (1977): In: Anorexia Nervosa, edited by R. A. Vigersky, pp.199-209. Raven Press, New York.
48. Wakeling, A., De Souza, V.F.A., Gore, M.B.R., Sabur, M., Kingstone, D. and Boss, A.M.B. (1979): Psychol. Med. 9:265-272.
49. Warren, M. P. (1977): In: Anorexia Nervosa, edited by R. A. Vigersky pp.189-198. Raven Press, New York.
50. Warren, M. P. (1980): J. Clin. Endocrinol. Metab. 51:1150-1157.
51. Yen, S.S.C., Rebar, R., Vandenberg, G. and Judd, H. (1978): J. Clin. Endocrin. Metab. 36:811-816.
52. Yoshimoto, Y., Moridera, K. and Imura, H. (1975): N. Engl. J. Med. 292:242-245.

Neuroendocrinology and Psychiatric Disorder,
edited by G. M. Brown, et al.
Raven Press, New York 1984.

Anorexia Nervosa: An Overview of Hypothalamic-Pituitary Function

Paul E. Garfinkel

Anorexia nervosa is characterized by exaggerated attempts to maintain a thin body, and by a phobia of weight gain and fat, even though the person may already be emaciated. Once considered a rare disorder, recent studies have confirmed that anorexia nervosa is relatively common. The prevalence in adolescent girls has been estimated at about 1/250 in high schools and about 5% of reported cases are male. While the usual age of onset is adolescence, the illness may first appear in patients during their twenties (48).

The anorexic's pursuit of thinness begins with dieting not unlike that of her peers. A particular part of her body such as the abdomen or thighs may feel too large. She then develops extreme rigidity in her eating habits in an effort to control her weight, usually selecting high protein low carbohydrate foods that are presumed to be low in calories. Certain foods become feared but this is secondary to the fear of weight gain.

Although the term anorexia implies a loss of appetite, the patient's appetite is often maintained until late in the starvation process. Most patients report a normal hunger awareness but also express a fear of giving in to the impulse to eat (48). By contrast, perception of satiety is extremely distorted. Patients report severe bloating, nausea and distension after even small amounts of food. In addition, they do not feel rested or satisfied after eating but feel guilty for having given in and are afraid of losing control and being unable to stop.

In spite of the progressive and severe weight loss, many anorexic women are unaware of their emaciation. They may deny many aspects of the disorder, especially the fact that their changed bodies are not healthy or beautiful. This disturbance of body image is of delusional proportions and usually takes one or two forms: either they deny the extent of weight loss or they feel that although they have lost weight, a particular body part is still much too large. This denial of illness extends to a lack of awareness of inner feelings, including fatigue. Thus anorexics often seen excessively energetic until rather late in the illness (71), though many limit their activities to exercise and schoolwork. In particular, they usually lose interest in their friends and by the time of medical intervention, may be socially isolated and spending their time totally on dieting, preoccupation with food, schoolwork and exercise.

Many patients with anorexia nervosa alternate between fasting and bulimia and may not be underweight (52). Often they have previously been obese and they have a history of obesity in the immediate family (43). Their moods can be quite labile and they feel out of control when overeating. Usually they restrict food intake when they are busy and overeat when alone. After gorging they may restrict food intake for several days and abuse laxatives or induce vomiting. A considerable amount of money may be spent on food and some patients begin to steal. This group of bulimic patients may also display other impulsive behaviour including misuse of alcohol and street drugs, suicide attempts and self-mutilation (43).

Our understanding of the evolution and perpetuation of the illness is incomplete but it is known that anorexia nervosa is the product of several interacting factors in the patient, her family and her culture. For a complete review of this see Garfinkel and Garner (48). Sociocultural factors are indicated by the fact that of all anorexics, 95% are women, most are aged 12-35 at onset and most are from upper or middle class families. In addition, there has been a dramatic rise in the number of patients during the last 15 years (see 48 for a review). Factors within the patient include a strong need for perfection and control, masking a sense of overall helplessness, and perceptual and conceptual disturbances. Premorbid obesity and early puberty have also been suggested as risk factors.

A confused sense of autonomy and identity appears to be at the root of the psychopathology (see 48 for a review). The patient feels a lack of self-control and a sense of personal mistrust of her body, and experiences conflict regarding her identity. This may be caused by a combination of constitutional factors and those learned from early parent-daughter interactions. It has been suggested that disturbances in body image and disturbances in the recognition of internal visceral and affective states are closely related to these general feelings of ineffectiveness.

Familial and cultural values play a part, perhaps creating excessively high expectations for the patient herself and causing her to have excessively high expectations of others (48). Alternatively the patient may find that those around her pay undue attention to weight and eating as symbols of self-control and success. For example, anorexia nervosa is significantly more common (a prevalence of 7%) in adolescents who must remain thin because they are dance students and the condition is most over-represented in dance groups in which there are very strong pressures to achieve.

Particular familial patterns may also make emotional and physical separation more difficult in adolescence thus making it more difficult for the girl to become autonomous. The disorder is then precipitated when she begins to face the issues of separation, autonomy and identity and the final precipitating events may therefore be quite varied and apparently minor.

However, the illness is precipitated, once it begins the starvation tends to perpetuate it, and this obviously has important therapeutic implications. For example, delayed gastric emptying may add to the feeling of bloating, and contribute to unrealistic dieting. In addition, depression, reduced concentration, anxiety, social withdrawal, obsessional preoccupation with food, food related dreams and difficulty stopping eating once started, all occur in starving people, whatever the cause. These factors all add to the anorexic's worries about lack of self-control, and the response may be to attempt to regain control by further calorie restriction.

The illness may be further perpetuated by the reduction in body size from an adult to pre-pubescent state, thereby relieving stress by avoidance of psychosexual maturity (28). Weight loss may also assume a functional role within a disturbed family.

Hypothalamic Function

Patients with anorexia nervosa have been found repeatedly to display abnormal hypothalamic function. Possibly pathogenic mechanisms underlying these disturbances include (1) hypothalamic changes which reflect weight loss or caloric deprivation; 2) emotional disturbance may be directly responsible for hypothalamic alterations, (3) both the emotional disturbance and the altered hormonal states may reflect a basic primary hypothalamic disorder. In the following review, we note that the various hormones are affected preferentially by weight, caloric intake and emotonal distress and that these factors account for what is currently known about the origin of hypothalamic disturbances.

In this chapter, the changes in growth hormone, thyroid, adrenal, prolactin, melatonin and testosterone secretion, carbohydrate metabolism, thermoregulation and water conservation and monoamine metabolism in anorexia nervosa will be reviewed. Changes in gonadotropins are reviewed in Chapter 23.

Growth Hormone

A number of investigators have reported that resting growth hormone (GH) levels are elevated in some patients with anorexia nervosa (19, 23, 42, 39, 67, 104). With recovery, plasma (GH) levels are normalized (19, 39, 42). This fall in (GH) levels occurs prior to weight gain and is unrelated to body weight. Rather, it is more closely tied to the patient's caloric intake (42). Change in plasma LH and in plasma GH are therefore related to two different factors, plasma LH changes are related to loss of body weight and are reversed by an increase in body weight, while GH levels are altered by caloric intake (19). Elevated basal levels of GH are found in a variety of states in which there is decreased food intake, including protein-caloric malnutrition, kwashiorkor and marasmus (82). In kwashiorkor, normalization of GH occurs after protein but not after carbohydrate refeeding. The observation, taken together with the lack of relationship of GH levels to the degree of weight loss (19) and the findings that GH levels in anorexics are elevated only in those with poor caloric intake strongly supports the contention that the elevation in GH is secondary to starvation.

Following a glucose load, patients with elevated resting GH levels have been reported to show a drop in GH (39, 42, 89), however a paradoxical rise following oral glucose has also been recorded (2, 91). The reason for this difference is not clear (23, 42). This paradoxical rise in GH does not occur after nutritional intake improves (23). Harrower, Yap, Nairn, Walton, Strong and Craig (56) described that in anorexia nervosa as well as in acromegaly, bromocriptine reduces the raised GH concentrations that occur during an oral glucose tolerance test. A reduced GH response to apomorphine has also been found in anorexia nervosa (23, 89); this response returns to normal following weight restoration (23). However the flattened response to L-dopa seen in anorexia nervosa may not revert to normal following weight gain (89). The GH response to insulin has also been described as attenuated in anorexia nervosa (18, 33). On the other hand, normal GH responses to arginine have been reported (80, 91).

In normal subjects GH secretion is unaltered by the administration of thyrotropin releasing hormone (TRH), while in anorexia nervosa a prompt release of growth hormone usually occurs (73). This response however, is not specific to anorexia nervosa. It has also been reported in acromegaly (37) and depression (72). A normal rise of growth hormone has been reported during sleep in anorexia nervosa (104).

The data on GH in anorexia nervosa suggest that the raised basal levels are related directly to starvation. However, GH responses to provocative tests have been variable. Reasons for this are not clear but may reflect studies of patients at various phases of the disorder or the clinical heterogeneity of patients, for example, with regard to bulimia (43).

Pituitary-Thyroid Function

Thyroxine (T4) levels in anorexia nervosa are usually within the normal range (19, 70) but may also be lower than normal (76, 106). Even when normal values are obtained, these are usually at the low end of the normal scale (60). Wakeling et al., (106) did not find a rise in T4 levels after 4-6 weeks of weight gain. A correlation of resting T4 and cortisol levels has been noted (19). Thyroxine binding protein, as assessed by T3 resin uptake, is also normal (19).

Serum triiodothyronine (T3) levels are reduced in anorexia nervosa (76, 60, 21, 78, 30). This decrease in T3 is associated with an increase in the inactive reverse form of T3 (21). Absolute levels of T3 are linearly correlated with weight expressed as a percentage of ideal weight and both reduced T3 and elevated reverse T3 are normalized by weight gain (69, 106). The identical alteration is seen in other forms of starvation (97). Reversible changes in the levels of thyroid hormones occur with acute starvation and caloric deprivation (24, 97) and with carbohydrate restriction (93). Spaulding et al., (93) have suggested that dietary carbohydrate is an important regulatory factor of T3 production. The alteration in T3 and reverse T3 is clearly related to fasting itself and it also occurs in obese subjects during fasting (98). Moshang and Utiger (78) have proposed that the low T3 in states of starvation serves an adaptive function. They suggest that the target cells for thyroid hormones have regulatory mechanisms based upon metabolic needs. If conversion of T4 to T3 at the cellular level is regulated by need, then deprivation of calories would alter cellular mechanisms involved in the control of deiodination of T4. This would reduce production of T3 and increase reverse T3 which is a much less calorigenic hormone. If these mechanisms also exist within the pituitary, the pituitary thyrotroph might not interpret low levels of T3 as being insufficient for needs and TSH levels would not increase. In accord with this, Gardner, Kaplan, Stanley and Utiger (41) have recently reported that fasting is associated with a lower set point of the pituitary thyrotrophs.

Resting levels of thyrotropin (TSH) appear to be within normal limits (11, 19, 70, 78, 104, 106), although there is one report that TSH is increased in anorexia nervosa (3) and Hurd et al., (60) found mean TSH levels to be less than the mean for control subjects. Wakeling et al., (106) have recently shown that TSH levels are not related to body weight. Normal TSH levels demonstrate that the thyroid changes are not due to a primary failure of the thyroid gland.

Thyrotropin responses to TRH are of normal magnitude in anorexia nervosa (70, 77, 11, 19), thus again demonstrating that the pituitary is intact. As in normal subjects, the response correlates with the resting TSH level (19). The maximal response to TRH has also been correlated with body weight (106). A delay in the TSH response to TRH with normal magnitude had been noted by several investigators (70, 3, 75, 104, 106). The delayed response occurs with simple weight loss (104) and returns to normal after weight gain (69). Delayed thyrotropin responses to TRH have been suggested to indicate hypothalamic dysfunction (55, 38) or altered TSH clearance. The increase in serum T3 which normally follows TRH administration is not diminished (21).

Low values of T3 and T4 together with normal TSH concentrations, have been shown to occur in euthyroid patients with a variety of chronic illnesses (22). In anorexia nervosa the changes in the hypothalamic-pituitary-thyroid axis are likely to occur as an adaptation to chronic illness and starvation, and are unlikely to be causally associated with the amenorrhea. Since these thyroid changes represent an adaptation to starvation, administration of thyroid hormone to correct these changes has no place in the management of anorexia nervosa.

Pituitary-Adrenal Regulation

Morning plasma cortisol levels have been found to be elevated in most cases of anorexia nervosa (74, 67, 99, 2, 60, 19) although normal levels have also been reported (103). A correlation between resting plasma morning cortisol and plasma thyroxine has been reported. This may be related to alterations in binding globulins (19). Although the binding globulins for thyroxine and cortisol are not identical, it is likely that factors that affect one globulin could also affect another, resulting in similar changes in both hormones. A decrease in cortisol binding in serum has previously been demonstrated in kwashiorkor (68).

The diurnal variation of plasma cortisol has been described as flattened (42, 17, 104). Boyar, Hellman, Roffwarg, Katz, Zumoff, O'Conner, Bradlow and Fukushima (16) found that the circadian rhythm for cortisol was preserved, but at a much higher level than that of normal controls. The absolute cortisol production rate (CPR) has been reported to be normal (16) but is increased, if cortisol production is calculated relative to body size (108). There is indirect evidence that CPR is normally proportional to body size (108) and therefore, in comparing the CPR's of emaciated patients with anorexia nervosa to those of normal weight controls, it may be appropriate to express the CPR relative to body size. These results show an increased rate in cortisol secretion in anorexia nervosa. Twenty-four hour excretion of urinary-free cortisol is also increased in anorexia nervosa (108, 16). The metabolic clearance rate of cortisol is significantly decreased and there is also a marked prolongation of the cortisol halflife (16). These results are consistent with a moderate impairment of cortisol metabolism.

Studies relying on urinary steroid excretion have generally reported 17 ketosteroids to be low (42, 32, 35, 88, 109), but 17-hydroxy and 17-ketosteroids have also been reported as normal (12). While responsiveness to dexamethasone may be normal (109), at least in some patients there is an incomplete failure of cortisol suppression (32, 108). Doerr, Fichter, Pirke and Lund (34) reported that almost all patients with emaciation showed a failure of suppression or an early escape from suppression. This reverted to normal after weight gain. ACTH stimulation tests generally result in normal to hyperactive adrenal responses (32, 109). Response to metapyrone has been reported on a small number of patients. These have been generally normal (109, 32) but Vanluchene, Aertsens and Vandekerckhove (100) found that while quantitatively normal, the metapyrone response was delayed. Several possibilities may account for these observations. On the one hand, the observed impairment of cortisol metabolism may be responsible for these changes. For example with cortisol synthesis blocked by metapyrone or dexamethasone, plasma levels will decrease more slowly because of the lowered metabolic clearance rate. Another possibility to explain the persistence of normal absolute rates of cortisol production with elevated plasma cortisol levels, the increased urinary-free cortisol excretion and the inconsistent responses to provocative tests is that the hypothalamic-pituitary mechanisms regulating adrenal activity are less sensitive than normal to negative feedback (108).

Several investigators (17, 100) have found that emaciated anorexic patients have an increased excretion of the cortisol metabolite, tetrahydrocortisol relative to tetrahydrocortisone. These abnormalties are also found in patients with hypothyroidism (16). As previously noted, starving anorexic patients show low T3 as do individuals with starvation from other causes. That these alterations in cortisol metabolism are likely related to the low levels of T3 has recently been demonstrated by Boyar et al., (16) who administered T3 to anorexic patients and found that the cortisol abnormalities (both the cortisol half-life and the tetrahydrocortisol/tetrahydrocortisone ratio) were reversed.

Many of the changes in adrenal function seen in anorexia nervosa have also been described for starvation from other causes. For example, decreased urinary excretion of adrenal corticosteroids, diminished rates of cortisol metabolism, elevated levels of plasma cortisol and incomplete suppression by dexamethasone (92, 83, 1) have all been described. However, unlike anorexia nervosa, in malnutrition, urinary-free cortisol is approximately normal and the cortisol production rate has been found to be reduced (92). The elevation of cortisol production rate relative to body size and the increased urinary-free cortisol in anorexia nervosa may indicate an increased activity of the hypothalamic-pituitary-adrenal system. A variety of poorly understood factors, including the patient's emotional distress, increased physical activity and sleep disturbance, may account for these alterations in the hypothalamic-pituitary-adrenal axis.

Prolactin

Since hyperprolactinemia is a common cause of secondary amenorrhea (40, 14), it is reasonable to determine whether abnormal prolactin secretion plays a role in the amenorrhea of anorexia nervosa. A series of studies have reported normal resting prolactin levels (10, 75, 102, 104, 106). In addition, Wakeling et al., (106) clearly demonstrated that there is no relationship between basal prolactin and body weight in anorexia nervosa. Similarly, there is no relationship between prolactin levels and those of the gonadotropins or estradiol (106). Chlorpromazine and other dopamine receptor-blockers are known to normally stimulate prolactin secretion (10), Hafner, Crisp and McNeilly (53) have shown that anorexic patients show a normal prolactin response to chlorpromazine. Moreover, TRH stimulation tests have resulted in normal increments in prolactin but a delayed response (104) and totally normal responses, not influenced by weight (106).

Normally in adults, plasma prolactin levels rise shortly after the onset of sleep at night. This is generally followed by a series of even larger secretory episodes resulting in progressively higher plasma concentrations during the night, with peak values occuring during the end of the sleep period (111). Kalucy and collaborators (64) found anorexic subjects to have low nocturnal prolactin levels. This absence of a sleep-induced rise in prolactin has been confirmed by Brown et al. (20)

and Tolis et al., (94). Since TRH can normally stimulate prolactin in these patients this suggests that the cause of the decreased prolactin secretion during sleep is of suprahypophyseal origin. This pattern of prolactin secretion may be due to dietary intake, since Hill and Wynder (58) found that changing 4 healthy non-obese nurses from a western diet to a vegetarian diet resulted in a reduction in nocturnal release of prolactin.

The data available on prolactin in anorexia nervosa strongly suggest that basal prolactin secretion is essentially normal, and prolactin responds to provocative tests normally. It is unlikely therefore, that prolactin plays a role in the amenorrhea of these individuals. The failure of patients to resume menstruation and cyclical output of gonadotropins after weight restoration is clearly not associated with high circulating prolactin. The one consistent prolactin abnormality low nocturnal levels, is likely the result of inadequate dietary intake.

Melatonin

Melatonin may be of interest in anorexia nervosa for two reasons: (1) blood levels of this hormone show a clearly defined diurnal rhythm and this may become altered as are LH and prolactin rhythms and (2) it is known to influence the reproductive hormones. Clearcut antigonadal and progonadal effects of the pineal can be demonstrated in the hamster (59, 81, 85). In the adult human female, a relationship between melatonin and the gonadotropins has been reported. Morning melatonin levels fluctuate throughout the menstrual cycle, being highest early in the follicular phase and late in the progestational phase (111). A marked 24-hour rhythm in blood melatonin exists in adult humans, with levels higher at night time than in the day (101). Jimerson et al., (62) have shown that this melatonin rhythm is preserved in patients with affective disorders, even when undergoing one night's sleep deprivation in constant light. Their data seem to indicate a close link between melatonin rhythms and a relatively stable circadian clock. Recently, Brown et al., (20) assessed the circadian rhythm of melatonin secretion in 5 emaciated subjects with primary anorexia nervosa and a sixth with both anorexia nervosa and Turner's syndrome. The latter patient was studied in order to determine if the characteristic hormonal changes of anorexia nervosa also occurred in someone with Turner's syndrome. All subjects showed a nocturnal rise in melatonin. By contrast, 3 of these subjects showed flattened nocturnal prolactin levels and all 5 primary anorexics displayed an immature circadian LH pattern.

Testosterone

Males with anorexia nervosa (especially of the restricting non-bulimic type) show complete impotence and absence of sexual activity and interest (26, 28, 48). Males with the bulimic variety are usually also impotent (28). Following weight restoration there is a gradual return of normal sexual activity.

Both reduced urinary testosterone in male patients (42, 39, 61, 9) and an elevated serum testosterone with a negative correlation to degree of weight loss in females (5) have been described. Both abnormalities tend to return to normal with weight restoration. In anorexia nervosa, the ratio of 5-alpha-reductase activity to 5-beta-reductase is significantly reduced such that the urinary metabolites of testosterone exhibit a preponderance of etiocholanolone at the expense of androsterone (15). A similar alteration is seen in hypothyroidism; that the thyroid abnormality is responsible for the changes in androgen metabolism is evident from the work of Boyar et al., (16) who showed that administration of exogenous T3 led to reversion of the adrenal androgen pattern to normal.

Carbohydrate Metabolism

The presence of fasting hypoglycemia varies considerably, for example, from Mecklenberg et al's (75) report in 100% of their patients to Vigersky et al's (102) in 56%. In response to a glucose load, anorexics may either have a flat or hyperglycemic response. A response similar to the anorexics is seen after 5 days of carbohydrate deprivation in normal subjects (54) and also in obese subjects starved for 14 days (8). Similar curves are seen in individuals with chronic wasting diseases (2). Russell and Bruce (86) have shown this impaired glucose tolerance in anorexia nervosa to be readily reversed by refeeding. Fasting insulin levels have been reported to be both elevated and lowered in anorexia nervosa and the insulin response to a glucose load may be sustained (65, 105, 26, 29). There is also an increase in insulin binding to erythrocytes which reverts to normal on refeeding (105). Similarly, insulin resistance has been reported in carbohydrate deprivation (54) in starvation (96) and in starvation of obese individuals (8). Mecklenberg et al., (75) by contrast, reported insulin sensitivity in anorexia nervosa.

The insulin resistance in anorexia nervosa has been shown to persist after weight restoration and resumption of menses in spite of normalization of the impaired glucose tolerance curve (29). This has been the basis for suggesting an inherent insulin resistance in anorexia nervosa (29); however, it is important to note that Hales and Randle (54) found a sustained insulin response in normal subjects for 14-35 days after carbohydrate deprivation. The occasionally high insulin levels, insulin resistance and hypoglycemia seen in anorexia nervosa all suggest that insulin is not a useful treatment for anorexia nervosa.

Water Conservation (Vasopressin) and Thermoregulation

Responses to heat and cold stimuli are abnormal (75, 102). These responses have been demonstrated to return to normal after weight gain (107) and the severity of the heat tolerance is significantly correlated with degree of weight loss (102). Moreover, Vigersky et al., (103) have demonstrated abnormal thermoregulation in individuals with amenorrhea and simple weight loss without anorexia nervosa.

Several investigators have demonstrated that a significant proportion of anorexics display impaired ADH secretion as inferred from failure to concentrate their urine maximally (86, 75, 102), but Vigersky et al., (103) have observed this in individuals with amenorrhea and simple weight loss without anorexia nervosa. Closely linked to disordered urine concentrating ability have been abnormalities in temperature regulation. There is a reduced basal temperature in anorexic patients (107).

Recently, investigators from the National Institute of Mental Health have measured arginine vasopressin (AVP) in both plasma and CSF (66, 49). They have reported an increase in the CSF to plasma ratio of AVP in anorexics, due to elevated CSF levels. These levels were further increased immediately on weight restoration. These findings may reflect alterations in catecholamine metabolism or they may be due to the fact that their weight-recovered patients were inducing vomiting; emesis is a potent stimulator of AVP.

Monoamine Metabolism

The neurotransmitter monoamines (MA) are of interest in anorexia nervosa for several reasons: (1) they exert significant control over the release of various hypothalamic hormones (36, 44) and (2) they exert significant regulatory control over eating behaviour. Several investigators (79, 84, 6) have recently implicated abnormalities in MA function in the pathophysiology of anorexia nervosa. However, it must be stressed that the evidence for this is indirect and the speculations have been varied. Mawson (79) suggested that the basis for anorexia nervosa may lie in a progressive depletion of subcortical brain norepinephrine and/or dopamine and that treatments which increase levels of these brain amines would be useful. He felt that ECT and chlorpromazine have proved useful because of their effects on these amines and further recommended L-dopa as a drug to correct the disorder. However, neither ECT nor chlorpromazine has actually been demonstrated to be superior to nonpharmacological therapies such as bed rest and high calorie diet, and both agents possess many other effects besides these on catecholamines. With regard to L-dopa, Johnson and Knorr (63) also suggested a possible brain dopamine deficiency and therefore administered L-dopa but without beneficial effects. Redmond et al. (84) focused on the abnormal satiety mechanism in anorexia nervosa and suggested that an increase in norepinephrine might be associated with this. Consistent with this, they described a single patient who was significantly helped by the α-adrenergic blocking agent phenoxybenzamine.

In contrast, Barry and Klawans (6) have suggested an increased brain dopamine synthesis or receptor sensitivity in the production of many of the symptoms of anorexia nervosa. Again the evidence for this is quite indirect. For example, amphetamine, which releases catecholamines at nerve endings, produces anorexia and hyperactivity (4). Apomorphine is also a dopamine agonist and results in signficiantly reduced food intake which is reversed by dopamine receptor blockade (7). Chlorpromazine, a dopamine receptor blocker, results in weight gain (13). Barry and Klawans (6) also linked the amenorrhea and decreased libido to a hyperdopaminergic state. Their hypothesis is based on indirect, largely psychopharmacological evidence.

There have been only a few evaluations of MA function in anorexic patients and those that are available have suffered from the methodological problems existing in other investigations in this field, in particular the source of the measured amines (i.e. from the brain or the periphery) (45, 46) and the influence of diet, weight and other factors must be taken into account. Halmi, et al., (57) have recently described reduced urinary 3,4-methoxy-hydroxyphenylglycol (MHPG) in anorexic patients. They linked this finding to depressive symptomatology and reduced MHPG is not uncommon in bipolar depression (47). However, their patients' MHPG levels increased with treatment so that it was not clear what effect reduced weight and low caloric intake play in the abnormality. Gross et al., (51) have confirmed this reduced urinary MHPG in emaciated anorexics but documented its increase on weight gain. Urinary homovanillic acid, an index of dopamine metabolism, and plasma dopamine were similarly reduced only in the starvation state (51). Dopamine beta-hydroxylase was normal throughout. Darby et al., (31) also found reduced plasma levels of dopamine and norepinephrine, which were weight-related. Using the probenecid test, Kaye et al., (66) reported reductions in both dopamine and serotonin turnover in emaciated anorexics. With weight restoration these tended to improve but CSF norepinephrine remained low, while patients were otherwise still symptomatic. Of importance, levels of neutral aminoacids were normal even when patients were seriously underweight. Earlier, Yap et al., (112) had reported reduced plasma tryptophan and neutral amino acids in three patients. Plasma-free tryptophan, an important serotonin precursor, has been reported to be low in anorexia nervosa, even after weight gain (25) and we have also observed this but only in emaciated patients. Also possibly linked to MA abnormalities is the recent finding and characterization of a peptide in the urine of some anorexia nervosa patients which when injected into mice produced a reduction of food intake (95).

While reductions in plasma-free tryptophan and CSF, plasma and urinary catecholamines have been documented, at present the mechanisms for these changes are not fully understood. In large measure they appear to be products of starvation. It is not yet known how these abnormalities relate to the changes in neuroendocrine secretion or anorexic symptoms.

SUMMARY

Disturbances in hypothalamic function in patients with anorexia nervosa are evident. These are mediated by several different mechanisms and are generally reversible. Certain disturbances relate directly to the degree of weight loss since they occur in starvation regardless of the cause. These include alterations in thermoregulation and water conservation, in TSH responses to TRH, in resting gonadotropin levels and LH responses to provocative tests. Other hypothalamic dysfunctions are secondary to caloric deprivation per se. Thus alterations in resting plasma growth hormone, plasma T3 and reverse T3 all appear to be directly related to food (carbohydrate) intake. Some variations in adrenal steroid and testosterone metabolism reflect these thyroid changes. Many of these disturbances in hypothalamic function are therefore secondary either to weight loss or to caloric restriction. Others (for example the elevated cortisol production rate) may in part reflect the emotional distress of the patient.

ACKNOWLEDGEMENT

The author wishes to acknowledge the Medical Research Council of Canada for their generous support.

REFERENCES

1. Alleyne, G.A.O., and Young, V. H. (1967): Clin. Sci. 33:189-200.
2. Alvarez, L. C., Dimas, C. O., Castro, A., Rossman, L. G., Vanderlaan, E. F., and Vanderlaan, W. P. (1972): J. Clin. Endocrinol. Metab. 34:400-409.
3. Aro, A., Lamberg, B. A. and Pelkonen, R. (1975): N. Engl. J. Med. 292:594-595.
4. Baldessarini, R. J. (1972): Pediatrics 49:694-701.
5. Baranowska, B. and Zgliczynski, S. (1979): Acta Encocrinol. (Copenh) 90:328-335.
6. Barry, V. C., Klawans, H. L. (1976): J. Neural. Transm. 38:107-122.
7. Barzaghi, F., Groppetti, A., Mantegassa, P. and Muller, E. F. (1973): J. Pharm. Pharmacol. 25:909-911.
8. Beck, P., Koumans, J.H.T., Winterling, G. A., Stein, M. H., Daughaday, W. H. and Kipnis, D. M. (1964): J. Lab. Clin. Med. 64: 654.

9. Beumont, P.J.V. (1970): In: Anorexia Nervosa: A Review. S. A. Med. J. August, pp.911-915.
10. Beumont, P.J.V., Friesen, H. G., Gelder, M. G., and Kolakowska (1974): Psychol. Med. 4:219-221.
11. Beumont, P.J.V., George, G.C.W., Pimstone, B. L. and Vinik, A. I. (1976): J. Clin. Endocrinol. Metab. 43:487-496.
12. Bethge, H., Nagel, A. M., Solbach, H. G., Weigelmann, W. and Zimmerman, H. (1970): Mat. Med. Nordm. 22:204-214.
13. Bobon, D. P., Jansen, P.A.J. and Bobon, J. (1970): In: The Neuroleptics: Modern Problems of Pharmacopsychiatry, edited by Basal, Karger.
14. Bohnet, H. G., Dehlen, H. G., Wutke, W. and Schneider, H. G. (1976): J. Clin. Endocrinol. Metab. 42:132-143.
15. Boyar, R. M., and Bradlow, H. L. (1977): In: Anorexia Nervosa, edited by R. A. Vigersky, pp.271-276. Raven Press, New York.
16. Boyar, R. M., Hellman, L. D., Roffwarg, H., Katz, J., Zumoff, B., O'Connor, J., Bradlow, L. and Fukushima, D. K. (1977): N. Engl. J. Med. 296:190-193.
17. Boyar, R. M. and Katz, J. (1977): In: Anorexia Nervosa, edited by R. A. Vigersky, pp.177-188. Raven Press, New York.
18. Brauman, H. and Gregoire, F. (1975): Eur. J. Clin. Invest. 5: 289-295.
19. Brown, G. M., Garfinkel, P. E., Jeuniewic, N., Moldofsky, H. and Stancer, H. C. (1977): In: Anorexia Nervosa, edited by R. A. Vigersky, pp.123-135. Raven Press, New York.
20. Brown, G. M., Kirwan, P., Garfinkel, P. and Moldofsky, H. (1979): 2nd International Symposium on Clinical Psychoneuroendocrinology in Reproduction, Venice. June (Abstract).
21. Burman, K. D., Vigersky, R. A., Loriaux, D. L., Strum, D., Djuh, Y-Y, Wright, F. D. and Wartofsky, L. (1977): In: Anorexia Nervosa, edited by R. A. Vigersky, pp.255-262. Raven Press, New York.
22. Carter, J. N., Corcoran, J. M., Eastman, C. J. and Lazarus, L. (1974): Lancet 2:971-974.
23. Casper, R. C., Davis, J. M. and Pandey, G. N. (1977): In: Anorexia Nervosa, edited by R. A. Vigersky, pp.137-227. Raven Press, New York.
24. Chopra, I. J., and Smith, S. R. (1975): J. Clin. Endocrinol. Metab. 40:221-227.
25. Coppen, A. J., Goupta, R. K., Eccleston, E. G., Wood, K. M., Wakeling, A. and Desousa, V.F.A. (1976): Lancet 1:961.
26. Crisp, A. H. (1965): Proc. Roy. Soc. Med. 58:814.
27. Crisp, A. H. (1968): Gut 9:270-372.
28. Crisp, A. H. (178): Inter. J. Obesity 2:17-32.
29. Crisp, A. H., Ellis, J. and Lowy, C. (1967): Postgrad. Med. 43: 97-102.
30. Croxson, M. S. and Ibbertson, H. K. (1977): J. Clin. Endocrinol. Metab. 44:167-174.
31. Darby, P. L., Vanloon, G., Garfinkel, P. E., Brown, G. M. and Kirwan, P. (1980): Presentation at the American Psychosomatic Society, New York.
32. Danowski, T. S., Livstone, E., Gonzales, A. R., Jung, Y. and Khurana, R. C. (1972): Hormones 3:105-118.
33. Devlin, J. G. (1975): Irish Med. J. 68:227-231.
34. Doerr, P., Fichter, M., Pirke, K. M. and Lund, R. (1980): Sixth International Congress of Endocrinology, Melbourne, p.630 (Abs.).

35. Emanuel, R. W. (1956): J. Clin. Endocrinol. Metab. 16:801-816.
36. Ettigi, P. G. and Brown, G. M. (1977): Am. J. Psychiatry 134: 493-501.
37. Faglia, G. P., Beck-Peccoz, B., Ambrosi, C., Ferrari, B. and Neri, V. (1973): J. Clin. Endocrinol. Metab. 33:99.
38. Faglia, G. P., Beck-Peccoz, P., Ferrari, C., Ambrosi, B., Spada, A., Travaglini, P. and Parocchi, S. (1975): J. Clin. Endocrinol. Metab. 37:596-601.
39. Frankel, R. J. and Jenkins, J. S. (1975): Acta Endocrinol. 78: 209-221.
40. Franks, S., Murray, M.A.F., Jequier, A.M., Stella, S. J., Nebarro, J.D.M. and Jacobs, H.S. (1975): Clin. Endocrinol. 4:597-607.
41. Gardner, D. F., Kaplan, M. M., Stanley, C. A. and Utiger, R. D. (1979): N. Engl. J. Med. 300:579-584.
42. Garfinkel, P. E., Brown, G. M., Moldofsky, H. and Stancer, H. C. (1975): Arch. Gen. Psychiatry 32:739-744.
43. Garfinkel, P. E., Moldofsky, H. and Garner, D. M. (1980): Arch. Gen. Psychiatry 37:1036-1040.
44. Garfinkel, P. E., Brown, G. M., Warsh, J. J. and Stancer, H. C. (1979): Psychoneuroendocrinology 4:13-20.
45. Garfinkel, P. E., Warsh, J. J., Stancer, H. C. and Sibony, D. (1976): Arch. Gen. Psychiatry 33:1462-1466.
46. Garfinkel, P. E., Warsh, J. J., Stancer, H. C. and Godse, D. (1977): Arch. Gen. Psychiatry 34:735-739.
47. Garfinkel, P. E., Warsh, J. J., and Stancer, H. C. (1979): Am. J. Psychiatry 136:535-539.
48. Garfinkel, P. E. and Garner, D. M. In: Anorexia Nervosa: A Multidimensional Perspective. Brunner-Mazel, New York (1982).
49. Gold, M. S., Kaye, W., Robertson, G., Goodwin, F. K. and Ebert, M. (1980): 133rd Annual Meeting of the American Psychiatric Assoc., Syllabus and Scientific Proceedings, p.326.
50. Gold, M. S., Pottash, A.L.C., Sweeney, D. R., Martin, D.M. and Davies, R. K. (1980): Am. J. Psychiatry 137:101-102.
51. Gross, H. A., Lake, C. R., Ebert, M. H., Zeigler, M. G. and Kopin, I. J. (1979): J. Clin. Endocrinol. Metab. 49:805-809.
52. Gull, W. W. (1874): Trans. Clin. Soc. Lond. 7:22-28.
53. Hafner, R. J., Crisp, A. H. and McNeilly, A. S. (1976): Postgrad. Med. J. 52:76-79.
54. Hales, C. N. and Randle, P. J. (1963): Lancet 1:790.
55. Hall, R., Besser, G. M., Ormston, G. J., Cryer, A. R. and McKendrick, M. (1972): Lancet 1:759-763.
56. Harrower, A.D.B., Yap, P. L., Nairn, I. M., Walton, H. J., Strong, J. A. and Craig, A. (1977): Brit. Med. J. 2:156-159.
57. Halmi, K. A., Dekirmenjian, J. H., Davis, J. M., Casper, R. and Goldberg, S. (1978): Arch. Gen. Psychiatry 35:458-460.
58. Hill, P. and Wynder, F. (1976): Lancet 2:806-807.
59. Hoffman, K. (1973): J. Comp. Physiol. 85:267-282.
60. Hurd, H. P., Palumbo, P. J. and Gharib, H. (1977): Mayo Clin. Proc. 52:711.
61. Ismail, A. A. and Harkness, R. A. (1967): Acta Endocrinol. 56: 469-480.
62. Jimerson, D. C., Lynch, H. J., Post, R. M., Wurtman, R. J. and Bunney, W. W. (1977): Life Sci. 20:1501-1508.
63. Johansen, A. J. and Knorr, N. J. (1977): In: Anorexia Nervosa, edited by R. A. Vigersky, pp.363-372. Raven Press, New York.

64. Kalucy, R. C., Crisp, A. H., Chard, T., McNeilly, A., Chen, C. N. and Lacey, J. H. (1976): J. Psychosom. Res. 20:595-604.
65. Kanis, J. A., Brown, P., Fitzpatrick, K., Hibbert, D. J., Horn, D. B., Nairn, I. M., Shirling, D., Strong, J. A. and Walton, H. J. (1974): Quart. J. Med. 43:321-338.
66. Kaye, W. H., Ebert, M. H. and Lake, C. R. (1980): 133rd Annual Meeting of the American Psychiatric Association. Syllabus and Scientific Proceedings, p.326.
67. Landon, J., Greenwood, F. C., Stamp, T.C.B. and Wynn, V. (1966): J. Clin. Invest. 45:437-449.
68. Leonard, P.L.J. (1973): In: Endocrine Aspects of Malnutrition, Marasmus, Kwashiorkor and Psychosocial Dwarfism, edited by L. I. Gardner and P. Amacher, pp.355-362. Kroc Foundation, Saint Ynez, California.
70. Lundberg, P. O., Walinder, J., Werner, I. and Wide, L. (1972): Eur. J. Clin. Invest. 2:150-153.
71. Lesegue, C. (1894): Arch. Gen. de Med. p.385.
72. Maeda, K., Kato, Y., Ohgo, S., Chihara, K., Yoshimoto, Y., Yamaguchi, N., Uromaru, S., and Imura, H. (1975): J. Clin. Endocrinol. Metab. 40:501-505.
73. Maeda, K., Kato, Y., Yamaguchi, N., Chihara, K., Ohga, S., Iwasaki, Y., Yoshimoto, Y., Moridera, K., Kuromaru, S. and Imura, H. (1976): Acta Endocrinol. (Kbh) 81:1-8.
74. Marks, V., Howorth, N. and Greenwood, F. C. (1965): Nature 686-687.
75. Mecklenberg, R. S., Loriaux, D. L., Thompson, R. H., Andersen, A. E. and Lipsett, M. B. (1974): Medicine 53:147-159.
76. Miyai, K., Yamamoto, T., Azukizawa, M., Ishibashi, I. and Kumahara, Y. (1975): J. Clin. Endocrinol. Metab. 40:334-338.
77. Moshang, T., Jr., Parks, J. S., Baker, L., Vaidya, V., Utiger, R.D., Bongiovanni, A. M. and Snyder, P. J. (1975): J. Clin. Endocrinol. Metab. 40:470-473.
78. Moshang, T., Jr., and Utiger, R. D. (1977): In: Anorexia Nervosa, edited by R. A. Vigersky, pp.263-270. Raven Press, New York.
79. Mawson, A. R. (1974): Psychol. Med. 4:289-308.
80. Neri, V., Ambrosi, B., Beck-Peccoz, P., Travaglini, P. and Faglia, G. (1972): Folia Endocrinol. (Roma) 25:143-152.
81. Orts, R. J., Kocan, K. M. and Wilson, I. B. (1975): Life Sci. 17:845-850.
82. Pimstone, B. L., Becker, D. J. and Hansen, J.D.L. (1972): In: Growth and Growth Hormone, edited by A. Pecile and E. E. Muller, pp.389-401. Excerpta Medica, Amsterdam.
83. Rao, K.S.J., Srikantia, S. G. and Gopalan, G. (1968): Arch. Dis. Child. 43:365-367.
84. Redmond, D. E., Jr., Swann, A., Heninger, G. R. (1976): Lancet 2:307.
85. Reiter, R. J., Vaughan, M. K., Blask, D. E. and Johnson, L. Y. (1974): Science 185:1169-1171.
86. Russell, G. F. M. and Bruce, T. (1964): Clin. Sci. 26:157-163.
87. Russell, G. F. M. and Bruce, J. T. (1966): Am. J. Med. 40:38-48.
88. Seidensticker, J. F. and Tzagournis, M. (1968): J. Chron. Dis. 21:361-367.
89. Sherman, B. M. and Halmi, K. A. (1977): In: Anorexia Nervosa, edited by R. A. Vigersky, pp.227-289. Raven Press, New York.
90. Simmonds, M. (1914): Arch. Path. Anat. 217:226-239.

91. Sizonenko, P. C., Rabinovitch, A., Schneider, P., Paunier, L., Wollheim, C. B. and Zhand, G. (1975): Pediatr. Res. 9:733-738.
92. Smith, S. R., Bledsoe, T., and Chhetri, M. K. (1975): J. Clin. Endocrinol. Metab. 40:43-52.
93. Spaulding, S. W., Chopra, I. J., Sherwin, R. S. and Lyall, S. S. (1976): J. Clin. Endocrinol. Metab. 42:197-200.
94. Tolis, G., Woods, I. and Guyda, H. (1979): Royal College of Physicians and Surgeons of Canada, p.40 (Abstract).
95. Trygstad, O., Foss, I., Edminson, P. D., Johansen, J. H. and Reichelt, K. L. (1978): Acta Endocrinol. (Copenh.) 89:196-208.
96. Unger, R. H., Eisenstant, A. M. and Madison, L. L. (1963): J. Clin. Invest. 42:1031.
97. Vagenakis, A. G. (1977): In: Anorexia Nervosa, edited by R. A. Vigersky, pp.243-252. Raven Press, New York.
98. Vagenakis, A. G., Burger, A., Portnay, G. I., Rudolph, M., O'Brian, J. I., Azizi, R., Arky, R., Nicod, P., Ingbar, S. H. and Braverman, L. E. (1975): J. Clin. Endocrinol. Metab. 41:191-194.
99. Vanderlaan, W. P., Parker, D. C., Rossman, L. G. and Vanderlaan, E. F. (1970): Metabolism 19:891-897.
100. Vanluchene, E., Aertsens, W. and Vandekerckhove, D. V. (1979): Acta Endocrinol. 90:133-138.
101. Vaughan, G. M., Pelham, R. W., Pang, S. F. Loughlin, L. L., Wilson, K. M., Sandock, K. L., Vaughan, M. K., Koslow, S. H. and Reiter, R. J. (1976): J. Clin. Endocrinol. Metab. 42:752-764.
102. Vigersky, R. A., Loriaux, D. L., Andersen, A. E., Mecklenburg, S. and Vaitukaitis, J. L. (1976): J. Clin. Endocrinol. Metab. 43: 893-900.
103. Vigersky, R. A., Andersen, A. E., Thompson, R. H. and Loriaux, D.L. (1977): N. Engl. J. Med. 297:1141-1145.
104. Vigersky, R. A. and Loriaux, D. L. (1977): In: Anorexia Nervosa, edited by R. A. Vigersky, pp.109-122. Raven Press, New York.
105. Wachslicht-Rodbard, H., Gross, H. A., Rodbard, D., Ebert, M. H. and Roth, J. (1979): N. Engl. J. Med. 300:882-887.
106. Wakeling, A., DeSouza, V. F. A., Gore, M.B.R., Sabur, M., Kingstone, D. and Boss, A.M.B. (1979): Psychol. Med. 9:265-272.
107. Wakeling, A. and Russell, G. (1970): Psychol. Med. 1:30-39.
108. Walsh, B. T., Katz, J. L., Levin, J., Kream, J., Fukushima, D. K., Hellman, L. D., Weiner, H. and Zumoff, B. (1978): Psychosomatic Med. 40:499-506.
109. Warren, M. P. and Vande Wiele, L. (1973): Am. J. Obstet, & Gynecol. 117:435-451.
110. Weitzman, E. D. (1976): Ann. Rev. Med. 27:225-243.
111. Wetterberg, L., Arendt, J., Paunier, L., Sizonenko, B. C., Van Donsellar, W. and Heyden, T. (1976): J. Clin. Endocrinol. Metab. 42:185-188.
112. Yap, S. H., Hafkenscheid, J.C.M. and Van Tongeren, J.H.M. (1975): Am. J. Clin. Nutr. 28:1356-1363.

Neuroendocrinology and Psychiatric Disorder,
edited by G. M. Brown, et al.
Raven Press, New York 1984.

Hypothalamic Control of the Menstrual Cycle: Implications for the Study of Anorexia Nervosa

Barry M. Sherman

The studies of hormonal changes in patients with anorexia nervosa were done in the expectation that they might lead to a better understanding of the neurochemical basis of both the behavioural and endocrine distrubances that characterize the syndrome. That hope has not been realized. The results cited by Dr. Vigersky (Chapter 23) strongly suggest that the abnormalities in hypothalamic-pituitary-ovarian regulation observed in anorexia nervosa are largely secondary to the nutritional changes that occur as a result of the altered behavioural state (35). Nevertheless, the study of anorexia nervosa has been an excellent model for the study of hormonal changes that occur during normal pubertal maturation and their relationship to growth and nutrition. As a result, clinical investigators and clinicians have been made aware of the importance of nutrition, weight loss, unusual dietary habits and exercise in reproductive disorders.

TABLE 1. A Summary of Changes in LH and FSH in Patients with Anorexia Nervosa

1. Low basal LH and FSH.
2. Greater depression of LH than FSH.
3. Correlation between basal LH and FSH and severity of weight loss.
4. Loss of pulsatile pattern of LH release.
5. Absence of nocturnal LH secretion associated with puberty.
6. Blunted or absent LH response to GnRH.
7. A greater FSH than LH response to GnRH.
8. Loss of LH and FSH response to clomiphene and estrogen.

Table 1 summarizes the major changes in gonadotropin regulation described in anorexia nervosa. The amenorrhea of anorexia nervosa represents the hormonal equivalent of the prepubertal state, in that there is an absence of spontaneous, pulsatile secretion of gonadotropin releasing hormone (GnRH) from the hypothalamus, a diminished pituitary synthesis and release of luteinizing hormone (LH) and follicle stimulating hormone (FSH) and depletion of the pituitary stores of those hormones. Amenorrhea is a consequence of the lack of gonadotropin stimulation of ovarian follicular maturation. The intermittent administration of exogenous GnRH to patients with anorexia nervosa can restore the pituitary secretion of LH and FSH, and of ovulation. Spontaneous recovery takes place with weight gain, recapitulating the hormonal changes that occur during normal puberty.

Regulation of the Menstrual Cycle

In order to fully appreciate the observations concerning gonadotropin

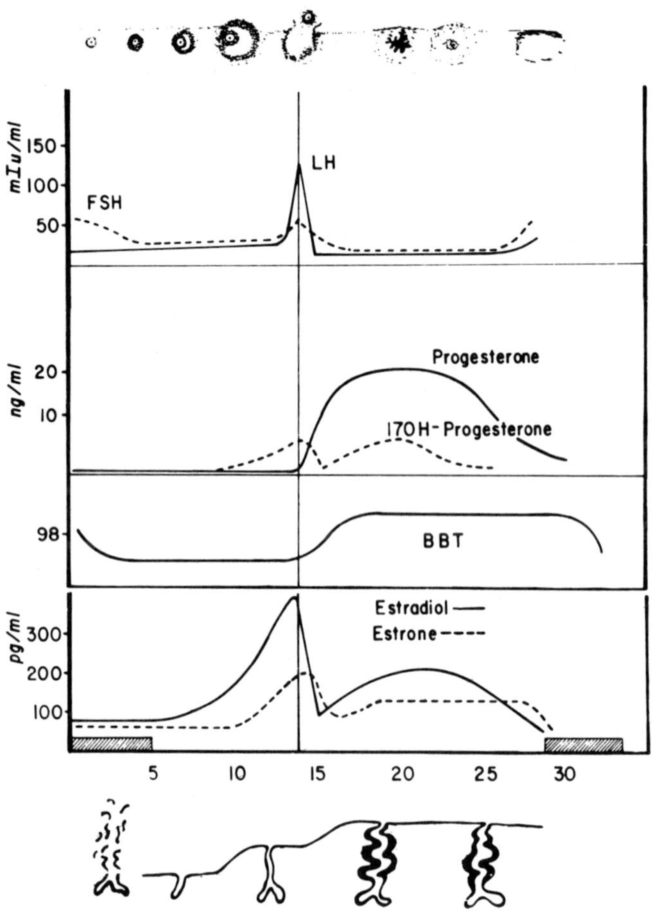

FIG. 1. Changes in concentrations of relevant hormones throughout the menstrual cycle illustrated and correlated with the sequential anatomic changes in the ovary and endometrium. BBT: basal body temperature. Follicular phase precedes day 14; luteal phase follows day 14.

regulation in anorexia nervosa, it is necessary to integrate the results of concurrent studies carried out in other model systems. For more than 10 years, Ernst Knobil and his colleagues at the University of Pittsburgh have been studying the control of the menstrual cycle in rhesus monkeys (18, 19). The menstrual cycle of the rhesus monkey has a periodicity and hormonal characteristics like that described for humans.

The principal features of the normal human adult menstrual cycle are illustrated in Figure 1. An increase in the plasma level of FSH begins late in the luteal phase and continues into the early follicular phase of the next cycle. This increase presumably initiates the maturation of multiple follicles, one of which is selected by mechanisms yet unknown for complete maturation and ovulation. Estradiol secretion increases during follicular maturation and reaches peak plasma concentrations of 300-500 picograms/ml, usually 24 - 48 hours before the mid-cycle LH surge.

This sequence represents a process of positive feedback in which the increasing estrogen concentrations sensitize the gonadotropes and result in a burst of LH secretion at a critical estrogen concentration. There is a second rise in estradiol concentration during the luteal phase, presumably reflecting synthesis by the corpus luteum. Plasma progesterone, which is in the 100 picogram/ml range during the preovulatory phase of the cycle, undergoes a 100-fold rise to levels of 10-30 ng/ml and is the principal secretion of the mature corpus luteum. Progesterone is responsible for the rise in basal body temperature and the change to the secretory state of the endometrium. If pregnancy does not occur, a fall in both estrogen and progesterone concentrations in the late luteal phase results in sloughing of the endometrium.

Dr. Knobil and his co-workers have used surgical and radiofrequency lesions of the central nervous system to localize the centers responsible for regulation of the menstrual cycle. Monkeys with complete surgical disconnection of the medial basal hypothalamus from higher control centers have normal basal levels of LH and retain the pulsatile pattern of LH release as well as the capacity to initiate a surge of LH and FSH after administration of exogenous estrogen (11). This experiment demonstrated that the medial basal hypothalamus was the only part of the nervous system necessary for operation of the complete menstrual cycle. The next step was to localize the critical area within the medial basal hypothalamus. To do this, bilateral radiofrequency lesions were placed in the arcuate region of the medial basal hypothalamus of ovariectomized monkeys with elevated serum gonadotropin levels. These lesions result in: 1) a sharp decline in serum LH and FSH concentrations to essentially undetectable levels; and 2) a loss of LH and FSH responsiveness to exogenous estrogen administration (Fig. 2)(28). The secretion of other pituitary hormones, including adrenocortical stimulating hormone, thyroid stimulating hormone, and prolactin, was unaffected by these discrete lesions.

The pulsatile administration of exogenous GnRH restored secretion of LH and FSH. Infusion of GnRH at a rate of 1 μg/minute for 6 minutes of each hour restored normal basal LH and FSH concentrations, and in monkeys with intact ovaries, the continuous administration of GnRH in this pattern for 4 - 6 months restored regular ovulatory menstrual cycles (Fig. 3)(19, 20). In a similar fashion, cyclic ovulatory menstrual cycles were induced in prepubertal monkeys by the hourly administration of GnRH for up to 8 months (19, 37). Cessation of GnRH treatment was associated with regression to the prepubertal state.

Monkeys with arcuate nucleus ablation fail to demonstate the positive feedback release of LH and FSH after exogenous administration of estrogen. This phenomenon is resotred if the estrogen challenge is administered to the lesioned monkeys during GnRH replacement. Figure 4 shows an initial fall in LH and FSH concentration (negative feedback), followed by a surge of LH and FSH secretion (positive feedback) (Fig. 4)(26). This experiment indicates that both the negative and postive feedback effects of estrogen are exerted at the pituitary rather than the hypothalamic level.

The data derived from Knobil's work in the monkey have led to fundamental conclusions regarding regulation of the menstrual cycle. Sustained secretion of LH and FSH is dependent on the permissive effect of an appropriate pattern of GnRH stimulation. Ovarian follicular development and estrogen production occur in response to gonadotropin stimulation. The pattern of pituitary LH and FSH secretion including the midcycle, preovulatory surge, occurs in response to ovarian steroid hormone secretion. Moreover, the timing of the menstrual cycle is dependent on the

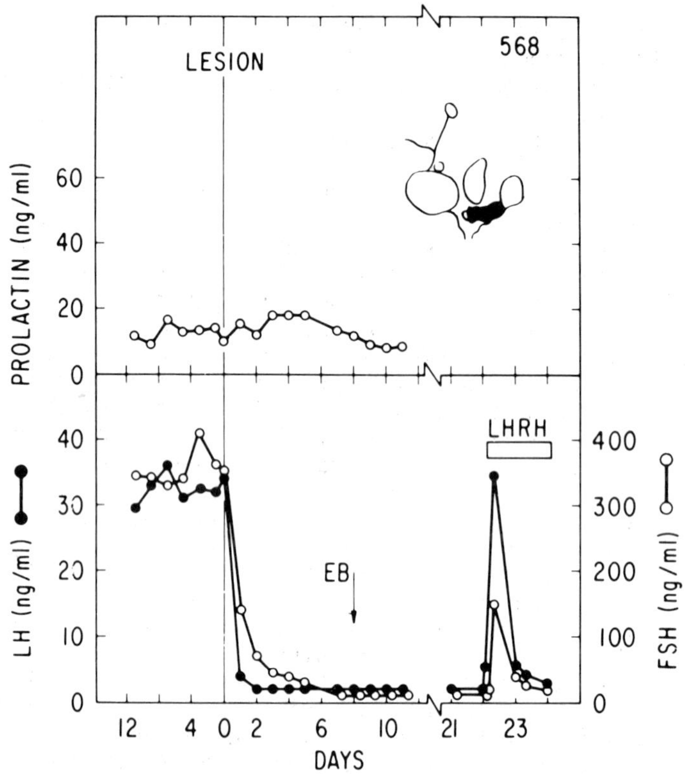

FIG. 2. Changes in serum LH and FSH concentrations in ovariectomized rhesus monkey after placement of a radiofrequency lesion in the arcuate region on day 0. The positive feedback action of estradiol benzoate administered on day 8 and indicated by an arrow was abolished by the lesion. The continuous infusion of GnRH caused a transient release of LH and FSH. From Plant et al. (28) with permission.

interval necessary for follicular maturation, approximately 14 days, and the duration of corpus luteum function, also about 14 days. In this view, the ovary rather than the central nervous system times the events of the menstrual cycle (19).

Implications for Anorexia Nervosa

The rhesus monkey with arcuate nucleus ablation has obvious similarities to amenorrheic patients with severe anorexia nervosa. Basal LH and FSH levels are low, there is loss of both pulsatile gonadotropin secretion and the positive feedback of estrogen on LH and FSH release. The repetitive administration of exogenous GnRH can restore gonadotropin secretion and ovulatory menses in patients with anorexia nervosa as in the lesioned monkeys (24, 27). The failure of LH and FSH to respond to estrogen administration in patients with anorexia nervosa is a manifestation of pituitary dependence on adequate GnRH priming. From these similarities, we can suggest that neither pituitary nor ovarian competence limits the resumption of cyclic menses in anorexia nervosa patients, and that the defect appears to reside in the failure of mechanisms loca-

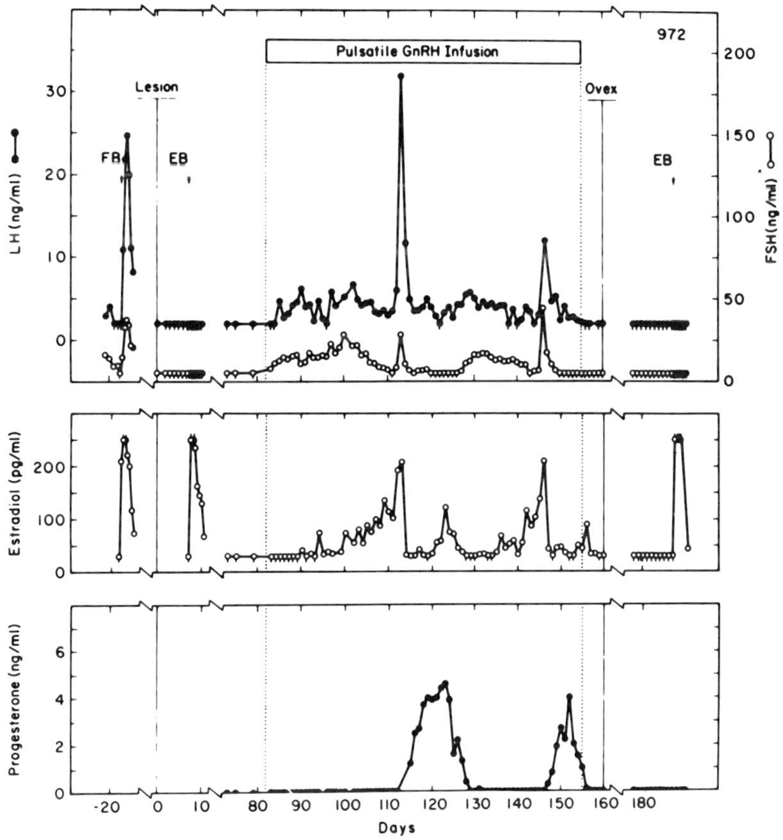

FIG. 3. The induction of ovulatory menstrual cycles in a rhesus monkey with a hypothalamic lesion administered pulsatile exogenous GnRH for approximately 75 days. The infusion consisted of 6 minute pulses of GnRH (1 μg/minute) each hour. From Knobil et al. (19, 20) with permission.

ted in the arcuate nucleus to initiate an appropriate pattern of GnRH secretion.

In patients with anorexia nervosa, serum FSH concentrations are generally less depressed and recover more promptly than LH levels (1, 33, 36). Throughout the reproductive biology literature, there are other examples of disparate patterns of LH and FSH secretion. These have been difficult to interpret, particularly in the context of information suggesting that there is but one releasing hormone for both LH and FSH and that both hormones arise from one pituitary cell type. The experiments in monkeys with arcuate nucleus ablation indicate that the pituitary release of LH and FSH is sensitive to the pattern of GnRH administration. Pulses at a frequency greater than once per hour caused a reduction in LH and FSH levels like that seen during continuous GnRH administration (19, 28). This phenomenon has been attributed to receptor down-regulation, but there is no direct confirmatory evidence for that. At a pulse frequency of less than once per hour, the LH and FSH response pattern becomes discordant with an inversion of the LH/FSH ratio. The

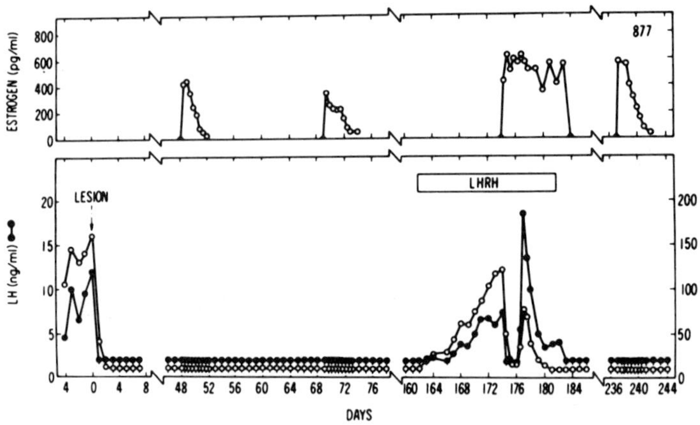

FIG. 4. The administration of estradiol benzoate before GnRH replacement in a lesioned monkey was ineffective. During GnRH replacement a sustained increase in circulating estrogen caused a biphasic effect on LH and FSH concentrations. From Nakai et al. (26) with permission.

explanation for this is not clear, but may be a result of differences in clearance rates for LH and FSH and the greater magnitude of the gonadotropin responses to low frequency pulses of GnRH (19). Thus, changes in the frequency of arcuate nucleus activity at different stages of anorexia nervosa, or during various stages of pubertal maturation might explain, in part, the disparate patterns of gonadotropin concentrations observed in those situations.

Neurochemical Regulation

If the amenorrhea of anorexia nervosa represents a functional abnormality in the area of the arcuate nucleus, it is important to appreciate the neurochemical regulators of GnRH. There is comparatively little information concerning this or the related question of the factor(s) that initiate spontaneous activity in the arcuate area.

The histochemical studies of Fuxe and colleagues indicate a close relationship of dopamine and GnRH containing cell bodies in the arcuate nucleus, and similarly staining nerve terminals in the external layer of the median eminence (12). There is also evidence for termination of norepinephrine containing neurons in the arcuate nucleus.

The administration of alpha adrenergic blocking agents, such as phenoxybenzamine to ovariectomized rhesus monkeys showed a decrease in basal serum LH concentrations and an abolition of the pulsatile pattern of gonadotropin secretion. Beta adrenergic blockade with propranolol had no effect (2). These studies have not been duplicated in humans, perhaps because of the limitation necessarily placed on the drug dose employed.

A more recent series of human studies showed that the infusion of dopamine lowers serum gonadotropin concentrations in man (14-16, 21, 22). There is a greater effect on LH than FSH levels, while for both hormones, the absolute magnitude of suppression is significantly correlated with the basal concentration. Studies done during the late follicular phase of the menstrual cycle when LH levels are elevated demonstrate a greater

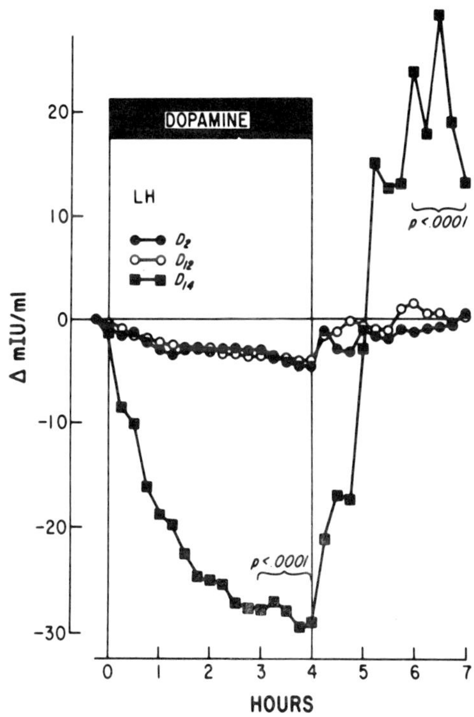

FIG. 5. The effect of infusion of dopamine at a rate of 4 μg/kg per minute on serum LH on days 2, 12, and 14 of the menstrual cycle. From Judd et al. (15) with permission.

absolute decrease, but the same percent decline as during the early follicular or luteal phases of the cycle (Fig. 5)(15, 16).

Interest in a possible role for endogenous opiates in the regulation of the reproductive cycle has led to the use of naloxone, an opiate antagonist in human studies. Administration of 8-10 mg of naloxone to adult women causes an increase in the serum LH concentration. As for dopamine, response to naloxone varies with the stage of the menstrual cycle (Fig. 6). In healthy, regularly cycling women, LH responses were elicited during the late follicular and luteal phases but not during the early follicular phase of the cycle (3, 30). There was no change in FSH after naloxone challenge during any part of the menstrual cycle.

At this time, it is difficult to integrate these observations concerning dopamine and endogenous opiates into a coherent model for neurochemical modulation of hypothalamic GnRH and pituitary gonadotropin synthesis and secretion. Their site(s) of action, whether hypothalamic, pituitary, or both, is unclear. The variable responses elicited at different phases of the menstrual cycle imply a role for estrogen and progesterone as modifiers of the effects of both agents, but this requires more study. While an intact medial basal hypothalamus may be sufficient for maintenance of the menstrual cycle, these observations support the notion of modulation by higher centers. Such neurochemical regulation is essential to explain the amenorrheic states related to stressful states. In some women with hypothalamic amenorrhea, administration of metoclopramide or naloxone results in a significant increase in LH.

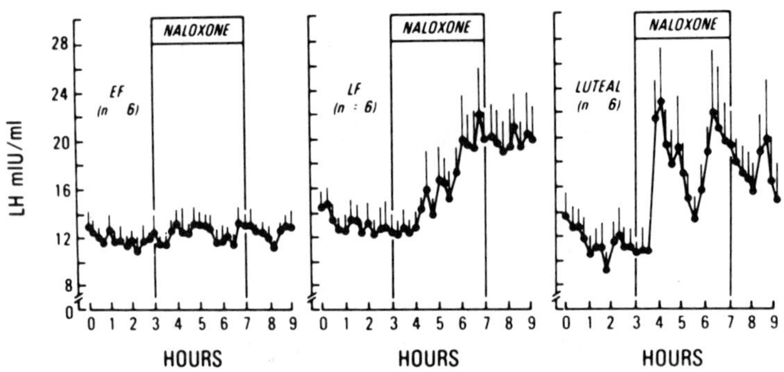

FIG. 6. The effect of an infusion of naloxone at a rate of 1.6 mg/hour for 4 hours during the early and late follicular phase and mid-luteal phases of the menstrual cycle. From Quigley and Yen (29) with permission.

These results have suggested increased hypothalamic opiate and/or dopamine activity in some amenorrheic syndromes (29).

Initiation of Hypothalamic Activity

A major piece of missing information relates to the characterization of the signal that triggers the onset of hypothalamic GnRH activity at puberty. It is here that the mechanisms for normal pubertal maturation and the amenorrhea of anorexia nervosa intersect. The secular change in menarcheal age and its relation to nutrition have dominated recent discussions regarding the onset of sexual maturation in women. Many studies have confirmed Tanner's observation that there has been a steady decrease in age at menarche averaging approximately 3-4 months per decade (34, 38). This secular change now observed in many different populations has been attributed to a general improvement in nutrition and is illustrated by contemporary studies which show that, within the same country, women residing in socio-economically deprived areas have a significantly later onset of menarche than those living in more affluent regions (23, 31, 32). During the recent social upheaval in Bangladesh, there was a significant delay in the onset of sexual maturation in women that was related to nutritional deprivation (4). The experiences with anorexia nervosa patients, those with amenorrhea associated with minimal weight loss, and those who have amenorrhea accompanying vigorous exercise, all lend support to the notion that nutrition and energy balance are in some way related to the initiation and sustenance of the hypothalamic mechanisms responsible for GnRH secretion.

Frisch and Revelle (5-8) emphasized the relationship of menarcheal age to the attainment of a critical nutritional state presumptively optimal for reproduction. Particular attention has been addressed to the issue of an average critical weight at the initiation of pubertal weight gain and at menarche for both early and late-maturing girls. This critical weight has been correlated with the ratio of lean body mass to fat, and with estimates of the percent body fat. This debate over whether the onset of puberty and menses is related to a specific body weight or percent fat may have obscured the overall evidence that links nutritional adequacy to the reproductive capacity of women (9, 10).

Some have challenged the conclusion that the gonadotropin abnormalities in anorexia nervosa are wholly explained by nutritional deficits. This challenge is often based upon observations that amenorrhea may precede marked weight loss and may not resolve even after restoration of near normal body weight (13, 17, 25). It must be remembered, however, that body height and weight and the estimates of body fat or body water extrapolated from height and weight are only indirect indicators of a postulated biologic signal that activates hypothalamic function. The nature of that signal, whether it arises inside or outside the central nervous system and how it is related to body mass, is completely unknown. Because there are changes in steroid hormone metabolism that accompany obesity, it has been tempting to postulate that the signal is related to change in androgen or estrogen metabolism.

SUMMARY

Concomitant studies in human and animal systems have greatly increased our appreciation of the complex regulation of the menstrual cycle and of the pathogenesis of certain disorders of female reproduction. The limits of our understanding of the pathogenesis and mechanisms underlying anorexia nervosa are, to an extent, the same that circumscribe our knowledge of normal physiology. Progress can be anticipated in both areas. As advances are made in other systems, anorexia nervosa will be an excellent model for further study of the relationship between nutritional status and mechanisms of activation and regulation of hypothalamic GnRH secretory capacity in man.

ACKNOWLEDGMENT

This work was supported in part by Grant RR59 from the General Clinical Research Center Program, NIH.

REFERENCES

1. Beumont, P.J.V., George, G.C.W., Pimstone, B. L. and Vinik, A. I. (1976): J. Clin. Endocrinol. Metab. 43:487-496.
2. Bhattacharya, A. N., Kierschke, D. J., Yamaji, T. and Knobil, E. (1972): Endocrinology 90:778-786.
3. Blankstein, J., Reyes, F. I., Winter, J.S.D. and Faiman, C. (1981): Clin. Endocrinol. 14:287-325.
4. Chowdbury, A.K.M.A., Huffman, S. L. and Curlin, G. T. (1977): Social Biology 24:316-325.
5. Frisch, R. E. and Revelle, R. (1970): Hum. Biol. 43:140-159.
6. Frisch, R. E. and Revelle, R. (1971): Arch. Dis. Child 46:695-701.
7. Frisch, R. E., Revelle, R. and Cook, S. (1973): Hum. Biol. 15: 469-483.
8. Frisch, R. E. and McArthur, J. W. (1974): Science 185:949-951.
9. Frisch, R. (1978): Science 199:22-30.
10. Frisch, R. E. (1980): Fed. Proc. 39:2395-2400.
11. Hess, D. L., Wilkins, R. H., Moossy, J., Chang, J. L., Plant, T. M., McCormack, J. T., Nakai, Y. and Knobil, E. (1977): Endocrinology 101:1264-1271.
12. Hokfelt, T., Elde, R., Fuxe, K., Johansson, O., Ljungdahl, A., Goldstein, M., Luft, R., Efendic, S., Nilsson, G., Terenius, L., Perez de la Mora, M., Possani, L., Tapia, R., Teran, L. and Palacios, R. (1978): In: The Hypothalamus, edited by S. Reichlin, R. J. Baldessarini and J. B. Martin, pp.69-135. Raven Press, New York.

13. Hsu, L.K.G., Crisp, A. H. and Hardin, B. (1979): The Lancet 1: 61-65.
14. Huseman, C. A., Kugler, J. A. and Schneider, I. G. (1980): J. Clin. Endocrinol. Metab. 51:209-214.
15. Judd, S. J., Rakoff, J. S. and Yen, S.S.C. (1978): J. Clin. Endocrinol. Metab. 47:494-498.
16. Judd, S. J., Rigg, L. A. and Yen, S.S.C. (1979): J. Clin. Endocrinol. Metab. 49:182-184.
17. Katz, J. L., Boyar, R., Roffwarg, H., Hellman, L. and Weiner, H. (1978): Psychosomatic Med. 40:549-567.
18. Knobil, E. (1974): In: Recent Progress in Hormone Research, edited by R. O. Greep, pp.1-36. Academic Press, New York.
19. Knobil, E. (1980): In: Recent Progress in Hormone Research, edited by R. O. Greep, pp.53-88. Academic Press, New York.
20. Knobil, E., Plant, T. M., Wildt, L., Belchetz, P. E. and Marshall, G. (1980): Science 207:1371-1373.
21. Lachelin, G.C.L., LeBlanc, H. and Yen, S.S.C. (1977): J. Clin. Endocrinol. Metab. 44:728-731.
22. LeBlanc, H., Lachelin, G.C.L., Abu-Facil, S. and Yen, S.S.C. (1976): J. Clin. Endocrinol. Metab. 43:668-674.
23. Malina, R. M., Chumlea, C., Stepick, C. D. and Lopez, F. G. (1977): Ann. Hum. Biol. 4:551-558.
24. Marshall, J. C. and Kelch, R. P. (1979): J. Clin. Endocrinol. 49: 712-718.
25. Morimoto, Y., Oishi, T., Hanasaki, N., Miyatake, A., Sate, B., Noma, K., Kato, H., Yano, S. and Yamamura, Y. (1980): Endocrinol. Japon 27:191-200.
26. Nakai, Y., Plant, T. M., Hess, D. L., Keogh, E. J. and Knobil, E. (1978): Endocrinology 102:1008-1014.
27. Nillius, S. J., Fries, H. and Wide, L. (1975): Am. J. Obstet. Gynecol. 122:921-928.
28. Plant, T. M., Krey, L. C., Moossy, J., McCormack, J. T., Hess, D. L. and Knobil, E. (1978): Endocrinology 102:52-62.
29. Quigley, M. E., Sheehan, K. L., Casper, R. F. and Yen, S.S.C. (1980): J. Clin. Endocrinol. Metab. 50:949-953.
30. Quigley, M. E. and Yen, S.S.C. (1980): J. Clin. Endocrinol. Metab. 51:179-181.
31. Roberts, D. F., Chiun, S., Girija, B. and Singh, H. D. (1977): Ann. Hum. Biol. 4:171-177.
32. Rona, R. and Pereiva, G. (1974): Hum. Biol. 46:33-42.
33. Sherman, B. M., Halmi, K. A. and Zamudio, R. (1975): J. Clin. Endocrinol. Metab. 41:135-142.
34. Tanner, J. M. (1962): Growth at Adolescence. Blackwell, Oxford.
35. Vigersky, R. (1981): In: this volume.
36. Warren, M. P., Jewelewicz, R., Dyrenfurth, I., Ans, R., Khalaf, S. and Vande Wiele, R. L. (1975): J. Clin. Endocrinol. Metab. 40: 601-611.
37. Wildt, L., Marshall, G. and Knobil, E. (1980): Science 207: 1373-1375.
38. Zacharias, L., Wurtman, R. J., Schatzoff, M. (1970): Am. J. Obstet. Gynecol. 108:833-846.

26

Neuroendocrinology and Psychiatric Disorder,
edited by G. M. Brown, et al.
Raven Press, New York 1984.

Neuronal and Endocrine Mechanisms Involved in the Control of Gonadotropin Secretion

L.C. Krey

Anorexia nervosa is accompanied by numerous abnormalities in endocrine and neuroendocrine function and these have been documented extensively in the foregoing chapters. Some abnormalities, in particular several of those involving growth hormone release and adrenal and thyroid function, have also been observed in normal individuals subjected to a decreased caloric input. Thus, they may be considered as compensatory, adaptive responses of the endocrine and neuroendocrine systems to chronic starvation (see Chapters 24 and 29 for references). Amenorrhea is another symptom which is presented by individuals with anorexia nervosa and this indication of reproductive dysfunction appears to be the result of a hypogonadotropism of presumably hypothalamic origin (see Chaper 23 for references). Significantly, this amenorrhea can develop in anorexia nervosa prior to the appearance of any behavioural or weight abnormality. Moreover, occasional patients with this psychiatric disorder present prior histories of amenorrheic episodes, suggesting a predisposition for irregulatiries in the neuroendocrine control of gonadotropin release. Such observations argue that one cannot attribute the appearance of the reproductive abnormality solely to declines in food intake or losses in body weight. Rather, they suggest that this symptomology may constitute a neuroendicrine reflection of the neural dysfunction(s) which generate the behavioural abnormalities associated with this disease.

In an effort to understand better the etiology of the abnormalities in reproductive neuroendocrinology which afflict individuals with anorexia nervosa, I will use this chapter to review our current knowledge about the neuronal and endocrine mechanisms controlling gonadotropin release. Most of the information that will be covered has been generated in recent studies in rhesus monkeys subjected either to neurosurgical isolation or electrolytic destruction of the arcuate, or infundibular, nucleus of the hypothalamus. The discussion will be in three sections. The first will review the neuroanatomic organization of the neuronal networks which control gonadotropin secretion and will compare the distribution of these networks with those that regulate the release of the other adenohypophysial hormones. The second section will discuss the neuronal and endocrine mechanisms which play a role in the regulation of basal, or tonic, luteinizing hormone (LH) and follicle stimulating (FSH) release. This is the mode of gonadotropin secretion which is responsible for gonadal development and maintenance. It is deficits in this mode of secretion which appear to be a primary cause of the amenorrhea observed in patients with anorexia nervosa. The final section will update our understanding of the neuroendocrine control of LH and FSH secretion during puberty. Such a review is appropriate considering the quantitative and qualitative similarities between the developmental patterns of gonadotropin secretion seen in children and those observed during the cachetic and treatment stages of anorexia nervosa.

A. Organization of the neuronal systems regulating the secretion of adenohypophysial hormones

In the past ten years, the hypothalamic neurohormones which regulate the secretion of LH, FSH, growth hormone, thyrotropin and prolactin have been identified and, in several instances, the patterns of secretion of these hormones into the pituitary portal system have been characterized (2, 12, 32, 34). Furthermore, immunocytochemical procedures and microdissection + radioimmunoassay techniques have been used to map the intrahypothalamic and extrahypothalamic distribution of the neurons containing these hormones (gonadotropin releasing hormone - GnRH, thyrotropin releasing hormone - TRH, somatostatin; dopamine) and neurophysiologic approaches have been employed to demonstrate that these neurons are involved in the control of pituitary function. Several of these latter studies are of relevance to this discussion, since they suggest that neuronal control of anterior pituitary function is "compartmentalized" in a fashion which may explain the neuroendocrine symptomology reported for anorexia nervosa.

GnRH-containing neurons have been identified within a limbic brain continuum extending from the septum to the retromamillary region of the hypothalamus. In primate and subprimate species, the neuron perikarya appear to be concentrated in the medial preoptic area and in the arcuate nucleus-retromamillary region of the hypothalamus (1, 6, 9, 26, 39, 61, 88). The relative contribution of these cells to the GnRH-terminals in the medial eminence appears to vary from species to species. For example in the rat, the preoptic cells supply about 80% of the median eminence GnRH (93). On the other hand, in the guinea pig and rhesus monkey, it is the GnRH neurons in the arcuate, or infundibular nucleus which are primarily responsible for the regulation of gonadotropin release. Such a conclusion is based on the observation that lesions which destroy this nucleus produce reductions of up to 80% of median eminence GnRH terminals and depress markedly the capacity of the adenohypophysis to secrete LH and FSH (48, 76). In contrast, lesions which destroy preoptic GnRH inputs to the median eminence have little effect on gonadotropin release (45, 48). In both monkeys and guinea pigs, the septal and preoptic GnRH neurons have been observed to send their axonal projections not only into the median eminence but also into other hypothalamic and extrahypothalamic areas (48, 61, 88). Little is presently known concerning the physiologic role of these extrahypothalamic projections.

Considering the similarities in the distribution of GnRH-containing neurons in humans and monkeys (6, 9, 61, 88), it is reasonable to assume at this time that the infundibular GnRH network plays the preeminent role in the regulation of pituitary gonadotropin secretion in man. Unfortunately, there is currently little anatomic information in man or experimental animals concerning the characteristics of the neuronal inputs which impinge on these cells. There is also little data to describe the other neuroendocrine characteristics of the GnRH cells - for example, do they possess steroid hormone receptors or receptors for specific neurotransmitters? Such information is essential if one is to devise rational neurophysiologic and neuropharmacologic strategies to explore the neuronal control of GnRH release under normal conditions and it alterations in diseased states.

The foregoing anatomic pattern of GnRH neuron networks differs from those reported for TRH, somatostatin and dopamine, neurohormones involved in the control of thyrotropin, growth hormone and prolactin secretion. In general, these neurohormones are distributed extensively throughout the brain with only a small intrahypothalamic network involved in the regulation of adenohypophysial function. For example, the TRH-neurons which regulate thyrotropin secretion in the rat appear to originate in the periventricular region of the anterior hypothalamus, in the vicinity of the dorsomedial nucleus (34). Such a conclusion is based on the findings that the destruction of the neuron perikarya in this region or the interruption of their projections to the median eminence reduce markedly the number of TRH nerve terminals in contact with the portal vasculature and induce chronic hypothyroidism (26, 81). However, such lesions have no influence on TRH inputs to other hypothalamic and extrahypothalamic regions (40). Although TRH networks have not been analyzed immunocytochemically in higher species, Okon and Koch (67) have utilized a detailed dissection-immunoassay approach to characterize the intrahypothalamic distribution of this peptide in man. They found that the highest TRH levels are present in the posterior nucleus of the hypothalamus and the region connecting this nucleus with the pituitary stalk. Thus, it would appear that the "thyrotropic area" of the brain may well occupy a more caudal position in primates than it does in rodents.

The somatostatin-containing neurons which regulate growth hormone (GH) secretion have also been localized immunocytochemically in laboratory mammals and in man (1, 20, 21, 24, 39, 71). These cells lie in the rostral periventricular hypothalamus extending from the level of the suprachiasmatic nucleus to the arcuate nucleus; occasional magnocellular neurons are present in the paraventricular nucleus. Once again, the physiologic importance of these somatostatin cells for normal GH secretion is highlighted by the findings that the electrolytic destruction of this region results in the disappearance of somatostatin-containing neuron terminals in the median eminence (19, 26, 27) and produces marked deficits in the control of GH release (19). However, such lesions do not influence somatostatin inputs to other hypothalamic and extrahypothalamic regions (26, 27). In humans, somatostatin has similarly been localized in parvicellular neurons in the periventricular regions of the anterior hypothalamus and the anterior pole of the arcuate nucleus and in the magnocellular cells in the paraventricular nucleus (20, 21).

Dopamine is also distributed extensively throughout the mammalian brain, but the dopaminergic neuron network which controls prolactin secretion is discrete and consists of cell bodies in the infundibular or arculate nucleus and their projections throughout the median eminence (1, 29, 69). These cells would appear to be located more anteriorly to those regulating GnRH release (76). In general, their projections overlay those of the other neurohormone-secreting neurons and direct contacts between dopaminergic and GnRH-containing terminals have been reported in the medial eminence (1, 39).

The foregoing descriptions of anatomically distinct neurohumural networks suggests that the neuroendocrine systems which control the release of the various pituitary hormones may be "compartmentalized" within the central nervous system. Neurosurgical studies in animals and clinical reports also provide evidence to support such an arrangement. For example, the complete transection of neuronal inputs to the medial basal hypothalamus (ventromedial nucleus + arcuate nucleus + median eminence) of the adult rhesus monkey with a Halasz-type knife does not result in any dramatic influences on LH and FSH release since the GnRH cells are within the confines of the cut; however, such a transection does suppress thyroid function dramatically, block stress-induced GH and cortisol release and abolish the diurnal pattern of adrenocorticoid release (47). A contrasting set of symptoms can be generated by subjecting rhesus monkeys to discrete electrolytic lesions in the region of the arcuate or infundibular nucleus. Such lesions destroy the GnRH cells located there and, as a result, the animals are incapable of LH and FSH secretion - but they do display normal circulating levels of thyroxine, prolactin, and growth hormone, as well as cortisol and growth hormone responses to insulin hypoglycemia and normal diurnal patterns of cortisol release (76). In general, this symptomology resembles that noted in clinical reports of hypothalamic hypogonadotropism and it is significant that, in both instances, the hypogonadotropic dysfunction can be corrected simply by the administration of GnRH (41, 50, 51, 52). This neuroendocrine profile also resembles that of patients with anorexia nervosa and, in fact, one may view these lesioned animals as an experimental "model" to study the hypogonadotropic dysfunctions characteristic of this disorder. Unfortunately, monkeys bearing arcuate nucleus lesions do not display any striking evidences of weight loss or aberrant feeding patterns and, thus, contribute little or no information toward understanding the behavioural disorders seen in anorexia nervosa. Curiously, one can produce chronic hyperphagia in rhesus monkeys by transecting lateral-medial hypothalamic interconnections at the level of the ventromedial nucleus, but such connections are not essential for normal reproductive function (47, 58).

B. Neuronal and endocrine mechanisms controlling basal gonadotropin secretion

Basal, or tonic, LH and FSH secretion is the low-level, day-to-day release responsible for the development of the ovaries and testes during puberty and the functional maintenance of these organs in adulthood. It has two components. The first appears to consist of a constant, very low-level release which has been hypothesized to reflect GnRH-independent activity of the gonadotrophs (86). The second component is episodic and is characterized by brief secretory discharges of LH and, on occasion, FSH which occur every 30 minutes - 3+ hours depending on the mammalian species studied and its hormonal state (11, 22, 86, 96). This ultradian mode of release appears to determine in large part the mean, absolute level of LH and FSH present in the cirulation, primarily via alterations in both the magnitude and frequency of the secretory discharges (30, 31, 86, 96). Parenthetically, patients with anorexia nervosa with very low levels of circulating LH and FSH have been reported to display very small and infrequent secretory discharges (86). However, some anorexic patients also present elevations in serum gonadotropins following sleep onset and one must speculate that, at these times, either the frequency or amplitude of the episodic discharges increase toward normal values.

The pulsatile rhythm of gonadotropin secretion depends in turn on the episodic release of GnRH into the portal circulation. GnRH discharges have been monitored directly in portal blood (2, 10) and their physiologic importance demonstrated in several model systems (45, 46, 68, 87). Perhaps the most productive of these models has been the female rhesus monkey bearing arcuate nucleus lesions which abolish endogenous GnRH release. Gonadotropin secretion can be restored in these animals by periodic GnRH infusion (6 min in length) and Knobil and colleagues (45, 46) have recently demonstrated that modulations in the amplitude and frequency of administration parameters of this GnRH therapy can have profound influences on the rate and ratio of LH and FSH release.

Significantly, the frequency of GnRH administration which most effectively elicited LH and FSH secretion was once every hour, the approximate frequency of endogenous GnRH release observed in non-lesioned monkeys (10, 22). When GnRH was administered more frequently (2-5 times every hour), circulating LH and FSH concentrations fell dramatically. This phenomenon has been attributed to a down-regulation of GnRH receptors which is precipitated by their internalization into the gonadotroph (36). Serum LH levels also fell following less frequent (once every 2-3 hours) stimulation with GnRH, but in contrast, FSH levels appeared to rise. This observation, which is attributable in part to the slower clearance rate of FSH (45), is important, since it suggests that one need not postulate specific FSH-releasing hormones to account for "selective" increases in circulating FSH. Such a conclusion is also supported by the observations that passive immunization with GnRH-specific antisera produce rapid declines in serum LH <u>and</u> FSH concentrations in the rhesus monkey (55).

Taken together, the foregoing experimental findings indicate that one can induce hypogonadotropism either by hyperstimulation or hypostimulation with GnRH. This consideration is an important one for the clinician, since it suggests that one cannot ascribe <u>a priori</u> hypothalamic hypogonadotropism to the absence of GnRH release. Clearly, patients presenting this syndrome should be tested with GnRH - those that lack GnRH should respond to such a treatment with gonadotropin release, whereas those with GnRH hypersecretion should not. Thus, the clinical observations that individuals with anorexia nervosa display elevations in gonadotropin levels following GnRH replacement therapies suggest that endogenous GnRH release in these individuals is deficient (see Chapter 23 for references).

In more recent work, Richardson, <u>et al</u>. (83) and Leyendecker and colleagues (52) have monitored the influences of amplitude and frequency modulations of episodic GnRH treatments on ovarian development and function. This work was performed on monkeys with arcuate nucleus lesions or in women with hypothalamic hypogonadotropism, respectively. In the lesioned monkeys, hourly treatments of GnRH restored ovulatory menstrual cycles, whereas treatments given every 120-180 minutes failed to stimulate follicular development to a level sufficient to elicit ovulatory LH release. In the hypogonadotropic women, variations in the amplitude of the intermittent (once every 90 minutes) treatments influenced dramatically the level of steroid hormone release, as well as the frequency of ovulation. Taken together, these data demonstrate in convincing fashion that the morphologic and endocrine status of the entire reproductive system can be determined directly by the secretory activity of the GnRH-neurons present in the infundibular region of the hypothalamus. This also appears to apply for anorexia nervosa as well, since GnRH replacement treatments will reinitiate ovarian and testicular activity in individuals with this disorder (see Chapter 23 for references).

One of the key mechanisms whereby episodic GnRH secretion determines an individual's reproductive status is by its trophic actions on the gonadotroph. It is well documented that this decapeptide not only stimulates the immediate release of LH and FSH, but also programs the gonadtroph for subsequent secretory activity. Both of these actions result from the interaction of GnRH with its receptor in the cell membrane of the gonadotroph (14, 16, 74). Perhaps the most striking demonstration of this programming action is "GnRH self-priming", a phenomenon which has been observed when GnRH infusions or multiple GnRH injections are administered to estrogentreated humans and animals (38, 73, 92). In such paradigms, large elevations in circulating GnRH tend to favour the release of LH and FSH, whereas small GnRH increments preferentially prime the gonadotrophs for a future gonadotropin discharge (38). The intracellular mechanisms underlying GnRH's programming action are potentially numerous and may include the stimulation of LH and FSH synthesis (54), the stimulation of the synthesis of other cell constituents necessary for gonadotropin release (16, 73, 75), the preparation of stored gonadotropins for release perhaps by reorganization of intracellular microfilaments (44, 75) and the self-regulation of available GnRH receptors (14). In view of these preparative actions, it is reasonable to assume that prolonged deficits in GnRH secretion can have long-term, deleterious consequences on gonadotroph function. One consequence should be a decline in gonadotropin stores. Such a decline has been observed in rhesus monkeys following destruction of the arcuate nucleus (72); curiously, under these experimental conditions, pituitary FSH content remains elevated long after LH has declined to very low values (Peckham, personal communication). Such a differential decline in gonadotropin stores provides a reasonable explanation for the blunted gonadotropin responses to single iv GnRH challenges observed in anorexics as well as the altered FSH:LH ratios initially observed in such individuals following more prolonged GnRH therapies (see Chaper 23 for references).

The information presented thus far suggests strongly that one may ascribe all of the clinical observations of reproductive dysfunction reported in individuals with anorexia nervosa to the absence of a "sufficient" (i.e. episodic) pattern of GnRH release by the brain. In view of this interpretation, it is appropriate to consider the physiologic inputs which influence the secretory activity of the GnRH neurons and speculate on the neuronal factors mediating their dysfunction in anorexia nervosa. Although we know from experimental studies in animals that episodic GnRH secretion need not require any extrahypothalamic inputs (47) and, most likely, reflects the activity of neurons within the medial basal hypothalamus (25, 46), we also know that under normal circumstances this system does not function as an "isolated island" but rather is subject to both hormonal (gonadal steroid, gonadotropin, GnRH) and neuronal influences. For example, there are numerous reports that the episodic secretion pattern of LH can be modulated by the activation or inhibition of a variety of intrahypothalamic and extrahypothalamic inputs. Electrical stimulation of various brain regions influences episodic GnRH release as does the administration of neuropharmacologic agents (e.g., α-adrenergic blockers in monkeys) which inhibit the neurotransmission of monoaminergic inputs from the midbrain (29, 45, 77). Furthermore, there are numerous physiologic states which can be explained only by extrahypothalamic regulation of GnRH neuron activity. These include suckling-induced amenorrhea (3, 79), seasonal stimulation and inhibition of gonadotropin secretion in domestic animals (53) and stress-induced amenorrhea (see Chapter 23 for references). Most likely, the sleep-induced patterns of episodic LH release reported in prepubertal children and patients with anorexia nervosa also reflect a particular profile of extrahypothalamic inputs reaching the GnRH neuron. Each of these phenomena may be mediated by one or combinations of neuronal networks which utilize neurotransmitters (epinephrine, norepinephrine, serotonin, dopamine, histamine, GABA, endorphins, acetylcholine) previously implicated in the control of GnRH release (see Chapter 23 for references).

The activity of the GnRH neurons may also be influenced by gonadal steroid hormones. Although some investigators have postulated that, in some instances, steroid feedback control of gonadotropin secretion may be explained by steroid-gonadotroph interactions (45, 64), there are numerous studies which suggest that steroids also modulate GnRH release. Microimplant studies have indicated that the selective uptake of steroids by the brain does eventuate in a change in gonadotropin release (13, 15) and steroid treatments have been demonstrated to influence hypothalamus and median eminence GnRH levels in rodents (89) and rhesus monkeys (Silverman and Krey, unpublished observations). In humans, testosterone and progesterone have been reported to influence the frequency of pulsatile LH release, whereas estradiol has been shown to modulate the amplitude of the gonadotropin discharges (85, 86, 96). Both of these actions could be explained by changes in the rate and amount of the GnRH release. There are a variety of potential mechansisms through which the gonadal steroids could alter GnRH release. For example, they could act directly on the GnRH-secreting neuron to influence the synthesis and packaging of its neurohormone. Alternatively, steroids could act to modify the neuronal input which impinges on the GnRH cell by one of a variety of neuronal mechanisms - modulation of neurotransmitter receptor levels, regulation of the levels of enzymes responsible for neurotransmitter synthesis and degradation and influences on high-affinity neurotransmitter uptake systems (56). Such mechanisms need not be restricted to the control of gonadotropin secretion - they may well play an important role in other aspects of brain function such as behaviour. In this regard, it is important to note that gonadal steroids can influence dietary preferences and food intake in small laboratory rodents (63).

Other hormones may also modulate the secretory activity patterns of GnRH secreting neurons. LH and GnRH have been reported to influence various parameters of brain function (56, 89, 91) and the gonadal peptide hormones - inhibins, folliculostatins and gonadocrinins (5, 20, 98) - may also play a role. As with the gonadal steroids, each of these hormones may also influence other aspects of brain function not directly involved in the regulation of GnRH release.

At the present time, it seems unlikely that the deficits in GnRH release associated with anorexia nervosa can be attributed to disruptions in gonadal steroid feedback control. This is especially so when one considers the exceptionally low levels of circulating steroids which are characteristic of this disorder (see Chapter 23 for references). Rather, it is not unreasonable to speculate that the absence of intermittent GnRH release is the result of disruptions in the pattern of neuronal input which impinges on these cells. Such a mechanism appears to take place during infancy and childhood when the neuroendocrine systems regulating gonadotropin release are undergoing maturation.

C. Maturation of the neuroendocrine control systems regulating gonadotropin release

Recent studies have revealed that there are three different phases of gonadotropin secretion which occur between birth and adolescence. During the initial phase - infancy (birth - 2 years) - gonadotropin secretion is elevated and gonadal steroid hormone levels are in the low-normal adult range (35, 84, 95). Curiously, the circulating levels of LH, FSH and the gonadal steroids are even higher in premature infants

(90). In stage two - childhood (2-11 years) - gonadotropin secretion is markedly suppressed despite very low circulating levels of gonadal steroids (33, 84). Stage three - puberty and adolescence (11 years and up) - is heralded by nocturnal sleep-induced elevations in gonadotropin release and gonadarche (7, 8, 43, 59, 70) and circulating levels of these hormones display a continuous rise until adult levels are achieved at the end of this stage. Such a maturational profile of gonadotropin secretion has also been reported in children with gonadal dysgenesis or subjected to castration early in life (17, 18, 33, 50). It has also been reported in the rhesus monkey (33, 97). In fact, recent studies by Plant and Hess (37, 78, 80) provide the most conclusive evidence to date that the neuroendocrine mechanisms controlling gonadotropin secretion in higher primates are highly mature at birth. In particular, infant male monkeys (3 months) display nocturnal elevations in serum LH and testosterone concentrations which resemble those seen in adult males. Furthermore, the castrated infant shows adult-like elevations in circulating LH and FSH concentrations with episodic discharges occurring every 60 minutes. However, at 3-6 months of age, this pattern of secretion ceases and serum LH and FSH levels decline to low values. Such low values persist for 2-3 years after which time, the approximate age of gonadarche in the male monkey, gonadotropin secretion recommences and elevated serum LH and FSH concentrations return.

GnRH replacement studies have also been conducted using rhesus monkeys to determine the etiology of the foregoing triphasic pattern of gonadotropin release. When intermittent GnRH therapies were administered to immature 13-month-old female rhesus monkeys, they were found to stimulate precocious gonadotropin release, gonadal development and ovulation (94). Similar GnRH treatments have also been reported to stimulate gonadotropin and gonadal steroid secretion in children with delayed adolescence (41). Thus, it would appear that the absence/presence of episodic GnRH release is the primary neuroendocrine mechanism that determines the changes in reproductive function observed during the transitions from infancy to childhood and childhood to puberty.

Both neuronal and endocrine hypotheses have been put forth to explain the changes in GnRH and gonadotropin secretion observed between infancy-childhood and childhood-puberty. The endocrine hypothesis suggests that the maturational changes in LH and FSH release can be attributed to a change in the sensitivity to the negative feedback actions of the gonadal steroids. Thus, the child is more sensitive to steroidal suppression of gonadotropin release and, as he or she matures, the set point for the expression of this feedback response is raised allowing for elevations in both gonadotropins and gonadal hormones to occur. There is extensive support for this hypothesis in prepubertal children and monkeys (23, 33). However, since the level of gonadotropin secretion is so low in these individuals, one must wonder if the increased sensitivity observed is but a secondary response to a low level of GnRH stimulation. Nonetheless, an increased responsiveness to estrogen feedback can also be demonstrated in early pubertal individuals which have regained the capacity for episodic GnRH release (28, 62). Thus, it may be that differential sensitivity to gonadal steroid negative feedback constitutes an important "fine tuning" control mechanism which establishes the time of onset of normal reproductive function following gonadarche (33).

The neuronal hypothesis suggests that, during maturation, central nervous system mechanisms which operate independently of gonadal steroid feedback selectively shut down and then resuscitate the episodic activity patterns of the GnRH-secreting neurons. The support for this hypothesis has consisted primarily of the observations that the alterations in gonadotropin secretion observed during infancy, childhood, puberty and adolescence also occur within a relatively normal time frame in agonadal individuals, such as children with gonadal dysgenesis or subjected to castration early in life (17, 18, 33, 42, 59). Moreover, such agonadal children also display evidence of intermittent nocturnal GnRH release at approximately 10-12 years of age followed by a later expansion of this release pattern throughout the day. Agonadal children also display the qualitative and quantitative patterns of pituitary responsiveness to GnRH test treatments which are characteristic of normal children. Such findings provide further support for the importance of the trophic actions of endogenous GnRH secretion on the secretory status of the anterior pituitary gland.

At the present time, we do not know the neuroendocrine mechanisms responsible for turning on/off episodic GnRH release and modulating responsiveness to gonadal steroid negative feedback during maturation. There are numerous clinical observations linking precocious puberty with neoplasms in the region of the tuber cinereum and mamillary bodies (4). These observations suggest that local influences on the GnRH neurons located in this brain region may play a key role in the attainment of reproductive competence. Such a conclusion is also suggested by the recent observations that the complete transection of neuronal inputs into the medial basal hypothalamus of the immature rhesus monkey has little appreciable influence on the age at which pubertal patterns of gonadotropin and gonadal steroid secretion develop (49, 66). However, one cannot conclude from these studies that extrahypothalamic input plays no role in determining the maturational changes in GnRH secretion, since neurohumoral or humoral inputs from the central nervous system or peripheral tissues would still be able to reach the isolated hypothalamic "islands" via the cerebrospinal fluid or the bloodstream.

In summary, the foregoing studies on the neuroendocrinology of puberty contributes two important pieces of information which are relevant to our understanding of the reproductive dysfunction seen in individuals with anorexia nervosa. First, they indicate that the patterns of regression/recovery of gonadotropin release observed during anorexia nervosa are not uncommon phenomena - we all have undergone similar phases of regression and recovery during the early years of our lives. Furthermore, in both the anorexic and the maturing child, the regressive/recovery patterns appear to reflect the absence/recurrence of episodic GnRH release. Secondly, the studies suggest that these changes in neuroendocrine activity need not be mediated by steroid feedback mechanisms but rather may be controlled by a neuronal mechanism(s) which shuts down/turns on the GnRH neuron. This last piece of information is of interest, particularly when one considers the correlations between the onset of GnRH and gonadotropin secretion and body weight which have been noted in children and individuals with anorexia nervosa. It was previously thought that these correlations may be attributed to the ability of body fat to metabolize gonadal steroids (see Chapter 23 for references). However, by ruling out steroid feedback as a factor influencing GnRH release, one must assume that there is some other physiologic "signal" which informs the brain to initiate GnRH release. Considering that there are no pronounced effects of hypothalamic disconnection on the timing of puberty onset in rhesus monkeys (49, 66), one must consider the possibility that the signal is processed within this region of the brain, perhaps by the GnRH-secreting cells themselves.

The identification of the neuronal mechanisms which suppress GnRH release in children and in individuals with anorexia nervosa is an important research problem for future study. There are several potential research approaches which could be used in such work. A neuropharmacologic approach could be used which is similar to that employed by Dr. Quigley and his colleagues in their studies on the neuronal control systems regulating GnRH secretion in women (see Chapter 30 for references). Such procedures could easily be extended to explore alterations in the activity of these systems in disorders like anorexia nervosa. A second research approach would be to study animal "models" which show reversible periods of activation and suppression of GnRH secretion. Although such "models" must be viewed with caution in view of prominent species-to-species variations in the neuronal control of GnRH release, they nonetheless may suggest some diagnostic and/or therapeutic hypothesis to be tested in individuals with anorexia nervosa. One such animal model might be a seasonal breeder, like the ram (53). These animals show light-induced suppression/recovery of GnRH release which can occur independently of steroid feedback and the neuronal mechanisms mediating these changes may be similar to those expressed during anorexia nervosa. A second type of animal model may be generated by neurosurgical manipulation of the central nervous system. For example, Dr. Leibowitz will discuss in a later chapter that discrete lesions in the brain of a rat will precipitate several of the feeding behaviours characteristic of anorexia nervosa. Such lesioned animals may also display transient alterations in GnRH and gonadotropin release.

SUMMARY

In primates, neurons present in the infundibular and retromamillary regions of the brain control hypophysial gonadotropic function via the secretion of the neurohormone GnRH into the portal circulation. This secretion is episodic in nature and can be influenced by extrahypothalamic inputs and gonadal steroid administration. Modulations in the frequency/amplitude of these intermittent GnRH discharges determine the physiologic status of the gonadotrophs of the adenohypophysis and alter the secretion rates of LH and FSH; these changes, in turn, influence the development and secretory activity of the gonads. Thus, episodic GnRH release plays a direct role to determine the physiologic status of the entire reproductive system. The presence/absence of episodic GnRH release appears to account in large measure for the maturational changes in gonadotropin secretion which occur from birth to adolescence and most likely explains the alterations in LH and FSH release observed during the onset and treatment of anorexia nervosa.

ACKNOWLEDGMENTS

LCK is supported by a grant from the Rockefeller Foundation (RF70095) and by a Career Scientist Award from the Irma T. Hirschl Foundation. The editorial assistance and patience of O. Wengerchuk is gratefully acknowledged.

REFERENCES

1. Ajika, K. (1980): In: Frontiers in Neuroendocrinology, Vol. 6,

edited by L. Martini and W. F. Ganong. Raven Press, New York.
2. Antunes, J. L., Carmel, P. W., Housepian, E. M. and Ferin, M. (1978): J. Neurosurg. 49:382-386.
3. Baird, D. T., McNeilly, A. S., Sawers, R. S. and Sharpe, R. M. (1979): J. Clin. Endocrinol. Metab. 49:500.
4. Barnes, N. D., Cloutier, M. D. and Hayles, A. B. 91974): In: Control of the Onset of Puberty, edited by M. M. Grumbach, G. D. Grave and F. L. Mayer, pp.213-228. John Wiley & Sons, New York.
5. Barraclough, C. A., Wise, P. M., Turgeon, J., Shander, D., DePaolo, L. and Rance, N. (1979): Biol. Reprod. 20:86-97.
6. Barry, J. (1976); Neurosci. Letters 3:287-291.
7. Beck, W. and Wuttke, W. (1980): J. Clin. Endocrinol. Metab. 50: 635-639.
8. Boyar, R. M., Rosenfeld, R. S., Kapen, S., Finkelstein, J. W., Roffward, H. P., Weitzman, E. D., Hellman, L. (1974): J. Clin. Invest. 54:609-618.
9. Bugnon, C., Bloch, B. and Fellmann, D. (1977): Brain Res. 128: 249-262.
10. Bugnon, C., Fellmann, D. and Bloch, B. (1977): Cell Tiss. Res. 183:319-328.
11. Butler, W. R., Malven, P. V., Willett, L. B. and Bolt, D. (1972): Endocrinology 91:793-801.
12. Carmel, P. W., Araki, S. and Ferin, M. (1976): Endocrinology 99: 243-248.
13. Cheung, C.Y. and Davison, J. M. (1977): Endocrinology 100:232-301.
14. Clayton, R. N. and Catt, K. J. (1981): Endocrine Reviews 2:186-209.
15. Chappel, S. C., Resko, J. A., Norman, R. L. and Spies, H. G. (1981): J. Clin. Endocrinol. Metab. 52:1-8.
16. Conn, P. M., Marian, J., McMillian, M., Stern, J., Roger, D., Hamby, M., Penna, A. and Grant, L. S. (1981): Endocrine Reviews 2:174-185.
17. Conte, F. A., Grumbach, M. M. and Kaplan, S. L. (1975): J. Clin. Endocrinol. Metab. 40:670-674.
18. Conte, F. A., Grumbach, M. M., Kaplan, S. L. and Recter, E. O. (1980): J. Clin. Endocrinol. Metab. 50:163-168.
19. Critchlow, V., Rice, R. W., Abe, K. and Vale, W. (1978): Endocrinology 103:817-825.
20. deJong, F. H. (1979): Molec. Cell Endocrinol. 13:1-10.
21. Desy, L. and Pelletier, G. (1977): Cell Tissue Res. 184:491-497.
22. Dierschke, D. J., Bhattacharya, A. N., Atkinson, L. E. and Knobil, E. (1970): Endocrinology 87:850-853.
23. Dierschke, D. J., Karsch, F. J., Weick, R. F., Weiss, G., Hotchkiss, J. and Knobil, E. (1974): In: Control of the Onset of Puberty, edited by M. M. Grumbach, G. D. Grave and F. E. Mayer, pp.104-114. John Wiley & Sons, New York.
24. Dubois, M. P. and Kolodziejczyk, D. (1975): C. R. Acad. Sci. (Paris) 281(D):1737-1740.
25. Dufy, B., Dufy-Barbe, L., Vincent, J. D. and Knobil, E. (1979): J. Physiol. (Paris) 75:105-108.
26. Elde, R. and Hokfelt, T. (1978): In: Neuroendocrinology, Vol. 5, edited by W. F. Ganong and L. Martini, pp.1-33. Raven Press, New York.
27. Epelbaum, J., Willoughby, J., Brazeau, P. and Martin, J. B. (1977): Endocrinology 101:1495-1502.
28. Foster, D. L., Rapisarda, J. J. and Bergmen, K. S. (1981): Proc.

63rd Annual Meeting of the Endocrine Society, Abs. 490.
29. Gallo, R. W. (1980): Neuroendocrinology 30:122-131.
30. Gallo, R. V. (1981a): Biol. Reprod. 24:100-104.
31. Gallo, R. V. (1981b): Biol. Reprod. 24:771-777.
32. Gibbs, D. M. and Neill, J. D. (1978): Endocrinology 102:1895-1901.
33. Grumbach, M. M., Roth, J. C., Kaplan, S. L. and Kelch, R. P. (1974): In: Control of the Onset of Puberty, edited by M. M. Grumbach, G. D. Grave and F. L. Mayer, pp.115-166. John Wiley & Sons, New York.
34. Guldesky, G. A. and Porter, J. C. (1979): Endocrinology 104:583-587.
35. Hammond, G. L., Koivisto, M., Kouvalainen, K. and Vihko, K. (1979): J. Clin. Endocrinol. Metab. 49:40-45.
36. Hazum, E., Cautrecasas, P., Marian, J. and Conn, P. M. (1980): Proc. Natl. Acad. Sci. USA 77:6692-6695.
37. Hess, D. L. and Plant, T. (1981): Proc. 63rd Annual Meeting of the Endocrine Society, Abs. 137.
38. Hoff, J. D., Lasley, B. L. and Yen, S.S.C. (1979): J. Clin. Endocrinol. Metab. 49:8-11.
39. Hokfelt, T., Elde, R., Fuxe, K., Johanssen, O., Ljungdahl, A., Goldstein, M., Luft, R., Efendic, S., Nilsson, G., Terenius, L., Ganten, D., Jeffcoate, S., Rehfeld, J., Sarel, S., Perez de la Mora, M., Possani, L., Tapia, R., Teran, L. and Palacios, R. (1978): In: The Hypothalamus, edited by S. Reichlin, R. Baldessarini and J. Martin, pp.69-135. Raven Press, New York.
40. Jackson, I.M.D. and Reichlin, S. (1977): Nature (Lond.) 267:853.
41. Jacobson, R. I., Seyler, L. E., Tamborlane, W. V., Gertner, J. M. and Genel, M. (1979): J. Clin. Endocrinol. Metab. 49:652-655.
42. Job, J. C., Garnier, P. E., Chan, J. L., Scholler, R., Toublanc, J. E. and Canlorbe, P. (1974): J. Clin. Endocrinol. Metab. 38: 1109-1115.
43. Judd, H. L. (1979): In: Endocrine Rhythms, edited by D. T. Krieger, pp.299-324. Raven Press, New York.
44. Khar, A., Kunnert-Radek, J. and Jutisz, M. (1979): FEBS Lett. 104: 410-414.
45. Knobil, E. (1980): Rec. Prog. Horm. Res. 36:53-88.
46. Knobil, E. (1981): Biol. Reprod. 24:44-49.
47. Krey, L. C., Butler, W. R. and Knobil, E. (1975): Endocrinology 96:1073-1087.
48. Krey, L. C. and Silverman, A. J. (1975): Brain Res. 157:247-256.
49. Krey, L. C., Hess, D. L., Butler, W. R., Espinosa-Campos, J., Lu, K-H., Piva, F., Plant, T. and Knobil, E. (1981): Endocrinology 108:1944-1948.
50. Leyendecker, G. (1979): Eur. J. Obstet. Gynec. Reprod. Biol. 9:175.
51. Leyendecker, G., Wildt, L. and Hansmann, M. (1980): J. Clin. Endocrinol. Metab. 51:1214.
52. Leyendecker, G., Wildt, L., Niesert, S. and Plotz, E. (1981): Proc. 63rd Annual Meeting of the Endocrine Society, Abs. 28.
53. Lincoln, G. A. and Short, R. V. (1980): Rec. Prog. Horm. Res. 36: 1-52.
54. Liu, T-C., and Jackson, G. L. (1977): Endocrinology 100:1294-1299.
54a. Liu, T-C. and Jackson, G. L. (1978): Endocrinology 103:1253-1263.
55. McCormack, J. T., Plant, T. M., Hess, D. L. and Knobil, E. (1977): Endocrinology 100:663-667.
56. McEwen, B. S. (1980): Molec. Cell Endocrinol. 18:151-164.
57. McEwen, B. S., Davis, P. G., Parsons, B. and Pfaff, D. W. (1979): Ann. Rev. Neurosci. 2:65-112.

58. McHugh, P. R. and Gibbs, J. (1972): Brain 95:279-292.
59. Marrama, P., Dellacasa, L. and Bonat, B. (1978): In: Recent Progress in Andrology, edited by A. Fabbrini and B. Steinberger, pp.85-97. Academic Press, London.
60. Marshall, J. C. and Kelch, R. P. (1979): J. Clin. Endocrinol. Metab. 49:712-718.
61. Marshall, P. E. and Goldsmith, P. C. (1980): Brain Res. 193:353-372.
62. Maruca, J., Kulin, H. E. and Santner, S. (1981): Proc. 63rd Annual Meeting of the Endocrine Society, Abs.492.
63. Nance, D. M. (1976): In: Advances in Psychobiology, Vol. 3, edited by A. H. Riesen and R. F. Thompson, pp.75-124. John Wiley & Sons, New York.
64. Nansel, D. D. and Trent, D. F. (1979): Endocrinology 104:532-515.
65. Nillius, S. J., Fries, H. and Wide, L. (1975): Amer. J. Obstet. Gynecol. 122:921-928.
66. Norman, R. L. and Spies, H. G. (1981): Endocrinology 108:1723-1729.
67. Okon, E. and Koch, Y. (1976): Nature (Lond.) 263:345-347.
68. Osland, R. E., Gallo, R. V. and Williams, J. A. (1975): Endocrinology 96:1210-1216.
69. Palkovits, M. (1979): International Review of Cytology 56:315-339.
70. Parker, D. C., Judd, H. L., Rossman, L. G. and Yen, S.S.C. (1975): J. Clin. Endocrinol. Metab. 40:1099-1109.
71. Parsons, J., Erlandsen, S. L., Hegre, O. D., McEvoy, R. and Elde, R. P. (1976): J. Histochem. Cytochem. 24:872-882.
72. Peckham, W. D. (1981): Proc. 63rd, Annual Meeting of the Endocrine Society, Abs.575.
73. Pickering, A. J. and Fink, G. (19760: J. Endocrinol. 69:373-379.
74. Pickering, A. M. and Fink, G. (1976): J. Endocrinol. 69:453-454.
75. Pickering, A. J. and Fink, G. (1979): J. Endocrinol. 81:223-234.
76. Plant, T. M., Krey, L. C., Moossy, J., McCormack, J. T., Hess, D.L. and Knobil, E. (1978): Endocrinology 102:52-62.
77. Plant, T. M., Nakai, Y., Belchetz, P., Keogh, E. and Knobil, E. (1978): Endocrinology 102:1015-1018.
78. Plant, T. M. (1980): Endocrinology 106:1451-1454.
79. Plant, T. M., Schallenberger, E., Hess, D. L., McCormack, J. T., Dufy-Barbe, L. and Knobil, E. (1980): Biol. Reprod. 23:760-766.
80. Plant, T. M. (1981): Proc. 63rd Annual Meeting of the Endocrine Society, Abs.488.
81. Reichlin, S. (1960): Endocrinology 66:340-354.
82. Renaud, L. P., Martin, J. B. and Brazeau, P. (1975): Nature (Lond.) 255:233-235.
83. Richardson, D. W., Hutchison, J. S., Pohl, G. R., Germak, J. A. and Knobil, E. (1981): Proc. 63rd Annual Meeting of the Endocrine Society, Abs.513.
84. Ryle, M., Stephenson, J., Williams, J. and Stuart, J. (1975): Clinical Endocrinology 4:413-419.
85. Santen, R. J. (1975): J. Clin. Invest. 56:1555-1562.
86. Santen, R. J. and Bardin, C. W. (1973): J. Clin. Invest. 52: 2617-2628.
87. Schuiling, G. A. and Gnodde, H. P. (1976): J. Endocrinol. 70: 97-104.
88. Silverman, A. J. and Krey, L. C. (1978): Brain Res. 157:233-246.
89. Simpkins, J. W., Kalra, P. S. and Kalra, S. P. (1980): Neuroendocrinology 30:94-100.
90. Tapanainen, J., Koivisto, M., Vihko, R. and Huhtaniemi, I. (1981):

J. Clin. Endocrinol. Metab. 52:235-238.
91. Van Loon, G. R. (1979): Nature (Lond.) 275:331-332.
92. Wang, C. F., Lasley, B. L., Lein, A. and Yen, S.S.L. (1976): J. Clin. Endocrinol. Metab. 42:718-728.
93. Weiner, R. I., Pattou, E., Kerdelhue, B. and Kordon, C. (1975): Endocrinology 97:1597-1600.
94. Wildt, L., Marshall, G. and Knobil, E. (1980): Science 107: 1373-1375.
95. Winter, J.S.D., Hughes, I. A., Reyes, F. I. and Faiman, C. (1976): J. Clin. Endocrinol. Metab. 42:679-686.
96. Yen, S.S.C., Tsai, C. C., Naftolin, F., Vandenberg, G. and Ajabor, L. (1972): J. Clin. Endocrinol. 34:671-675.
97. Yeoman, R., Terasawa, E. and Bridson, W. (1981): Proc. 63rd Annual Meeting of the Endocrine Society, Abs.491.
98. Ying, S-Y., and Guillemin, R. (1980): Proc. 63rd Annual Meeting of the Endocrine Society, Abs.114.

27

Neuroendocrinology and Psychiatric Disorder,
edited by G. M. Brown, et al.
Raven Press, New York 1984.

Summary Overview: Anorexia Nervosa—Endocrine Findings

Francesca Brambilla

Anorexia Nervosa (AN) is the most typical example of the strict interdependence between neuroendocrine and mental disorders. Described in the late XIX century as a psychosis, it has since been considered sometimes to be a pure neuroendocrine and sometimes a pure mental disease. Even though its psychopathological origin and characteristics are now well defined and described, the constant presence of specific hormonal alterations as part of the disease indicates that it might be a psycho-endocrine disorder.

The papers presented in the first part of the symposium were strictly metabolic, illustrating the organic aspects of the disease. The first speaker Dr. R. A. Vigersky (Chapter 23) reported on studies investigating the influence that weight loss, type of food consumption, exercise and stress exert on the appearance, duration and response to therapy of the secondary amenorrhea which is the most typical and earliest neuroendocrine abnormality observed in AN.

With regard to fat loss and food consumption, it has been proposed that amenorrhea arises when a standard critical low weight (or weight for height) is reached, and disappears spontaneously when the weight for a normal mean population is resumed, but this does not seem to hold true. Each patient may have her own critical body weight for menstruation, and the quality as well as the caloric quantity of food may be important.

Moreover, strenuous exercise which requires prolonged energy expenditure, often practiced by these patients, can lead to the appearance of amenorrhea. As an example of this phenomenon, the analogy to amenorrhea in ballet dancers and long-distance runners, without signs of AN and without significant reduction of food consumption, was drawn.

The third point, stressful events, frequently induces, per se, secondary amenorrhea, and may intervene also in AN.

The type of neuroendocrine impairment which underlies the amenorrheic process includes low basal FSH and LH levels which is correlated with the severity of the weight loss. The response to LHRH stimulation may be either normal or delayed or blunted or paradoxical (normal or increased secretion of FSH and blunted response of LH as in puberty). There is no response to Clomiphene or to acute estrogen administration. The circadian pattern of LH secretion is impaired. The same phenomena occur in men with AN, together with reduced testosterone levels.

From the above mentioned data, it is evident that the origin of the phenomenon is hypothalamic, and according to the researcher is correlated with the gravity of the disease, the weight loss and the nutritional deprivation.

Excessive energy expenditure seems to induce amenorrhea through a mechanism which is, in part, similar to that of AN, being probably related to the loss of weight and body fat in these subjects, even though the underlying hormonal pattern has not yet been fully clarified.

The pathogenesis of stress-induced amenorrhea is even less well known, since no endocrine studies of a pure "stress-induced" amenorrhea group exist.

Dr. P. Garfinkel, then reviewed the hormonal abnormalities in anorexia nervosa (Chapter 24).

Growth hormone (GH) is generally increased in AN and normalizes with recovery. The phenomenon is not correlated with body weight but is linked to the specific caloric intake. Often the GH response to a glucose load shows a paradoxical rise which can be prevented by bromocriptine. The responses to apomorphine, L-Dopa and insulin stimulation are generally blunted, while an unexpected increase of GH after IV TRH administration is sometimes reported. The reasons for these abnormal responses to provocative tests are unclear.

The function of the pituitary-thyroid axis is also impaired, with low basal levels of T3, high levels of rT3, low to normal T4 levels, and normal-to-high TSH levels, with a delayed response to TRH stimulation. These phenomena seem to be related to starvation, and especially to carbohydrate deficiency.

Basal plasma cortisol levels are generally elevated, possibly due to alterations in binding globulin, with a circadian rhythm that is flattened at higher levels, an increased production rate, a decreased metabolic clearance rate and a prolonged half-life of the hormone. Urinary 17-ketosteroids and 17-hydroxycorticoids have been reported to be either low or normal. The response to Dexamethasone inhibition is incomplete, either with a total failure of suppression or with early escape. ACTH and Metopirone tests are generally normal to-hyper-reactive or delayed. Tetrahydrocortisol and tetrahydrocortisone are often increased. Many of these changes, but not all of them, have been described in other forms of starvation not related to AN.

Basal prolactin(PRL) levels are normal, with a normal but somewhat delayed response to TRH or chlorpromazine stimulation and an absent or reduced sleep-induced rise. This phenomenon has been observed in other forms of reduction of caloric intake.

Melatonin circadian rhythm is generally preserved, a few cases showing a flattened curve with no nocturnal rise.

In anorectic women, basal testosterone levels tend to be high, while in men they are low, with reduced 5-alpha-reductase activity.

Glucose levels after a glucose load are low, with a tendency toward hypoglycemia. Insulin levels are variable, from elevated to low, with a sustained response to glucose load and increased binding. The insulin resistance is not correlated with weight loss and persists after weight restoration.

With regard to thermoregulation, it has been observed that the basal temperature is low, does not rise normally after acute hypothermia or fall after heat stimulus. These impairments are significantly correlated with the degree of weight loss.

Partial diabetes insipidus is often observed in anorectic patients. The ratio between cerebrospinal fluid and plasma arginine vasopressin (AVP) is generally increased.

For monoaminergic metabolism in the brain, whose alterations might underly the neuroendocrine impairments typical of AN, it has been suggested the noradrenalin (NE) and dopamine (DA) are low. Thus, treatment with electric shock and L-Dopa has been given to correct any such abnormality, without clearcut effects. In contrast, because of the type of symptomatology, it has been proposed that the disease is linked to a DA hypertonus in the brain, and therefore treatment should be with neuroleptics. Low levels of urinary 3-methoxy-4-hydroxy-phenylglycol (MHPG), urinary homovanillic acid, plasma DA, plasma NE, plasma free tryptophan and neutral aminoacids have been reported. Using the probenecid test,reductions in both DA and serotonin turnover have been shown.

Dr. B. Sherman presented data on hypothalamic control of the menstrual cycle (Chapter 25). Dr. Sherman suggested that the impairments in both gonadotropins and ovarian hormones in AN are similar to those observed by Dr. E. Knobil in rhesus monkeys with various types of lesions of the medial basal hypothalamus, and in particular of the arcuate nucleus. In fact, both models include reduced FSH and LH secretion, with loss of pulsatility and of the positive feedback of estrogens on LH and FSH release. Repetitive administration of GnRH restores normal endocrine patterns in both rhesus monkeys and in patients with AN. The impairments in the latter might be linked to alterations in the metabolic pattern of the neurotransmitters on which the secretion of the releasing hormone depends.

Noradrenaline, dopamine and endogenous opiates are all involved in this regulation, the first stimulatory and the last two inhibitory. It has been suggested that increased hypothalamic opiates and/or dopamine are responsible for some amenorrheic syndromes, but it is still unclear which alteration may underlie the metabolic dysfunction in AN. The syndrome has been repeatedly compared to the physiological situation of prepuberty. Information is lacking about the mechanism that triggers the onset of increased hypothalamic GnRH activity at puberty and, in the same way, modifies its secretion in AN. However, it has been suggested that there is a relationship between body weight, or body fat, and the onset of puberty or of the appearance of amenorrhea in AN. Thus, the author suggests that the endocrine impairments of the syndrome are due only to the malnutrition and emaciation.

Dr. L. C. Krey's paper dealt with the neuronal and endocrine mechanisms involved in the control of gonadotropin secretion in relation to AN (Chapter 26). First, analysis of the anatomical organization of the neuronal system that regulates the secretion of the adenohypophysial hormones, and in particular the localization and distribution of the neurons secreting GnRH, reveals that it is possible to distinguish between areas, limited to the hypothalamus, which strictly influence the pituitary function and other, randomly distributed over the entire brain, which still secrete GnRH but have extrapituitary effects. Considering the neuronal and endocrine mechanisms which control FSH and LH secretion in AN, the author suggests that the function of the entire reproductive system depends on the secretory activity of the tuberoinfundibular neurons. In fact, GnRH stimulation of the pituitary induces not only an immediate release of both gonadotropins, but also programs the gonadotroph for subsequent secretory activity, especially through a "self-priming" phenomenon. Large quantities of GnRH tend to favour FSH and LH release, small quantities prime the gonadotrophs for future hormonal discharge. That would explain why a GnRH deficiency results in a decline in gonadotroph activity, and suggests that in AN the reproductive dysfunction is linked to the absence of a sufficient episodic pattern of GnRH release by the brain. GnRH secretion may be regulated by all the classical neurotransmitters and neuromodulators in the hypothalamus and may be influenced also by extrahypothalamic neurons and peripheral hormones.

At the moment, it is difficult to say which of these different regulatory systems is primarily impaired and responsible for the GnRH deficiency in AN.

Secondly, another set of data would indicate that the hypothalamic GnRH secretion has major responsibility for the impairment in AN. It has been demonstrated that during the period from birth to adolescence in normal humans and in rhesus monkeys there are phases of regression/recovery of gonadotropin release exactly similar to those observed in AN, and that these phases are strictly related to the pattern of GnRH secretion. Numerous studies suggest that these changes in neuroendocrine activity need not be mediated by a steroid feedback mechanism, but rather appear to be controlled by a neural mechanism(s) which shuts down/turns on the GnRH neurons. Therefore, the author suggests that the disease is not simply related to the starvation and emaciation of the patients, but involves primarily an impairment of the hypothalamic/suprahypothalamic neurons responsible for the regulation of the reproductive system.

On the whole, the controversy on the pathogenesis of the metabolic alterations of AN is still unresolved. However, even though nobody can deny the relevant relationship between starvation and development of the neuroendocrine disorders, the above-mentioned studies show that these disorders, and in particular those related to the reproductive system, are linked to evident alterations of hypothalamic/suprahypothalamic centers. The influence of mental disorders on the functioning of these centers remains to be investigated.

Neuroendocrinology and Psychiatric Disorder, edited by G. M. Brown, et al. Raven Press, New York 1984.

Discussion: Anorexia Nervosa—Endocrine Findings

Gregory M. Brown

Gregory M. Brown, Chairman

A number of questions deserve further examination. Which endocrine changes seen in anorexia nervosa are simply due to nutritional changes and which might be related to the basic process of anorexia nervosa itself? We have heard that amenorrhea can precede dietary changes and that it can also precede weight change. Does this mean that there is a primary CNS abnormality underlying amenorrhea? What would the mechanism be? How good is the evidence for preexisting amenorrhea? Does persistent amenorrhea after weight restoration mean that there is a primary CNS disorder? Are there any other abnormalities which persist? We have heard that the urinary free cortisol abnormalities persist and also that dexamethasone suppression abnormalities persist. What does this mean? Is that related to the syndrome itself? Even if the majority of these endocrine changes seem primarily related to nutritional factors or to weight loss - are they nevertheless useful in diagnosis and for monitoring response to treatment or are they simply complicating phenomena which should be ignored?

Francesca Brambilla

We have heard a lot about the physical factors like weight loss and endocrine abnormalities, but little about the deep psychological abnormalities which characterize anorexia nervosa. Weight loss is one of the symptoms of the disease, and gaining weight is the expression of recovery from a very peculiar psychopathology. To say that the weight changes are largely responsible for the endocrine abnormalities we see - may be just to avoid the possible influence of the psychopathology behind it. It is very difficult to discriminate between what is due to weight changes per se and what is due to psychopathology. There are certainly a few things which make one think that the psychopathology is responsible for at least some of the endocrine symptomatology. For instance, patients can resume weight gain while having psychological treatment such as psychoanalysis and psychotherapy but not drug therapy and the psychological impairment can remain in the sense that they will still refuse to fit into their family background for their particular age and sex. This is probably the most important psychological characteriztic of anorexia nervosa, namely the denial of being an adult, or denial of being female, and the denial of a normal relationship with the family. While this psychopathology remains, the girl will not resume spontaneous menstruation, and especially spontaneous ovulation, and clomiphene stimulation will remain negative and can go on being negative for as long as the psychopathology remains - possibly for one or two years. Even though the weight will be fairly normal and feeding sufficiently normalized to keep up the weight, the endocrine changes will persist. So, in this respect we cannot just talk about weight loss, as we would malnutrition. This weight loss is significantly different.

Dr. P. Garfinkel

These are extremely important points. Many of the manifestations of anorexia nervosa classically thought of as anorectic symptoms of anorexia patients, were evident in Keyes' study of Minnesota's starving normal men. The obsession and food pre-occupations, food dreams and indecisiveness, thought by many to be anorexia symptoms, are in a psychological sense related to starvation. But after weight restoration, many psychological issues remain. They continue to be concerned around a drive for fitness, fear of losing control, trust in one's self and one's body, trust in other people, concern about the body, body sensitivity and negative feelings. What you have raised is extremely important. Could these be some of the effects, say of chronic overproduction of cortisol, on some of these psychological factors - or of low levels of monoamines, leading to a persistence - or is altered arginine vasopressin related to some of the cognitive changes? There are very curious cognitive patterns, in terms of what has been called dichotomist thinking. Patients don't see things in between. They see all or none and they personalize situations - having marked difficulties in autonomy. I think a lot of these psychological changes have been 'separated' from the process of starvation, but we still don't know what the physiological basis of the response is.

Dr. Vigersky

I would like to introduce another possibility or a confounding factor - whether or not an anorexic having lost weight and regained it, incurs some permanent damage in anatomic structures or even functional relationships of the anatomic structures. These may take some time to recover or may never recover. There is very little data on this. We studied a few patients after they recovered weight and presumably had normal feeding behaviour, and they still had thermoregulatory abnormalities. Basic experiments need to be done to see what kind of changes occur as the result of prolonged weight loss and if they persist after weight gain. As far as I know, there have been no histochemical or histopathological studies of the hypothalamus or neuroendocrine evaluations in anorexia patients.

Barry Sherman, Iowa City

There is no reason to believe that there are not other influences. Clinicians see patients with amenorrhea who resemble in every way recovered anorexia patients - those who have regained weight but don't yet menstruate, and this seems to be related to environment, stress or some unknown factors. And they show no weight change when they begin to menstruate so there must be other factors. In some patients hard data are not always extensive. Height, weight and other parameters of nutritional assessment are obviously hard to come by for patients entering this syndrome - nor are they very prevalent in patients who are recovering. Height and weight are the crudest methods for assessing nutritional status, but we need to sharpen our techniques, especially in terms of looking at recovered patients. We need to concentrate on doing more detailed endocrine studies on the earliest phases of the syndrome, and compare them with patients with other types of hypothalamic amenorrhea.

Benjamin Rusak, Halifax, N.S.

I would like to take time to go back to very basic methodological issues. Dr. Garfinkel told us that basal prolactin levels were normal and that prolactin responses were unchanged. He then showed us a slide with the most spectacular difference in prolactin I can imagine - a most beautiful slide with no nocturnal rise. It was flat and that is not normal. Basal levels are irrelevant, because the critical aspect of prolactin is the functional pattern through time. A good analogy would be to compare a comatose and a normal sleeping person at night, and concluding that their basal activity levels were similar. Comparisons during the day however, would lead us to conclude that there is a significant difference between these individuals. If you believe that the functional unit of prolactin secretion is the pattern, then these people are far from normal. They are very, very abnormal.

It is always necessary to consider the pattern of secretion of hormones in the real animal, and ask why it is there? Evolution didn't put them there just to confound you. When you mimic the normal pattern, you get physiological effects. When you do something non-physiological, you get pathological effects. The same is true of prolactin, in that a group of experts should look at the prolactin pattern and say 'Does that look normal?' In terms of the physiological importance of prolactin, they would recognize that the nocturnal peak <u>is</u> the pattern of patterns - and if it is not there, something is desparately wrong. The most important functional consideration in the endocrine system, in physiology in general and in behaviour, is the pattern through time. If Einstein has not convince you, Knobil should - that spatio-temporal patterns are all one and that you cannot study levels independently of their change through time. The dynamic pattern of the endocrine system defines the endocrine system, and not a single cross-sectional examination at any one time. I would like to make exactly the same point about noradrenergic mechanisms. We heard that the MHPG levels seem to be slightly depressed. I did not see anything significant in the pattern of noradrenergic activity throughout the day. Margolis published a paper in 1972 in which he injected norepinephrine into the brain of rats during the light phase and induced anorexia. The rats stopped eating. He injected exactly the same dose during the dark phase and got no decrease in food intake - same site in the brain, same chemical, two different animals, and just because you look at them 12 hours apart. So the critical question in these patients is not whether MHPG is decreased or increased, but when is it increased, how is it increased and how does it change through time? If norepinephrine can have an anorexic effect at some time in the circadian cycle and not at others, then an integrated daily assessment of its levels is irrelevant to the question. So before we can answer Dr. Brown's questions, we must collect the endocrine and neural data which is relevant and then go back and try to address those questions which we think are the most important but which cannot be answered in ingnorance.

<u>Peter E. Stokes, New York, N.Y.</u>

I did not hear an explanation of why there are elevated urine free cortisol levels when, in fact, the diurnal curves or circadian rhythms were essentially normal or low. No information was given about low corticosteroid binding globulin (CBG), which in fact has been looked at and is generally normal. There was no reported evidence of high pulses, but in fact I think there are high pulses, and the accumulated data suggests that one explanation for the high urine free cortisol is based on episodes of over-saturation of CBG. This is related to cycle change and to activity, and should be examined further.

Katherine A. Halmi, White Plains N.Y.

In many of the studies, all of the endocrine changes have been related to change in weight, but in fact very few people have systematically assessed changes in behaviour - and to ignore something such as this doesn't mean it doesn't exist. If observations are related only to weight, the question of relationship to behaviour cannot be answered.

The other issue that one of the panelists mentioned is exceedingly important, namely, that if a patient is significantly below normal weight for a long period of time - I mean 60-70% below normal weight for several years, it is reasonable to assume that there may be some irreparable damage. In a recent one-year follow-up on 40 patients, we found that those patients who maintained low weight for a long period of time were those who at the one year follow-up did poorly.

Dr. Vigersky made a point about critical weight for the onset of menses. We also have some data on this. There may be a critical point for each individual, but I am not certain we should generalize. We have analyzed data on 105 patients - 15 with primary amenorrhea, with two of them only 10 years of age when illness developed. Thirteen were between the ages of 15 and 17 when they developed the illness, and 10 of the 13 were well above Frisch's 10% critical line for a long period of time before they developed symptoms of anorexia. So they had ample time for onset of menses. The onset of menses is complicated and nutrition is, I am sure, important but certainly not the sole factor and probably has been receiving too much emphasis. Another observation was that eight people in that sample regained their menses or recovered from the secondary amenorrhea, and five of the eight started cycling below the 10% crucial line.

Robert A. Vigersky, Washington, D.C.: May I add to that. Michele Warren, in her paper on ballet dancers, reported that their menarche is delayed, and even after they have been at or above the critical weight for up to a year, they still do not begin menstruating. In ballet dancers, onset of menses is not a simple matter of weight. In their case, it may be exercise, the diet or stress.

John R. Sutton, McMaster University

I would like to follow up on an issue that Dr. Vigersky raised earlier, and that is the relationship of activity to secondary amenorrhea, and perhaps whether or not the secondary amenorrhea that occurs in athletes is really a reflection of part of the broader spectrum of Anorexia Nervosa. Certainly, from clinical situations where we have observed it, it is very difficult to be certain that patients coming to you as athletes with secondary amenorrhea don't have anorectic features. Many of them have altered their diet. As people become more physically active, there may be subtle changes in diet. They don't necessarily reduce their calories to a major extent, but they may change from a predominantly red meat diet to more poultry and fish, and sometimes actually become vegetarians. What is the impact of this diet change? Being an athlete, in fact, seems etiologically related to the production of secondary amenorrhea. Epidemiologists would laugh at us, because there have not been any true prospective studies, appropriately stratified by premenstrual conditions, menstrual history, rigidity of diet, control and maintenance of body weight, body fat, etc. - so, in fact, the evidence is indeed limited that there is a prima facie case for athletes developing secondary amenorrhea on that basis alone. Would Dr. Vigersky like to speculate, on the answer to the question? Is it possible that in highly trained individuals with a vigorous and very active life-style, this life-style alone can give rise to secondary amenorrhea? What of metabolic hormonal responses in the trained state, and can the episodes of activity per se give rise, on a mechanistic basis, to secondary amenorrhea? Also, I would be delighted to know why there is such a female versus male preponderance. Can anyone shed new light on this issue?

Robert A. Vigersky: I did not mention the very scanty data available at the moment on hormonal changes in athletes - but there are some. McArthur and Beitins, in Endocrine Research Communications last year, studied pulsatile LH and FSH, the response to LRH and the response to naloxone as well, in three of their runners. And similar findings were reported by Warren. That is, LH and FSH are low, they did not seem to have the adult pattern of gonadotrophin secretion and they did respond to LRH. One of the three patients responded to naloxone with an LH spike. At the Endocrine Society meetings last week there was an intriguing paper, which Dr. Quigley might be able to comment on, about an anticipatory rise in LH before the beginning of exercise, in a group of women.

Dr. M. E. Quigley, San Diego

We have two bits of information. The first relates to baseline sampling. One of our medical students, for her fourth-year thesis, elected to draw a single sample in a group of female joggers and to do a very detailed dietary and jogging history. Contrary to anticipation, she documented that in the small percentage of female joggers that were amenorrheic, the baseline LH levels, based on a single sample, correlated positively with the number of miles the female jogged per week.

The more miles per week she jogged, the higher the LH levels were. As opposed to anorexia nervosa patients, who have very low gonadotropin levels, the amenorrheic joggers studied in this population had high basal levels. I can only speak for this small group of women, but this may bring new light to what we are going to discuss later. As Dr. Vigersky has discussed this morning, the one thing we know about anorexia nervosa is that there is hypo-gonadotropism. Especially in California, where jogging is such a part of everyday life, I think we are going to see more patients with anorexia nervosa with high basal gonadotrophin levels - that is, patients for whom exercise is a major part of their means for maintaining low body weight.

In the paper presented last week at the Endocrine Society meeting, we demonstrated an anticipatory increase in both LH and testosterone in a group of normal women and in trained joggers. This was demonstrated at the zero point just prior to undergoing bicyle exercise in which we monitored numerous parameters. This is very similar to the data presented by Dr. Rose (see Chapter 7).

Another interesting factor in the initial study done by the medical student was the fact that when the women were asked the simple question "How stressed are you?" (on a score of 0 - 10), amenorrheic women scored themselves much higher than the joggers going the same distance. We did not find any difference between the women who did and did not develop amenorrhea, based on distance - that is, we had an equal number of women jogging greater than 60 miles who were amenorrheic and who were normal.

Dr. J. R. Sutton; The gonadotropin data seem to be slightly at variance with the findings of Dale, in similar subjects in Atlanta, so presumably there is a very wide variation.

Sarah F. Leibowitz, New York, N.Y.

I want to underscore the questions Dr. Brown posed at the beginning. I have been concerned that we have perhaps studied anorexia nervosa as a model for studying gonadotropin and other hormonal abnormalities, rather than using these hormones as markers to better understand the etiology of anorexia nervosa. We have tried to determine whether these changes are a function of body weight, but perhaps even more important is the question of diet and feeding patterns. My interest is in understanding the neurochemical and anatomical basis for feeding behaviour - to see perhaps if it can be used as a model for anorexia nervosa. To underscore Dr. Brown's question, I would like to ask if we are studying anorexia nervosa in these endocrine studies, and how can we use them to understand its etiology, and how does it relate to feeding behaviour. Can we study these issues in anorectic animals and simply put them through a protocol, studying endocrine changes, as well as putting the monoamines directly into the brain, to see what impact they have on the various hormonal changes?

Dr. Krey

I will comment on that. A key consideration is the type of animal used. Certainly the easiest preparation to use is the rat, but control of gonadotropins in the rat is tremendously different from that in higher mammalian forms - especially in man. Some people may say this is a bias on my part, but if you are going to do this type of study, I would restrict it to one of the higher primates - rhesus monkey or baboon, showing distinct endocrine similarities, in terms of control, to what is seen in man.

Neuroendocrinology and Psychiatric Disorder,
edited by G. M. Brown, et al.
Raven Press, New York 1984.

Endocrine Changes in Anorexia Nervosa: An Interpretation Based on the Metabolic Adaptation to Caloric Restriction

Lewis Landsberg and James B. Young

The starving mammalian homeotherm has two major metabolic requirements: On the one hand metabolic rate or energy expenditure must be reduced so that calories are not wasted at a time of restricted caloric intake; on the other hand substrates need to be mobilized to support the vital functions of the organism. Substrate mobilization, however, to be maximally effective must proceed without increased energy expenditure and with the greatest conservation of muscle protein stores. The metabolic adaptation to starvation involves neural and humoral mechanisms that appear to address these requirements. In anorexia nervosa, in which starvation is the central physiological alteration, a variety of changes in endocrine function have been described and are well summarized in other chapters of this volume. The significance of these changes, however, as they relate to the pathogenesis and clinical course of anorexia nervosa, is less clear. Many of the endocrine-metabolic features of anorexia nervosa appear to depend upon alterations in hypothalamic function. A major question, therefore, is whether the involvement of the hypothalamus is primary. A primary abnormality in the hypothalamus could conceivably account for both the eating disturbance and the endocrine abnormalities in anorexia nervosa. Alternatively, it is possible to view the hypothalamic alterations and the changes in endocrine-metabolic function that ensue as a consequence of starvation. If starvation is responsible for the endocrine-metabolic alterations, either diminished body mass or caloric deprivation may be responsible. In this paper the possibility that the endocrine changes in anorexia nervosa reflect the metabolic adaptation to caloric deprivation will be explored.

THE SYMPATHETIC NERVOUS SYSTEM IN STARVATION AND ANOREXIA NERVOSA

Role of the sympathetic nervous system in the regulation of thermogenesis

The sympathetic nervous system has a major role in the regulation of metabolic rate and metabolic heat production. The critical role of the sympathetic nervous system in the mammalian defense against cold exposure has long been recognized. In the absence of a functioning sympathetic nervous sytem body temperature cannot be maintained against a temperature gradient. When the temperature falls, receptors in the skin and central nervous system are stimulated and give rise to neural impulses integrated in the anterior and posterior hypothalamus; hypothalamic connections with the brainstem sympathetic centres result in a net increase in sympathetic nervous system activity. The physiological result of sympathetic activation is two-fold: on the one hand sympathetically mediated vasoconstriction in the subcutaneous tissues limits heat dissipation; on the other, stimulation of metabolic heat production, a process referred to as non-shivering thermogenesis, also occurs and contributes importantly to the maintenance of body temperature (11, 17, 27, 44).

Although changes in thermogenesis (or oxygen consumption) in response to changes in dietary intake have been well documented (14, 21), only recently has the sympathetic nervous system been recognized as potentially important in the relationship between thermogenesis and dietary intake. The role of the sympathetic nervous system in the regulation of diet-induced changes in thermogenesis has been deduced from two lines of evidence. The studies of Young and Landsberg (25, 26, 51, 52) demonstrating that fasting suppresses while overfeeding sucrose stimulates sympathetic nervous system activity, as described more fully below, provided evidence that changes in dietary intake influence the activity of the sympathetic nervous system. The studies of Rothwell and Stock (37, 38) provided evidence of an essential similarity between thermogenesis in response to cold (non-shivering thermogenesis) and thermogenesis in response to caloric intake (diet-induced thermogenesis). If, therefore, diminished metabolic rate is an important adaptive response to caloric restriction, the activity of the sympathetic nervous system in starvation and anorexia nervosa is of considerable interest.

The sympathetic nervous system in starvation

Opinions to the contrary notwithstanding, it is reasonably clear that starvation is associated with a decrease in sympathetic nervous system activity in the experimental animal and in man. Thus, diminished norepinephrine turnover attributable to a diminuation in central sympathetic activity has been demonstrated in a variety of organs in the rat and mouse (24, 51, 52, 54, 55). In obese human subjects, semi-starvation has been shown to result in a fall in the excretion of catecholamine metabolites and a decrease in plasma norepinephrine levels (9, 18). In normal weight human subjects the urinary excretion or norepinephrine similarly falls during a brief fast (Rosa, Young and Landsberg - unpublished observations). Evidence in the experimental animal suggests that suppression of sympathetic activity during fasting is a consequence of an integrated hypothalamic response that results in suppression of the brainstem sympathetic centres. Thus, mice treated with gold-thioglucose, an agent that destroys portions of the ventromedial hypothalamus, fail to suppress sympathetic activity during a fast (55). Similarly, decerebration reverses starvation induced suppression of thermogenesis in newborn rats exposed to cold (3). These observations suggest that diminished caloric intake is sensed at the level of the hypothalamus, and that an inhibitory pathway between the hypothalamus and the brainstem is stimulated, thus resulting in diminished central sympathetic outflow (55).

How does the hypothalamus sense the diminished caloric intake or assess the nutritional state of the organism? One signal that couples changes in dietary intake with changes in sympathetic activity appears to be intracellular glucose metabolism within the central nervous system. In the rat both hypoglycemia and 2-deoxy-glucose administration have been shown to suppress sympathetic nervous system activity (23, 35, 53) while sucrose overfeeding has the opposite effect (51). Under most circumstances, however, the circulating glucose level would not appear to be a sufficient signal, in and of itself, since changes in plasma glucose level are rather small despite considerable changes in caloric or carbohydrate intake. Studies in human subjects have raised the possibility that insulin may be involved in coupling changes in dietary intake with changes in sympathetic nervous system activity (39). With starvation insulin levels, as well as glucose levels, are known to fall (31). The available data are thus consistent with the following mechanism: during starvation a decrease in insulin-mediated glucose utilization within certain critical neurons (perhaps in the ventromedial portion of the hypothalamus) results in suppression of central sympathetic outflow.

A decrease in sympathetic nervous system activity may contribute to the decrease in oxygen consumption that accompanies starvation. Studies consistent with such an interpretation have been reported by Shetty and coworkers (41); in obese subjects consuming a low energy diet (semi-starvation) a fall in resting metabolic rate (oxygen consumption) of about 18% was noted after three weeks. The administration of L-dopa, an agent which has a mild peripheral sympathomimetic effect, completely prevented the fall in oxygen consumption (41). This observation does not prove, but is consistent with diminished sympathetic nervous system activity as the underlying factor responsible for the decrease in oxygen consumption. The hypotension and bradycardia of chronic starvation (20) may also be secondary to suppression of sympathetic activity.

Sympathetic nervous system activity in anorexia nervosa

Although few studies of sympathetic activity in patients with anorexia nervosa have appeared (15, 16) convincing evidence of diminished sympathetic activity has been provided by Gross and associates (15). Diminished plasma norepinephrine levels with diminished plasma norepinephrine response to upright posture and isometric hand grip were noted by these workers along with a decrease in the urinary excretion of catecholamine metabolites. After refeeding and weight gain the changes in plasma norepinephrine and catecholamine metabolite excretion returned to normal levels. Similarly, pulse rate and blood pressure, both supine and upright, were reduced in the patients with anorexia nervosa but returned toward normal after weight gain. These data are consistent with suppression of sympathetic nervous system activity in patients with anorexia nervosa. Likewise, the defect in thermoregulation (29) in patients with anorexia nervisa is consistent with an impairment in sympathetic nervous system activity. Thus, the evidence suggests that in anorexia nervosa, like starvation, the sympathetic nervous system is suppressed.

In neither anorexia nervosa nor starvation can changes in plasma tyrosine level (the catecholamine precursor) explain the documented changes in sympathetic activity, since plasma tyrosine levels are unchanged in anoretic patients and in obese subjects fasted for forty days (10, 15).

Weight loss vs decreased caloric intake

Is the effect of starvation on sympathetic activity secondary to weight loss per se (loss of body mass) or does it reflect a response to diminished caloric intake? In the experimental animal suppression of sympathetic nervous system activity is demonstrable within the first 24 hours of a fast before appreciable loss of weight occurs (34). In human subjects the data are less decisive but a fall in catecholamine and catecholamine metabolite excretion can be demonstrated early in a fast before significant change in body mass has occurred (18) (Rosa, Young and Landsberg - unpublished observations). The mechanism described above, namely diminished glucose utilization within critical central neurons is also consistent with an effect of caloric restriction. This is supported by human studies in which caloric restriction with a carbohydrate free diet has been shown to suppress sympathetic activity while the same caloric intake with 50% calories given as sucrose was without effect (9).

Most of the data therefore are consistent with a primary effect of caloric (or carbohydrate) restriction on sympathetic activity during starvation rather than change in body mass.

THYROID HORMONES IN STARVATION AND ANOREXIA NERVOSA

The thyroid-pituitary axis in starvation

In 1974 Portnay and associates (33) demonstrated a striking fall in plasma concentration of total and free triiodothyronine (T_3) in obese subjects after a four week fast. This observation, which has been widely confirmed, occurs in normal weight individuals following caloric restriction and has been shown to result from a decrease in the peripheral conversion of thyroxine (T_4) to T_3 (30, 43, 45, 46, 49). Since T_3 is believed to be the major active thyroid hormone in most peripheral tissues exclusive of the pituitary, a fall in T_3 level is an effective way of reducing thyroid hormone action. The evidence suggests, moreover, that this fall in circulating T_3 reflects a physiological adaptation to starvation. TSH levels in starvation have been reported as both normal (30, 33) or low (1, 7) rather than elevated as they are when the T_3 level is depressed in hypothyroidism. Furthermore, several investigators have shown that the TSH response to TRH is not enhanced during starvation (12, 33) and may even be diminished (1, 5) in distinction to the augmented response in hypothyroidism due to thyroid failure. The fact that the TSH response to TRH is increased after thyroid hormone output is reduced by potassium iodide in fasting subjects indicates that the hypothalamic-pituitary-thyroid axis is reset during starvation to maintain a lower circulating level of triiodothyronine (12) which cannot be explained by a nonspecific suppression of hypothalamic function.

The central connections and the signals involved in mediating decreased peripheral conversion of T_4 have not been clearly established. It is known, however, that carbohydrate has a particularly important effect on peripheral conversion of T_4 to T_3 so that glucose feeding rapidly reverses the fall in the peripheral level of T_3 (1, 5). A possible role for insulin is indicated by the fact that peripheral conversion of T_4 to T_3 is inhibited in diabetic patients (32) and in the tissues of diabetic animals (2). Thus, there may be an underlying similarity between the regulation of peripheral thyroid hormone action and sympathetic nervous system activity, with both systems dependent upon carbohydrate utilization within the central nervous system, and both systems dependent upon circulating insulin levels. This is consistent with the observation that insulin is the major signal to tissues outside the central nervous system that calories, especially carbohydrates, have been assimilated and it would be parsimonious for insulin to serve a similar function for the central nervous system as well.

The fall in circulating T_3 levels would result in a reduction in the metabolic rate since thyroid hormones and catecholamines are synergistic in their effects on heat production (22, 40). In addition, the fall in thyroid hormone may exert a protein sparing or anti-catabolic effect. T_3 administration during fasting has been shown to antagonize the fall in urea production that occurs during a fast without T_3 replacement (12), an effect not noted with small doses of T_3 in the fed state. Furthermore, 3-methyl histidine excretion, a measure of skeletal muscle breakdown, is also increased by T_3 administration in fasting (but not in fed) subjects (47). Thus, the diminution in T_3 during fasting may be associated with a decrease in metabolic rate and an enhancement of muscle protein conservation.

Thyroid-pituitary axis in anorexia nervosa

As is well documented in this volume (13) anorexia nervosa is associated with a low T_3 level similar to that found in starvation (8). Furthermore, the TSH response to TRH is normal resembling the response seen in chronic starvation and inconsistent with that seen in primary hypothyroidism (8). A decrease in the speed of the Achilles' tendon reflex has also been noted in patients with anorexia nervosa presumably a peripheral manifestation of diminished thyroid hormone effect (8). Biochemical evidence of diminished thyroid hormone action in anorexia nervosa has appeared as well. Thyroid dependent alterations in the metabolism of cortisol (4) (see below) and testosterone (4a) have been demonstrated in patients with anorexia nervosa.

Caloric restriction vs. reduction in weight

The decrease in peripheral conversion of T_4 to T_3 in starvation (and presumably anorexia nervosa) is due to a reduction in caloric intake rather than a loss of body mass. Significant decrease in T_3 is noted during the second day of a fast before appreciable change in body mass occurs (12); the rapid increase in T_3 levels after carbohydrate feeding in fasting subjects (5) is also incompatible with a change in body mass as an explanation for the alterations in peripheral conversion of T_4 to T_3.

OTHER ENDOCRINE CHANGES IN STARVATION AND ANOREXIA NERVOSA

The changes in both sympathetic nervous system activity and in the hypothalamic-pituitary-thyroid axis in anorexia nervosa and in starvation therefore, may be viewed as an adaptive response to caloric restriction. While these changes appear to be the most important and most pronounced of the endocrine changes in anorexia nervosa, changes in growth hormone cortisol, and insulin also occur.

Growth hormone

Growth hormone levels are modestly elevated in many patients with anorexia nervosa (13) and in some patients with starvation (6). The mechanisms involved in stimulation of growth hormone under these circumstances are not known with certainty. The plasma glucose level is low in patients with anorexia nervosa (29) and in normal subjects during a fast (31). The ventromedial nucleus of the hypothalamus plays an important role in the regulation of growth hormone secretion (28) and this region is believed to be sensitive to glucose and insulin, raising the possibility that diminished plasma glucose during starvation is related to the increase in growth hormone. The role of plasma glucose in the mediation of increased growth hormone levels during starvation, however, has been questioned and attention directed to decreased somatomedin levels as an explanation. Fall in somatomedin level, which has been documented in some patients with anorexia nervosa (36), would increase growth hormone concentration by disrupting the negative feedback normally exerted by somatomedin on growth hormone release. The fact that growth hormone levels rise and then fall during a prolonged fast suggests an important role for caloric restriction rather than change in body mass (6).

Cortisol

In patients with anorexia nervosa there is an alteration in cortisol metabolism (4). Although plasma cortisol levels are elevated diurnal variation is preserved and cortisol production rate is not increased. Metabolic clearance rate of cortisol is markedly diminished as is the plasma cortisol half life (4). These alterations in plasma cortisol level may reflect the low circulating levels of T_3 since administration of T_3 has been shown to restore the abnormalities in cortisol metabolism towards normal in anorectic patients (4). Similar alterations in cortisol metabolism have been described in patients with protein-calorie malnutrition (42).

Insulin

Insulin levels are suppressed in both patients with anorexia nervosa (50) and in normal weight subjects during a fast (31). As noted above the low levels of insulin, in conjunction with the low glucose levels, may be an important signal to the central nervous system that caloric intake is diminished. Since insulin exerts a strong restraining influence on the processes of fuel mobilization, the fall in insulin level also plays an important adaptive role in starvation. As a consequence of the low circulating level of insulin, therefore, both gluconeogenesis and lipolysis are potentiated and substrate mobilization for support of vital functions is enhanced.

In both starvation and anorexia nervosa the insulin response to a glucose challenge is altered. The insulin level rises more slowly and stays elevated longer in association with prolonged elevation of the plasma glucose level (19). Peripheral sensitivity to insulin, however is maintained or even enhanced (29, 50) during caloric restriction.

SUMMARY AND CONCLUSIONS

The thesis is developed that many, if not all, of the endocrine abnormalities in anorexia nervosa can be explained as part of an integrated metabolic adaptation to reduced caloric intake. Suppression of sympathetic nervous system activity and diminished peripheral conversion of T_4 to T_3 are probably involved in the fall in metabolic rate that occurs when caloric intake is diminished. The decrease in T_3 and possibily the increase in growth hormone may be important in preserving muscle protein during the substrate mobilization that occurs in starvation. Carbohydrate utilization within the hypothalamus may be an important signal that caloric intake is diminished and may therefore trigger this adaptive response. Changes in the pituitary-adrenal axis may be entirely secondary to changes in cortisol metabolism induced by the fall in T_3. Impaired thermoregulation, hypotension, and bradycardia are probably related to suppression of sympathetic nervous system activity. There appears to be no decisive evidence for a distinct primary hypothalamic or endocrine abnormality in anorexia nervosa.

ACKNOWLEDGEMENT

The excellent secretarial assistance of Mrs. Edith Cusher is gratefully acknowledged.

REFERENCES

1. Azizi, F. (1978): Metabolism 27:935-942.

2. Balsam, A. and Ingbar, S. H. (1978): J. Clin. Invest. 62:415-424.
3. Bignall, K. E., Heggenes, F. W., Palmer, J. E. (1975): Exp. Neurol. 49:174-188.
4. Boyar, R. M., Hellman, L. D., Roffwarg, H., Katz, J., Zumoff, B., O'Connor, J., Bradlow, H. L. and Fukushima, D. K. (1977): N. Engl. J. Med. 296:190-193.
4a. Bradlow, H. L., Boyar, R. M., O'Connor, J., Zumoff, B. and Hellman, L. (1976): J. Clin. Endocrinol. Metab. 43:571-574.
5. Burman, K. D., Dimond, R. C., Harvey, G. S., O'Brian, J. T., Georges, L. P., Burton, J., Wright, F. D. and Wartofsky, L. (1979): Metabolism 28:291-299.
6. Cahill, G. F., Jr., Herrera, M. G., Morgan, A. P., Soeldner, J. S., Steinke, J., Levy, P. L., Reichard, G. A., Jr. and Kipnis, D. M. (1966): J. Clin. Invest. 45:1751-1769.
7. Croxson, M. S., Hall, T. D., Kletzky, O. A., Jaramillo, J. E. and Nicoloff, J. T. (1977): J. Clin. Endocrinol. Metab. 45:560-568.
8. Croxson, M. S. and Ibbertson, H. K. (1977): J. Clin. Endocrinol. Metab. 44:167-174.
9. DeHaven, J., Sherwin, R., Hendler, R., Felig, P. (1980): N. Engl. J. Med. 302:477-482.
10. Felig. P., Owen, O. E., Wahren, J. and Cahill, G. F., Jr. (1969): J. Clin. Invest. 48:584-594.
11. Gale, C. C. (1973): Annu. Rev. Physiol. 35:391-430.
12. Gardner, D. F., Kaplan, M. M., Stanley, C. A. and Utiger, R. D. (1979): N. Engl. J. Med. 300:579-584.
13. Garfinkel, P. E. (1981): Chapter 24, this volume.
14. Garrow, J. S. (1978): In: Energy Metabolism and Obesity in Man. Elsevier, Amsterdam.
15. Gross, H. A., Lake, C. R., Ebert, M. H., Ziegler, M. G. and Kopin, I. J. (1979): J. Clin. Endocrinol. Metab. 49:805-809.
16. Halmi, K. A., Dekirmenjian, H., Davis, J. M., Casper, R., Goldberg, S. (1978): Arch. Gen. Psychiatry 35:458-460.
17. Himms,-Hagen, J. (1976): Annu. Rev. Physiol. 38:315-351.
18. Jung, R. T., Shetty, P. S., Barrand, M., Callingham, B. A., Hames, W.P.T. (1979): Br. Med. J. 1:12-13.
19. Kanis, J. A., Brown, P., Fitzpatrick, K., Hibbert, D. J., Horn, D. B., Nairn, I. M., Shirling, D., STrong, J. A. and Walton, H. J. (1974): Quarterly J. of Med. 43:321-338.
20. Keys, A., Brozek, J., Henschel, A., Mickelsen, O., Taylor, H. L. (1950): In: The Biology of Human Starvation, Vol. 1, pp.303-339.
21. Keys, A., Brozek, J., Henschel, a., Mickelsen, O., and Taylor, H.L. (1950): In: The Biology of Human Starvation, Vol. 1, pp.607-634.
22. Landsberg, L. (1978): In: The Thyroid, edited by S. C. Werner and S. H. Ingbar, pp.791-799. Harper & Row, Hagerstown, MD.
23. Landsberg, L., Greff, L., Gunn, S. and Young, J. B. (1980): Metabolism 29:1128-1137.
24. Landsberg, L., Saville, E., Young, J. B., Rothwell, N. J. and Stock, m. J. (1981): Clin. Res. 29:542A.
25. Landsberg, L. and Young, J. B. (1978): N. Engl. J. Med. 298:1295-1301.
26. Landsberg, L. and Young, J. B. (1981): Life Sci. 28:1801-1819.
27. Landsberg, L. and Young, J. B. (1981): Obesity and Metabolism 1: 3-39.
28. Martin, J. B. (1973): N. Engl. J. Med. 288:1384-1393.
29. Mecklenburg, R. S., Loriaux, D. L., Thompson, R. H., Anderson, A. E. and Lipsett, M. B. (1974): Medicine 53:147-159.

30. Merimee, T. J. and Fineberg, E. S. (1976): Metabolism 25:79-83.
31. Merimee, T. J. and Tyson, J. E. (1974): J. Engl. J. Med. 291: 1275-1278.
32. Pittman, C. S., Suda, A. K., Chambers, J. B., Jr. and Ray, G. Y. (1979): Metabolism 28:333-338.
33. Portnay, G. I., O'Brain, J. T., Bush, J., Vagenakis, A. G., Azizi, F., Arky, R. A., Ingbar, S. H. and Braverman, L. E. (1974): J. Clin. Endocrinol. Metab. 39:191-194.
34. Rappaport, E. B., Young, J. B. and Landsberg, L. (1980): Endocrinology 106(Suppl):183.
35. Rappaport, E. B., Young, J. B. and Landsberg, L. (1980): Clin. Res. 28:403A.
36. Rappaport, R., Prevot, C., Czernichow, P. (1980): Acta Paediatr. Scand. 69(1):37-41.
37. Rothwell, N. J. and Stock, M. J. (1979): Nature (Lond.) 281:31-35.
38. Rothwell, N. J. and Stock, M. J. (1980): Can. J. Physiol. Pharmacol. 58:842-848.
39. Rowe, J. W., Young, J. B., Minaker, K. L., Stevens, A. L., Pallotta, J. and Landsberg, L. (1981): Diabetes 30:219-225.
40. Sellers, E. A., Flattery, K. V., Steiner, G. (1974): Am. J. Physiol. 226:290-294.
41. Shetty, P. s., Jung, R. T., James, W.P.T. (1979): The Lancet 1: 77-79.
42. Smith, S. R., Bledsoe, T. and Chhetri, M. K. (1975): J. Clin. Endocrinol. Metab. 40:43-52.
43. Suda, A. K., Pittman, C. S., Shimizu, T. and Chambers, J. B., Jr. (1978): J. Clin. Endocrinol. Metab. 47:1311-1319.
44. Thompson, G. E. (1977): In: International Review Physiology, Environmental Physiology, edited by D. Robertshaw, Vol. 15. University Park Press, Baltimore.
45. Vagenakis, A. G., Burger, A., Portnay, G. I., Rudolph, M., O'Brian, J. T., Azizi, F., Arky, R. A., Nicod, P., Ingbar, S. H. and Braverman, L. E. (1975): J. Clin. Endocrinol. Metab. 41:191-194.
46. Vagenakis, A. G., Portnay, G. I., O'Brian, J. T., Rudolph, M., Arky, R. A., Ingbar, S. H. and Braverman, L. E. (1977): J. Clin. Endocrinol. Metab. 45:1305-1309.
47. Vignati, L., Finley, R. J., Hagg, S. and Aoko, T. T. (1978): In: Transactions of the Association of American Physicians, Vol. 91, pp.169-179.
48. Vigersky, R. A. (1981): Chapter 23, this volume.
49. Visser, T. J., Lamberts, S.W.J., Wilson, J.H.P., Docter, R. and Hannemann, G. (1978): Metabolism 27:405-409.
50. Wachslicht-Rodbard, H., Gross, H. A., Robard, D., Ebert, M. H., Roth, J. (1979): N. Engl. J. Med. 300:882-887.
51. Young, J. B. and Landsberg, L. (1977): Nature 269:615-617.
52. Young, J. B. and Landsberg, L. (1977): Science 196:1473-1475.
53. Young, J. B. and Landsberg, L. (1979): J. Clin. Invest. 64:109-116.
54. Young, J. B. and Landsberg, L. (1979): Am. J. Physiol. 236:E524-E 533.
55. Young, J. B. and Landsberg, L. (1980): J. Clin. Invest. 65:1086-1094.

Neuroendocrinology and Psychiatric Disorder,
edited by G. M. Brown, et al.
Raven Press, New York 1984.

Hypothalamic Inhibitory Influences on Gonadotropin Secretion in Normal Cycling and Hypogonadotropic Amenorrheic Women

M.E. Quigley

Anorexia nervosa is an intriguing psychoneuroendocrine disorder occurring predominantly in young females. The salient features of this disorder are voluntary weight loss, a distorted behaviour towards food and body image, and amenorrhea in the absence of other medical or psychiatric disease (29). In their unrelenting pursuit of thinness, these young women regress biologically to a pubertal or even prepubertal state. This regression has been postulated to be an attempt to avoid the increasing psychological and social responsibilities of adolescence (17). The initiation and persistence of the amenorrhea in patients with anorexia nervosa often involves various interrelated psychogenic and physical stresses (Figure 1). Environmental, psychological, social and psychosexual factors are common psychogenic stresses that frequently interrupt normal menstrual cyclicity (51, 53). In addition, physical stress or caloric drain, such as decreased caloric input (33, 92) or increased expenditure of calories e.g. exercise (24, 28, 96) have also been associated with menstrual irregularities. Although the effect of these factors on the menstrual cycle varies markedly with each individual, it is clinically apparent that their impact is greatest during the psychoneuroendocrine transition from childhood to adulthood. The onset of amenorrhea in anorexia nervosa may precede, occur concomitant with, or follow significant weight loss (32, 94). Weight gain may be associated with resumption of normal menstrual cyclicity in many patients with anorexia nervosa. However, Boyar and Katz have documented the persistence of "immature" LH secretory patterns despite adequate weight gain in patients with prolonged, unchanged states of anorexia nervosa (15), indicating that factors other than weight gain (i.e. psychogenic stress and/or exercise) are also important in the eventual resumption of normal menstrual cyclicity. This probably explains why almost 50 percent of patients fail to resume spontaneous menses despite apparent adequate weight gain (9, 84).

The amenorrhea with anorexia nervosa is associated with decreased basal gonadotropin levels, attenuated or normal but delayed gonadotropin responses to exogenous GnRH (2, 11, 31, 37, 62, 87, 91, 95), and decreased frequency and magnitude of LH pulsatile activity (2, 14, 60, 85). These gonadotropin dysfunctions are restored and indeed ovulation occurs following the administration of exogenous GnRH (60, 69, 100), strongly suggesting that decreased endogenous hypothalamic GnRH release plays an important role in the pathophysiology of the amenorrhea in this complex disorder. Additional evidence for hypothalamic dysfunction includes abnormalities in temperature and water regulation (62, 91), hypercholesterolemia (23, 52, 68), sleep disturbances and delayed serum TSH responses to TRH (65, 91).

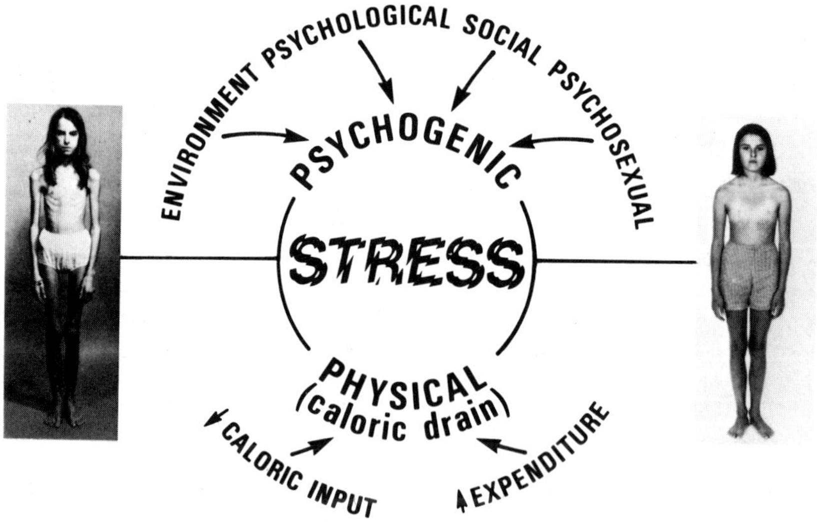

FIG. 1. Various psychogenic and physical stresses contributing to the amenorrhea in patients with anorexia nervosa.

The co-existence of obvious psychic and hypothalamic dysfunctions suggests the possibility of an underlying neurotransmitter abnormality.

Evidence for a Neurotransmitter Dysfunction in Anorexia Nervosa

Various investigators have implicated an increase in dopamine (7) or norepinephrine (79) or a decrease in dopamine (45) and/or norepinephrine (61) in the pathophysiology of anorexia nervosa based on a review of symptoms or on uncontrolled studies assessing response to pharmacologic therapies. Two double-blind studies to determine the efficiency of cyproheptadine, a serotonin antagonist, in treating patients with anorexia nervosa, have shown cyproheptadine to be effective only in treating the more seriously affected patients with the greatest weight loss, in excess of 30-40 percent ideal body weight (39, 93). Whether this suggests that an excess of serotonin plays a role in the pathophysiology of anorexia nervosa in general or only in the more severe stages of the disease remains to be determined. Although controversy exists as to whether serotonin stimulates (98) or inhibits GnRH-LH release in rodents (20, 36), human data is lacking. In addition, low circulating or urinary monoamines (norepinephrine, epinephrine and serotonin), or their precursor/metabolites (22, 25, 40, 43) have been reported in patients with anorexia nervosa; however, whether these changes accurately reflect central neuronal activity, casts doubt on their interpretation.

Based on a review of the pathophysiology of major symptoms, Barry and Klawans proposed that increased central dopamine (and norepinephrine) may occur in anorexia nervosa (7). They noted that the psychologic disturbances of anorexia nervosa are similar to those seen in amphetamine abusers (27). Amphetamines are indirect catecholamine agonists and act by blocking the re-uptake of catecholamines into neurons, thus, increasing the amount of available catecholamines (dopamine and/or norepinephrine) in the synaptic clefts to act at the postsynaptic receptor (4). They noted that increased central dopamine could account for the anorexia, weight loss and hypothermia; however, human data to suggest the role of an excess of hypothalamic dopamine to account for the hypogonadotropinism in patients with anorexia nervosa was lacking. During the last few years we have studied the role of 2 hypothalamic neurotransmitters, dopamine and endogenous opioids, in the regulation of GnRH-LH release in both normal cycling women and various amenorrheic states.

The Effect of Dopamine on Gonadotropin Secretion

Both GnRH (6) and dopamine (12) neurons have cell bodies in the arcuate nucleus which project into the lateral palisade zone of the median eminence where GnRH is believed to be released in pulses from the hypothalamus (3, 18, 67) into portal vessels. GnRH then travels via the portal circulation to the pituitary where it stimulates LH and FSH release. Since administration of antiserum to GnRH in ovariectomized rhesus monkeys abolishes the pulsatile gonadotropin release (58), the frequency and/or magnitude of the LH pulses probably reflects endogenous GnRH pulsatile activity.

In contrast to dopamine which functions as a neuro-hormone in inhibiting PRL release from the lactotropes (10, 19, 38), the dopaminergic regulation of GnRH-LH release appears to occur at the level of the hypothalamus (34, 35, 42, 57, 64, 82, 86) via an axoaxonal interaction (1, 59). Although conflicting data based on studies in rodents exists as to whether dopamine inhibits (8, 34, 35, 42, 57, 64) or stimulates (82, 86) GnRH release, we and other (50, 55) have accumulated data to suggest that dopamine inhibits GnRH release in humans.

Following preliminary dose-response studies, dopamine (4 μg/kg/min i.v.) has been shown to inhibit circulating LH levels in humans (50, 54, 55). In an attempt to determine whether the dopamine inhibition of circulating LH levels varied with different basal gonadotropin or steroid levels, dopamine (4 μg/kg/min x 4 h) was then infused into normal women at various stages of the menstrual cycle (48) as well as hypergonadotropic subjects with either polycystic ovarian syndrome (PCO)(77) or hypogonadism (49). Dopamine infusion resulted in a significant decrease in circulating LH in hypergonadotropic and normal cycling women (Fig. 2). In hypergonadotropic, hyperestrogenic women at mid-cycle (D_{14}) or with PCO, the dopamine infusion resulted in a sustained decrease in LH and attenuation of the LH pulsatile activity; however, in the hypogonadal/agonadal subjects, although there was an initial significant decline in circulating LH levels, a diminished LH pulsatile activity persisted and this accounts for the apparent increase in LH levels in these women (Ag) prior to discontinuing the dopamine infusion (Fig. 2). In midcycle subjects and PCO patients the relationship between the maximum net decrease in LH during the 4 h dopamine infusion and basal LH levels, revealed the same linear curve ($r = 0.995$); whereas, that for the hypogonadal/agonadal subjects followed a distinctly different curve ($r = 0.75$) with a statistically significant ($p < 0.01$) lower slope. Although the maximum net decrease in LH during the 4 hour dopamine infusion was greater in all 3 forms of hypergonadotropinism compared to early follicular control women, when their data was expressed as the maximum percent decrease from basal concentrations, the hyper-estrogenic, hypergonadotropic groups (the midcycle and the PCO patients) had similar (60 + 3% and 59 + 4%) but significantly greater decrements in LH than the hypoestrogenic hypogonadal women whose maximum

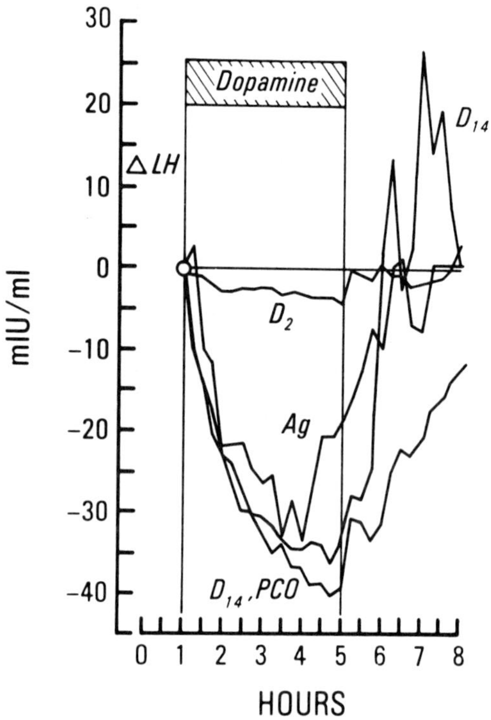

FIG. 2. Net change in serum LH from basal concentrations (mean of 5 samples) during and for 3 h following the infusion of dopamine 4 μg/kg/min for 4 h in 6 normal women studied on day 2 of the cycle (D_2), 12 hypo or agonadal women (Ag), 8 patients with polycystic ovarian syndrom (PCO) and 6 women studied on the day of the midcycle LH surge (D_{14}). (Data modified from Judd et al. 1976 and Quigley et al. 1981).

percent decrement during the 4 h dopamine infusion was comparable to that seen in early follicular (D_2) subjects (35 + 3% vs 42 + 5%). These data suggest that the estrogenic feedback on the GnRH-LH system may, in part, involve a dopaminergic mechanism.

In an attempt to determine whether endogenous dopamine inhibition of GnRH-LH release plays a physiological role during the normal menstrual cycle, we have administered a dopamine receptor antagonist, metoclopramide (26, 47, 71) 10 mg i.v. bolus, to 6 normal women during the early and late follicular, as well as the mid-luteal phase of the menstrual cycle (78). The dopamine antagonist induced a small but significant increase in circulating LH levels in subjects during the late follicular phase (Fig. 3). The acute LH increments, expressed as either the maximum percent increment or the area under the curve for percent change in LH during the first hour following metoclopramide (MCP) administration, were significantly ($p < 0.01$) greater in mid-luteal compared to late follicular subjects. These data provide evidence for an increased dopaminergic inhibition of the GnRH-LH system during the high estrogen and estrogen-progesterone phases of the menstrual cycle.

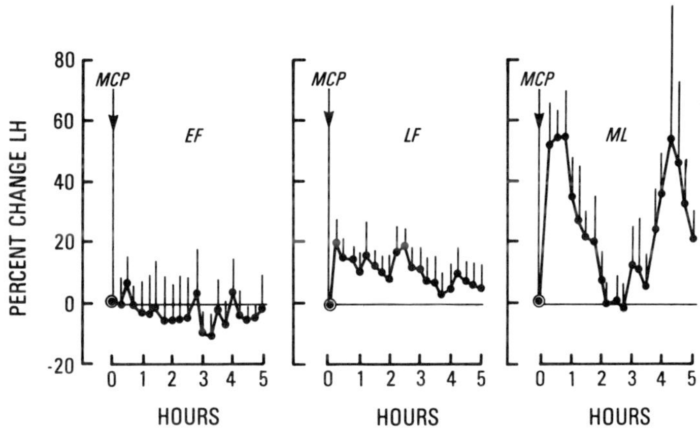

FIG. 3. The mean (± SE) percent change in serum LH from basal concentrations (mean of 5 samples), in response to a dopamine receptor antagonist, metoclopramide (MCP) administered as a 10 mg i.v. bolus to normal women during the early follicular (EF, n = 6), late follicular (LF, n = 6) and mid-luteal (ML, n = 6) phases of the menstrual cycle.

The Effect of Endogenous Opioids on Gonadotropin Secretion

Recent evidence indicates that opioid substances inhibit GnRH-LH release in rodents (5, 13, 16, 21, 46, 70) and humans (66, 80, 88, 89). The arcuate nucleus-median eminence region of the hypothalamus contains the greatest β-endorphin concentration in the human brain (97). Since GnRH and dopamine are also aggregated in this region (1, 6, 56, 59), we postulated the potential interaction of their neuronal networks in the inhibition of GnRH-gonadotropin secretion. Following determination of an LH dose response curve in humans, for a specific opioid receptor antagonist, naloxone, we elected to determine whether endogenous opiates exerted a tonic inhibitory effect on gonadotropin secretion in normal cycling women by examining the LH changes in responses to naloxone infused at a constant rate of 1.6 mg/hr for 4 hrs at various stages of the cycle (76). Naloxone failed to exhibit any discernible acute effect on LH release in early follicular subjects; however, LH levels increased significantly in women studied during both late follicular and mid-luteal phases (Fig. 4). During the late follicular phase, subjects exhibited a slow, steady increase in LH, while prompt, episodic and quantitatively greater LH increments were exhibited in mid-luteal phase subjects. In addition, there was a significant linear correlation between basal estradiol levels and the net LH increment during naloxone infusion in subjects in the late follicular phase. These data suggest that endogenous opiates may be involved in the GnRH-LH release in normal cycling women or that endogenous opiates may modify the endogenous dopamine inhibition of GnRH-LH release.

Since the short term (4 hour) naloxone infusion appeared to be associated with an increased LH pulsatile release during the mid-luteal phase (Fig. 4), we then investigated whether endogenous opiates may participate in the neuroendocrine mechanisms accounting for the reduced frequency of LH pulses during this high estrogen-progesterone phase of the menstrual cycle (63, 85, 99). When six normal cycling women underwent sequential 6 hour infusions of equal volumes of normal

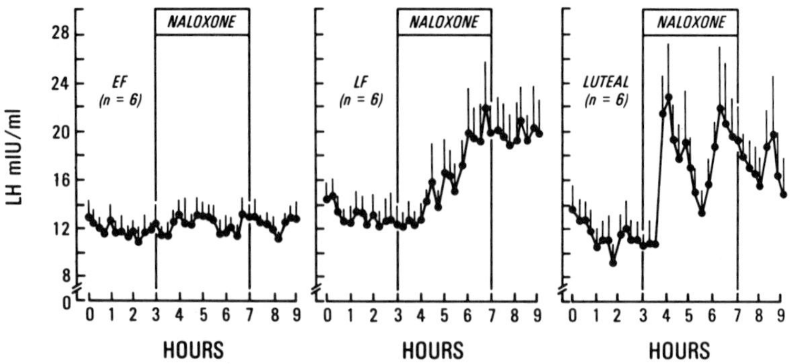

FIG. 4. The mean (+SE) serum LH levels 3 hours before, during and for 2 hours following the infusion of a specific opioid receptor antagonist, naloxone, at a rate of 1.6 mg/hr for 4 h in 6 women during the early (EF) and late (LF) follicular and mid-luteal (LUTEAL) phases of the menstrual cycle. (Reproduced from Quigley et al. 1980, J. Clin. Endocrinol. Metab. with permission).

saline and naloxone (1.6 mg/hr), a significant ($p < 0.01$) increase in both the frequency of LH pulses and amplitude of the first LH pulse was observed during the naloxone infusion compared to saline control studies (81). The naloxone-induced LH increases were associated with a concomitant increase in circulating FSH levels. These data strongly suggest that endogenous opiates inhibit hypothalamic GnRH release in humans and that an increased opioid inhibition of GnRH during the mid-luteal phase may participate in events leading to the low frequency of episodic LH secretion which are characteristic of this phase of the menstrual cycle.

Similar trends in the magnitude of LH increments at various phases of the menstrual cycle following the administration of both dopamine and opioid receptor antagonists (Figures 3 and 4), together with rodent data suggesting a functional link between endogenous opioid and dopaminergic activity (30, 41, 72, 90) which may then modify GnRH release (83), lead us to examine the effect of concomitant infusion of dopamine and naloxone during the mid-luteal phase of the cycle when the LH response to naloxone alone was found to be greatest (Figure 4). Dopamine infused together with naloxone 1.6 mg/hr, completely abolished the naloxone-induced increments in gonadotropins suggesting that endogenous opioids may modulate the GnRH-LH system in humans by interfering with dopaminergic inhibition; however, this does not eliminate the possibility that endogenous opiates may act directly on GnRH neurons.

The Role of Dopamine and Opioids in Hypogonadotropinism

When dopamine was infused (4μg/kg/min for 4 h) into 9 hypogonadotropic patients with later surgical documentation of prolactinoma, their LH inhibition to exogenous dopamine was less than that seen in early follicular women (D_2, Figure 5), suggesting that the hypogonadotropinism may, in part, be secondary to increased endogenous dopamine inhibition of GnRH-LH release. This hypothesis is strengthened by the fact that 5 moderately hyperprolactinemic patients (basal PRL $<$ 125 ng/ml) with their moderately depressed basal LH levels had a significant but

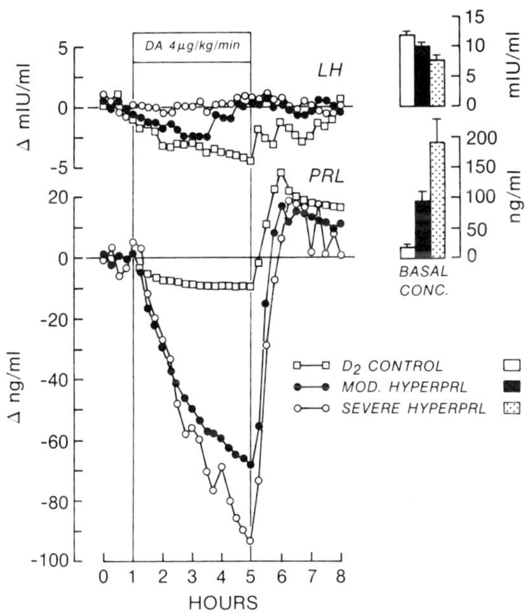

FIG. 5. Mean (+SE) basal serum LH and PRL concentrations and the mean (+SE) net change before, during and following a 4 h infusion of dopamine (DA) 4 µg/kg/min in 5 moderately (PRL < 125 ng/ml, ●—●) and 4 severely (PRL > 125 ng/ml, ○—○) hyperprolactinemic patients with subsequent documentation of prolactinoma. The moderately hyperprolactinemic patients with their moderately depressed basal LH levels had a significant decrease in serum LH during the DA infusion, but less than that seen in day 2 control subjects, while severely hyperprolactinemic patients with their significantly lower basal LH levels had no further LH inhibition with exogenous DA administration.

reduced LH decrement during dopamine infusion compared to D_2 control subjects (Figure 5) while the 4 severely hyperprolactinemic patients with basal PRL levels > 125 ng/ml, had significantly lower basal LH levels and no further LH inhibition to the exogenous dopamine administration (Figure 5). More recently, we have further strengthened this hypothesis by demonstrating that although these same 9 prolactinoma patients failed to respond to 2.5 mg of metoclopramide (unpublished data), 6 subsequent prolactinoma patients had a significant acute increment in LH levels following the administration of metoclopramide 10 mg i.v. bolus (Figure 6), while normal cycling women studied during the early follicular phase failed to exhibit any significant LH change (73). This suggests that much larger doses (at least 10-fold) of the dopamine antagonist, metoclopramide, are required to elicit an LH response compared to PRL when the drug is given intravenously to humans. The difference in the in vivo dose response curves for LH and PRL following metoclopramide administration may partly be explained by the fact that dopamine is believed to function as a neurotransmitter in its modulation of hypothalamic GnRH-LH release; whereas, dopamine acts as a hormone in inhibiting PRL release from the lactotropes.

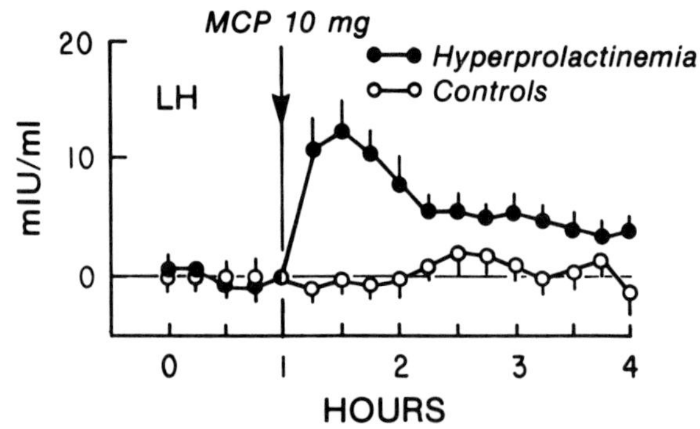

FIG. 6. Mean (± SE) net change in serum LH following administration of a dopamine receptor antagonist, metoclopramide (MCP) 10 mg i.v. bolus to 6 patients with hyperprolactinemia with later surgical documentation of prolactinoma and 6 normal control women studied during the early follicular phase of the menstrual cycle.

More recently, we have administered the opioid receptor antagonist, naloxone 1.6 ng/hr for 4 hours to 10 patients with prolactinoma (74) and we observed 2 distinct group responses (Figure 7). The 4 most severely hyperprolactinemic patients with prolactinoma had significantly lower basal LH levels, in the prepubertal range, attenuated LH pulsatile release suggesting a severe GnRH deficiency and they failed to exhibit any significant LH response to naloxone. Meanwhile the moderately hyperprolactinemic tumor patients with hypogonadotropinism exhibited an obvious increase in both the frequency and amplitude of LH pulses (Figure 7) strongly suggesting that an endogenous GnRH deficiency plays an important role in their hypogonadotropinism. In contrast, early follicular subjects failed to demonstrate any changes in circulating gonadotropins during the naloxone infusion. The decreased LH response to exogenous dopamine and the increased LH response to both MCP and naloxone suggest an increased dopamine and/or opioid inhibition of GnRH-LH in prolactinoma patients.

Similarly, we have studied the possible role of an excess dopaminergic or opioid inhibition in patients with hypogonadotropic hypothalamic amenorrhea (75), a condition which has many of the same factors, contributing to the amenorrhea (psychogenic stress, weight loss, exercise), as patients with anorexia nervosa (Figure 1). When patients with hypogonadotropic hypothalamic amenorrhea were infused with dopamine, there was a decreased LH inhibition compared to early follicular control subjects (unpublished data), suggesting that an excess dopamine inhibition of GnRH-LH release may play a role in the pathophysiology of the hypogonadotropinism in this common but heterogeneous disorder. In addition, when the dopamine receptor antagonist (metoclopramide) and the opioid receptor antagonist (naloxone) were both given to the same hypogonadotropic patients with hypothalamic amenorrhea in separate studies 1 week apart, again patients with prepubertal gonadotropin levels failed to have an LH response to either receptor antagonist while the remaining patients exhibited significant increases in LH to both metoclopramide (MCP) and naloxone (Figure 8).

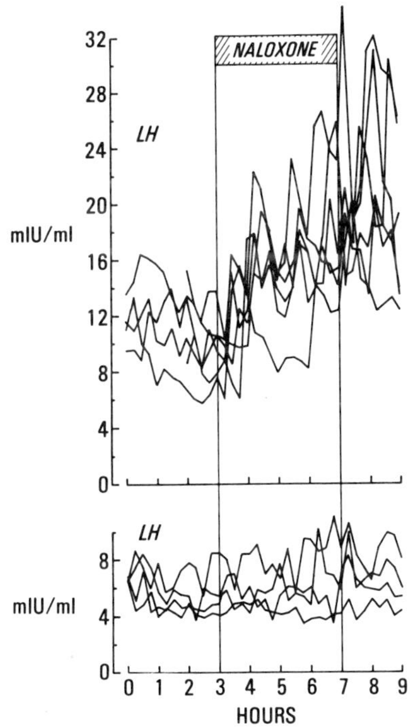

FIG. 7. The individual pattern of LH levels in 10 patients with prolactinoma before, during and 2 h following the administration of a specific opioid receptor antagonist, naloxone, infused at a rate of 1.6 mg/hr for 4 h. The six LH responders exhibit an increase in the pulsatile pattern of LH release (upper panel), while there is no change in the small LH auscillations in the LH non-responders who had significantly lower, prepubertal LH levels (lower panel). (Reproduced from Quigley et al. 1980, J. Clin. Endocrinol. Metab. with permission).

Again, naloxone resulted in both an increase in both the magnitude and the frequency of LH pulses. Whether the lack of an LH response to either receptor antagonist is due to decreased endogenous GnRH priming of gonadotrophs (44) or whether the LH responders and non-responders represent 2 separate psychoneuroendocrine disorders remains to be determined.

If indeed anorexia nervosa represents a more severe form of hypogonadotropic hypothalamic amenorrhea, we would predict that a transitory LH response may occur following metoclopramide and/or naloxone in patients with anorexia nervosa as they improve their ability to cope with their various stresses and gain weight (Figure 1). We would anticipate no LH response to naloxone or metoclopramide in the severe stages of this disorder when basal gonadotropin levels are in the prepubertal range and patients lack a gonadotropin response to GnRH.

The present data suggesting that dopamine and endogenous opioids are potent inhibitors of GnRH-LH release in humans and that they may interact through a common pathway, together with the clinical evidence for excess dopaminergic activity in patients with anorexia nervosa (7)

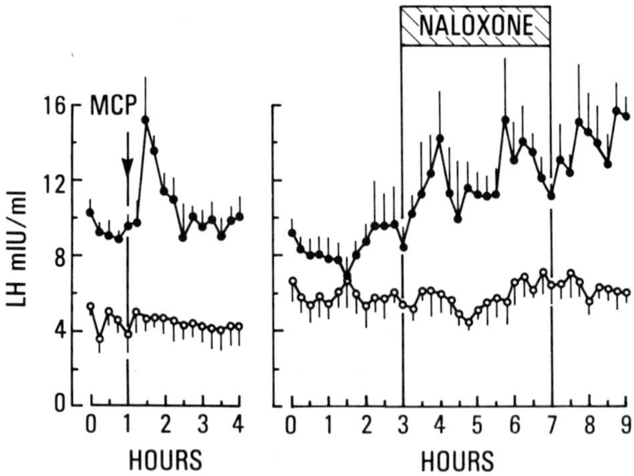

FIG. 8. Mean (+SE) serum LH levels and their responses to a dopamine receptor antagonist, metoclopramide (MCP) 10 mg i.v. bolus, and an opioid receptor antagonist, naloxone 1.6 mg/hr infused for 4 h, in 2 separate studies one week apart. A clear increment in LH was observed to both receptor antagonists in 4 patients (●-●), with an increase in both the number and frequency of LH pulses during naloxone, while the other 4 patients, with prepubertal gonadotropin levels, showed no response (○-○) to either receptor antagonist. (Modified from Quigley et al. 1980, J. Clin. Endocrinol. Metab. with permission).

strengthens the hypothesis that an excess dopaminergic inhibition of GnRH release may play a role in the hypogonadotropinism and resulting amenorrhea in patients with anorexia nervosa. Disturbances in other neurotransmitters may exist but they have not as yet been characterized.

ACKNOWLEDGEMENTS

I am indebted to Dr. Samuel S. C. Yen for his continued guidance and support and to Drs. S. Judd, J. F. Ropert, K. Sheehan and J. Rakoff who contributed to the data presented in this chapter. In addition, I wish to thank P. Malcom, the nurses in the GCRC, J. Aurand, A. Latham, K. Holcomb, M. Reck and B. Hopper for their technical help and D. Crowe for her secretarial assistance. This research was funded by Rockefeller Foundation Grant RF-75029, National Institute of Health Grant HD-12303 and the Mellon Foundation. STudies were conducted in the General Clinical Research Center in the University Hospital UCSD supported by RR-00827. I thank A. H. Robins and Endo Laboratories for providing metoclopramide and naloxone respectively. Radioimmunoassay materials were supplied by NIAMDD-NIH.

REFERENCES

1. Ajika, K. (1980): In: Frontiers in Neuroendocrinology Vol. 6, edited by L. Martini and W. F. Ganong, pp.1-32. Raven Press, New York.

2. Aono, T., Kinugasa, T., Yamamoto, T., Miyake, A. and Kurachi, K. (1975): Acta Endocrinologica 80:630-641.
3. Baker, H. W., Santen, R. J. and Burger, H. G. (1975): J. Steroid Biochem. 6(5):793-801.
4. Baldessarini, R. J. (1972): Pediatrics 49:694-700.
5. Barraclough, C. A. and Sawyer, C. H. (1955): Endocrinology 57: 329-337.
6. Barry, J. (1976): Neuroscience Letters 3:287-291.
7. Barry, V. C. and Klawans, H. L. (1976): J. Neural Transm. 38: 107-122.
8. Beck, W., Hancke, J. L. and Wuttke, W. (1978): Endocrinology 102: 837-843.
9. Bell, E. T., Harkness, R. A., Loraine, J. A. and Russell, G.F.M. (1966): Acta Endocrinologica 51:140-148.
10. Ben-Jonathan, N., Oliver, C., Winer, H. J., Mical, R. S. and Porter, J. C. (1977): Endocrinology 100:452-458.
11. Beumont, P.J.V., George, G.C.W., Primstone, B. L. and Vinik, A. I. (1976): J. Clin. Endocrinol. Metab. 43:487-496.
12. Bjorklund, A., Moore, R.Y., Nobin, A. and Stenevi, U. (1973): Brain Res. 51:171-191.
13. Blank, M. S., Panerai, A. E. and Friesen, H. G. (1979): Science 203:1129-1131.
14. Boyar, R. M., Katz, J., Finkelstein, J. W., Kapen, S., Weiner, H., Weitzman, E. G. and Hellman, L. (1974): N. Engl. J. Med. 291: 861-865.
15. Boyar, R. M., and Katz, J. (1977): In: Anorexia Nervosa, edited by R. A. Vigersky, pp.177-187. Raven Press, New York.
16. Bruni, J. F., Van Vugt, D. A., Marshall, S. and Meites, J. (1977): Life Sci. 21:461-466.
17. Brush, H. (1977): In: Anorexia Nervosa, edited by R. A. Vigersky, pp. 1-10. Raven Press, New York.
18. Carmel, P. D., Araki, S. and Ferin, M. (1976): Endocrinology 99: 243-248.
19. Caron, M. G., Beaulieu, M., Raymond, V., Gagné, B., Drouin, J., Lefkowitz, R. J. and Labrie, F. (1978): J. Biol. Chem. 253: 2244-2253.
20. Charli, J. L., Rotsztejn, W. H., Pattou, E., Kordon, C. (1978): Neurosci. Lett. 10:159-163.
21. Cicero, T. J., Badger, T. M., Wilcox, C. E., Bell, R. D. and Meyer, E. R. (1977): J. Pharmacol. Exp. Ther. 203:548-555.
22. Coppen, A. J., Gupta, R. K., Eccleston, E. G., Wood, K. M., Wakeling, A., and Desousa, V.F.A. (1976): Lancet 1:961.
23. Crisp, A. H., Blendis, I. M. and Parvan, G.L.S. (1968): Metab. Clin. Exptl. 17:1109-1118.
24. Dale, E., Gerlach, D. H., Wilhite, A. L. (1979): Obstetrics Gynecology 54:47-53.
25. Darby, P. L., VanLoon, G., Garfinkel, P. E., Brown, G. M. and Kirwan, P. (1980): Presented at the American Psychosomatic Society, New York.
26. Dolphin, A., Jenner, P., Marsden, C. D., Pycock, C. and Tarsy, D. (1975): Psychopharmacologia 41:133-138.
27. Ellinwood, E.H.J., Sudilovsky, A. and Nelson, L. M. (1973): Am. J. Psychiatry 130:1088-1093.
28. Erdelyi, G. J. (1976): Phys. Sportsmed. 4:79-81.
29. Feighner, J. P., Robins, E., Guze, S. B., Woodruff, R. A.,Jr., Winokur, G. and Munoz, R. (1972): Archives of Gen. Psych. 26: 57-63.

30. Ferland, L., Fuxe, K., Eneroth, P., Gustafsson, J. A. and Skett, P. (1977): European J. Pharmacol. 43:89-90.
31. Frankel, R. J. and Jenkins, J. S. (1975): Acta Endocrinologica 78:209-221.
32. Fries, H. (1977): In: Anorexia Nervosa, edited by R. A. Vigersky, pp.163-176. Raven Press, New York.
33. Frisch, R. E. (1977): In: Anorexia Nervosa, edited by R. A. Vigersky, pp.149-161. Raven Press, New York.
34. Fuxe, K., Hökfelt, T. and Nilsson, O. (1972): Acta Endocrinol. 69: 625-639.
35. Fuxe, K., Hökfelt, T., Agnati, L., Lofstrom, A., Everitt, B. J., Johansson, O., Jonsson, G., Wuttke, W. and Goldstein, M. (1976): In: Neuroendocrine Regulation of Fertility, edited by T. C. Anand, pp.124-140. Kumar, Karger, Basel.
36. Gallo, R. V. (1980): Neuroendocrinology 30:122-131.
37. Garfinkel, P. E., Brown, G. M., Moldofsky, H. and Stancer, H. C. (1975): Arch Gen. Psychiatry 32:739-744.
38. Gibbs, D. M. and Neill, J. D. (1978): Endocrinology 102:1895-1900.
39. Goldberg, S. C., Halmi, K. A., Eckert, E. D., Casper, R. C. and Davis, J. M. (1979): Brit. J. Psychiat. 134:67-70.
40. Gross, H. A., Lake, C. R., Ebert, M. H., Zeigler, M. G. and Kopin, I. J. (1979): J. Clin. Endocrinol. Metab. 49:805-809.
41. Gudelsky, G. A. and Porter, J. C. (1979): Life Sci. 25:1697-1702.
42. Hall, T. R., Advis, J. P., Bruni, J. F., Hodson, C. A. and Meites, J. (1977): Fed. Proc. 36:321.
43. Halmi, K. A., Dekirmenjian, H., Davis, J. M., Casper, R. and Goldberg, S. (1978): Arch. Gen. Psychiatry 35:458-460.
44. Hoff, J. D., Lasley, B. L. and Yen, S.S.C. (1979): J. Clin. Endocrinol. Metab. 49:8-11.
45. Johanson, A. J., Knorr, N. J. (1977): In: Anorexia Nervosa, edited by R. A. Vigersky, pp.363-372. Raven Press, New York.
46. Johnson, J. G. and Rosecrans, J. A. (1978): Res. Commun. Chem. Pathol. Pharmacol. 19:435-444.
47. Judd, S., Lazarus, L. and Smythe, G. (1976): J. Clin. Endocrinol. Metab. 43:313-317.
48. Judd, S. J., Rigg, L, A. and Yen, S.S.C. (1978): J. Clin. Endocrinol. Metab. 47:494-498.
49. Judd, S. J., Rigg, L. A. and Yen, S.S.C. (1979): J. Clin. Endocrinology Metab. 49:182-184.
50. Kaptein, E. M., Kletzky, D. A., Spencer, C. A., Nicoloff, J. T. (1980): J. Clin. Endocrinol. Metab. 51:488-491.
51. Klinefelter, H. F., Albright, F., Jr., and Griswold, G. C. (1943): J. Clin. Endocrinol. 3:529-544.
52. Klinefelter, H. F. (1965): J. Clin. Endocrinol. Metab. 25:1520-1521.
53. Lachelin, G.C.L. and Yen, S.S.C. (1978): Am. J. obstet. Gynecol. 130:825-831.
54. Leblanc, H., Lachelin, G.C.L., Abu-Fadil, S. and Yen, S.S.C. (1976): J. Clin. Endocrinol. Metab. 43:668-674.
55. Leebaw, W. F., Lee, L. A. and Woolf, P. D. (1978): J. Clin. Endocrinol. Metab. 47:480-487.
56. Löfström, A., Jonsson, G. and Fuxe, K. (1976): J. Histochem. Cytochem. 24:415-429.
57. Löfström, A., Eneroth, P., Gustafsson, J. A. and Skett, P. (1977): Endocrinology 101:1559-1569.
58. McCormack, J. T., Plant, T. M., Hess, D. L. and Knobil, E. (1977): Endocrinology 100:663-667.

59. McNeill, T. H. and Sladek, J. R., Jr. (1978): Science 200:72-74.
60. Marshall, J. C. and Kelch, R. P. (1979): J. Clin. Endocrinol. Metab. 49:712-718.
61. Mawson, A. R. (1974): Psychol. Med. 4:289-308.
62. Mecklenburg, R. S., Loriaux, D. L., Thompson, R. H., Andersen, A. E. and Lipsett, M. B. (1974): Medicine (Baltimore) 53:147-159.
63. Midgley, A. R., Jr. and Jaffe, R. B. (1971): J. Clin. Endocrinol. Metab. 33:962-969.
64. Miyachi, Y., Mecklenburg, R. S. and Lipsett, M. B. (1973): Endocrinology 93:492-496.
65. Miyai, K., Yamamoto, T., Azukizawa, M., Ishibashi, K. and Kumahara, Y. (1975): J. Clin. Endocrinol. Metab. 40:334-338.
66. Morley, J. E., Baranetsky, N. G., Wingert, T. D., Carlson, H. E., Hershman, J. M., Melmed, S., Levin, S. R., Jamison, K. R., Weitzman, R., Chang, R. J. and Varner, A. A. (1980): J. Clin. Endocrinol. Metab. 50:251-257.
67. Neill, J. D., Patton, J. M. and Tindall, G. T. (1977): Endocrinology 101:430-434.
68. Nestel, P. J. (1974): J. Clin. Endocrinol. Metab. 38:324-328.
69. Nillius, S. J. and Wide, L. (1979): Ups. J. Med. Sci. 84:21-35.
70. Pang, C. N., Zimmerman, E. and Sawyer, C. H. (1977): Endocrinology 101:1726-1732.
71. Peringer, E., Jenner, P., Donaldson, I. M. and Marsden, C. D. (1976): Neuropharmacology 15:463-469.
72. Pollard, H., Llorens-Cortes, C. and Swartz, J. C. (1977): Nature 268:1745-1747.
73. Quigley, M. E., Judd, S. J., Gilliland, G. B. and Yen, S.S.C. (1979): J. Clin. Endocrinol. Metab. 48:718-720.
74. Quigley, M. E., Sheehan, K. L., Casper, R. F. and Yen, S.S.C. (1980): J. Clin. Endocrinol. Metab. 50:427-430.
75. Quigley, M. E., Sheehan, K. L., Casper, R. F. and Yen, S.S.C. (1980): J. Clin. Endocrinol. Metab. 50:949-954.
76. Quigley, M. E. and Yen, S.S.C. (1980): J. Clin. Endocrinol. Metab. 51:179-181.
77. Quigley, M. E., Rakoff, J. S. and Yen, S.S.C. (1981): J. Clin. Endocrinol. Metab. 52:231-234.
78. Quigley, M. E. and Yen, S.S.C.: Life Science (submitted).
79. Redmond, D. E., Jr., Swann, A. and Heninger, G. R. (1976): Lancet 2:307.
80. Reid, R. L., Hoff, J. D., Yen, S.S.C. and Li, C. H. (1981): J. Clin. Endocrinol. Metab. 52:1179-1184.
81. Ropert, J. F., Quigley, M. E. and Yen, S.S.C. (1981): J. Clin. Endocrinol. Metab. 52:583-585.
82. Rotsztejn, W. H., Charli, J. L., Pattou, E. and Kordon, C. (1977): Endocrinology 101:1475-1483.
83. Rotsztejn, W. H., Drouva, S. V., Pattou, E. and Kordon, C. (1978): European J. Pharmacol. 50:285-286.
84. Russell, G.F.M. (1977): In: Anorexia Nervosa, edited by R. A. Vigersky, pp.277-289. Raven Press, New York.
85. Santen, R. J. and Bardin, C. W. (1973): J. Clin. Invest. 52: 2617-2628.
86. Schneider, H.P.G. and McCann, S. M. (1969): Endocrinology 85: 121-132.
87. Sherman, B. M., Halmi, K. A. and Zamudio, R. (1975): J. Clin. Endocrinol. Metab. 41:135-142.
88. Stubbs, W. A., Delitala, G., Jones, A., Jeffcoate, W. J., Edwards,

C.R.W., Ratter, S. J., Besser, G. M., Bloom, S. R. and Alberti, K.G.M.M. (1978): Lancet 2:1225-1227.

89. Tolis, G., Hickey, J. and Guyda, H. (1975): J. Clin. Endocrinol. Metab. 41:797-800.
90. Van Vugt, D. A., Bruni, J. F., Sylvester, P. W., Chin, H. T., Ieiri, T. and Meites, J. (1979): Life Sci. 24:2361-2368.
91. Vigersky, R. A., Loriaux, D. L., Andersen, A. E. and Lipsett, M. B. (1976): Clinics in Endocrinol. and Metab. 5:517-535.
92. Vigersky, R. A., Andersen, A. E., Thompson, R. H., Loriaux, D. L. (1977): N. Engl. J. Med. 297:1141-1145.
93. Vigersky, R. A., Loriaux, D. L. (1977): In: Anorexia Nervosa, edited by R. A. Vigersky, pp.349-356. Raven press, New York.
94. Warren, M. P. and Vande Wiele, R. L. (1973): Am. J. Obstet. Gynecol. 117:435-449.
95. Warren, M. (1977): In: Anorexia Nervosa, edited by R. A. Vigersky, pp.189-198. Raven Press, New York.
96. Warren, M. P. (1980): J. Clin. Endocrinol. Metab. 51:1150-1157.
97. Wilkes, M. M., Watkins, W. B., Stewart, R. D. and Yen, S.S.C. (1980): Neuroendocrinology 30:113-121.
98. Wuttke, W., Hancke, J. L., Höhn, K. G., Baumgarten, H. G. (1978): Ann. N.Y. Acad. Sci. 305:423-436.
99. Yen, S.S.C., Tsai, C.C., Naftolin, F., Vandenberg, G. and Ajabor, L. (1972): J. Clin. Endocrinol. Metab. 34:671-675.
100. Yoshimoto, Y., Moridera, K. and Imura, H. (1975): N. Engl. J. Med. 292:242-245.

Neuroendocrinology and Psychiatric Disorder,
edited by G. M. Brown, et al.
Raven Press, New York 1984.

Experimental Psychological Aspects of Anorexia Nervosa

Joel A. Grinker

The following discussion will explore several experimental-phychological areas of research. The psychological aspects of anorexia, although not of major interest in recent research, appear to be the prominent among the diagnostic criteria for primary anorexia nervosa: substantial weight loss, a refusal to maintain normal weight, disturbance in body image, an almost pathological fear of being obese, and amenorrhea in women (17). The majority of the criteria are either behavioural or psychological, and yet current research is focused on neuroendocrine abnormalities which are, in the main, returned to normal when the patient has regained an appropriate amount of weight and maintained it (36).

The lack of adequate control or contrast groups remains a problem in this kind of clinical research. Data collected only on anorectic individuals in treatment are difficult to interpret. The issue of an appropriate control group, however, is far from clear. Previously well-nourished subjects who are victims of malnutrition or individuals eating equivalent types of diets are difficult to obtain. Studies have attempted to correct these deficiencies by utilizing other strategies, e.g. assessing the patient samples with pre and post-measures and making within-group comparisons (34, 38, 42, 57).

It has been suggested in several studies that appropriate comparison groups include those high in risk factors such as dieting or decreased body fat and that anorexia might even be induced by inappropriate dieting or loss of weight and obsessiveness with food (24, 25, 35). In some cases, trained athletes or exercisers such as dancers or runners with reduced body fat have served as appropriate contrast groups (25, 28). Animal models provide an additional means to assess the regulation of body fat (52). In the majority of cases of naturally occuring animal anorexias, the animals spontaneously stop eating in order to attend to other behaviours that involve continuity of the species: raising the young, breeding, etc. (52, 56). Thus, during incubation and hatching or feeding the young, different species often refrain from feeding for long periods of time. Prior to hibernation or migration, many species increase body fat to carry them through periods without food (52, 56). During hibernation or migration, body fat is severely depleted. These animal anorexias occur despite the wide availability of food. This anorectic behaviour is adaptive, appropriate and self limiting. Thus, the mechanism which produces this behaviour is of interest but direct applicability is doubtful.

Diagnosis and Prevalence

Anorexia nervosa has become a common and serious disease of modern affluent societies (49). The disorder is more frequent among higher socioeconomic class females than among lower class females (11). A British study estimated the prevalence rate of 1.7 per thousand among females in independent schools under the age of 16, and 10.5 per thousand for females over the age of 16 (14). Coupled with these figures are data suggesting that eating disorders or weight phobias are increasingly common among female adolescents (43). Nevertheless, not all dieting adolescents develop anorexia.

Bruch identified primary anorexia nervosa as a struggle for identity or competence represented by the struggle for thinness (4). Bruch also emphasized the distortions in body image, faulty perception of internal body stimuli, and a sense of ineffectiveness which prompted the dieting. Other criteria have included the "relentless" pursuit of thinness, the aversion to regaining weight, the denial of the severity of weight loss (including a weight loss of 80% standard) and, in females, amenorrhea of at least three months' standing (2). The most recent diagnostic criteria emphasizes a descriptive approach and focuses on the behaviour associated with fasting or bulimia while minimizing the intrapsychic components (1). An initial diagnosis usually requires that the patient show marked fat or weight loss, obsessive concern with body weight and size, as well as very marked abnormalities in eating behaviour, including fasting and/or binging and vomiting (7, 17).

The socioeconomic, age and sex-linked characteriztics of this disease have argued in favour of psychological or psychiatric theories. Unfortunately, theories based on pscyhodynamic or interpersonal conflicts have not proven useful in understanding mechanisms or prevalence rates, while providing some basis for successful treatment. Consequently, new diagnostic criteria have been developed based on observable behaviours rather than intrapsychic conflict. Neuroendocrine profiles have been examined to provide a basis for diagnosis and to estimate treatment effectiveness as well as to elucidate possible mechanisms.

It has been suggested that anorexia nervosa, like obesity, is not a single disease entity, since both have nutritional and psychological as well as endocrine manifestations. In both syndromes, food intake and behaviours related to feeding play significant roles. Another complexity in common is that the majority of symptoms, including endocrine disorders, appear to be conseuqences of food consumption or restriction, starvation, or changes in body fatness - in other words, consequent or correlated phenomena. Many neuroendocrine abnormalities are reversed following weight gain or maintenance of stable weight in anorexia, or are actually produced by alterations in metabolism following caloric restriction or by frank malnutrition (36, 45). Thus, a 24-hour "pubertal" pattern of luteinizing hormone secretion has been shown to be related to dietary inadequacy and weight loss, rather than anorexia nervoza per se (44). Other hormonal abnormalities, including blunting of LH and TSH release to appropriate stimuli have also been related to the metabolic consequences of caloric restriction (e.g. decreasing fatness or dietary inadequacy and weight loss) (36).

Behavioural Indices

Behavioural indices have usually been employed to predict successful treatment completion and have met with varying degrees of success (6, 58, 61, 63). Questionnaires, interviews and self-rating procedures as well as ratings by trained observers have been used. Several studies report that longer duration, older age of onset, and impaired family relations are related to a poor prognosis or to greater weight loss, and that less denial of illness, no previous obesity and normal sexual development are related to a more favourable prognosis (10, 42).

The appropriate control group, e.g. other hospitalized adolescents, age-matched normal adolescents or the recovered anorectic must be carefully considered. For example, in one study the only comparison group was working, normal weight women at least five years older than the hospitalized anorectic group (65). Recent scales have focused on behaviours directly related to weight loss, e.g., behaviours during hospitalization such as depression or hyperactivity as well as specific kinds of eating behaviours, rather than more generalized affective disturbances. In one study, changes in endocrine patterns over treatment were correlated with decreased depression ratings by nurses (40). Pre and post-measures require a careful definition of successful treatment termination. These have included restoration of normal menses, stable weight or the achievement of normal weight, regardless of treatment duration.

Recently, a range of eating behaviours have been characterized in anorectic individuals. Some individuals reduce body weight through fasting and food restriction while other engage in periodic gorging and binging (2, 8, 21). It has been reported that individuals with dietary rather than bulimic symptomatology are less disturbed and have a more favourable prognosis (21). These individuals are usually younger and have fewer other related symptomatology. A high prevalence of bulimic symptoms in a normal college population has been reported, suggesting an almost epidemic-like occurrence of weight phobias and food obsessions (37).

Body Image

A marked symptom of the anorectic individual, which has attracted sizable research attention, is the distortions in body image or body size. Body image refers to attitudes and feelings of the individual towards his or her own body as well as the individual's pictorial representation of "physical appearance" (18, 64). Thus, body image need not be synonymous with reality. In contrast, body size refers to objective estimations of physical appearance. Recently, investigators have reported disturbed body size perception in patients with abnormal body composition - the massively obese and the anorectic (27, 30, 32, 59). Clinicians have long suggested that not only is the anorectic patient unconcerned or unaware of her extreme thinness, she often denies that this problem exists. Thus, marked overestimations in body size have been reported (60) and related to the degree of weight loss (60, 9, 20). Yet, one study reported that body size overestimations existed in only 31% of anorectic patients compared to 6% of the normal group, but that variability across subjects in the anorectic group was significantly higher (22).

Several different techniques for measuring body size (calipers to estimate the width of various body parts, or the distorting anamorphic lens using current photographic slides) have been used in these studies of anorectic individuals (23, 29). The failure to find significant overestimations in all subjects may also be interpreted in terms of whether the task requires perceptual accuracy or an affective response: e.g. some subjects may be able to "size" themselves correctly, yet still report "feeling" fat (9). These subjects do not overestimate the sizes of control female subjects or of neutral objects. The results from one study strongly suggest that age-matched controls are essentially no different from the anorectic individuals (5). In another study, not only did approximately 50% of the adolescent anorectic females overestimate body size with the anamorphic lens technique, but age-matched controls did so as well (9). However, overestimation was positively correlated with both increased depression and with lesser feelings of control, and may therefore be of clinical usefulness.

Nonetheless, it is clear that a marked component of the behavioural response of some anorectic individuals is a disturbed body image; e.g., the greater the overestimation of body size, the greater the denial and the worse the prospects for recovery (9, 13, 20). A potentially useful correlation might be established between changes in body size estimation and changing neuroendocrine profiles.

New Applications

Other perceptual abnormalities, including cognitive or perceptual responses to food items, have not been explored in detail. Chronic eating disorders or abnormal food preferences resulting in malnutrition may be reflected in perceptual distortions regarding the sensory or nutritional values of different foods or in distorted hedonic preferences. The misperceptions by anorectic individuals regarding their perceived fatness or body size have been extensively studied, but little effort has been made to document systematically perceptual distortions with respect to foods. This issue is of particular interest since it appears that misconceptions about the caloric or nutritional values of foods can affect subsequent generations: there is preliminary evidence that the "anorectic-like" individual may well interfere with the nutrition of her children.

Powerful quantitative methods borrowed from marketing research now allow the study of the perception of food items and its relationship to food preferences. The major premise of the mathematical technique known as multidimensional scaling (MDS) (31) is that judgments of psychological similarity between pairs of objects reflect the location of these objects in the subject's perceptual space. Specifically, objects that are perceived as similar to one another are located proximally in the attribute space, whereas objects perceived as less similar are located further apart. In addition, the principal dimensions of the attribute space are taken to reflect those attributes of the scaled objects that the subject perceives as most salient. Scaling procedures have been used to establish perceptual maps for different types of food products as a function of the subjects' sex, degree of overweight, or the extent of dietary restraint (54, 15), without asking the subject any overt questions about the nature of the food products studied. This indirect approach should prove especially useful in studies of food intake in anorexia since self reports of food preferences or actual food intake are normally contaminated by sociocultural pressures and subject bias.

There is some evidence that greater perceptual distortions (including errors inthe estimation of body size) as well as the presence of bulimic systoms can identify those individuals that respond less well to treatment. Similarly, it may be useful to know whether the perceptions of specific food products (e.g. "high calorie" or 'fattening" ones) are modified as a consequence of weight regain. Appropriate modification of the perceptual space following weight regain may be the difference between long-term successful and unsuccessful treatment.

A first study employing these techniques is reported below and is preliminary; it should be regarded solely as a demonstration of this new methodology. The subjects were a group of normal-weight individuals (mean weight: 145 lbs), an outpatient group of obese subjects (mean weight: 400 lbs.), and a group of young women hospitalized for anorexia nervosa (mean weight: 91 lbs.). The study employed proximity judgments followed by multidimensional scaling analysis to provide an estimate of the degree of preceived similarity among different food items, e.g., soft drinks, presented verbally by brand name. Other techniques of cognitive and psychological methodology (Semantic Differential and the Hedonic Preference ratings) are normally employed in conjunction with scaling techniques to provide verbal "labels" for the principal perceived attributes of the food objects under study. It appeared that the subjects distinguished between the several soft drinks on the basis of their three chief attributes - naturalness, flavour intensity and sweetness; in other words, a three-dimensional solution was sufficient to describe the attribute space. The perceptions of both obese and anorectic individuals were the same as that of the normal weight individuals in terms of the principal dimensions of the attribute space. However, preference ratings differed among the groups. Anorectic individuals reported a lower preference for items perceived as sweet. Obese individuals, on the other hand, tended to prefer items which were high in flavour, whereas normal-weight individuals like natural tasting items. These techniques, of course, cannot answer the question as to whether these cognitive differences are merely the consequences of the disordered weights, or whether they play a direct role in producing them. The former anorectic or the reduced obese may be studied to provide information as to whether the sam differences remain after normal weight is achieved.

We have begun a pilot project to examine the effect of parental (usually maternal) attitudes on nutrition to the child's growth and development. A new subpopulation of children are now being referred to at least one pediatric-endocrinology clinic for evaluation for "failure to thrive". "Failure to thrive" includes children who do not grow in stature for a variety of reasons, including the primary endocrine abnormalities as well as psychogenic factors. The children that are relevant to this discussion do not fit either of these categories. These children are referred for failure to grow in stature, but for some very specific reasons - namely, the deliberate intervention on the part of the parents, usually the mother, to limit caloric intake or carbohydrate consumption in order to insure optimum growth or prevent the development of obesity. The mother is generally responsible for limiting food intake as a consequence of deviant attitudes, beliefs or perceptions about food or diet. There are no pathological disturbances in mother-child interactions or aberrant behaviours by the child.

These children are referred for failure to grow appropriately in height but appear well nourished: in no case do they appear to lack adequate subcutaneous deposits of fat. Intervention consists solely of hospitalization in the clinical research centre at the Department of Pediatrics, Endocrinology Unit, New York Hospital and appropriate refeeding and nutritional counseling to the family. In all case, these children proceed to grow appropriately following nutritional intervention. The mothers in these cases were previously either anorectic or underweight, and had been models, dancers, etc., for whom thinness was particularly important.

Risk Factors

The marked increase in bulimia (binging, gorging and associated vomiting) in college students, coupled with obsessive concerns for thinness and appearance now prevalent may produce a heightened risk for the development of anorexia (24, 26, 37). It has further been suggested that anorexia might be induced by inappropriate dieting or loss of weight and obsessiveness with food in other populations (28). Thus, models or dancers who are low in weight/fat may be at a higher risk, as might normal or underweight people who control their weight through dieting or bulimic episodes or who score high on a scale of 'restrained" eating (25, 41). It has been suggested that appropriate comparison groups include those high in these risk factors. One study has reported that modeling and ballet students display several behaviours similar to that of anorexia nervosa patients (morbid fear of fatness, amenorrhea), and score high on the scale of "eating disorders" (26). Others (16, 62) have commented on the existence of eating abnormalities in highly motivated school-age athletes and the need for guidance in weight management. These studies suggest that the pressure to perform well, to be slim, and to achieve highly may be sociocultural risk factors in the development of anorexia nervosa. These sociocultureal determiners should thus be added to the list of potential determining factors which include individual, familial and personality factors (12).

Regulation of Body Fat

Both obesity and anorexia nervosa are accompanied by dramatic changes in body composition (increased or decreased fat with possible reductions in lean body mass), altered endocrine status, aberrant dietary intake, the additional complexity of disturbed emotional states, and high rates of relapse. Increasingly, some investigators now consider massive obesity as a regulatory disorder and focus on individual susceptibility. Paradoxically, with weight reduction a number of parameters may not be improved, including metabolic rate and emotional status (30, 32). The behavioural responses of the reduced obese individual have been compared to those of volunteers undergoing experimental starvation (32, 53). Other data suggest that severe obesity is not an easily available state for the normal-weight individual. Normal-weight volunteers have shown a resistance ot weight increments during overfeeding by changing basal metabolic rate and increasing activity (57). Thus, the suggestion has been made that some individuals may be "protected" from obesity producing diets.

"Susceptibility" to anorexia has not been well defined, nor are data available on the ability of anorectic individuals to defend against weight changes in either direction. In contrast to individuals undergoing experimental starvation, anorectic individuals are reported to disregard hunger signals and show marked hyperactivity (7). Garfinkel et al. have reported that anorectic individuals have an impaired ability to respond to satiety stimuli (22). Thus, the ability to tolerate weight loss needs to be considered in terms of regulation.

Animal models offer an important perspective in any discussion of the regulation of body fat. Both obesity and anorexia have been produced by surgical lesions of different brain centres or pathways. A second animal model is that of the naturally occurring animal anorexias.

Animal Models

Many neural manipulations change body weight, adipocity and food intake in animals. Until recently, it was thought that the electrolytic lesions and knife cuts of the ventro-medial hypothalamus (VMH) produce hyperphagia and obesity and that similar lesions of the lateral hypothalamus (LH) produce aphagia, anorexia and weight loss in rats. It now appears that neither the LH or VMH is the central site of action. Investigators using studies based on lesions, knife cuts and intracranial injections of 6-hydroxydopamine now attribute the aphagia and adipsia associated with LH lesions to insult to the dopaminergic nigrostriatal bundle (NSB) rather than to LH neurons (33). Other aspects of motivated behaviour, including arousal and motor disfunction are also produced by these lesions. In contrast, intrahypothalamic injections of kainic acid, which damage LH neurons but do not affect the fibres of the passage procude aphagia without the associated behavioural abnormalities (33, 55). Dorsomedial hypothalamic (DMN) lesions in rats also produce hypophagia and reduced body weight, but without effects on body composition (55). Trigeminal deafferentiation (loss of taste) produces a rat with behaviours similar to that seen in the rats with lateral hypothalamic (LH) lesions (67). These feeding deficits are actually greater than those produced by severing of the gustatory or olfactory nerve. Thus, it is clear that many neural manipulations can reduce body weight, adiposity, or food intake in rats. Their importance as model systems for the study of a disease as deverse as anorexia nervosa is often unclear. Nevertheless, they raise some interesting questions for the study of anorexia nervosa in humans which are explored below.

Lateral Hypothalamic Lesions: Regulation of Body Fat

Lesions of the laterial hypothalamus produce hypophagia, sensory neglect and weight loss (66). In the classic case, the rat refuses to eat or drink for long periods of time and may, in extreme cases, starve to death. Depending on the size (smaller) and the placement (mid-lateral) of lesions, the rat begins to accept wet, palatable foods and, finally, maintain weight at a reduced level. Other associated abnormalities include impairment in water balance and an exaggerated rejection of dry or unpalatable foods.

At least one investigator has actually proposed that the LH rat shows a chronic reduction in body weight not because of continued problems in feeding abilities but because of a hypothesized alteration in "set point" or regulation of body fat (46). Experimental data suggest that a reduced level of body weight/fat is not only maintained by the LH rat but defended when challenged by force-feeding (47) or by underfeeding (50). In the first case, force-feeding produced an initial increment in body weight. Once the force-feeding was discontinued, the lowered body weight was quickly reachieved. In the second case, following lesioning, rats maintained their body weight at approximately 86% of control rats. Following additional restriction to 80% of control levels, animals were allowed to refeed ad libitum and, again, weight quickly returned to the previous level (86% of controls).

Changes in basal metabolism have been implicated in this so-called regulation (19). A recent study (48) showed that the food intake of the LH rat was close although slightly less than that of normal controls. They also reported normal oxygen consumption and increased efficiency of food utilization during post-starvation weight recovery. The LH rat did not lose weight faster than the non-lesioned rat, nor did it show an inability to regain weight following weight loss or fail to respond to changes in diet palatability.

The interpretation of these results is controversial and has been criticized as nothing more than a restatement of a phenomenon rather than evidence for a mechanism or an active regulator. Some investigators view the data as evidence for a mechanism or an active regulator. Some reservations about this model concern the existence of hunger awareness. Decreased hunger or appetite is inferred from the behaviour of the LH rats, whereas some investigators suggest hidden or denied hunger in anorectic individuals (7).

Animal Anorexias

The naturally occuring animal anorexias or adaptive changes in body weight occur in many species regularly and predictably. They are related to the animals' life history and ecological adaptation. The anorexias typically occur at at time when eating can only be engaged in at the sacrifice of other essential behaviours involved in reproduction and survival. Furthermore, most data suggest that these changes in weight are under strict endogenous control rather than being consequences of changes in food availability (52). The animals' complete abstinence from feeding is carried out in the face of a high degree of food availability. Such an adaptive weight loss is well illustrated by the incubation behaviour of the red jungle fowl (56). Sitting on the egg is done almost full time by the female, alone, and has two advantages: the correct thermal environment and protection from predators. During the 20-day course of incubation, food intake is reduced to 20% of baseline levels and body weight falls by 20%. In one experiment, jungle fowl were completely deprived of food during short periods while incubating: following return to _ad lib_ feeding, intake increased above control levels until weight had resumed a value near that of other birds at the same stage of incubation.

Other animals also manifest weight loss and reduced food intake in the face of plentiful food. Hibernators begin hibernation even with food available. The "regulation" of body weight has not been suspended but reoccurs under new rules. These data in animals are in accord with a model suggesting changes in a "set point" for body weight or body fat. Set point here is meant not as a neural reference, but as an equilibrium among many physiological processes.

These animal states are distinguished by several major differences between them and human anorexia nervosa. The psychological components of anorexia nervosa play marked and significant roles. The body image disturbances, disturbed family interactions, and preoccupations with food are impossible to duplicate completely in animal models. These analogies reinforce what would appear to be a major problem in the study of the complex state of anorexia nervosa - the difficulty in determining the primary disorder from the secondary manifestations.

Conclusions

Current research in anorexia nervosa emphasizes the physiological or neuroendocrine profile and explanation rather than the psychological - the fear of fatness, the body image disturbances, etc., all of which play a major part in diagnosis. This review has examined recent studies and outlined several new areas of investigation. Current cognitive techniques to assess attitudes and perceptions of food items have been reported. The existence of a special population of mothers who have been anorectic or thin and who are concerned about preventing obesity in their children has been documented. These mothers have deprived their children calorically and the children are now referred for failure to grow in height. Recovered anorectic patients, in whom extreme endocrine abnormalities or psychological or psychiatric syndromes have been eliminated, may be the most appropriate group in which to study this disease. Unfortunately, the marked behavioural deficiencies (distortions in body image, concern with control, family problems, associated bulimia and the preoccupation with food) are not reflected in animal anorexias. Nevertheless, studies of animal models and the hypothalamic mechanisms by which animals migrate or hibernate and breed may provide some clues as to the appropriate mechanisms in human anorexia.

ACKNOWLEDGMENTS

This study has been supported in part by grant NIH AMHD 27980.

I am indebted to Drs. Maria I. New and Lenore Levine of the Department of Pediatrics, New York Hospital, and to Dr. Adam Drewnowski of the Rockefeller University for allowing me to comment on experiments in progress.

REFERENCES

1. American Psychiatric Association Task Force on Nomenclature and Statistics (1980): Diagnostic and Statistical Manual of Mental Disorder, 3rd edition. American Psychiatric Association, Washington, D.C.
2. Beumont, P.J.V., George, G.C.W. and Smart, D. E. (1976): Psych. Med. 6:617-622.
3. Booth, D. A. (1978): In: The Psychiatric Clinics of North America, Vol. 1, edited by A. J. Stunkard, pp.545-579. W. B. Saunders Company, Philadelphia.
4. Bruch, H. (1973): Eating Disorders. Basic Books, New York.
5. Button, E. J., Fransella, F. and Slade, P. D. (1977): Psych. Med. 7:235-243.
6. Cantwell, D. P., Sturnzenberger, S., Burroughs, J., Salkin, B. and Green, J. K. (1977): Arch. Gen. Psychiatry 34:1087-1093.
7. Casper, R. C. and Davis, J. M. (1977): Am. J. Psychiatry 134: 974-978.
8. Casper, R. C., Eckert, E. D., Halmi, K. A., Goldberg, S. C. and Davis, J. M. (1980): Arch. Gen. Psychiatry 37:1030-1035.
9. Casper, R. C., Halmi, K. A., Goldberg, S. C., Eckert, E. D. and Davis, J. M. (1979): Brit. J. Psychiatry 134:60-66.
10. Casper, R. C., Offer, D. and Ostrov, E. (1981): J. Pediatrics 98: 656-661.
11. Crisp, A. H. (1965): Proc. Roy. Soc. Med. 58:814-820.
12. Crisp, A. H. (1970): World Review of Nutrition and dietetics 12; 452-504.
13. Crisp, A. H. and Kalucy, R. S. (1974): Brit. J. Med. Psych. 47: 349-361.
14. Crisp, A. H., Palmer, R. L. and Kalucy, R. S. (1976): Brit. J. Psychiat. 128:549-554.
15. Drewnoski, A., Gruen, R. and Grinker, J. A. (1982): In: Basic Symposium on Food Carbohydrates, edited by D. R. Lineback and G. E. Inglett. AVI Publishing Co. (in press).
16. Druss, R. G. and Silverman, J. A. (1979): In: General Hospital Psychiatry.
17. Feighner, J. P., Robins, E. and Guze, S. B. (1972): Arch. Gen. Psychiatry 26:57-63.
18. Fisher, S. (1964): Arch. Gen. Psychiatry 10:519-529.

19. Forbes, E. G., Kriss, M. and Miller, R. C. (1934): J. Nutrition 8:535-552.
20. Fries, H. (1977); In; Anorexia Nervosa, edited by S. Vigersky, pp.163-176. Raven Press, New York.
21. Garfinkel, P. E., Moldofsky, H. and Garner, D. M. (1980): Arch. Gen. Psychiatry 37:1036.
22. Garfinkel, P. E., Moldofsky, H., Garner, D. M., Stancer, H. C. and Coscina, D. V. (1978): Psychosomatic Medicine 40:487-498.
23. Garner, D. M. and Garfinkel, P. E. (1982): Unpublished Manuscript.
24. Garner, D. M. and Garfinkel, P. E. (1978): The Lancet, Letter to the Editor.
25. Garner, D. M. and Garfinkel, P. E. (1979): Biological Medicine 9: 273-279.
26. Garner, D. M. and Garfinkel, P. E. (19800: Psych. Med. 10:647-656.
27. Garner, D. M., Garfinkel, P. E. and Moldofsky, H. (1978): Canadian Psychiatric Association Journal 4:249-262.
28. Garner, D. M., Garfinkel, P. E., Schwartz, D. and Thompson, M. (1980): Psychological Report 47:483-491.
29. Garner, D. M., Garfinkel, P. E., Stancer, H. C. and Moldofsky, H. (1976): Psychosom. Med. 38:327-337.
30. Glucksman, M. L. and Hirsch, J. (1969): Psychosom. Med. 31:1-6.
31. Green, P. E. and Carmore, I. J. (1970): In: Multidimensional Scaling and Related Techniques in Marketing Analysis. Allyn and Bacon, Boston.
32. Grinker, J. (1973): J. Am. Diet. Assoc. 62:31-34.
33. Grossman, S. P. (1975): Psych. Rev. 82:200-224.
34. Halmi, K. A. (1974): J. Nervous and Mental Disease 158:222-225.
35. Halmi, K. A. (1981): In: The Proceedings of the American College of Psychiatrists Meeting.
36. Halmi, K. A. and Falk, J. R. (1981): International Journal of Eating Disorders 1:16-27.
37. Halmi, K. A., Falk, J. R. and Schwartz, E. (1982): Psychological Medicine (in press).
38. Halmi, K. A., Goldberg, S. C., Casper, R. C., Eckert, E. D. and Davis, J. M. (1979): Brit. J. Psychiatry 134:71-77.
39. Halmi, K. A., Goldberg, S. C. and Cunningham, S. (1977): Psychological Medicine 7:253-257.
40. Halmi, K. A. and Sherman, B. M. (1979): In: Biological Psychiatry Today, edited by J. Obiols, et al., pp.609-614. Elsevier North Holland Biomedical Press.
41. Herman, C. P. (1978): In: Psychiatric Clinics of North America, Vol. 1, edited by A. J. Stunkard, pp.545-579. W. B. Saunders Co., Philadelphia.
42. Hsu, L. K. G., Crisp, A. H. and Harding, B. (1979): The Lancet 2: 61-65.
43. Hueneman, R. L. (1966): Am. J. Clin. Nutr. 18:325-338.
44. Kapen, S., Sternthal, E. and Braverman, L. (1981): Psychosom. Med. 43:177-182.
45. Katz, J. L., Boyar, R., Roffwarg, H., Hellman, L. and Weiner, H. (1978): Psychosomatic Medicine 40:549-567.
46. Keesey, R. E. (1978): In: The Psychiatric Clinics of North America Vol. 1, edited by A. J. Stunkard, pp.523-543.
47. Keesey, R. E., Boyle, P. C., Kemnitz, J. W. (1976): In: Hunger: Basic Mechanisms and Clinical Implications, edited by D. Novin, W. Wyrwicka and G. A. Bray, Raven Press, New York.

48. Keesey, R. E., Boyle, P. C. and Storlien, L. H. (1978): Physiol. Behav. 21:261-270.
49. Kendell, R. E., Hall, D. J., Hailey, A. and Babigian, H. M. (1973): Psychological Medicine 3:200-203.
50. Mitchel, J. S. and Keesey, R. E. (1977): Physiol. Behav. 18:1121-1125.
51. Morgan, H. G. and Russell, G.F.M. (1975): Psychol. Med. 5:355-371.
52. Mrosovsky, N. and Sherry, D. F. (1980): Science 207:837-842.
53. Schiele, B. C. and Brozek, J. (1948): Psychosom. Med. 10:31-50.
54. Schiffman, S. S., Musante, G. and Conger, J. (1978): Physiol. Behav. 21:417-422.
55. Sclafani, A. (1981): In: The Body Weight Regulatory System: Normal and Disturbed Mechanisms, edited by L. A. Cioffi, W.P.T. James and T. B. Van Itallie, pp.153-160. Raven Press, New York.
56. Sherry, D. (1981): In: The Body Weight Regulatory System: Normal and Disturbed Mechanisms, edited by L. A. Cioffi, W.P.T. James and T. B. Van Itallie. Raven Press, New York.
57. Sims, E.A.H., Danforth, E., Jr., and Horton, E. S. (1973): Recent Prog. Hormone Res. 29:457-496.
58. Slade, P. D. (1973): Brit. J. Psychiat. 122:83-85.
59. Slade, P. D. and Russell, G.F.M. (1973): Psych. Med. 3:188-199.
60. Slade, P. D. and Russell, G.F.M. (1973): Psychother. Psychosom. 22:359-363.
61. Smart, E. D., Beaumont, P.J.V. and George, G.C.W. (1967): Brit. J. Psychiat. 128:57-60.
62. Smith, N. J. (1980): Pediatrics 66:139-142.
63. Stonehill, E. and Crisp, A. H. (1977): J. Psychosom. Res. 21: 187-193.
64. Stunkard, A. and Mendelson, M. (1967): Amer. J. Psychiat. 123:10.
65. Russell, G.F.M., Campbell, P. G. and Slade, P. G. (1975): Psychoneuroendocrinology 1:45-56.
66. Teitelbaum, P. and Epstein, A. N. (1962): Psychol. Rev. 69:74-94.
67. Ziegler, H. P. (1975): J. Comp. and Phys. Psych. 89:827-844.

Neuroendocrinology and Psychiatric Disorder,
edited by G. M. Brown, et al.
Raven Press, New York 1984.

Brain Monoamine Projections and Receptor Systems in Relation to Food Intake, Diet Preference, Meal Patterns, and Body Weight

Sarah Fryer Leibowitz

While the two syndromes, anorexia nervosa and obesity, are commonly placed at opposite ends of a continuum, recent elaboration of the components of these eating disorders has led investigators to link them on several grounds (5, 52). A significant number of anorexia nervosa patients, prior to loss of weight, are pudgy or obese; furthermore, on body weight recovery, these patients frequently return to a greater than ideal level. Anorexia nervosa and obese patients share other features in common, such as distortion of body image, preoccupation with food, binge eating, food preferences (in particular, preferences for sweets), menstrual and sleep disturbances. Each of these disorders is marked by hormonal changes (such as insulin, cortisol, growth hormone, and luteinizing hormone), some of which are the product of decreased or increased body mass, chronic illness, or nutritional deprivation.

Anorexia nervosa, like obesity, is a complex, probably heterogeneous disorder which is characterized by a wide range of social, psychological psychiatric, and hormonal deviations. It occurs most frequently in adolescent and young adult women (as many as 1% of the population), and is frequently associated with a stressful life situation. While a considerable amount of information about its manifestations, psychopathology, and pathophysiology has been accumulated in the past decade, the etiology of anorexia nervosa, its pathogenetic mechanism, and rational treatment remain unknown. The operational criteria used for the diagnosis of anorexia nervosa are as follows (14): 1) age of onset prior to 25 years; 2) anorectic behaviour, with accompanying loss of at least 25% of original body weight; 3) a distorted, implacable attitude toward eating, food, or weight that overrides hunger, admonition, reassurance, or threats, i.e., a) denial of illness with failure to recognize nutritional needs, b) apparent enjoyment in losing weight, with overt manifestation that food refusal is pleasurable indulgence, c) a desired body of extreme thinness with overt evidence that it is rewarding to the patient to achieve and maintain this state, d) unusual hoarding or handling of food; e) no known medical illness that could account for the weight loss; f) no other known major psychiatric disorder, e.g., affective illness, schizophrenia; g) at least two of the following manifestations: amenorrhea, bradycardia, periods of overactivity, episodes of bulimia, vomiting.

In addition to changes in eating behaviour and body weight, there are a variety of endocrine and metabolic disturbances which are commonly associated with anorexia nervosa (4, 8, 16, 21, 26, 34, 36, 38, 52, 53). The primary symptoms of this disorder may be summarized as follows:

1) Eating behaviour: Decrease in food consumption, meal size, and rate of eating; preferential decrease in carbohydrate ingestion; and consequent body weight loss.

2) Body fluid homeostasis: Increase in fluid intake and urine excretion.

3) Pituitary-gonadal function: Hypogonadism which is due to hypogonadotropism, as suggested by normal pituitary and ovarian function and abnormal brain regulation of gonadotropin release.

4) Pituitary-adrenal function: Increased adrenal activity, as indicated by increased plasma cortisol concentration; increased cortisol concentration; increased cortisol production rate (if calculated as a function of body size); hyperresponsiveness to adrenocorticotropin; lack of sensitivity to negative feedback from dexamethasone; and increased urinary free cortisol excretion.

5) Pituitary-thyroid function: Hypothyroidism, as reflected by low or below normal serum thyroxine and triiodothyroxine levels.

6) Growth hormone: Elevated resting growth hormone levels and loss of growth hormone release response to L-DOPA and apomorphine (but normal response to arginine).

7) Vasopressin: Partial diabetes insipidus.

8) Thermoregulation: Decreased basal temperature associated with cold and heat intolerance.

9) Carbohydrate metabolism: Impaired glucose tolerance and alterations in insulin sensitivity.

10) Cholesterol metabolism: Elevated serum cholesterol levels.

11) Catecholamine (CA) metabolism: Decreased plasma CA levels; decreased CA and serotonin (5-HT) turnover; decreased urinary CA metabolites (3,4-methoxyhydroxyphenylglycol and homovanillic acid); and decreased levels of norepinephrine (NE) and of dopamine (DA) and 5-HT metabolites in cerebrospinal fluid.

These changes in eating behaviour and in endocrine and metabolic processes have led scientists to consider seriously the possibility that anorexia nervosa may have, amongst other disturbances, an underlying anterior hypothalamic dysfunction. This hypothesis is based on extensive evidence in the literature which reveals a primary (although not exclusive) role of the hypothalamus in control of these processes. A major obstacle to this hypothesis is the fact that a large number of the above symptoms associated with anorexia nervosa are reversed by refeeding and weight gain and thus may be secondary to malnutrition. If this is the case, the symptoms observed may provide little information concerning the etiology of the malady. There is evidence to suggest, however, that a few of the changes manifested in anorexia nervosa occur independently of body weight and, in some cases, diet intake. These symptoms include: the increased cortisol production rate (25); decreased growth hormone release response to L-DOPA (21); decreased NE concentration in the cerebrospinal fluid (27); hypercholesterolemia (9, 28, 41); insulin resistance (10); and immature circadian pattern for luteinizing hormone secretion (26). Since these symptoms appear to be at least partially independent of body weight, the possibility of a primary hypothalamic disorder becomes more reasonable and deserves investigation.

The traditional view of anorexia nervosa holds that hypothalamic dysfunction is itself a consequence of a primary psychiatric disturbance. Indeed, psychological stress is known to alter hypothalamic function, and anorexic patients exhibit symptoms of depression, affective disorders, and stress (6, 22, 42, 48). While it will be difficult to establish the sequence of events in the pathogenesis of anorexia nervosa, the constellation of symptoms associated with this disorder has provided the foundation for several hypotheses based on hypothalamic (as well as extrahypothalamic) function, specifically in relation to monoamine neurotransmitter activity. Mawson (36) and Johanson and Knorr (24) proposed that anorexia nervosa results from a progressive depletion of brain CA and L-DOPA, by raising the levels of these amines in the brain, should lead to a reversal of the symptoms. This hypothesis was based on the findings that: hypothalamic NE injections stimulate feeding in rats (20); nigrostriatal DA lesions suppress feeding in rats (51); and anorexic patients exhibit Parkinson-like symptoms (rigid, obsessive-compulsive, stereotyped behaviour involving eating and movement in general). (See ref. 49 for a discussion of this proposed relationship between extrahypothalamic DA and anorexia nervosa). Barry and Klawans (1) and Redmond et al. (44), in contrast, have suggested that the opposite may be the case, namely, that anorexia nervosa involves an increase in activity within brain CA neuronal systems. Barry and Klawans focused on DA and based their hypothesis primarily on the findings that: DA agonists decrease food intake and body weight in rats (see 30); the DA blocker chlorpromazine produces the opposite effect (31); and amphetamine psychosis manifests symptoms similar to those of anorexia nervosa (e.g., distortion of body image and perception, hyperactivity, and obsessive-compulsive activities). Thus, these investigators suggested that symptomatic treatment of anorexia should be directed toward antagonism of activity of dopaminergic synapses, through the use of "pure" neuroleptics (ideally, ones specifically screened for action on hypothalamic DA receptors). Redmond et al. (44) focused instead on NE and based their hypothesis on the finding that locus ceruleus lesions, which cause a major depletion of forebrain NE, produce hyperphagia and weight gain in monkeys. These investigators proposed that hyperactivity of postsynaptic noradrenergic receptors may be associated with pathological satiation in humans and that pharmacological blockade of these receptors may reverse this process, as well as alleviate certain symptoms of anorexia nervosa.

While each of these hypotheses is reasonable and has some predictive value, the confusion reflected in their diverging assumptions is believed to be based in part upon the misconception that anorexia nervosa is a homogeneous disorder, with a primary symptom of appetite loss, and that brain monoamines have only one effect on eating behaviour. From the evidence presented below, it becomes clear that several monoamine systems, in different brain areas, are involved in regulating eating patterns, appetite for specific foods and body weight. Furthermore, recent evidence indicates that anorexia nervosa is clearly a complex and heterogeneous syndrome, which involves a disturbance in the experience of satiety perhaps more than in hunger.

Garfinkel (15) has reported that anorexic patients, unlike control subjects, frequently fail to describe satiety in terms of gastric fullness. They perceive hunger in a manner similar to controls, but they are more preoccupied with thoughts of food, have a stronger urge to eat, and are more anxious when hungry. Their continual fight against the urge to eat frequently gives way to binge eating at night (binge eating occurs in up to 50% of anorexic patients (52)). Mawson (36) has described these periodic over-eating episodes in anorexia nervosa as attempts toward re-equilibration of grossly disturbed biological mechanisms. These episodes, which also occur in manic-depression, with which anorexia nervosa has sometimes been compared, are associated with greatly increased subjective hunger, and are frequently accompanied by breathlessness, sweating, tachycardia, racing pulse, and inflated metabolic rate, suggesting a general increase in sympathetic activation (7, 17, 36). During the binge, a large amount of food is rapidly consumed in a discrete period of time, and a specific preference for high caloric, sweet-tasting foods is exhibited. The episode is terminated either by abdominal pain, sleep, social interruption, or self-induced vomiting, and results in depressive moods, feelings of guilt and remorse, and a continuation of the severely restrictive diets typical of the anorexic individual. (While symptomatic of anorexia nervosa, binge eating, or bulimia as it is called, also occurs in normal weight as well as obese individuals).

From this brief description of alternate binges and fasts, we become acutely aware that anorexia nervosa is not so much a disorder of appetite loss but appears to be one of increased desire to eat (perhaps of specific foods) associated with a profound and over-compensatory inhibition of this desire and then periodic breakdown of this inhibition. While anorexia nervosa clearly involves a host of other disturbances (as described above), these extreme fluctuations in eating patterns underscore the need to examine separately the different components of this disorder. With this appraoch, any potential relationship between anorexia nervosa and the different brain monoamine systems, or any possible interventions for treatment of anorexia nervosa, would appear to be more open to discovery.

Evidence obtained in a variety of mammalian species suggests the existence of several different monoaminergic systems in the brain which influence food-related behaviours in a variety of ways. Ultimately, each of these systems, as well as their interaction, will need to be considered in detail to establish a reasonable foundation for understanding the brain's control of normal eating behaviour, in addition to determining the relationship of these brain systems to the development of abnormal eating patterns. The evidence summarized below is derived predominantly from studies conducted in our laboratory on the albino rat. For these studies, a variety of techniques have been employed to investigate adrenergic, dopaminergic, and serotonergic systems of the brain in relation to eating behaviour, with a focus on the chronic cannula technique for administering drugs directly into discrete brain sites of freely-moving animals. The results of these and related studies are described in detail in a recent review chapter (30) and in references cited therein, and thus will be presented only in outline form below. The evidence suggests the existence of four distinct monoaminergic systems within the brain which modulate eating patterns, appetite, and body weight (see Table 1). These systems are: 1) <u>α-noradrenergic systems</u> within the medial hypothalamus, in particular <u>the paraventricular nucleus</u>, which stimulates eating and is believed to be involved in the appetite-stimulating action of clonidine and antidepressant drugs; 2) <u>serotonergic system</u> within the medial hypothalamus which inhibits eating and participates in the appetite-suppressant effects of anorectic drugs such as fenfluramine (FENF); 3) <u>β-adrenergic system</u> within the lateral hypothalamus, in particular the <u>mid-lateral perifornical area</u>, which inhibits eating and participates in the appetite-suppressant effects of amphetamine (AMPH); and 4) <u>dopaminergic system</u> within the lateral hypothalamus which also <u>inhibits eating and mediates</u> anorexia induced by AMPH, mazindol, and L-DOPA, and possibly the appetite-stimulating action of antipsychotic drugs. These studies reveal that drugs injected directly into these hypothalamic areas produce effects very similar to those observed with peripheral drug injections, in humans as well as in rats.

TABLE 1. Summary of Monoamine Regulation of Eating Behaviour*

	Stimulation	Suppression	
Brain Area	Medial PVN	Medial PVN	Lateral PFH
Neurotransmitter	NE	5-HT	EPI DA
Receptor Type	α	5-HT	β_2 DA
Presynaptic-Acting Drugs	Antidepressants	FENF CIMIP	AMPH L-DOPA
Receptor Antagonist Effect	↓	↑	↑
Bodyweight Change			
Chronic Stimulation	↑	↓	↓
Chronic Deficit	↓	↑	↑
Meal Patterns			
Meal Size	↑	↓	↓
Meal Frequency			↓
Rate of Eating	↑	↓	↑
Nutrient Selection			
Carbohydrate	↑	↓	
Protein			↓
Neuroendocrine Interactions	Glucocorticoids Insulin		Insulin
Cell Bodies of Origin	Dorsal Pons	Raphe	Medulla Ventral Midbrain

*Summary of evidence obtained through experiments in the rat, as reviewed by Leibowitz (30). Abbreviations: α, α-noradrenergic; AMPH, D-amphetamine; β_2, β_2 -adrenergic; CIMIP, chlorimipramine; DA, dopamine; L-DOPA, L-3,4-dihydroxyphenylalanine; EPI, epinephrine; FENF, fenfluramine; 5-HT, 5-hydroxytryptophan; NE, norepinephrine; PFH, perifornical hypothalamus; PVN, paraventricular nucleus.

In view of the similarities between the effects in these two species, it appears that the rat may indeed provide an appropriate physiological model for examining central neurochemical systems regulating eating behaviour. As will be described, the anatomical focus of the central injection studies is on the hypothalamus. Whereas this structure is consistently found to be most sensitive to the feeding modulating effects of monoaminergic agonists and antagonists, this evidence does not imply that other brain areas are not also involved in regulating food intake. The unique sensitivity of the hypothalamus may simply reflect its more direct role in actually triggering or inhibiting the eating response, in contrast to a modulating influence of extra-hypothalamic forebrain areas which mediate motivational, emotional, and cognitive effects on eating behaviour.

See Table 1 for a summary of the findings described below.

B. Medial Hypothalamic α-Noradrenergic System Stimulates Eating

1. Description of main effect

Hypothalamic injection of NE into the satiated rat produces an eating response which is remarkably similar to the spontaneous eating exhibited by rats under normal conditions (30). The response is dose-dependent and can be observed at a dose (1 to 4 ng) near physiological levels. A similar stimulatory effect on food intake can be observed with the adrenergic agonist, clonidine.

2. Sensitive brain area

Analyses of 30 different sites within the brain have revealed no eating effect with extra-hypothalamic or lateral hypothalamic NE injections and a progressively larger effect with movement of the drug cannula towards the medial paraventricular nucleus (PVN).

3. Type of monoamine receptors

Tests with PVN injection of a variety of monoaminergic receptor blockers demonstrate a selective blockade of the NE response with α-adrenergic receptor antagonists, such as phenoxybenzamine and phentolamine (30). These antagonists, when injected at higher doses, are found to have an effect of their own on food consumption, namely, an inhibition of eating.

4. NE effects on body water homeostasis

In addition to stimulating eating behaviour, PVN injection of NE alters water ingestion, as well as urine excretion (30). Immediately after NE administration, a brief "preprandial" drinking response can be observed. This response, which lasts for only a few minutes, is followed by a strong inhibition of water consumption which is apparent throughout the period in which eating is exhibited, as well as after the eating terminates. Also associated with PVN injection of NE is a decreased urine excretion and increased urine osmolarity, which is apparently due to the release of antidiuretic hormone. These effects of NE on water intake and urine excretion can be observed at very low doses of NE (between 1 and 10 ng) and are blocked by α-adrenergic receptor antagonists.

5. Antidepressant drugs

Antidepressant compounds, which are known to block neuronal uptake of NE and thereby enhance the synaptic availability of the endogenous neurotransmitter, are found to stimulate eating behaviour when injected directly into the PVN (30). This effect can be observed with desipramine, protriptyline, tranylcypromine, and amitriptyline, and is found to be antagonized by α-adrenergic receptor blockers. It is also blocked by central injection of NE synthesis inhibitors, suggesting that these antidepressants are acting presynaptically through endogenous NE.

6. Analyses of endogenous NE metabolism

Biochemical studies conducted in other laboratories (see ref. 30 for review) have distinguished the medial region of the rostral hypothalamus, specifically the PVN, dorsomedial and ventromedial nuclei, as exhibiting the most dramatic changes in NE turnover or release as a function of changes in eating behaviour.

7. Effect of chronic NE and phenoxybenzamine administration

Recent studies have revealed that chronic injections of NE into the PVN are effective in producing a significant increase in daily food intake and body weight gain (33). The opposite effects, namely decreased eating and body weight, are produced by chronic injection of the α-adrenergic antagonist phenoxybenzamine.

8. NE effects on meal patterns

Work conducted in this laboratory (Leibowitz, Marinescu and Grinker, unpublished data), as well as by others (45), indicate that the stimulatory effect of PVN NE injection on food intake is attributed primarily to an increase in meal size (and duration) rather than meal frequency. In addition, NE causes a marked increase in the animals' rate of eating.

9. NE effects on diet selection

Studies with the self-selection feeding paradigm (where 2 or 3 dishes of food are simultaneously available) demonstrate that PVN injection of NE increases the animals' preference for a specific dietary constituent, namely carbohydrate (30, 50). Norepinephrine induces the rats to consume sugar, sugar water or sweet milk (but not saccharin) and increases their preference for pure carbohydrate (sweet or non-sweet) over protein or fat.

10. Effects of antidepressants and clonidine on diet selection

LIke NE, injection of desipramine into the PVN causes a preferential increase in consumption of carbohydrate. The same effect is also observed with peripheral, as well as central, injection of the α- adrenergic agonist clonidine (13, 50).

11. Eating induced by glucose deprivation

Evidence reviewed in ref. 30 suggests that eating induced by the nonmetabolizable glucose analogue 2-deoxy-D-glucose (2-DG), which inhibits glucose utilization, may be mediated, at least in part, by hypothalamic noradrenergic neurons. Eating induced by 2-DG is blocked by α- adrenergic blockers and CA synthesis inhibitors. This 2-DG response is associated with an increase in the efflux and turnover of endogenous NE, and stress-induced depletion of hypothalamic NE leads to a decrease in responsiveness to 2-DG. Injection of 2-DG is also found to induce a specific preference for carbohydrate.

12. Glucocorticosteroids and NE-induced eating

The eating response elicited by PVN injection of NE is found to be dependent upon adrenal hormones, in particular corticosterone (30). Adrenalectomy abolishes the NE eating response, which is restored selectively by injections or subcutaneous implants of corticosterone (as opposed to a variety of other hormones tested).

13. Insulin and NE-induced eating

Eating induced by PVN injection of NE is abolished by subdiaphragmatic vagotomy and significantly attenuated by dissection specifically of the coeliac branch of the vagus nerve (46). The NE eating response which has been associated with an increase in release of insulin (12), is also antagonized by peripheral injections of the cholinergic antagonists, atropine and scopolamine (30, 46).

14. PVN lesions and alterations in eating

Electrolytic lesions of the PVN, where NE is most effective in stimulating eating, are themselves found to induce overeating and ultimately cause obesity. This evidence suggests that endogenous NE may stimulate eating by inhibiting the firing of "satiety" neurons located within the PVN. Other laboratories have demonstrated that wire knife cuts in the vicinity of the PVN are also effective in producing hyperphagia and weight gain. (see ref. 30 for review.) A recent study has demonstrated that discrete lesions of the PVN attenuate or abolish the eating response induced by ventricular NE injection (32).

15. Effects of NE depletion within the medial hypothalamus

Neurotoxin lesions which damage noradrenergic innervation to the medial hypothalamus (including the PVN) produce the following constellation of effects (30); a) a loss of the eating reponse induced by injection of the antidepressant drugs; b) an increase in noradrenergic receptor sensitivity within the PVN; c) a small reduction of daily food intake and body weight, associated with an increase in water intake; d) a loss of eating in response to glucoprivation; e) a decrease in sucrose consumption; f) a failure to increase eating in compensation for food deprivation; and g) a disruption of the nocturnal pattern of eating.

16. Cell bodies of origin

Pharmacological and histochemical analyses of ascending noradrenergic projections to the hypothalamus suggest that the NE cell bodies which mediate the PVN stimulation of eating phenomenon, as well as antidepressant drug effects on this system, are located in the dorsal pons and may exist within the nucleus of the locus ceruleus (23, 30).

C. Medial Hypothalamic Serotonergic System Suppresses Eating

1. Description of main effect

Peripheral drug injection studies have demonstrated that serotonergic agonists reduce food consumption and serotonergic antagonists enhance food consumption (2). Work conducted in our laboratory has revealed similar effects with medial hypothalamic injection of these drugs (30). While PVN injection of 5-HT is effective in suppressing eating induced by food deprivation, it is considerably more effective in blocking the eating response elicited by PVN NE injection. This inhibitory effect of 5-HT on NE eating is dose dependent and can occur at a dose at least as low as 100 ng.

2. Type of monoamine receptor

Serotonin's inhibitory action within the PVN is antagonized by local injection of the 5-HT antagonists, e.g. cinanserin and cyproheptadine (30). It is also reversed by α-adrenergic and dopaminergic antagonists which are known to interact with 5-HT receptors but is unaffected by other dopaminergic and cholinergic antagonists which have little impact on these receptors.

3. FENF and related compounds

Peripheral injection of drugs which enhance the synthesis or release of endogenous 5-HT or block its neuronal uptake have been shown to cause a suppression of food intake and ultimately body weight. (2) The opposite effect, namely increased appetite and body weight, has been associated with 5-HT antagonists, in particular cyproheptadine (2). Studies conducted with central drug injections in the rat confirm these findings and suggest that the medial hypothalamus may be one central site of action (30). Injection of the 5-HT stimulants, FENF, fluoxetine, norfenfluramine, quipazine and chlorimipramine (CIMIP), into the PVN inhibits the eating response induced by NE injection. This effect is dose dependent and occurs at doses 3 to 4 orders of magnitude lower than effective peripheral doses. A similar dose-dependent suppression of food intake has been observed with the 5-HT precursor, 5-hydroxytryptophan, and this phenomenon is blocked by prior central injection of decarboxylase inhibitors, which prevent the synthesis of endogenous 5-HT.

4. 5-HT effects on meal patterns

Drugs which inhibit food intake through their action on serotonergic systems are found to affect meal patterns in a manner distinct from that exhibited by CA drugs (3, 30). Peripheral injection of FENF appears to have little or no effect on the initiation of eating or the frequency of meals but instead acts to decrease meal size as well as decrease rate of eating (3). This pattern is similar to what this laboratory has observed with PVN injection of 5-HT and norfenfluramine (Leibowitz, Marinescu and Grinker, unpublished data) and is precisely opposite to what occurs with PVN injection of NE (see above). This suggests that 5-HT mechanisms may activate a satiety process, whereby food intake is suppressed specifically through an early termination of eating. There is extensive evidence for a function of the medial hypothalamus in the mediation of satiety (30), and whereas NE may be acting to inhibit this satiety area (disinhibit eating through increasing meal size), 5-HT may be activating this area (decreasing meal size) through antagonism of noradrenergic function.

5. 5-HT effects on diet selection

Using the self-selection feeding paradigm to examine drug effects on dietary choice, Wurtman and Wurtman (56) have shown that peripherally injected serotonergic stimulants, namely FENF and fluoxetine, cause a selective decrease in calorie intake, while preserving (or possibly potentiating) protein intake. Studies in this laboratory conducted with PVN drug injection (Leibowitz and Tretter, unpublished data) similarly demonstrate that 5-HT and to a lesser extent norfenfluramine selectively decrease consumption of sweet or non-sweet carbohydrate and have minimal effect on fat or protein intake. Once again, this effect of 5-HT in the PVN is precisely opposite to what has been observed with NE injection (see above).

6. Cell bodies of origin

While there is not a great deal of evidence regarding the location of the serotonergic cells which control eating behaviour, the evidence which exists points to the cell bodies located in the midbrain raphe nuclei which are known to be a primary source of forebrain 5-HT (2, 30).

D. Lateral Hypothalamic β-Adrenergic and Dopaminergic Systems Suppress Eating

1. Description of main effect

Peripheral drug injection studies have demonstrated that adrenergic and dopaminergic agonists are generally inhibitory towards eating behaviour (30). Studies conducted in this laboratory indicate that central injections of either epinephrine (EPI) or DA are effective in inhibiting the eating response of food-deprived, pargyline-pretreated rats (30). This response is dose dependent and can occur at doses as low as 30 to 100 ng. Other CA agonists, such as apomorphine, epinine and isoproterenol, are also effective in reducing eating when injected into the hypothalamus.

2. Sensitive brain area

Mapping studies of this inhibitory effect of the CA have demonstrated little or no response with injection of EPI or DA into extra-hypothalamic, medial hypothalamic or far-lateral hypothalamic sites. In contrast, the midlateral perifornical region (PFH) is found to be most responsive, where the CA produce a 50 to 70% suppression of eating. This effect is potentiated by drugs which block the neuronal uptake of the CA.

3. Type of monoamine receptors

Tests with PFH injection of a variety of monoaminergic receptor blockers demonstrate that the inhibitory effect of DA on eating is selectively blocked by dopaminergic antagonists, and the effect of EPI on eating is blocked by β-adrenergic blockers, as well as by dopaminergic blockers (30). When these antagonists are administered at somewhat higher doses into the PFH, they are found to have an effect of their own on food intake. The β-adrenergic blocker propranolol and the dopaminergic blockers chlorpromazine, haloperidol and clozapine, are effective in potentiating the eating response of hungry rats, as well as eliciting eating in satiated rats (30).

4. CA effects on body water homeostasis

Hypothalamic injections of EPI and DA are found to have a predominantly inhibitory effect on water intake (30). Whether this is primary or secondary to their effect on food intake is not known. When injected into the PVN, as well as the supraoptic nucleus, DA has a potent inhibitory effect on urine excretion (30). This effect occurs at very low doses (1 ng) and is blocked by dopaminergic receptor antagonists.

5. AMPH and L-DOPA

Consistent with reports that peripheral injection of AMPH, mazindol and L-DOPA suppress food ingestion, this laboratory has demonstrated that hypothalamic administration of these compounds produces a similar suppressant effect (30). Mapping studies indicate that the PFH is the most sensitive brain area for this phenomenon, and pharmacological analyses demonstrate that these drug effects are attenuated or blocked by β-adrenergic and dopaminergic receptor antagonists. They are also reversed by prior central injection of CA synthesis inhibitors, indicating that these drugs are acting presynaptically through endogenous CA.

6. Effects of chronic CA administration

In recent studies (Leibowitz, Roossin and Rosenn, unpublished data), this laboratory has demonstrated that chronic DA or AMPH injection into the PFH is effective in inhibiting daily food intake, as well as suppressing daily body weight gain.

7. CA effects on meal patterns

Detailed analyses of various parameters of eating suggest that DA, apparently in the lateral hypothalamus, is specifically involved in adjusting the rate of eating and that its anorexic effect may be attributed to an effect on meal frequency and to some extent meal size. Peripheral injection of AMPH and mazindol reduce the number of meals taken by the animals and, surprisingly, increase the rate of eating (3). Dopaminergic antagonists, in contrast, cause the opposite effect, namely a decrease in rate of eating. Work conducted in this laboratory (Leibowitz, Marinescu and Grinker, unpublished data) reveal a similar effect with PFH injection of AMPH, namely a decrease in meal frequency and increase in rate of eating, but in addition, demonstrate a suppressive effect on meal size. These effects with AMPH contrast with those obtained with the serotonergic stimulant FENF, which is found to suppress eating by reducing meal size and rate of eating (see above).

8. CA effects on diet selection

Studies with the self-selection feeding paradigm reveal that PFH injection of DA or EPI have similar and specific effects on nutrient selection (Leibowitz and Tretter, unpublished data). These two neurotransmitters are found to preferentially decrease consumption of protein while leaving unaffected or possibly stimulating ingestion of carbohydrate or fat. This pattern of effects may occur in the absence or presence of a significant alteration of total food consumption. This effect of CA stimulation in the PFH contrasts with that observed with 5-HT stimulation in the PVN where its suppressive effect on eating is associated with a preferential decrease in consumption of carbohydrate (see above).

9. Effects of AMPH and chlorpromazine on diet selection

Similar to DA and EPI, injection of AMPH into the PFH causes a selective decrease in consumption of protein (Leibowitz and Tretter, unpublished data). Preliminary studies with peripheral injection of chlorpromazine indicate that this DA receptor antagonist produces an increase in consumption of protein and to some extent fat, while leaving unaffected or actually inhibiting consumption of carbohydrate. This contrasts with the stimulatory effect of PVN NE injection on eating, which is associated with a selective increase in consumption of carbohydrate. Thus, medial hypothalamic neurotransmitter systems appear to be involved in regulation of carbohydrate ingestion, whereas the perifornical lateral hypothalamus appears to participate in regulating protein ingestion.

10. Glucocorticosteroids, insulin and CA suppression of eating

Very few studies have investigated the interaction of hormones with CA systems which inhibit eating behaviour. Preliminary studies in this laboratory suggest that anorexia induced by PFH injection of AMPH or DA is unaffected by adrenalectomy. In contrast, there is evidence that the eating suppressant effect of peripheral AMPH injection is attenuated in diabetic animals and restored by administration of insulin (35).

11. PFH lesions and alterations of eating

Electrolytic lesions of the PFH, where AMPH and the CA are most effective in suppressing eating, are found to result in hypophagia and reduction in body weight gain (30). This evidence suggests that the endogenous CA may suppress eating by inhibiting the firing of "feeding-stimulatory" neurons located within the PFH. Preliminary studies indicate that PFH lesions or knife cuts in the area of the PFH significantly attenuate or abolish the anorexic effect of peripheral or central injection of AMPH and central injection of DA (37).

12. Effects of CA depletion within the perifornical lateral hypothalamus

Experiments with neurotoxin lesions which damage CA innervation to the midlateral hypothalamus (including the PFH) have revealed the following constellation of effects: 1) a loss of the anorexic effect induced by injection of AMPH; b) an increase in dopaminergic and β-adrenergic receptor sensitivity within the PFH; and c) an increase in daily food intake and body weight gain.

13. Cell bodies of origin

Pharmacological and histochemical analyses of ascending dopaminergic and adrenergic projections to the hypothalamus have provided some evidence to suggest that the DA cell bodies, which innervate the PFH to suppress feeding, are located in the ventral midbrain (30). Potential EPI cell bodies which mediate β-adrenergic suppression of eating exist further posteriorly, within the dorsal and ventral medulla.

E. Discussion

These monoaminergic systems identified in the rat brain provide a basis for examining and explaining various drug effects on eating behaviour in humans, as well as in other mammalian species. They help us to understand the appetite stimulating action of such drugs as clonidine, antidepressants, antipsychotics and cyproheptadine, and the appetite suppressant action of such drugs as amphetamine, L-DOPA, and FENF. They indicate where these drugs might be acting and characterize the mechanism through which they act.

Drug studies conducted on patients with anorexia nervosa have met with limited success but have revealed some promising effects which are generally similar to those described above for the rat. The antidepressant drug, amitriptyline, has been shown in some patients to reverse the anorexia and body weight loss, perhaps independent of its effect on depression, and in addition, cause a preferential increase in consumption of carbohydrate independent of any changes in plasma glucose or insulin tolerance (29, 39, 40, 43). In addition to increasing body weight, this compound is also effective in reducing the number of episodes of binge eating and self-induced vomiting exhibited by anorexic patients (39), as well as these individuals' general preoccupation with food (40). The 5-HT antagonist cyproheptadine also appears to have some therapeutic effect in anorexic patients, particularly in the most severely ill (18). The CA precursor, L-DOPA has been found to increase body weight in one study on anorexia nervosa (24), and two other studies have revealed a potentiating effect of the DA antagonist, chlorpromazine, on both food intake and body weight (11, 36). Dally (11) noted that chlorpromazine may actually have the adverse effect of increasing the patients' chances of ultimately developing compulsive overeating and overweight.

In addition to seeking information regarding the therapeutic effects of drugs on anorexia nervosa, we are also interested to determine whether this information obtained provides a clue as to the basic neurochemical mechanisms underlying the syndrome. The similarities in the drug effects observed in humans and in rats (see above) strengthen the rationale for applying what we know about brain-behavioural neurochemical systems in rats to our understanding of normal and pathological neurochemical function in humans. Unfortunately, at this point the abnormal neuroendocrine profile established in anorexia nervosa provides us with limited information regarding the etiology of this malady, since most symptoms are reversed by refeeding and increased body weight. In light of our present knowledge of hypothalamic monoamine control of eating behaviour in animals, it may be fruitful at present simply to focus on the oscillating eating patterns exhibited in some anorexic patients.

Based on the evidence described above in the rat, the neurochemical substrate(s) for these oscillating feeding patterns may be postulated to be: for anorexic behaviour, either decreased medial hypothalamic α-noradrenergic activity, increased medial hypothalamic serotonergic activity, or increased lateral hypothalamic dopaminergic and β-adrenergic activity; and for binge eating behaviour, either increased medial hypothalamic α-noradrenergic activity, decreased medial hypothalamic serotonergic activity, or increased lateral hypothalamic dopaminergic or β-adrenergic activity. The few symptoms described in the Introduction, which appear to occur in anorexic patients independent of food intake and body weight changes, are at least consistent with such alterations in brain monoamine metabolism, which if not primary to the illness, may be primary for inducing the oscillating eating patterns. There has been some suggestion in the past that certain symptoms of anorexia nervosa may in part be manifestations of pathological sympathetic neuronal function (36). The neuropharmacological evidence obtained in the rat focuses our attention in particular on a possible relationship between abnormal consummatory behaviour in anorexia nervosa and fluctuations in α-noradrenergic function within the paraventricular and periventricular hypothalamus. Specifically, during the anorexic state, the symptoms include: a decrease in total food intake (carbohydrate in particular), body weight, meal size, rate of eating, insulin responsiveness, and deprivation-induced eating; an increase in fluid intake and urine output; a disturbed diurnal pattern of eating; hyperactivity; and increased propensity to rebound toward overeating. This constellation of events appears identical to what we observe in the rat with a <u>decrease</u> in noradrenergic activation (via pharmacological blockade or irreversible damage to specific noradrenergic projections to the paraventricular hypothalamus) and is opposite to what we observe with an increase in noradrenergic activation (through medial hypothalamic injection of NE). During the bulimic episode, in contrast, many of these symptoms become reversed by a sudden increase in α-noradrenergic activation, perhaps evoked by stress or drug administration. While these dramatic oscillations between anorexia and bulimia may theoretically involve simply this noradrenergic projection to the medial hypothalamus, it is more likely that active, reciprocal interactions between the different hypothalamic monoamine systems are required to achieve the over-compensatory or homeostatic switch in eating patterns. That is, during the anorexic state, α-noradrenergic activity may be in a depressed state through active inhibition from medial hypothalamic serotonergic or lateral hypothalamic dopaminergic fiber systems; in the bulimic state, in contrast, symptoms of extreme noradrenergic activation (peripherally as well as in the medial hypothalamus) may be a consequence of attenuated serotonergic or dopaminergic function.

There is direct evidence obtained in our laboratory (see above) which indicates that chronic disturbances in brain monoamine activity may have profound and long-term impact on eating patterns and body weight in the rat. For example, chronic administration of NE into the medial paraventricular hypothalamus produces increased daily food intake and body weight gain. During the first few days of stimulation, a consequent decrease in α- adrenergic receptor sensitivity is detected. Preliminary biochemical analyses of CA receptors in the hypothalamus have demonstrated that, after two days of food deprivation, a significant change in the receptor population may occur. In particular, a decrease in specific radioligand binding to α-adrenergic receptors is detected in the medial hypothalamus, in contrast to an increase in specific radioligand binding to β-adrenergic and dopaminergic receptors in the lateral hypothalamus (Jhanwar-Uniyal, Makman and Leibowitz, unpublished data). Hypothalamic receptor changes have also been observed after chronic depletion of medial hypothalamic NE due to neurotoxin damage to specific ascending noradrenergic projections. Such lesions are found to cause a dramatic increase in the eating response to direct NE receptor stimulation, associated with a loss of responsiveness to antidepressant drugs which depend upon endogenous NE synthesis. The syndrome associated with NE depletion also includes additional symptoms, such as a 10 to 15% decrease in daily food intake; a 4% decrease in body weight; a decrease in consumption of carbohydrate and responsiveness to insulin; and a loss of compensatory eating which normally occurs in response to food deprivation. This syndrome, which bears close similarities to anorexia nervosa, may be reversed, possibly towards overeating and bulimia, by direct NE administration into the medial hypothalamus and theoretically by stress (which releases endogenous NE) and by drugs (e.g., cyproheptadine, amitriptyline or chlorpromazine) and hormones (e.g. corticosterone) which shift the balance towards increased noradrenergic activation. It is interesting that chlorpromazine has been reported to increase a patients' chances of ultimately exhibiting compulsive overeating and overweight (11).

While any such comparisons as these, between a clinical syndrome of anorexia nervosa and neurochemical-behavioural changes in the rat, are clearly simplistic, they may provide a first step towards understanding an extremely complex constellation of phenomena. The above pattern may possibly be extended to incorporate hormonal changes (such as the increase in cortisol and decrease in T_3 and gonadotropins) which occur in anorexia nervosa and may eventually be associated with changes in mood state (e.g , depression and increased activity) which also occur in anorexia nervosa and have been linked with changes in adrenergic activation. For the moment, however, it appears most fruitful to focus simply on the changes in eating behaviour which may not only be symptoms of psychiatric disturbance but may also have profound repercussions on the overall progress of the syndrome. In this light, focusing on the bulimic episode may be particularly helpful since it involves a discrete series of events (generally lasting two to three hours) and is therefore subject to more systematic experimental manipulation and short-term study. Furthermore, the bulimia may be more susceptible to manipulation since, to the anorexic patient, it appears to represent the most troublesome feature of the syndrome, in contrast to the anorexia which is denied as being a problem and is actually welcomed and actively enforced.

While bulimia appears to be a major symptom of anorexia nervosa and also occurs in normal weight as well as obese individuals, it has received relatively little attention with regard to its neurochemical basis and its pharmacological properties. Based on the suggestion that bulimia has an underlying neurophysiological dysfunction, investigators have examined the effectiveness of the anti-epileptic drug Diphenylhydantoin in reducing the intensity of the compulsive eating episode (19, 55). Using this drug, Green and Rau (19) have reported success of treatment in 9 out of 10 bulimic patients. In a double-blind crossover study, however, Wermuth et al. (55) achieved a more moderate, but statistically significant, reduction in binge eating. While the pharmacological effects of Diphenylhydantoin are numerous and complex, its interaction with brain monoamine systems would suggest that increased serotonergic function (and thus possibly decreased adrenergic activity) may contribute to its effectiveness in treating bulimia.

Bulimia occurs in as many as 50% of anorexic patients. Understanding the bulimic episode, therefore, should enchance our appreciation of anorexia nervosa in general and the anorexic state in particular, which seems in part to reflect an over-reaction to the bulimia. Unfortunately studies of drug treatment of anorexia nervosa have met with limited success, and the difficulties encountered may be partially attributed to the patients' denial of their condition and their strong desire to maintain their low body weight. It may also be attributed to a focus of scientists on anorexia nervosa as a unitary syndrome, frequently viewed as a deficiency in stimulation of hunger and appetite. In recent years, it has become clear that anorexia nervosa is characterized by intense hunger and preoccupation with food, apparently with the bulimic episode representing a culmination of these features. Thus, particularly in the case of the bulimic anorexic, it appears that the cyclical components of the disorder warrant separate attention and more focused treatmnt, at least until our present limitations in understanding of drug action no longer exist. Based on extensive work conducted in animals, it is proposed that specific drugs which are known to suppress appetite through hypothalamic monoaminergic systems might be helpful in alleviating this eating disorder, particularly the bulimic episode. In view of the anorexic patients' strong denial and desire to work towards a low body weight, it would appear that (pharmacological) assistance in dealing with the bulimic aspect of the anorexia nervosa syndrome, its most troublesome feature for the patient, may be more favourably received and my have positive impact on the disorder as a whole.

ACKNOWLEDGMENTS

This research was supported by USPHS grant MH 22879 and by funds from the Whitehall Foundation.

REFERENCES

1. Barry, V. C. and Klawans, H. L. (1976): J. Neural Trans. 38:107-122.
2. Blundell, J. E. (1977): Int. J. Obesity 1:15-42.
3. Blundell, J. E. and Latham, C. J. (1978): In: Central Mechanisms of Anorectic Drugs, edited by S. Garattini and R. Samanin, pp.83-109. Raven Press, New York.
4. Brown, G. M. (1980): In: Handbook of Biological Psychiatry, Part III, edited by H. M. Van Praag, pp.217-240. Marcel Dekker, New York.
5. Bruch, H. (1973): Eating Disorders. Basic, New York.
6. Cantwell, D. P., Sturzenberger, S., Burroughs, J., Salkin, B. and Green, J. K. (1977): Arch. Gen. Psychiat. 34:1087-1093.
7. Casper, R. C., Eckert, E. D., Halmi, K. A., Goldberg, S. C. and Davis, J. M. (1980): Arch. Gen. Psychiat. 37:1030-1035.
8. Crisp, A. H. (1976): J. Psychosom. Res. 11:117-131.
9. Crisp, A. H., Blendis, L. M. and Pawan, G.L.S. (1968): Metabolism 17:1109-1118.
10. Crisp, A. H., Ellis, J. and Lowy, C. (1967): Postgrad. Med. 43: 97-102.
11. Dally, P. and Sargant, W. (1966): Brit. Med. J. 2:793-795.
12. deJong, A., Strubbe, J. H. and Steffens, A. B. (1977): Amer. J. Physiol. 233:E380-E388.
13. Fahrbach, S. E., Tretter, J. R., Aravich, P. F., McCabe, J. and Leibowitz, S. F. (1980): Neurosci. Abstr. 6:784.
14. Feighner, J. P., Robins, E., Guze, S. B., Woodruff, R. A.,Jr., Winkokur, G. and Munoz, R. (1972): Arch. Gen. Psychiat. 26:57-63.
15. Garfinkel, P. E. (1974): Psychol. Med. 4:309-315.
16. Garfinkel, P. E. (1983): This volume.
17. Garfinkel, P. E., Moldofsky, H. and Garner, D. M. (1980): Arch. Gen. Psychiat. 37:1036-1040.
18. Goldberg, S. C., Halmi, K. A., Eckert, E. D., Casper, R. C. and Davis, J. M. (1979): Brit. J. Psychiat. 134:67-70.
19. Green, R. S. and Rau, J. H. (1974): Amer. J. Psychiat. 131:428-432.
20. Grossman, S. P. (1962): Amer. J. Physiol. 202:872-882.
21. Halmi, K. A. (1978): Annu. Rev. Med. 29:137-148.
22. Halmi, K. A., Dekirmanjian, H., Davis, J. M., Casper, R. and Goldberg, S. (1978): Arch. Gen. Psychiat. 35:458-460.
23. Halperin, R., Brown, L. L. and Leibowitz, S. F. (1979): Neurosci. Abstr. 5:218.
24. Johanson, A. J. and Knorr, N. J. (1977): In: Anorexia Nervosa, edited by R. Vigersky, pp.363-372. Raven Press, New York.
25. Katz, J. L., Boyar, R., Roffwarg, H., Hellman, L. and Weiner, H. (1978): Psychosom. Med. 40:549-567.
26. Katz, J. L., Boyar, R. M., Weiner, H., Gorzynski, G., Roffwarg, H. and Hellman, L. (1976): In: Hormones, Behavior and Psychopathology, edited by E. J. Sachar, pp.263-283. Raven Press, New York.
27. Kaye, W. H., Ebert, M. H., Raleigh, M. and Lake, C. R. (1983): Am. J. Psychiat. 3 (in press).

Scientific Proceedings, p.326 (Abstract).
28. Klinefelter, H. F. (1965): J. Clin. Endocrinol. Metab. 25:1520-1521.
29. Kupfer, D. J., Coble, P. A. and Rubinstein, D. (1979): Psychosom. Med. 41:535-544.
30. Leibowitz, S. F. (1980): In: Handbook of the Hypothalamus, Vol. 3, edited by P. J. Morgane and J. Panksepp, pp.299-437. Marcel Dekker, New York.
31. Leibowitz, S. F. and Miller, N. E. (1969): Science 165:609-611.
32. Leibowitz, S. F., Hammer, N. J. and Chang, K. (1981): Physiol. Behav. 27:1031.1040.
33. Leibowitz, S. F., Roossin, P. and Rosenn, M. (1984): Pharmacol. Biochem. Behav. (in press).
34. Lupton, M., Simon, L., Barry, V.and Klawans, H. L. (1976): Life Sci. 18:1341-1348.
35. Marshall, J. F., Friedman, M. I. and Heffner, T. G. (1976): Brain Res. 111:428-432.
36. Mawson, A. R. (1974): Psychol. Med. 4:289-308.
37. McCabe, J. and Leibowitz, S. F. (1980): Neurosci. Abstr. 6:784.
38. Mecklenburg, R. S., Loriaux, D. L., Thompson, R. H., Andersen, A. E. and Lipsett, M. B. (1974): Medicine 53:147-159.
39. Moore, D. C. (1977): Amer. J. Psychiat. 134:1303-1304.
40. Needleman, H. C. and Waber, D. (1977): In: Anorexia Nervosa, edited by R. Vigersky, pp.357-362. Raven Press, New York.
41. Nestel, P. J. (1974): J. Clin. Endocrinol. Metab. 38:325-328.
42. Paykel, E. S. (1977): J. Psychosom. Res. 21:401-407.
43. Paykel, E. S., Mueller, P. S. and DeLaVergna, P. (1973): Brit. J. Psychiat. 123:501-507.
44. Redmond, D. E., Jr., Huang, Y. H., Baulu, J., Snyder, D. R. and Maas, J. W. (1977): In: Anorexia Nervosa, edited by R. Vigersky, pp.81-96. Raven Press, New York.
45. Ritter, R. C. and Epstein, a. N. (1975): Proc. Natl. Acad. Sci. USA 72:3740-3743.
46. Sawchenko, P. E., Gold, G. M. and Leibowitz, S. F. (1981): Brain Res. 225:249-269.
47. Sherman, B. M. and Halmi, K. A. (1977): In: Anorexia Nervosa, edited by R. Vigersky, pp.211-224. Raven Press, New York.
48. Shopsin, B., Friedman, E. and Gershon, S. Arch. Gen. Psychiat. 33:811-819.
49. Stricker, E. M. and Andersen, A. E. (1980): Life Sci. 26:1927-1934.
50. Tretter, J. R. and Leibowitz, S. F. (1980): Neurosci. Abstr. 6:532.
51. Ungerstedt, U. (1971): Acta Physiol. Scand., Suppl. 367:95-122.
52. Vigersky, R. A. (editor) (1977): In: Anorexia Nervosa. Raven Press, New York.
53. Vigersky, R. A. (1983): This volume.
54. Walsh, B. T., Katz, J. L., Levin, J., Kream, J., Fukushima, D. K., Hellman, L. D., Weiner, H. and Zumoff, B. (1978): Psychosom. Med. 40:499-506.
55. Wermuth, B. M., Davis, K. L., Hollister, L. E. and Stunkard, A. J. (1977): Amer. J. Psychiat. 134:1249-1253.
56. Wurtman, J. J. and Wurtman, R. J. (1977): Science 198:1178-1180.

Neuroendocrinology and Psychiatric Disorder,
edited by G. M. Brown, et al.
Raven Press, New York 1984.

Discussion: Anorexia Nervosa—Neural and Psychological Mechanisms

Gregory M. Brown

Regina C. Casper, Chicago, Ill.

I want to congratulate you, Dr. Leibowitz, on developing a model of anorexia nervosa. Based on primate studies, we have used clonidine in the treatment of anorexia nervosa. In monkeys, we found an increase in eating and an increase in weight, and looking in the literature, found that some of your work seemed to confirm this. We have started a pilot study in anorexia nervosa patients administering clonidine, using doses which are probably equivalent to yours and presumably having a stimulatory effect on appetite. The study is a placebo cross-over with clonidine. Clonidine is used at 7 mg for up to 3-4 weeks, then taking them off slowly and putting them on placebo for an equivalent period and followed by clonidine again. In the first three patients studied we have not been able to see a greater weight gain on clonidine than during the placebo period in anorectic patients. The only thing we have seen is a rebound effect after taking them off clonidine. They lose weight unexplicably, one pound or so. When you look at the curve, it is obvious that they drop in weight when taken off clonidine, but we do not see an increment in weight or increased eating while on clonidine.

Sarah F. Leibowitz

You might mention the side effects that you are seeing with clonidine.

Regina C. Casper: The side effects are worth mentioning, because I would discourage anyone from using clonidine in anorexia nervosa patients. That is why we kept it a pilot study. Clonidine is an uncomfortable drug for patients. There is an observable drop in blood pressure, which they tolerate fairly well, because they are chronically in a bradycardia and hypotensive state. There is also some increased sleepiness. I had one patient who reproached me, saying, 'I have not taken a nap in the past seven years, and all of a sudden I feel like taking a nap in the afternoon'. There is reporting of headaches, similar to tension headaches. I think before we have a better model for clonidine as an adrenergic agonist, it should not be used as a drug for treating anorexia nervosa.

Lewis C. Krey, New York, N.Y.

We know how the brain operates in general - it take sensory inputs, analyzes them and gives an efferent output. What I am not sure about is what is the afferent pathway through which the brain assesses body size and knows that everything is all right? Looking at this issue in terms of the onset of puberty, we thought we had the answer a while ago because fat has been shown to produce alterations in steroid metabolism and these changes in steroid metabolism could have accounted for the changes in gonadotropin observed. It is however apparent in recent human studies from Grumbach's laboratory and from Tony Plant's work on rhesus monkeys that gonadotropin secretion develops normally in agonadal individuals - agonadals and humans with gonadal dysgenesis, or in monkeys castrated at birth and which do not have steroids. Obviously, then, it is not working through changing the steroids. The brain gets the information somewhere else, and I would like to find out what information it is getting. We seem to know what it is doing with it, but what is coming in? Are there any speculations?

Sarah F. Leibowitz: There's obviously a body weight set point, and it is a very complicated mechanism. Looking at it neurologically has been a big problem, and it is not known what part of the brain regulates the set point. It was thought to be the ventromedial hypothalamus - but this is no longer held to be true.

Benjamin Rusak, Halifax, N.S.

As I am sure you are aware, a number of years ago Silverman and Zucker showed that hamsters completely failed to show any post-fast compensation and in addition, hamsters were completely incapable of responding to a 2-deoxyglucose (2-DG) stress with increased food intake. I wonder if you know anything about the locus coeruleus-paraventricular hypothalamic connections in the hamster, or whether any other features resembled the rat with medial hypothalamic lesions. With the very different eating patterns of hamsters and rats - do you think this is a model worth exploiting?

Sarah F. Leibowitz: There are several symptoms that are shown by the medial hypothalamic lesioned rat that are exactly the same as hamsters. Not only are they deficient in insulin and 2-DG feeding response, but their nocturnal patterns are disrupted and they also decrease their carbohydrate intake - the hamsters showing a diminution in eating carbohydrates. Because of this response, hamsters will not restore themselves with food deprivation, and will just kill themselves even if the food is right there. So there are several similarities. I have not looked at a hamster's locus coeruleus so I really couldn't say, but it certainly is a promising model to work on.

Laurence S. Jacobs, Rochester, N.Y.

The patterns of feeding in the rodent are relatively dissimilar to feeding patterns in humans. My impression is that rodents tend to nibble over longer periods of time at night when they are active, rather than consolidating their total daily food needs into several more discrete time periods. If that is right, perhaps we should question whether these very elegant and quite refined studies showing monoamine effects in the rat, despite similarities in external symptomatology or manifestations, really have any relevance for primates or humans. In the medial basal disconnection that Dr. Krey talked about, what happens is that the animals eat and eat and gain weight, so that, if anything, the predominant influence in these animals which are disconnected from inputs may not be that they are lacking a noradrenergic eating drive as the dominant effect, but rather being deprived of the serotonergic input that is inhibitory.

Sarah F. Leibowitz: The eating patterns of rodents are actually not dissimilar. A rat has a discrete number of meals, maybe seven or eight. At nighttime rats may have three main meals. So it is not as if the rat had twenty meals or something - they do have discrete meals. So, on this point I don't believe they are that dissimilar. In fact, they drink first and they drink after, and actually it is not so different from the human. With respect to the medial basal cut, I think it goes above the ventromedial nucleus. But before that, I want to emphasize that there are many different feeding mechanisms. It may just be affecting one here. Whether it is serotonergic or whether it has anything to do with the noradrenergic system is unclear. Before I move on to another point, perhaps you wish to further clarify your question.

Laurence S. Jacobs: What I was driving at was, which of the neurotransmitter systems you described do you believe has a more important physiological regulatory influence on feeding behaviour?

Sarah F. Leibowitz: As I said at the beginning, I really don't know. I know more about the noradrenergic system and feel more comfortable talking about it, but I think all three neurotransmitters may be involved here. Let me emphasize again that the ventromedial hypothalamus is not the centre for controlling the food intake and body weight. Lesions in the paraventricular nucleus, very minute lesions, will produce an obese animal, and there is no impact from the ventromedial hypothalamus. So you need to be careful - the ventromedial nucleus has nothing to do with feeding behaviour. In fact, you can do quite a lot of damage there and still get no changes in food intake and body weight. So to answer the question of which systems are involved, I can only say that they may all be.

M. A. Quigley, La Jolla, California

I wonder if somebody on the panel or in the audience could help me answer the question: why do we see anorexia nervosa so predominantly in the young age group - in the transition from childhood to adulthood? What do we know about normal brain maturation and synaptic development - the hypothalamic and suprahypothalamic interconnections?

Sarah F. Leibowitz: We are doing anatomical studies on these systems and find that the noradrenergic system for stimulation of feeding behaviour appears to develop first and the inhibitory systems develop later. In the rat, this is a matter of about thirty days. I am not certain what that would be in terms of years for the human. It doesn't necessarily coincide with puberty - there is a difference in the pattern of development of the functional activity of these systems. It is possible that hormonal changes are triggering the functional activity of a system which is not developing normally. In a growing infant stimulatory actions are going full speed, and the inhibitory mechanisms are downplayed. But at some point an inhibitory mechanism comes into play - and that is where you may get into trouble, because they may now become hyperactive, depending on hormonal effects.

M. A. Quigley: That is quite interesting, because it is opposite to what we see with gonadotropins. At birth in humans, gonadotropins are high, and then they decrease very rapidly. Our current belief (we don't have much to back it up) is that during childhood there may be an inhibitory influence and that during puberty we may have a release from inhibition. This is something we are currently working on, but it seems to be different from what you are saying - that initially, you get the stimulatory system going and then you add the inhibitory. Perhaps in utero, we develop the stimulatory systems and then it is with birth that we see the development of inhibitory mechanisms.

Eugenio E. Muller, Milan, Italy

My first question is for Dr. Casper. When you were doing the clonidine studies, did you evaluate growth hormone secretion? As I discussed earlier, clonidine is a more specific drug for investigation of release of growth hormone. Incidentally, stimulation of the locus coeruleus in the rat, and also I think in the monkey, induces an increase in growth hormone release, and growth hormone is regulated (although we don't know the exact mechanism) at the level of the limbic system an area which may be involved in the psychopathology of anorexia nervosa.

As far as drugs are concerned, Dr. Leibowitz has reported the inhibitory effect of indirectly acting dopamine agonists to be at the level of the perifornical area. We have extensively studied a series of direct dopaminergic agonists of the ergot series, and they are quite potent inhibitors of food intake, in fooddeprived animals at doses which barely have any direct CNS activity. In other words, stereotyped behaviour is induced only at very high doses. From the clinical viewpoint, these data are interesting because there are scattered reports in the literature that in hyperprolactinemic subjects the administration of bromocriptine or lisuride is capable of decreasing food intake. Therefore, I wonder if anyone in the audience has studied the action of antidopaminergic drugs on anorexia nervosa patients?

Sarah F. Leibowitz: I have looked at them centrally and peripherally, and they do stimulate food intake.

Regina C. Casper: We have not studied dopaminergic blockers, but I know Dr. Katherine Halmi is studying them.

Katherine A. Halmi, White Plains, N.Y.

We are not studying them now. There has been no doubleblind study of chlorpromazine, although I should mention that it was the first drug that was used in the treatment of anorectic patients, and is still the drug most frequently used in England and Germany when drugs are used. In those patients who are severely ill the most severely obsessive compulsive and preoccupied with losing weight and having difficulties holding food all of them respond to high doses of chlorpromazine in a structured environmental situation. It was the first drug used by Sargeant and Morelli and I think it is still used as the drug of choice in their severely ill patients.

Eugenio E. Muller: Do you know if there are any studies of treatment of anorexia nervosa with diazepam?

Katherine A. Halmi: No doubleblind studies have been done. I am not very enthusiastic about using diazepam, for a number of reasons. Its effects wear off and the patient's anxiety increases. Even at high doses of benzodiazepines you get the same results, and then after 34 weeks of steady, chronic usage, an opposite kind of effect sets in - patients tend to get irritable and the drug is no longer effective. Some of my colleagues use benzodiazepines, giving a dose to the patient just before eating, because they want to reduce the anxiety of thinking she should eat a larger meal. But I would predict that the effect cannot be sustained over the 2-3 month period required to get the patient up to normal weight. Clinically I still recommend the use of chlorpromazine in severely ill patients but it needs to be studied further.

Sarah F. Leibowitz: The benzodiazepines show differential tolerance. There is development of tolerance to their sedative, quietening and anti-anxiety properties, but not to the food intake stimulation properties of benzodiazapines. We have used it quite extensively and in animals for periods of up to six weeks at least, no tolerance to stimulation of the feeding phenomenon is seen.

Katherine A. Halmi: The effect in animals may be very different than that found in humans.

Regina A. Casper: I wanted to briefly respond to Dr. Muller's question, as to whether we studied growth hormone. We have not. We have measured LH in the urine and have also done behavioural measurements including an anxiety and depression scale, and we will also be able to comment on carbohydrate preference. But these studies have not been fully evaluated.

I would also like to add a note of caution about using anti-depressant medications. I think Dr. Leibowitz's work shows very clearly that we might induce a preference for carbohydrates. We see this of course in patients who are not necessarily on anti-depressants, but patients with anorexia nervosa typically deprive themselves of carbohydrates for long periods of time, and on refeeding, a large proportion of them do prefer carbohydrates to any other foodstuffs and can sometimes consume very large quantities - such as a gallon or a couple of gallons of ice cream, and we should be more aware of the composition of their diet and perhaps use some of Dr. Grinker's work to tap the behavioural dimension of this.

John R. Sutton, Hamilton, Ontario

I wished to raise the tantalizing question Dr. Levine left us with about pioneering societies, where the women worked particularly hard and were obviously able to have fairly large families. I wonder if there are any biological lessons to be learned from these observations, both in terms of activity levels and caloric restrictions. In the Australian aborigines, for instance, there would be times when the whole tribe would go hungry for weeks and months at a time. Presumably, from a biological point of veiw, this would not be the ideal time to conceive and to rear young. And I wonder whether we are now seeing in anorexia nervosa a reflection of the broader biological implications of food restriction, on the one hand, and increased activity on the other.

M. A. Quigley: With respect to your point about the effect of weight loss or forced starvation in hunters, there was a very nice paper in the Journal of Clinical Endocrinology and Metabolism in 1978 looking at this. What they showed was a marked increase in the weight of the women in a particular tribe during the hunting season - as you would expect, and then a dramatic decline after the four month hunting season. And what was interesting was that nine months after the dramatic increase in weight at the start of the hunting season was the time for their peak number of births, and it was a very short-lived time - the majority of their babies being born within 2-3 month time interval.

Concluding Remarks

Gregory M. Brown

Anorexia nervosa can be viewed as an ideal model system for the study of neuroendocrine systems in relation to psychiatric disorder. This condition has a number of neuroendocrine abnormalities, for which there is no single explanation. The neuroendocrine approach has been described as a "window on the brain" and this window gives a hazy picture. Nonetheless, it is a window and it give valid information. The problem is how do we interpret this information? We have heard of a wide variety of factors that can produce endocrine changes; these include psychological factors, aberrant hypothalamic function, dietary factors - both calorie intake and the carbohydrate vs. protein mix, the effect of weight loss and effects of exercise.

Which of these factors are crucial to anorexia nervosa? Clearly, related to altered diet, there are changes in catecholamines, gonadotropins, thyroid function, and in growth hormone as well as considerable and poorly understood variability in cortisol secretion - all clearly related to diet, with evidence that some of these may persist when diet is normal.

While these hormone changes are all influenced by diet, there are a number of other changes that are related more closely to weight loss - notably the amenorrhea and related reproductive hormone changes such as changes in the 24-hour pattern of LH and FSH secretion and changes in LH and FSH responsivity to various stimuli. A variety of studies in monkeys and humans show that control of LH and FSH by the hypothalamus is both frequency-modulated and amplitude-modulated. This is a very interesting phenomenon - how the height of the LH secretory bursts have one effect, and how the interval between bursts has another effect. The fact that reproductive function in anorexia nervosa resembles puberty or the pre-pubertal state may be more apparent than real. It may be that any situation in which the LHRH release is reduced or significantly altered may result in a similar state. So puberty may not really be a model of anorexia nervosa. I think this needs exploration, because we have been pushing the puberty explanation pretty hard in the past, and it may not be valid.

There is evidence that dopamine and opiates are intimately involved in the control of LH (and FSH) secretion in man, and these systems deserve further exploration in patients with anorexia nervosa.

Although diet is intimately involved in some of these changes, and weight loss in other changes, the nature of the mechanisms involved is not clear. Diet, of course, may not just influence hormone regulation by altering metabolic events - it also produces effects on behaviour in its own right, and what do those effects do in turn to hormone regulation? Is behaviour the intermediate link? Prolonged dietary restriction in an anorectic patient might also lead to permanent changes in neural function, which in turn could lead to persistent endocrine abnormalities, and we have heard of the persistent endocrine abnormalities in patients with anorexia nervosa even after recovery to ideal body weight. What do they mean? Are they something basic to anorexia nervosa or are they induced by diet? The weight loss issue is not as clear as it first appeared - the concept of a critical weight and critical percentage body fat at which normal menstrual function and normal control of gonadotropins ceases may not be so simple. There may be a critical weight, but it may be very different in different individuals, and it is probably influenced by several other factors. There is a 16% incidence of amenorrhea preexisting prior to weight loss in patients with anorexia nervosa. What causes that? There is persistent amenorrhea in another fraction of patients despite normal weight. What is this due to? Is that related to something specific in the disorder? Are those with persistent amenorrhea the same individuals who have amenorrhea preceeding significant weight loss? Factors such as exercise, stress and diet change may be responsible for persistent amenorrhea, but this has to be studied systematically - and the behavioural correlates as well.

There are a number of behavioural factors that throw new light on the simple explanations we once had of the endocrine abnormalities. What about athletes who change their diet - is that why they get altered endocrine function? There are changes in body image, perceptual changes and food preference changes. There are interesting issues with respect to body fat regulation. What is the set point - how is it regulated? An interesting distinction has been recently made between patients who are bulimic and anorectic patients who have never been bulimic. They have a very different clinical course with a different outcome and a different response to treatment. Are they different endocrinologically? Nobody knows. That should be studied. Satiety, specific eating patterns and the fact that these patients really do have reduced or aberrant eating patterns, despite increase in food intake should be evaluated.

We heard about an animal model for anorexia nervosa. A very interesting and stimulating concept was developed based on increased noradrenergic activity involving the paraventricular hypothalamus as well as the possibility of a decreased serotonergic influence in that area (they go in opposite directions) and dopamine involvement in the perifornical region. Three different transmitters are involved, each of which, with the proper manipulation, could be involved in a model in which there is alternating anorexia and bulimia.

There are questions arising from this concept. How do the brain areas involved in appetite phenomena relate to the brain areas which are involved in neuroendocrine control? How do the substances - the transmitters, which are involved in appetite behaviour relate to the transmitters involved in neuroendocrine regulation? Dopamine can cause a decrease in food intake in the rat and when administered in the human, causes a decrease of LH. Is there a relationship here? And what about the food preference changes - dopamine being related to protein intake and the ratio of noradrenaline to serotonin being related to carbohydrate intake.

We have to conclude there is still a lot yet to be learned both about this disorder and from it. It is a model psychoendocrine disorder, and clearly a mixture of primary and secondary phenomena which are difficult to sort out. We can learn a great deal from the search which will be of tremendous use in studies on other psychoendocrine conditions.

Neuroendocrinology and Psychiatric Disorder,
edited by G. M. Brown, et al.
Raven Press, New York 1984.

Summary and Conclusions

Gregory M. Brown

One of the most important biological models of psychiatric illness in modern times was developed from the studies of Selye, who described the syndrome of adaptation to non specific stress and emphasized the importance of pituitary-adrenal activation as a measure of the adaptive response. The concept of using hormonal changes as an indicator of stress has been extended to the study of many different kinds of experimental and naturalistic stress, and of disorders such as anorexia nervosa in which endocrine abnormalities are clearly manifest. Development of modern concepts of hypothalamic control of the pituitary, and the recognition that the secretions of the pituitary are also influenced by central neurotransmitters has led to the development of psychoneuroendocrine strategies to elucidate the nature of central neurotransmitter abnormalities in the major psychiatric disorders, depression and schizophrenia. This approach has become one of the most active areas of biological psychiatry. In order to evaluate the relevance of these endeavors and to assess their importance as potential tools for elucidating the nature of psychiatric disease a critical review of the assumptions and approaches of psychoendocrinology was initiated. A panel of experts in the endocrinology of mental disorder has been assembled, and asked to prepare comprehensive reviews of selected areas that are now the most active. These reviews were analyzed and evaluated by endocrinologists and neuroendocrinologists who were asked to approach these questions from the standpoint of methodology and basic brain science. In a setting of active debate and discussion a number of critical issues were raised and evaluated. This volume presents the formal papers given at this meeting, and much of the informal discussion that took place over a three day period.

Our purpose in publishing this volume is to share with a larger readership our assessment of the status of psychoneuroendocrine approaches to the understanding of psychological dysfunction and psychiatric disease.

Schizophrenia

Abnormalities which have been reported in prolactin, growth hormone and gonadotrophin regulation in schizophrenia were reviewed by Meltzer. Although baseline growth hormone and amphetamine stimulated growth hormone levels are reported as normal, aberrent responses to apomorphine have been described. Responses are variable; a proportion of acute schizophrenic patients show increased growth hormone responses while some show hypo-responsivity. In contrast most chronic schizophrenic patients show greatly reduced growth hormone responses. Meltzer cited evidence that decreased growth hormone response to apomorphine is related to the duration of illness both in schizophrenic and non-schizophrenic patients so that these changes are not specific to schizophrenia. Paradoxical growth hormone responses to gonadotrophin releasing hormone have been reported in a proportion of adolescent male schizophrenic patients: a response which does not occur in normal subjects. In a small number of subjects a reduced growth hormone rise during sleep has been reported. With few exceptions studies indicate normal resting prolactin in schizophrenia.

Resting testosterone and luteinizing hormone levels, exaggerated LH responses to LHRH and decreased or absent LH and testosterone increase following clomiphene citrate is reported in some chronic schizophrenic patients. These abberations are of interest but only a few studies have been done. Whether they are secondary to neuroleptic treatment or chronic institutionalization rather than to a primary abnormality remains to be determined.

John Davis and co-workers reviewed pharmacoendocrine research in schizophrenia. Drugs with anti-psychotic activity stimulate prolactin secretion although the potency for effects on prolactin is greater than for the anti-psychotic effect. The locus of action of anti-psychotic drugs in elevating prolactin is external to the blood-brain barrier. Tolerance to the prolactin elevating effect occurs after several months whereas tolerance to the anti-psychotic effect does not develop. On the other hand in tardive dyskinesa in which there is a presumed hyper-sensitivity of striatal dopamine receptors, there is no alteration in prolactin. Growth hormone responses to a variety of stimuli are blunted by administration of neuroleptic drugs but there is no major effect on plasma luteinizing hormone follicle, stimulating hormone or TSH. In general, anti-psychotic drugs have pronounced effects only on prolactin.

Thorner and Evans examined the relationship of prolactin to brain dopamine function. Because circulating prolactin varies throughout the day, accurate representation requires repeated sampling. Dopamine has been shown to inhibit prolactin release by a direct action on receptors on the anterior pituitary cells. Studies using a perfused cell column with rat anterior pituitary cells show an extremely rapid and reversible effect of dopamine in inhibiting prolactin release. Current evidence argues that the various dopaminergic pathways of the central nervous system are functionally independent. The fact that prolactin secretion appears normal in schizophrenia suggests intact function of the tuberoinfundibular dopamine system but neither proves nor discounts the possibility of abnormal function in one or more of the higher dopaminergic systems.

Neuropharmacologic strategies in schizophrenia were evaluated by Dr. L. A. Frohman. Interpretation of findings of decreased growth hormone responses to various stimuli in both schizophrenic and other psychiatric populations is complicated by the fact that there are two hypothalamic factors controlling growth hormone secretion, a growth hormone releasing factor and a growth hormone inhibiting factor (somatostatin). Somatostatin secretion is stimulated by dopamine and hence cannot account for the net stimulatory effect of dopamine on growth hormone release. Somatostatin also has an inhibiting effect on basal and TRH stimulated TSH secretion. However, TSH secretion does not differ in schizophrenics and normal controls.

Drs. K. E. Moore and K. T. Demarest evaluated neuropharmacologic strategies as applied to prolactin secretion and dopaminergic neurons.

Several different groups of dopamine neurons are recognized. The tuberoinfundibular dopamine neurons play an important role regulating prolactin, luteinizing hormone and possibly growth hormone. Many properties of these tuberoinfundibular dopamine neurons are unique. In contrast to other brain dopamine neurons this system is selectively stimulated by prolactin, shows no acute response to administration of dopamine agonists or antagonists and lack a high affinity amine uptake system. Reports that there are no major differences between prolactin responses in schizophrenics and normal controls, therefore probably have little bearing on the possible role of dopamine in the psychopathology of schizophrenics. Furthermore, differences between tuberoinfundibular and other dopamine neurons suggest that it may be possible to develop compounds which interact specifically with mesolimbic dopamine neurons, those neurons which are thought to be involved in the schizophrenic process. Such selective compounds would be expected to have minimal side effects and would be without effect on prolactin.

Dr. O. Hornykiewicz opened the discussion by describing findings on growth hormone and prolactin regulation in Parkinson's patients. No correlation is found between resting or stimulated levels of growth hormone or prolactin and the patients status. It can be concluded that if we know nothing about the state of dopamine receptors in the forebrain of such patients, from neuroendocrinological data alone we would not be able to determine that these receptors were in a state of increased sensitivity. Evidence was also cited that increases in brain dopamine activity are associated with exacerbation of schizophrenic symptoms. On the other hand, dopamine supersensitivity as indicated by tardive dyskinesia develops in schizophrenic patients receiving chronic neuroleptic treatment. However, this supersensitivity in itself is not sufficient to produce schizophrenic symptomatology. The implication of this is that neuroleptics may well influence secondary biochemical phenomena rather the primary biochemical disturbance in schizophrenia. Dr. Hornykiewicz raised two issues with respect to the dopamine hypothesis of schizophrenia. There is evidence that the elevation in cortical homovanillic acid found in neuroleptic treated schizophrenic patients is not contained in dopamine neurons but in noradrenergic neurons where dopamine functions as an intermediate in the biosynthesis of noradrenaline. This finding would point to a role of noradrenaline in psychosis. A final point is the question of withdrawal psychosis. This type of response seen on withdrawal of neuroleptic drugs indicates that dopamine receptor supersensitivity develops as a consequence of chronic treatment and implies that tolerance to dopamine develops in the brain related to the anti-psychotic effects of the neuroleptic drugs.

Two alternative future directions in neuroendocrine research in schizophrenia were discussed. Dr. Meltzer suggested that future studies should be targeted on those abnormalities which have been already described in a few studies. One major problem in schizophrenia may be that of heterogeneity. The strategy would be to look at larger samples and use the tests as screening devices to define sub populations. On the other hand, the logic of continuing with neuroendocrine studies in schizophrenia as a way to understand the illness was questioned by several investigators. There is lack of parallelism between the systems, there is a tremendous variation in responses and specific hypotheses are lacking. There could therefore be great difficulties in distinguishing subgroups using this approach.

Stress

The psychoendocrinology of stress was reviewed by Robert M. Rose. The definition of the word stress was discussed. The word stress is used in different ways by different people: by some as a characteristic of the environment, by others as the response of the individual and by yet others as the interaction of the individual's perception of the environment with his response. In using the term, it is important to specify its meaning in context. Most studies of endocrine responses to stress relate to exposure to acute events and in the vast majority of cases, there is a rapid loss of responsivity which probably reflects adaptation. Serious questions can therefore be raised about the utility of studying most endocrine systems to assess differential risk for future illness. Significant activation of the adrenal cortex occurs when individuals are exposed to important changes of their environment. However, rapid adaptation of this response occurs, a crucial variable being the individual's perception of the event as stress. Individuals who employ psychological defences such as isolation and denial often experience little cortisol elevation. The majority of individuals engaged in difficult tasks to which they have been exposed for some time fail to demonstrate any significant endocrine responses. In fact, in some studies, certain individuals suppress hormone levels below base line during chronic exposure to stimuli. Detailed investigation on endocrine systems other than adrenal cortical responses is not yet available. Recent advances in the assay of circulating catecholamines cast doubt on the validity of most earlier data. Recent work supports the concept that uncertainty plus vigilance are associated with increased catecholamine levels particularly epinephrine. There is evidence that catecholamine responses do not extinguish or adapt to chronic stimulation as rapidly as cortisol. Another difference is that catecholamines show significant increases in positively arousing or stimulating situations whereas cortisol does not. Growth hormone is also a stress response hormone which requires a somewhat higher threshold of stimulus intensity. Differences in coping style and in intensity appear to explain why growth hormone is not always elevated along with cortisol in stressful situations. Prolactin is also stress responsive, and requires a more intensely provocative stimulus than cortisol or the catecholamines. Testosterone is also responsive to stress, the usual response being a drop. Modification of endocrine responses by circadian variation was discussed as a factor responsible for difficulties in adapting to shift work and jet travel.

The classification and description of stress were critiqued by Drs. H. Ursin and R. C. Murison. Use of the term 'activation' rather than 'stress' was urged to help clarify which processes are being described. According to this concept relevant stimuli converge on a single activation process which then diverges to a variety of processes. A distinction is made between phasic and tonic activation. Phasic activation is a short lasting fast acting activation as is observed in heart rate and epinephrine. This response shows little attenuation with progressive training. In contrast, the longer lasting activation characteristic of cortisol and several other hormones is markedly dampened by repeated experience. Moreover, two different endocrine factors a catecholamine factor and a cortisol factor were described which emerged from multivarate analysis of stress endocrine data. The cortisol factor correlated consistently with effectiveness of defense or coping operations while the catecholamine factor related significantly to performance in intellectual tasks and physical tasks.

Neurotransmitter mechanisms underlying stress responses were reviewed by Dr. W. F. Ganong who used ACTH as an example. The resting output of ACTH is stabilized by a negative feedback effect of cortisol on the anterior pituitary. Converging neural pathways provide an emergency override by which stress via corticotrophin releasing hormone (CRH) produces prompt increases in ACTH secretion. Central but not intravenous administration of norepinephrine causes inhibition of ACTH. Therefore the site of action of norepinephrine is inside the blood brain barrier. Effects appear to operate via α-2 adrenergic receptors as they are restricted to drugs which act at such receptors. It is possible that this noradrenergic system mediates the inhibition of ACTH which is produced by stimulation of arterial baroreceptors. On the other hand, it is unlikely that the increased CRH secretion in response to stressful stimuli is mediated by a decrease in norepinephrine secretion. Possible excitatory mediators include dopamine, acetylcholine, histamine, serotonin and angiotensin 2. Many other neurotransmitters could be excitatory or inhibitory mediators as the functional and morphological mapping of the controlling pathways is incomplete.

Discussion of issues related to stress was moderated by Dr. S. Levine. There was some objection to the notion of categorizing stress. To define stress in terms of its responses is both inappropriate and inadequate, moreover there are specific endocrine responses which may be associated with specific classes of stimuli so that the concept of a generalized stress response may not be tenable. Two major functional issues were discussed. Endocrine responses are important in telling us how the brain works in adaptation. The notion that stress causes disease has to some extent detracted from the study of activation of the pituitary adrenal system in its relationship to perfectly normal functions. If a diseased organ is activated it is easy to document that this may cause functional disorder. The issue is whether activation can produce disease in healthy individuals. This has been pursued in animal studies. Sustained activation has been shown to be related to the formation of ulcers, hypertension and mild myocardial infarction. On the other hand, of the many hormonal changes resulting from stressful stimuli most have never been shown to be important in human illness and probably never will be.

Affective Disorder

Pituitary-adrenocortical and pituitary-gonadal function in affective disorder were reviewed by Drs. Rubin and Poland. Many studies have shown that adrenocortical activity is increased in depressed as compared with manic or normal individuals. Although subjectively experienced anxiety and dysphoria result in an adrenocortical stress response, most investigators postulate that the change in mood and increased corticosteroid secretion are secondary to an underlying disturbance of brain function. This latter explanation is likely as changes occur in apathetic as well as in anxious depressives and because they occur throughout the entire 24 hours especially during sleep. A phase advance in cortisol secretion is also described. A specific indicator of the hyperactivity of this axis in depression is the early escape from dexamethasone suppression. In the dexamethasone suppression test dexamethasone is given in a dose of one or two milligrams at midnight and normally suppresses ACTH and cortisol for a full twenty-four hours. Endogenously depressed patients often show an early increase in serum cortisol between sixteen and twenty-four hours post dexamethasone. The dexamethasone suppression test has about 85% to 95% specificity for endogenous depression and a sensitivity of 50% to 70%. Abnormal dexamethasone suppression usually normalizes as the illness remits. Bipolar depressed patients are reported to have a higher incidence of abnormality than unipolar depressed patients and within the unipolar group, familial pure depressives are more likely to show non-suppression as compared to nonfamilial sporadic depression. Furthermore, only a small percentage of depressive spectrum disease patients show an abnormality. A few reports of plasma gonadotropin concentration suggest reduced diurnal and nocturnal circulating LH and possibly FSH levels in depressed patients.

Studies on growth hormone, prolactin and melatonin in patients with affective illness were reviewed by Stuart Checkley and Josephine Arendt. Depressed patients are relatively resistant to the hypoglycemic effect of insulin and although they tend to have smaller GH responses, they have less hypoglycemia. In one study where patients were matched individually with controls for age, sex and degree of hypoglycemia a decreased response was found. Responses to clonidine, an alpha adrenoceptor agonist, are significantly less in patients with endogenous depression, as are responses to desipramine. Reduced responses are also seen following 5-hydroxytryptophan and thermal stimulation. An anomalous GH response to TRH has also been reported in depressed patients. Baseline prolactin levels have been reported as normal, low or elevated and the majority of studies show normal prolactin responses to TRH. A variety of studies suggest that depressed patients have significantly lower night time melatonin.

Findings in the thyroid axis in affective disorder were reviewed by Drs. A. J. Prange Jr. and P. T. Loosen. The vast majority of depressed patients are euthyroid by presently accepted criteria. The thyrotropin response to thyrotopin releasing hormone is blunted in approximately 25% of patients with primary depression. The abnormality is not a function of increasing age, previous drug intake or severity of illness. A blunted response is both a trait marker and a state marker. Increased responsivity during treatment appears to predict a favourable clinical outcome. TSH blunting may also occur in alcoholism, mania and anorexia nervosa. In the majority of reports there is no difference between primary and secondary depressed patients or between unipolar and bipolar patients.

Dr. John W. Kendall evaluated pituitary-adrenocortical dysfunction in affective disorder from an endocrinologist's perspective. The derangements in cortisol seen in pituitary-dependent Cushing's Syndrome and in depressive illness are qualitatively similar but quantitatively differ in that the derangement is more intense in Cushing's disease. Furthermore peripheral clinical features of cortisol excess are not present in severe depressive illness. In depressive disorder normalization of cortisol occurs with remission while in Cushing's disease this is uncommon. "Escape" from suppression should be regarded as an operational description of a difference rather than as a phenonomen unique to depression as this is also seen in Cushing's disease. Exclusion criteria for this test include pregnancy, high dose estrogens, severe weight loss, hepatic enzyme inducing states (drugs in particular), uncontrolled diabetes mellitus, major physical illness and of course any other states of cortisol excess including chronic renal failure and excess alcohol intake. The dexamethasone test must be employed in a rigidly standardized fashion both with respect to the dose of dexamethasone and time points for blood sampling and drug administration and interpreted in relation to data obtained in a appropriate local population.

Dr. G. Tolis evaluated the clinical neuroendocrine findings in affective disorder. The dexamethasone test alone may be a useful auxiliary diagnostic test for endogenous depression and may possibly help predict remission or relapse. Multiple blood sampling over time is also useful as a marker of sleep-wake cycle disturbance. In patients with non-suppressability of dexamethasone it is necessary to exclude the diagnosis of Cushing's syndrome. In terms of accuracy and small false negative result yield, insulin induced hypoglycemia, apomorphine and desipramine are the best tests of GH reserve. With respect to the reported paradoxical growth hormone response to TRH its significance is difficult to interpret and investigators should attempt to find out whether TRH responders are more responsive to particular neuropharmacologic or therapeutic agents.

Dr. Tolis suggested evaluation of TSH release by TRH and by anti-dopaminergic agents in circadian fashion and the correlation of these findings with endogenous cortisol values and with dexamethasone testing to help understand the control of thyrotropin function in affective disorders. There is a need for a collection of age and sex adjusted normative data for the TSH response to TRH. To determine whether the blunted response is indicative of a genetic disorder, this response should be examined in familial pure depressives and their relatives together with simultaneous assessment of genetic markers.

Dr. Donald S. Gann discussed pituitary-adrenal regulation in affective disorders in the light of understanding of the brain stem pathways involved in the control of ACTH. Specific areas in the medulla, pons, midbrain and hypothalamus are associated with facilitation or inhibition of ACTH release. These regions have been related to the distribution of neurons which are responsive to hemodynamic and to pain stimulation. Areas of the forebrain limbic system including the amygdala have been implicated both in affective disorders and in the modulation of stress induced pituitary-adrenal function. Neural structures in the limbic system have also been shown to participate in the steroid feedback control of ACTH secretion. Ascending pathways from the brain stem arise from areas where there are cell bodies containing epinephrine, norepinephrine, acetylcholine and serotonin. There is evidence that both norepinephrine and serotonin may be associated with either facilitation or inhibition of ACTH release. Epinephrine appears likely to be associated only with inhibition of ACTH release. Vasopressin also plays a facilitory role. The physiologic interrelationships of these transmitters remain to be elucidated.

Dr. L. Cass Terry assessed catecholamine regulation of growth hormone and thryotropin in patients with mood disorder. In general most of the stimuli that cause release of GH in man appear to be mediated by central α-adrenoceptors. Some are also mediated by dopaminergic stimulatory pathways and inhibitory β-adrenergic pathways are also present. Blunting of growth hormone responses to hypoglycemia, desipramine and clonidine in some depressed patients provides compelling evidence supporting the hypothesis that α-adrenergic neurotransmission is decreased in this disorder. At present it is difficult to provide a precise localization of this defect. There is little evidence for a physiologic role of norepinephrine in TSH regulation in man. Dopamine appears to have an inhibitory effect that is most evident when negative feedback effects of thyroid hormones are reduced. Several theories are offered to explain the decreased TSH response of depression: the most attractive one being altered pituitary receptor sensitivity.

Dr. I.M.D. Jackson reviewed the role of the hypothalamic regulating hormones in producing the neuroendocrine dysfunction in affective disorders. Alteration in one or more of the multiple factors that impinge on TRH-TSH interaction is the probable underlying cause of the reduced TSH rise seen following TRH in depressed patients. These factors include peripheral hormone levels (cortisol, sex steroids, GH), neurotransmitter milieu (dopamine or related chemicals), hypothalamic dysfunction (altered TRH, somatostatin, neuotensin, dopamine, prostaglandin secretion). At this time it is not possible to specify which of these factors are involved. The aberrent growth hormone response to TRH is probably due to defective central aminergic or peptidergic control of the pituitary which unmasks a weak stimulatory effect of TRH on growth hormone. A releasing hormone, in addition to its effects on the pituitary, directly or indirectly influences the actions of the established neurotransmitters in the CNS. Dr. Jackson proposed the hypothesis that TRH may form an endogenous brain ergotropic system and that alteration of this system could be responsible for disturbed biogenic amines and the resulting pituitary abnormalities seen in depression.

Dr. Benjamin Rusak assessed the significance of rhythm disruptions in affective illness. Endocrine rhythms are physiologically significant. The circadian system is comprised of multiple oscillators and rhythm disruptions reflect a lack of normal integration among these oscillators. Studying rhythms clinically is difficult; a detailed long term record is required from both patients and controls. Biological rhythms may be important in the pathogenesis of bipolar affective illness. Symptoms shown by these patients show cyclicity and lithium salts which reduce the endogenous mood swings also slow circadian oscillations. Another treatment that transiently improves symptoms of depression is total or selective sleep deprivation. It has been postulated that this treatment may produce the resetting of an abnormally phased circadian oscillator although as yet there is no definitive evidence for this. There is also evidence that anti-depressant drugs modify basic features of circadian organization. Further investigation should be aimed at monitoring a large number of rhythms in patients and control subjects over long periods of time. This information should permit development of treatments which aim as exclusively as possible at the regulators of the identified aberrent rhythms.

In the discussion period the issue of normative data was discussed extensively. Many "normal" subjects have aberrent responses and are discarded as unsuitable. Fifteen to forty percent of normal individuals fail to respond to one or another provocative stimuli to growth hormone release and about five percent demonstrate TRH blunting. If individuals with such abnormal values are eliminated from a normal control group a systematic error is created which will inevitably lead to a statistically significant difference.

Another possible problem is the presence of occult pituitary disease. About 25 percent of adult patients have been found to have pituitary tumours at autopsy.

Discussion also centred on the application of neuroendocrine strategies in affective disorder patients. Dr. Carroll described a study demonstrating that the sensitivity of the dexamethasone test was improved by repeating it. He also described the present phase of investigation of this test as a dialectic phase in which we are redefining diagnostic categories on the basis of biological indices. Eventually we should emerge with a small group of biologic markers that can be added to clinical criteria to provide a comprehensive definition of illness. In contrast to dexamethasone testing there is little doubt that the deranged growth hormone response to TRH and LHRH seen in patients with affective disorder is mediated at the level of the anterior pituitary and is an indicator of "deranged" neurotransmission in the CNS.

There was discussion about the dexamethasone suppression abnormality being present in only some depressed patients. Two alternate viewpoints were expressed. One was that there are both trait and state factors involved. Certain patients manifest the abnormality and in those patients, there would be a quantitative relationship between the degree of depression and the degree of abnormality in dexamethasone tests. Other patients would not show any abnormality despite the intensity of depression. An alternate point of view is that this test is only an indirect test of disturbance in the limbic system. There is therefore a lack of a direct relationship to severity. Whichever viewpoint is correct it is evident that in individual patients there is some parallelism between severity and the dexamethasone test.

Anorexia Nervosa

Dr. Robert A. Vigersky reviewed the hypogonadotropism that is seen in weight loss associated amenorrhea. Amenorrhea is a prominent symptom of women with anorexia nervosa. Although in the majority of patients amenorrhea coincides with the beginning of abnormal eating behaviour and weight loss, in fifteen to twenty percent of patients amenorrhea preceeds weight change. Furthermore, in some women, weight gain does not result in return of menses, suggesting that the development of the amenorrhea is multifactorial and not solely associated with weight loss. There is general agreement that the amenorrhea is due to hypogonadotropic hypogonadism. But, the mechanism of a critical body weight requirement for menstruation has not been elucidated. Increasing weight and fatness is necessary for menstrual recovery but may not be sufficient for menses to return. Other factors such as stress and exercise may be important. Serum luteinizing hormone and follicle stimulating hormone are reduced in anorexia nervosa and respond to luteinizing hormone releasing hormone with the pre-pubertal pattern, that is the FSH response is greater than the LH. There is a delayed peak in LH and FSH after LRH, an abnormal response of LH to clomiphene citrate and abnormalities of temperature regulation and water regulation. All these changes are reversed as patients gain weight. Why some women who gain weight do not resume menses is not clear. Physical exertion itself can produce amenorrhea and it has been proposed that there must be a positive "energy" balance in order for normal menses to occur.

Hypothalamic-pituitary function in anorexia nervosa was reviewed by Paul E. Garfinkel. A variety of hypothalamic abnormalities are reported in anorexia nervosa. Raised basal levels of growth hormone in anorexia nervosa are directly related to starvation and are rapidly reversed when caloric intake is increased. Serum triiodothyronine (T3) levels are reduced in anorexia nervosa in association with an increase in the inactive reverse form of T3. This alteration is clearly related to fasting intself and may be related directly to caloric deprivation and especially to carbohydrate restriction. The circadian rhythm for cortisol is preserved but at a higher level than normal controls. In many patients there is a failure to suppress following dexamethasone. Alterations in cortisol metabolism are likely related to the low levels of T3. Morning prolactin levels are normal however there is a failure of the night time rise in some patients. Fasting hypoglycemia may occur and impaired glucose tolerance, both of which are rapidly reversed by refeeding. Insulin resistance is also seen together with reduced circulating levels of plasma dopamine and norepinephrine. Alterations in resting plasma growth hormone, plasma T3 and reverse T3, and changes in adrenal steroid and testosterone metabolism which are secondary to the changes in T3 are all reversed rapidly with refeeding.

Dr. B. M. Sherman reviewed hypothalamic control of the menstrual cycle in relation to the findings in anorexia nervosa. The sequence of endocrine events which characterize the normal adult human menstrual cycle are dependent on the permissive effect of an appropriate pattern of stimulation by luteinizing hormone releasing hormone from the hypothalamus. In anorexia nervosa basal LH and FSH levels are low, there is a loss of episodic gonadotropin secretion and repetitive administration of exogenous luteinizing hormone releasing hormone restores gonadotropin secretion and ovulatory menses. We can conclude that the defect in anorexia nervosa resides in the failure of hypothalamic mechanisms to initiate an appropriate pattern of luteinizing hormone releasing hormone secretion. The signal by which alteration in nutritional status or body weight leads to changes in hypothalamic mechanisms is unknown, although it has been postulated that the signal may be related to changes in androgen or estrogen metabolism.

Dr. L. C. Krey reviewed the neuronal and endocrine mechanisms involved in control of gonadotropin secretion in relation to the abnormalities seen in anorexia nervosa. In the monkey, LHRH containing neurons come predominantly from the arcuate nucleus and lesions of this region producing a reduction of LH and FSH secretion with normal output of thyrotropin, prolactin, growth hormone and cortisol. LH and FSH secretion are released in a pulsatile manner which in turn depends upon pulsatile release of LHRH into the portal circulation. In lesioned animals, gonadotropin secretion can be restored to normal by LHRH infusion once every hour. If LHRH is administered more frequently, circulating LH and FSH drop dramatically, an effect which is attributed to down regulation of LHRH receptors. LH levels also fall following less frequent stimulation with LHRH but in contrast FSH levels rise. Hypogonadotropism can therefore be related to either hyperstimulation or hypostimulation by LHRH. Since individuals with anorexia nervosa show elevated gonadotropins following LHRH replacement therapy, one can presume that endogenous LHRH release in these individuals is deficient. Thus, one may ascribe all the clinical observation of reproductive dysfunction in anorexia nervosa to an absence of "sufficient" pattern of LHRH secretion. The patterns of regression and recovery of gonadotropin release observed during anorexia nervosa are not unique. The recovery pattern seen in anorexia nervosa is quite similar to the maturation process which occurs during puberty.

Dr. L. Landsberg and J. D. Young reviewed the metabolic adaptation to starvation and its relationship to the endocrine changes in anorexia nervosa. A primary abnormality in the hypothalamus could conceivably account for both the eating disturbance and endocrine abnormlaities in anorexia nervosa. Alternatively both the hypothalamic alterations and endocrine changes could be a result of starvation itself. The sympathetic nervous system, which has a major role in regulation of metabolic rate and heat production, shows a reduction of activity in starvation. There is evidence that during starvation a decrease in insulin-mediated glucose utilization within certain critical neurons results in a suppression of the sympathetic outflow. This effect is demonstrable within the first 24 hours of the fast before appreciable weight loss and hence is consistent with a primary effect of caloric restriction on sympathetic activity. The signals responsible for mediation of the decreased peripheral conversion of T4 to T3 have not been conclusively established. However, there is evidence that carbohydrate and insulin are involved, thus there may be a similarity between the regulation of peripheral thyroid hormone conversion and sympathetic nervous system activity. Furthermore, the decrease in peripheral conversion of T4 to T3 in starvation is related to a reduction in caloric intake rather than a loss in body mass. Increased growth hormone levels during starvation may be related to a fall in somatomedin which would increase growth hormone concentration by disrupting negative feedback. These growth hormone changes also appear to be related to caloric restriction rather than change in body mass. Alterations in cortisol may reflect the low circulating levels of T3. Thus many of the endocrine abnormalities in anorexia nervosa can be explained as part of an integrated metabolic adaptation to reduced caloric intake.

Dr. M. E. Quigley evaluated the hypothalamic inhibitory influences on gonadotropin secretion in normal cycling women and those with hypogonadotropic amenorrhea. In anorexia nervosa there is strong evidence that decreased endogenous hypothalamic LHRH release plays a role in the pathophysiology of amenorrhea. Various investigators have proposed that increased central dopamine and norepinephrine may occur in anorexia nervosa and that this may account for the alteration in LHRH release. Dopamine infused intravenously has been shown to inhibit circulating LH and the dopamine receptor antagonist metoclopramide causes a rise in circulating LH during the late follicular and mid luteal phases. The specific opioid receptor antagonist naloxone also causes a rise in circulating LH during the late follicular phase or the mid luteal phase. This data would suggest that endogenous dopamine and endogenous opioids are potent inhibitors of LHRH release in the human and that they interact through a common pathway. Together with clinical evidence for excess dopaminergic activity in patients with anorexia nervosa, this supports the hypothesis that excess dopaminergic inhibition of LHRH release plays a role in the hypogonadotropinism and amenorrhea that occurs in patients with anorexia nervosa.

Dr. J. A. Grinker reviewed experimental psychological aspects of anorexia nervosa. Psychological aspects of anorexia are prominent among the diagnostic criteria for primary anorexia nervosa. Anorexia nervosa is a disease of modern affluent societies which is more frequent among higher socioeconomic class females than lower class females. Longer duration, older age of onset, and impaired family relations are all related to a poorer prognosis and greater weight loss. On the other hand, lesser denial of illness, no previous obesity and normal sexual development are related to a more favourable prognosis. Individuals who engage in periodic gorging and binging are more disturbed and have a less favourable prognosis. Many anorectic individuals significantly over estimate their body size. There is evidence that anorectic individuals have a lower preference for items which are perceived as sweet. Modelling and ballet students as well as highly motivated school age atheletes may display feeding behaviour similar to those of anorexia nervosa patients.

Dr. S. F. Leibowitz evaluated the brain neurotransmitter projections and receptor systems in relation to food intake, dietary preference, meal patterns and body weight. Anorexia nervosa involves a disturbance in the experience of satiety more than in hunger. There is frequently an increased desire to eat associated with a profound inhibition of eating. Several monoamine systems in the brain influence food related behaviours. A medial hypothalamic α-noradrenergic system stimulated eating with a preferential increase in consumptio of carbohydrates. A medial hypothalamic serotonergic system suppresses eating, causing a selective decrease in consumption of sweet and non-sweet carbohydrate with minimal effect on fat or protein intake. Lateral hypothalamic β-adrenergic and dopaminergic systems suppress eating. These two neurotransmitters preferentially decrease consumption of protein leaving unaffected the ingestion of carbohydrate or fat. Thus anorexic behaviour could be related to a decreased medial hypothalamic α-noradrenergic activity, increased medial hypothalamic serotonergic activity or increased lateral hypothalamic dopaminergic and β-adrenergic activity. The converse would be expected in binge eating behaviour. A shift between bulimia and anorexia may well be related to a shift in neurochemical substrates. Furthermore based on extensive work in animals specific drugs which are known to suppress appetite through hypothalamic neurotransmitter systems may be helpful in alleviating this eating disorder.

Two major themes emerged in the discussion. First the role of factors other than weight loss and caloric deprivation were discussed. Patients with anorexia nervosa characteristically show a denial of being adult, a denial of being female and a denial of normal relationships with the family. The relationship of these characteristic changes to the endocrine abnormalities is unknown as is the physiologic basis of these psychological changes. The relationship of the gonadotropin changes to those seen in athletes were also discussed. Although some athletes show low LH and FSH levels, others show high levels, furthermore there is an anticipatory rise in luteinizing hormone and testosterone in women prior to exercise. Such high levels of gonadotropins have not been reported in patients with anorexia nervosa to this point. The issue of the persistence of amenorrhea and other endocrine findings in some patients following weight gain raises the question whether there may be persisting alterations in neural function which are secondary to weight loss or perhaps related more to environmental or stress factors. The second major theme that emerged in discussion was that it was essential to collect the right kind of data. Considering endocrine function the spatial temporal patterning is a most important consideration For exampl, prolactin levels and responses are normal during the day but a flattened night time rise has been reported in anorexia nervosa. Similarly with respect to the gonadotropins the crucial alteration in anorexia nervosa appears to be the change in the episodic patterning of LHRH secretion.

The question of which neurotransmitter system was the most important regulatory influence on feeding behaviour was discussed. Present evidence suggests that all of the monoamines could be involved. Related to that issue is the question of drug therapy. At this point there is no evidence that specific drugs such as alpha-adrenergic agonists, benzodiazepines or neuroleptics are of any use.

Subject Index

D

Q

R

S

T